THE BIOLOGY OF
IMMUNOLOGIC DISEASE

Dedication

The editors affectionately dedicate this volume to

SAMUEL C. BUKANTZ, M.D.

With this dedication we wish to acknowledge the friendship and guidance of a physician who perceived the breadth of the bonds that united the immunology laboratory and clinical medicine at a time when such perceptions were still prophetic.

Adapted from
Hospital Practice

Illustrated by
Nancy Lou Gahan
and
Albert E. Miller
(charts and graphs)
and other contributing artists
For complete illustration and data source credits, see page 399.

Cover painting by George V. Kelvin

Designed by
Robert S. Herald

THE BIOLOGY OF IMMUNOLOGIC DISEASE

Edited by
Frank J. Dixon, M.D.
Director
Research Institute of the Scripps Clinic
La Jolla, California

and

David W. Fisher
Editorial Director
HOSPITAL PRACTICE

A HOSPITAL PRACTICE BOOK
Published by

Sinauer Associates, Inc. • Publishers • Sunderland, Massachusetts

The Biology of Immunologic Disease

The material in this book has been updated through spring of 1983.
Copyright © 1983 by HP Publishing Co., Inc., New York, N.Y.

All rights reserved. No part of this book may be reproduced or transmitted in any form or by any means, electronic or mechanical, including photocopying, recording, or storage retrieval system, without written permission from the publisher.

For information, address:
Sinauer Associates Inc., Publishers
Sunderland, MA 01375

Printed in the United States of America

ISBN 0-87893-148-1

Library of Congress Cataloging in Publication Data
      Main entry under title:

The Biology of Immunologic Disease.

      (A Hospital Practice book)
      Collection of updated articles, originally published
      in Hospital Practice.
         Includes index.
         1. Immunologic diseases—Addresses, essays, lectures.
      2. Immunology—Addresses, essays, lectures.
      I. Dixon, Frank J. (Frank James), 1920-
      II. Fisher, David W.   III. Hospital Practice.   IV. Series.
      [DNLM: 1. Immunologic diseases.   WD 300 B615]
      RC582.B56   1983   616.9   83-4780
      ISBN 0-87893-148-1

9   8   7   6   5   4   3   2   1

Contents

Section I
IMMUNOREACTIVE CELLS, THEIR PRODUCTS, AND THEIR REGULATION

Section III
DISEASE-SPECIFIC IMMUNOPATHOLOGIC PROCESSES

Contributing Authors

K. FRANK AUSTEN — Theodore B. Bayles Professor of Medicine, Harvard Medical School; Chairman, Department of Medicine, Robert B. Brigham Division; and Chairman, Department of Rheumatology and Immunology, Brigham and Women's Hospital, Boston

BARUJ BENACERRAF — George Fabyan Professor of Comparative Pathology and Chairman, Department of Pathology, Harvard Medical School, Boston

EDWARD A. BOYSE — Head, Field of Cell Surfaces, Memorial Sloan-Kettering Cancer Center, New York

HARVEY CANTOR — Associate Professor of Medicine, Harvard Medical School and the Sidney Farber Cancer Institute, Boston

JEAN-CHARLES CEROTTINI — Director, Lausanne Unit of Human Cancer Immunology, Ludwig Institute for Cancer Research, Epalingessur-Lausanne, Switzerland, and Professor of Immunology, Faculty of Medicine, University of Lausanne

EUGENE D. DAY — Professor of Immunology and of Experimental Surgery, Duke University Medical Center, Durham, N.C.

MARIA DE SOUSA — Director, Laboratory for Cell Ecology, Memorial Sloan-Kettering Cancer Center, New York

FRANK J. DIXON — Director, Research Institute of the Scripps Clinic, La Jolla, Calif.

EDWARD C. FRANKLIN — Professor of Medicine, New York University School of Medicine; Director, Irvington House Institute; and Chairman, Rheumatic Diseases Study Group, New York University Medical Center, New York (deceased)

HENRY GEWURZ — Coogan Professor and Chairman, Department of Immunology/Microbiology, Rush Medical College, Chicago

ROBERT A. GOOD — Member and Head of the Cancer Program, Oklahoma Medical Research Foundation; Professor of Pediatrics, University of Oklahoma College of Medicine; Head, Clinical Immunology Service, Oklahoma Children's Memorial Hospital, Oklahoma City

NICOLA GREEN — Scientific Associate, Immunopathology Department, Research Institute of the Scripps Clinic, La Jolla, Calif.

JOHN A. HANSEN — Associate Professor of Medicine, University of Washington School of Medicine, and Director, Histocompatibility Laboratories, Puget Sound Blood Center and Fred Hutchinson Cancer Research Center, Seattle

RONALD B. HERBERMAN — Chief, Biological Development Branch, Biological Response Modifiers Program, National Cancer Institute at the Frederick Cancer Research Facility, Frederick, Md.

KIMISHIGE ISHIZAKA — O'Neill Professor of Immunology and Medicine, Johns Hopkins University School of Medicine, Baltimore, Md.

DAVID H. KATZ — President and Director, Medical Biology Institute, La Jolla, Calif.

HENRY G. KUNKEL — Professor of Immunology and Medicine, The Rockefeller University, New York

PHILIP LEDER — John Emory Andrus Professor of Genetics and Chairman, Department of Genetics, Harvard Medical School, Boston

RICHARD A. LERNER — Member, Immunopathology Department and Committee for the Study of Molecular Genetics, Research Institute of the Scripps Clinic, La Jolla, Calif.

HANS J. MÜLLER-EBERHARD — Chairman, Department of Molecular Immunology, and Green Investigator in Medical Research, Research Institute of the Scripps Clinic, La Jolla, Calif.

JOHN S. NAJARIAN — Professor and Chairman, Department of Surgery, University of Minnesota Medical School, Minneapolis

HERBERT F. OETTGEN — Member, Memorial Sloan-Kettering Cancer Center; Attending Physician and Chief, Clinical Immunology Service, Memorial Hospital; and Professor of Medicine, Cornell University Medical College, New York

MICHAEL B. A. OLDSTONE — Member, Department of Immunology, and Head of a viral immunobiology unit, Research Institute of the Scripps Clinic, La Jolla, Calif.

ARTHUR OLSON — Senior Staff Scientist, Immunopathology Department, Research Institute of the Scripps Clinic, La Jolla, Calif.

PHILIP Y. PATERSON — Chairman and Professor of Microbiology-Immunology, Northwestern University Medical School, Chicago

SUSAN ROBERTS — Supervisor, Hybridoma Facility, Albert Einstein College of Medicine, Bronx, N.Y.

JANE G. SCHALLER — Professor of Pediatrics, University of Washington School of Medicine, and Director, Division of Rheumatic Diseases, Children's Orthopedic Hospital, Seattle

MATTHEW D. SCHARFF — Professor and Chairman, Department of Cell Biology, Albert Einstein College of Medicine, Bronx, N.Y.

ROBERT S. SCHWARTZ — Professor of Medicine, Tufts University School of Medicine, Boston

THOMAS SHINNICK — Assistant Member, Immunopathology Department, Research Institute of the Scripps Clinic, La Jolla, Calif.

FREDERICK P. SIEGAL — Associate Professor of Medicine, Mount Sinai School of Medicine of the City University of New York; Head, Division of Immunology, Mount Sinai Medical Center; and Associate Scientist, Memorial Sloan-Kettering Cancer Center, New York

JOHN D. STOBO — Associate Professor of Medicine, University of California, San Francisco, and Head, Section of Rheumatology and Clinical Immunology, Herbert C. Moffitt Hospital, San Francisco

SAMUEL STROBER — Associate Professor of Medicine and Chief, Division of Immunology, Department of Medicine, Stanford University School of Medicine

J. G. SUTCLIFFE — Assistant Member, Immunopathology Department, Research Institute of the Scripps Clinic, La Jolla, Calif.

ENG M. TAN — Director, Autoimmune Disease Center, and Head, Division of Rheumatology, Research Institute of the Scripps Clinic, La Jolla, Calif.

PALLAIAH THAMMANA — Research Associate, Department of Cell Biology, Albert Einstein College of Medicine, Bronx, N.Y.

ARGYRIOS N. THEOFILOPOULOS — Associate Member, Department of Immunopathology, Research Institute of the Scripps Clinic, La Jolla, Calif.

EMIL R. UNANUE — Mallinckrodt Professor of Immunopathology, Harvard Medical School, Boston

WILLIAM O. WEIGLE — Member, Department of Immunopathology, Research Institute of the Scripps Clinic, La Jolla, Calif.

GERALD WEISSMANN — Professor of Medicine and Director, Division of Rheumatology, New York University School of Medicine, New York

MARC E. WEKSLER — Wright Professor of Medicine and Director, Division of Geriatrics and Gerontology, Cornell University Medical College, New York

CURTIS B. WILSON — Member, Department of Immunopathology, Research Institute of the Scripps Clinic, La Jolla, Calif.

ROLF M. ZINKERNAGEL — Institute of Pathology, University of Zurich, Switzerland

Introduction

When the extended series of articles in *Hospital Practice* upon which this volume is based was initiated more than six years ago, the introductory editorial noted that over the prior decades, the discipline of immunology "had been enjoying a period of investigative prosperity" that had "brought it to the borders of clinical application, with a number of salients into significant areas of medical practice."

These initial "beachheads have been consolidated and expanded tremendously," the editorial noted. It went on to cite the impressive increase in the sophistication with which the "laboratory scientist is able to probe the extraordinarily diverse facets of the immune response, enhancing our knowledge of how it operates in disease as well as in health."

It was then suggested that "given this accumulation of knowledge, the time appears ripe to bring together those aspects of recent immunologic advances most relevant to our understanding of human disease."

In the years during which this volume has been in preparation, the pace of progress has accelerated dramatically. What has been most striking has been the diversity of the sources of this acceleration. Major contributions to our understanding of both immunologic disease processes and the prevention, diagnosis, and treatment of specific disorders have been derived from geneticists, biochemists, cell biologists, oncologists, and computer scientists, as well as from "traditional" immunologists and immunopathologists.

Certainly there has been no greater contribution to our understanding of the complexity of the immunologic systems than that which has come from integration of genetics with immunology. This is nowhere better exemplified than in the presentation by Leder on the remarkable sequence of events that takes place in the genome in order to produce immunoglobulin. It has been impressively demonstrated that one of the most puzzling aspects of the immune response—the combination of exquisite specificity with almost unlimited diversity—can be explained fully by these genetic events.

In the same vein, we have come to understand that genes control the cellular interactions involved in every aspect of humoral and cell-mediated immunity. As described in the chapters by Katz, by Boyse and Cantor, and by Zinkernagel, among others, we have learned a great deal about those gene products on the surfaces of immunoreactive cells that determine the cellular roles in immunologic actions and interactions. These surface molecules also serve as invaluable markers in analysis of lymphoid malignancies, as discussed by Siegal and by Oettgen, and in permitting us to identify those disease states in which imbalances of various subpopulations of lymphocytes account for pathologic expressions. Those phenomena are central to the discussions by Schaller and Hansen of a wide array of diseases that have been associated with antigens coded for in the major histocompatibility gene complex, by Kunkel on the immunopathology of systemic lupus erythematosus, by Tan on antinuclear antibodies, and by Zinkernagel on the major histocompatibility antigens in host responses to infection.

A parallel expansion of understanding has occurred with respect to the cellular participants in immunologic activities. Whereas a decade ago, we were impressed by the recognition that there were two major and interrelated aspects of the immune response, one expressed through B lymphocytes, the other through T lymphocytes, we now know that the cellular cast of characters is far more diverse than we could have suspected. The suppressor T cell, discussed in this volume by Benacerraf, has joined the helper T cell and the cytolytic T cell as a major modulator of the immune response. Two populations of non-T, non-B cells have come to the fore. The K cells of antibody-dependent cytotoxicity are described by Cerottini, and the NK cells, which function without prior sensitization, are discussed by Herberman. In addition, much has been learned that permits assignment of a major role to the macrophages in regulating lymphocyte function, the subject of Unanue's chapter. Finally, we have achieved a fuller and more accurate understanding of the role of tissue mast cells in immediate hypersensitivity responses, as discussed by Austen.

Even as our understanding of the cellular components has grown, we have witnessed a parallel expansion of knowledge about the roles played by soluble factors. The effector functions subserved by complement, C-reactive protein, and the various mediators of inflammation have been intensively analyzed, as described here by Müller-Eberhard, Gewurz, and Weissmann respectively. With regard to complement, relationships to specific diseases and disorders have been amplified. However, beyond these long-recognized mediators, we have had added to our growing list of soluble effectors and modulators a host of factors that not only mediate cellular events but in many cases appear capable of replacing the relevant cells: the suppressor factors, the interleukins, the leukotrienes, etc. These discoveries take on particular importance for clinicians since they suggest immense possibilities for pharmacologic intervention in immunologic diseases.

It would undoubtedly be an exaggeration to say that our diagnostic and therapeutic capacities have kept pace with the explosive growth of underlying knowledge. However, it is fair to say that the roads to such clinical progress have been opened. We now have sophisticated methods for the detection of the immune complexes that are central to the pathology of a wide array of diseases, and some of those methods are described in this volume by Theofilopoulos and Dixon. Monoclonal and hybridoma technology, described by Scharff and colleagues, promises to provide an almost limitless source of specific antibodies for analysis and treatment of diseases. Computers have been employed to design specific synthetic vaccines free from the problems of biologic contamination, as reported by Lerner and his colleagues. And we have learned to manipulate the immune system by pharmacologic suppression and enhancement, by cellular engineering, and by targeting radiation. These developments are described in chapters by Schwartz, Najarian, Good, and Strober.

In encompassing all of those developments, along with a variety of chapters dealing with specific clinical disorders, we have been fortunate in having as participants in this volume many of the laboratory and clinical scientists who have contributed significantly to the acquisition of the vast body of knowledge. All have been generous not only in contributing their chapters over the years but also in updating them prior to publication in an effort to provide as far as possible a state-of-the-art overview.

We have also been fortunate in being able to call on the talents of a highly skilled group of medical illustrators, whose contributions are credited elsewhere in this book. Finally, an expression of appreciation is due to the staff members of *Hospital Practice*, whose editorial skills were invaluable in the preparation of this material for publication both in the journal and in this volume. Particular mention certainly is appropriate for Robert S. Herald, the Art Director, Audrey H. Redding, the Managing Editor, and David W. Fisher, my coeditor.

FRANK J. DIXON, M.D.

La Jolla, California
September 1983

Section I
IMMUNOREACTIVE CELLS, THEIR PRODUCTS, AND THEIR REGULATION

Genetics of Immunoglobulin Production

PHILIP LEDER   *Harvard University*

The ability to differentiate highly similar entities in the face of vast diversity is one of the most impressive endowments of genetic programming. Perhaps nowhere in nature is this capacity more impressive or more central to physiologic function than in B lymphocytes, each of which is genetically precommitted to respond to specific antigens by producing specific antibodies.

Higher animals, as we know, are preprogrammed to defend themselves against a virtually limitless array of foreign substances. It has been estimated that the immune system has the potential to produce between 10^6 and 10^8 different antibody specificities. For many years, one of the central questions related to the generation of antibody diversity—and specificity—was: Which aspects of these attributes are inherent in the antibody molecule and which are acquired in the wake of antigen encounter? It is now well established that virtually all of the tremendous diversity encoded in the immune system can be accounted for in genetic terms. After nearly two decades of inquiry, we seem to be very close to forming a complete picture of the structure of immunoglobulin genes and of the events controlled by these genes as they relate to the structure and the function of antibody molecules.

Each immunoglobulin molecule is composed of heavy and light polypeptide chains, with two chains of each type linked by disulfide bonds in each monomeric molecule. The familiar antibody structure includes, of course, antibody-combining sites (the variable regions) and a constant portion that subserve a host of biologic functions. The variable regions are formed from the approximately 100 amino-terminal amino acids of the heavy chains and the 100 amino-terminal amino acids of the light chains. These amino acids have been found to vary widely in sequence from immunoglobulin molecule to immunoglobulin molecule. Such variable regions, of course, provide antigen specificity. In contrast, the remainder of the immunoglobulin chains consist of amino acids that are invariant from molecule to molecule within an immunoglobulin class (or subclass). These constant regions contain in their heavy-chain moieties the class determinants for the immunoglobulin as well as the determinants of various class-associated immunologic functions (complement fixation, opsonization, etc).

During the 1960s and 1970s a profusion of general and detailed models were described to account for the generation of antibody diversity. The most popular of these was the germ-line theory. This model advanced the idea that every immunoglobulin subunit must be represented intact in the genome of each cell of an organism and that every antibody gene must be encoded colinearly with the structure of an immunoglobulin unit. There would consequently be thousands of genes for heavy chains and thousands for light chains. This argument required no unprecedented biochemical events to generate a larger antibody gene repertoire. Gene duplication, amplification, and the general mechanisms that accomplish divergence among other genes would allow evolution alone to provide amplification of variable region diversity.

This model had a basic flaw that was first pointed out by W. J. Dreyer and J. C. Bennett in 1965. They were troubled by the idea that evolution could have permitted such a multiplicity of mutations in the variable region sequence while tightly holding the constant region under control. There was, after all, no evidence to suggest a strong selection mechanism to keep the constant region stable. Consequently, thousands of discrete segments would have had to be divided by some unexplained mechanisms so that the initial portion of each could vary while the terminal portion was held absolutely constant.

Faced with this paradox, Dreyer and Bennett developed a radical hypothesis that turned out to be substantially correct. They proposed that the variable region must be constructed according to a genetic code contained in one of many genes, while the constant region was the product of a single gene. This arrangement implied that a single constant-region gene must be capable of being joined to any one of these variable-region genes. They therefore contended that immunologically competent cells must have evolved a pattern of somatic genetic behavior radically different from anything normally found in molecular genetics. They suggested that the genetic material in B cells must undergo a "scrambling" process to make this possible.

Although Dreyer and Bennett established a sound theoretical and intellectual framework for investigation of immunoglobulin genetics, nearly a dozen years elapsed before knowledge of molecular genetics and DNA chemistry and enzymology evolved sufficiently to permit conclusive testing of their hypothesis (see J. D. Baxter, "Recombinant DNA and Medical Progress," Hosp Pract, February 1980).

One of the first attempts to provide indirect proof of the Dreyer-Bennett hypothesis was made in 1974, when our group used newly developed hybridization kinetic analysis techniques to confirm the model's prediction that there was only one copy of the constant region sequence (a copy is a sequence of nucleotides that encodes a particular region). Our experiment showed that there were indeed only one or two copies of constant-region genes per haploid genome in immunoglobulin light-chain genes. Hybridization techniques could not specifically address the claim that there must be many copies of variable-region sequences (since variable regions are by definition different from each other). Still, we could infer from this incomplete evidence that there must be either some important genetic mechanism for generating diversity, or many copies of the variable region, or both.

The discovery of restriction endonucleases and their application to the mapping of gene sequences allowed N. Hozumi and S. Tonegawa to test the Dreyer-Bennett model in a more direct fashion in 1976. They employed a restriction endonuclease to cleave DNA from both murine embryonic cells and plasma cells derived from an immunoglobulin-producing plasmacytoma. They then separated the cleaved fragments according to size by electrophoresis and assayed for variable- and constant-region segments, using corresponding cDNA probes. Constant (C)- and variable (V)-region segments were found to reside on different fragments of DNA derived from embryonic tissues. The pattern of tumor DNA showed a single component that hybridized with both C and V sequences and was smaller than either of the components in embryo DNA. They interpreted this to mean that C and V segments, which are located some distance from each other in embryo cells, are joined to form a contiguous polynucleotide stretch during lymphocyte differentiation.

In the 1970s, rapid gains were made in understanding the nature of immunoglobulin-chain types and the events occurring during B-cell commitment that were to be indispensable in putting together the pieces of our genetic puzzle.

Every individual has the genetic potential to produce two types, or isotypes, of light chain that have interchangeable biologic functions. They are known as κ and λ chains and are defined by their constant regions, which are different in structure. There are eight types of heavy chains, known as μ, δ, ε, α, and four subtypes of γ. Heavy-chain isotype is the basis for the definition of antibody classes IgM, IgD, IgE, IgA, and IgG. A given B cell can only produce antibodies with either κ or λ chains (never both) and in its ultimate form, as a plasma cell, one type of heavy chain. This phenomenon is known as isotypic exclusion. Furthermore, most lymphocytes only produce heavy and light chains that correspond to one of their two chromosomal alleles (known as allelic exclusion).

The B cell has as its progenitor a postulated stem cell, which, according to existing evidence, is fully committed to all of the differential steps that eventuate in the antibody-secreting plasma cell. Moreover, it has all of the genetic information that will restrict its responsiveness to only one or very few antigens. Parenthetically, it might be noted that the ability of a single antibody species to interact with several antigens is incompletely understood in the sense that in some cases, the antigens involved do not always have discernibly common characteristics. At any rate, the genetic endowment of specificity to the B cell in the human requires contributions from genes located on at least three different chromosomes, as will be discussed.

Thus, one is confronted with something of a paradox. The Dreyer-Bennett hypothesis predicts that antibody diversity and specificity are achieved because the variable region is the product of many genes, while each constant region is the product of a single gene. However, a given B lymphocyte can ultimately express only a single set of variable-region gene segments. On the other hand, each cell can potentially express two light-chain constant-region isotypes (κ and λ) and eight different heavy-chain constant-region isotypes (μ, δ, α, ε, and γ1 through 4).

The steps of immunoglobulin formation during B-cell differentiation are shown in Figure 1, at right. The first step in this process is the appearance in the cytoplasm of a

Figure 1   Immunoglobulin Genetics

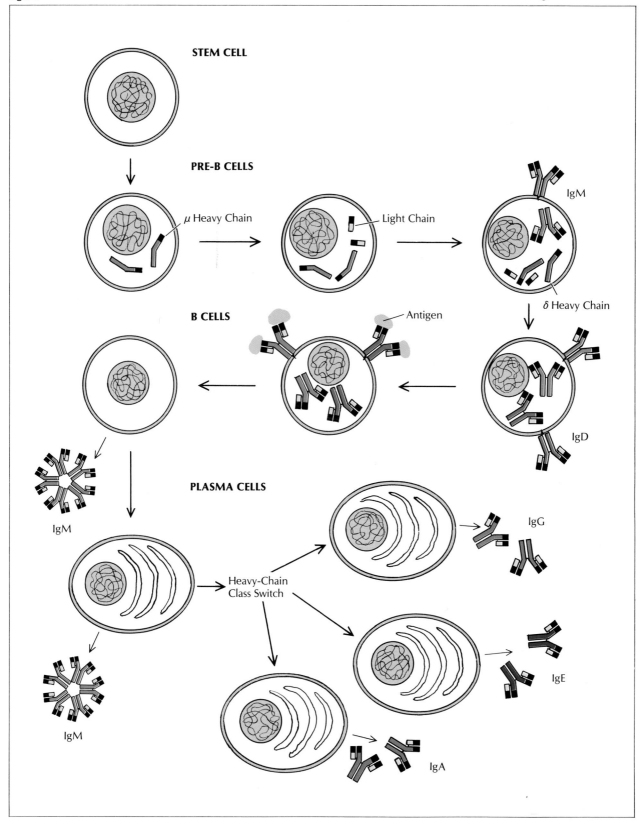

First step in B-cell differentiation is appearance of μ heavy chain, followed by light chain. These unite to form cytoplasmic, then membrane-bound, IgM. Subsequent synthesis of cytoplasmic and membrane IgD qualifies cell as specific, competent B cell. After antigen encounter, membrane IgM and IgD disappear and cell initiates synthesis of IgM and differentiation to plasma cell, which continues IgM production or undergoes heavy-chain switch to produce IgG, IgE, or IgA.

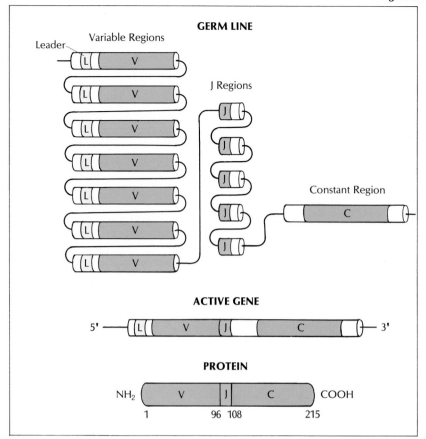

GERM LINE

Leader — Variable Regions

L V
L V
L V
L V
L V
L V
L V

J Regions

J
J
J
J
J

Constant Region

C

ACTIVE GENE

5' — L V J C — 3'

PROTEIN

NH₂ V J C COOH
1   96 108   215

Assembly of an active light-chain gene involves a recombination event that joins one of 100 to 200 different variable (V) regions, which encode amino acids 1 to 96 to one of five joining (J) regions (amino acids 96 to 108). The V region consists of a leader (L) segment separated from the V segment by a noninformational sequence encoding a signal peptide spliced off during light-chain formation. Variable region of light chain is encoded from L, V, and J segments; constant region is encoded from a C segment located 3 to 4 kilobases to the 3' side of the J. Noninformational DNA between V and C regions is removed during light-chain formation by RNA processing.

heavy chain of the μ type. Next, a light chain appears, which interacts with this heavy chain to form an IgM molecule, expressed first in the cytoplasm and subsequently on the surface of the cell where it is embedded in the cell membrane. Immediately thereafter in the cell, which at this point is considered a pre-B lymphocyte, a parallel interaction between δ heavy chains and light chains results in synthesis of cytoplasmic and membrane IgD. Both the IgM and IgD have the same specificities, i.e., the same variable-region sequences, as indeed will all immunoglobulins synthesized by the cell and its clonal progeny. At this point, the cell is a specific, competent B cell, ready to interact with an antigen.

On first encountering its "intended" antigen, the IgD and IgM on the cell surface disappear, and the cell begins to synthesize and secrete IgM. While there is some dispute as to the fate of IgD, the weight of evidence is that it simply disappears. The cell also undergoes division and amplification, with ultimate differentiation to plasma-cell form. This clone of cells may continue to produce IgM or, alternatively, may switch over to one of the other heavy-chain classes. This mechanism, through which a single variable region can occur in association with several different heavy chains, is known as the heavy-chain switch.

Since 1978, our group, along with many others, has applied recombi-

nant DNA technology to further elucidate the mechanism of genetic rearrangement during immunoglobulin production. Cloned genes are easily visualized by electron microscopy; thus, the different configurations appearing in antibody-producing cells can be visually compared with those in other cells. Nucleotide sequencing techniques have also permitted us to directly determine the structure of these genes.

Such studies have consistently demonstrated that V and C regions are separately encoded and that light-chain gene formation involves a somatic recombination event. Detailed sequencing studies of murine and human κ-chain genes have revealed interesting and unexpected features of their structure. In earlier studies, the germ-line V segment of the κ-chain gene had been associated with amino acid positions 1 to 108. However, we have since learned that this element (the V segment) only encodes amino acids through position 95. Electron microscopic and sequence analyses have shown that the remaining 13 amino acids (96 to 108) found at the terminal portion of the V region closest to the C region are encoded by one of four or five separate segments found approximately 3 to 4 kilobases to the 5' side of the C region. These are called joining, or J, segments.

The formation of an active immunoglobulin light-chain gene involves a recombination event that joins one of many variable-region sequences to one of these four or five J sequences (as illustrated in Figure 2, above). There are in the range of 100 to 200 different V-region sequences, each of which consists of a leader segment separated from the body of the V-region segment by a noninformational sequence. The leader segment encodes the hydrophobic amino acids, which form a signal peptide that is later spliced off during light-chain formation.

Hence the variable region of a light immunoglobulin chain is encoded from three segments: leader,

V, J. The constant region of the chain is encoded from a C segment located nearby on the same chromosome. The noninformational DNA occupying the area between the V and C regions is therefore incorporated into precursor RNA as it is formed to transmit the code for polypeptide synthesis. This precursor RNA is apparently processed to remove the intervening sequences and rejoin the structural sequences to form an intact light-chain code (known as RNA splicing).

Considerable study has been devoted to elucidating signals that might guide V–J recombination. Investigations by E. Max and others comparing V and J region sequences surrounding the recombination site failed to reveal any extensive regions of homology such as would be required to mediate homologous or generalized recombination. Instead, in the case of the κ light chain, two short complementary sequences appear to be conserved on the 3' side of each V segment and on the 5' side of each J segment (as illustrated in Figure 3, at right). There is a palindromic heptanucleotide sequence on the 5' side and a T (thymine)-rich sequence about 21 bases distant from the palindrome in all J segments sequenced thus far. V segments appear to have inverted repeats of this palindrome, as well as complementary A (adenine)-rich segments in an analogous position to the T-rich segments. The spacing between these, however, is 11 to 12 bases. V segments seem to be drawn to J complements that are presumably thousands of bases away. We can envision the two sets of sequences as a stemlike structure, pulling a V and a J segment together across its base. The A-rich and T-rich regions might provide an additional element of stability to the stem. Given the validity of this model, the DNA lying between the V segments and J segments must logically be deleted during V–J recombination. Our group recently used hybridization techniques to show that such deletions do indeed occur, although other mechanisms—such as more complicated genetic

crossovers—may be involved.

In our quest for diversity-generating mechanisms, we already have considerably amplified the mathematical possibilities. One hundred V-region sequences and five J-region sequences able to be connected in every possible combination afford us 500 different permutations for light chains alone. This figure is further expanded by diversity-producing mechanisms intrinsic to the recombination event.

When the first J-segment sequences were determined and compared with the known amino acid sequences in the corresponding light-chain region, it was found that amino acid position 96 was

often at variance with codons at position 96 in the germ-line J sequence. This suggested that V and J segments must be capable of joining at one of several crossover points, a notion that was confirmed by cloning and determining the nucleotide sequences of several rearranged κ-light-chain genes (see Figure 4, page 8). The region immediately surrounding position 96, referred to as a hypervariable region, seems to be involved in formation of the antibody-antigen combining site. Its variation must logically contribute to physiologic diversity by altering antibody specificity.

Recombination sometimes causes deletion of up to six nucleotides

Figure 3

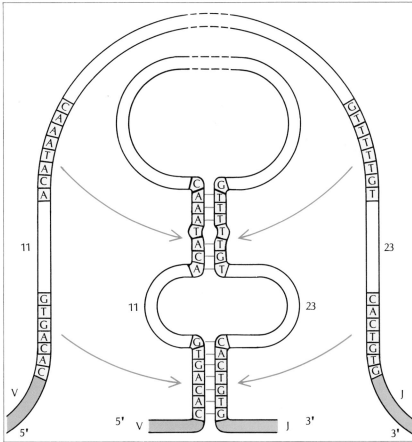

Hypothetical stem structure formed during V–J recombination is thought to consist of inverted repeat nucleotide sequences next to germ-line V and J segments. In the κ-light-chain series, J regions have a palindromic heptanucleotide sequence to their 5' side and a thymine-rich sequence about 21 to 23 bases distant from the palindrome. V segments have inverted repeats of palindrome and complementary adenine-rich sequences, but the space between these is generally 11 to 12 nucleotides. Inverted palindromes are postulated to draw V and J segments across the base of the stem; adenine-rich and thymine-rich regions appear to add stability. Looped regions represent the noncomplementary nucleotide sequences.

from the germ-line region. Although the codon is often preserved, this deletion sometimes throws the remaining portion of a segment into a nonsense translation frame, producing nonsense genes unable to function in the immune response. "Wasted" recombinants appear to be the price the organism pays for this additional diversity-generating mechanism.

Yet another source of diversity is provided by single-point mutations (targeted changes of single bases and, hence, single amino acid codewords) that are known to occur in the V region. The nature and molecular function of these mutations are not understood.

Recent experiments on mouse and human genes have helped to elucidate the mechanisms of isotypic and allelic exclusion. Early work with the mouse gene had shown that in many B cells, the silent allele remains in germ-line configuration and does not undergo somatic V–J rearrangement necessary for active gene formation. In other cells, however, it was observed that the inactive gene had been arranged in an aberrant manner. Such genes are, in fact, those that have been "pushed out of phase" in a failed recombination. In yet other cells, *both* alleles are rearranged into nonsense genes. The basis for selection and control of these pro-

cesses remains unclear.

Since λ genes are expressed at low frequency in the mouse, it has been difficult to study λ–κ expression in this species. However, in recent studies of three long-established λ-chain-producing mouse myeloma lines, F. Alt and co-workers found that κ genes had been aberrantly rearranged in two lines and possibly lost in a third. This led them to postulate the existence of a hierarchy of light-chain gene rearrangements in which the first attempt is always to produce a κ chain, the next a λ chain. They also suggested that the appearance of a functional light-chain product precludes further rearrangement.

Recent studies conducted by our group on human immunoglobulin genes (approximately one third of which are expressed as λ chains) showed that in each light-chain-producing B cell, at least one light-chain gene has undergone rearrangement, while its allelic partner has either remained in germ-line configuration, undergone a second rearrangement, or been lost. In all κ-chain-producing cells, λ genes were found in germ-line configuration. On the other hand, in all λ-chain-producing cells, κ genes had been either rearranged or deleted. These experiments support a κ–λ serial order.

It seems likely that cells with both classes of light-chain alleles aberrantly rearranged do not survive as expanded clones (with the exception of malignant cells, as will be discussed). In genes where a functional light chain has been formed, it is reasonable to assume that the presence of germ-line or aberrantly rearranged genes, or both, is in some way responsible for both the allelic and isotypic exclusion mechanisms.

Our findings suggest a scheme for light-chain production in which a pre-B cell makes an initial attempt to successfully produce an active κ-chain gene (see Figure 5, at right). Failing this, it switches to the other allele for a second try. If both κ alleles are rearranged or deleted, the next rearrangement attempt involves one of the λ alleles.

Figure 4

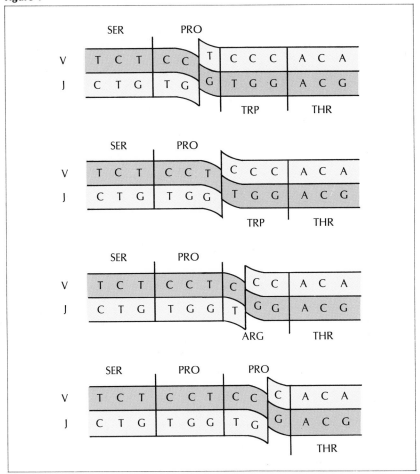

The variability of amino acids corresponding to position 96 in the germ-line J sequence can be accounted for by the existence of several possible crossover points during somatic recombination of V and J segments. When several rearranged κ-light-chain genes were cloned and sequenced, it was found that frame shifts occurring during recombination altered the codon sequence and, consequently, the amino acid content of the light-chain gene product. Variable crossover points depicted for κ-chain genes show altered coding for tryptophan, arginine, and proline.

The second λ allele represents the last resort: A failure here produces a null set. This system can be thought of as an error-compensating cascade that finally creates an active gene while experimenting with flexible joining rules that allow optimum diversification.

Although the structure and rearrangement of heavy-chain and light-chain genes are similar in many important ways, there are a number of differences that add interesting complexities to the heavy-chain system. The heavy-chain variable region is constructed by joining not two but three distinct segments of DNA: a V segment; a D, or diversity, segment; and a J segment. Heavy-chain J segments are separated by approximately 300 to 350 nucleotide sequences, occurring in regular tandem array. D-region segments, which encode only about 10 amino acids, are separated by about 10,000 bases. How these tiny islands of genetic information required for heavy-chain formation came to be placed adrift in a sea of nucleotide sequences remains a mystery.

Various cloning experiments have suggested that there are probably six active copies of J-region sequences and a reasonably large family of D and V segments. If, hypothetically, we projected 100 V, 50 D, and six J segments, we would have the potential to create 30,000 different combinations. Since each of these combinations allows for crossover-point variations and since there may be single-point mutations, it seems that hundreds of thousands of different genes can be created.

This finding nicely ties up the mathematical side of our puzzle. A system that can combine hundreds of thousands of different heavy-chain genes with thousands of different light-chain genes is clearly capable of constructing millions of immunoglobulins, each with a unique antigen-binding site.

Antibody class determination, as mentioned earlier, is controlled by a heavy-chain constant-region switching mechanism. Analysis of the heavy-chain locus of both hu-

Figure 5

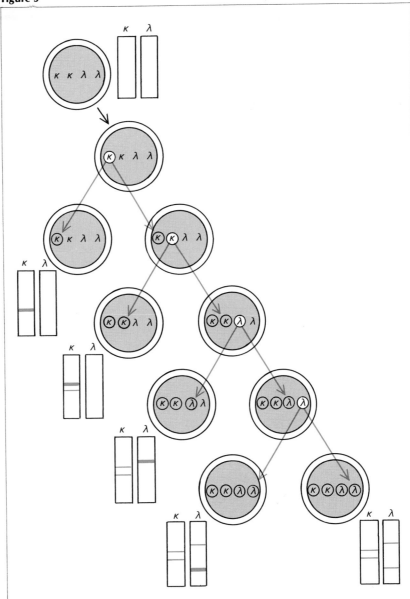

Mature B lymphocytes produce light immunoglobulin chains of either κ or λ isotype, but never both. F. Alt and co-workers have provided good experimental evidence for a hierarchy of light-chain gene rearrangement in which initial attempt is always to produce an active κ-chain gene. Failing this, an attempt is made with the second κ allele. With aberrant rearrangement or deletion of both κ alleles, recombination is attempted with a λ allele. Failure with both λ alleles results in an immunologically incompetent cell. Electrophoretic assay of gene fragments from each type of active light-chain gene shows characteristic fragment patterns. Black represents germ-line allele, blue is a failed recombination, and red is an active light-chain gene.

mans and mice by many groups, including our own, has indicated that the eight different types of heavy-chain constant-region genes are encoded on a single stretch of DNA, perhaps 100,000 bases in length. The μ- and δ-heavy-chain constant segments (which are expressed simultaneously in the initial stage of B-lymphocyte differentiation) lie in a 5' to 3' orientation approximately 2 kilobases from each other (see Figure 6, page 10). Two kilobases to the 5' side of the μ segment is a strip of six active J segments. To the 3' side of the δ segment are located, successively, the four γ segments, the ε segment, and the α segment.

The first step in the expression of a heavy-chain gene is a recombination event that associates a V segment with a J and a D segment close to the μ segment. This recombination is thought to involve the same kind of signals that play a role in light-chain V–J recombination (formation of a stemlike structure). The simultaneous expression of μ-chain and δ-chain genes is regulated by an RNA processing mechanism that alternatively splices or terminates the code. A μ chain is produced by straightforward transcription of the code from its 5' side with termination at the end of the μ-chain sequence. The original δ-chain transcript, however, includes both the μ-chain and δ-chain codes; a splicing mechanism then "cuts out" the μ-chain segment and joins the active V–D–J segment directly to the δ-chain segment.

The heavy-chain switch that frequently occurs during lymphocyte maturation from IgM to either IgA, IgG, or IgE must be accounted for in other terms. It has been determined, first by hybridization kinetic analyses and later by cloning studies, that the heavy-chain gene undergoes a recombination event in which the V–D–J sequence is switched to another site along the chromosome. In contrast to the relatively precise nature of V–J recombination, heavy-chain switch seems to occur at a variety of recombination sites included within the intervening sequences of the μ-, γ-, or α- germ-line sequence. This event usually deletes any intervening DNA. For example, in the formation of an active IgG gene, the V–D–J sequence is moved from its position adjacent to the μ-chain sequence to the area next to the γ-chain sequence, slicing out the μ and δ regions in the process. In the formation of IgE, the μ, δ, and γ regions are deleted, and so forth. This deletion can occur by a recombination event between sequences on the same strand of DNA (deleting what lies between them) or between

sequences on different strands of DNA (resulting in an unequal crossover and an apparent, rather than real, deletion).

The precise signals responsible for heavy-chain class switch are not understood, but the occurrence of runs of repeated sequences around certain switching sites suggests that homologous recombination may be responsible. Extensive areas of homology found at the switch region of the μ–α switch are particularly suggestive of such a mechanism. The fact that such homology is lacking between μ and γ genes implies that the two class switches may involve different mechanisms and depend on somewhat different enzyme systems.

Of course, the mature B cell may continue producing IgM rather than making the switch. It is interesting to note that the membrane-anchored form of IgM contains a short peptide chain at its C terminal not found in the secreted form, which appears to secure it to the cell membrane. The germ-line μ segment contains a code corresponding to this membrane-bound protein. A splicing event during RNA transcription that eliminates a termination code is responsible for determining whether an anchor peptide is synthesized. If this RNA processing step does not occur, the transcript fails to reach the anchor peptide code, and the secreted form, rather than the membrane form, of IgM is produced. Thus the immune system not only uses various sequence combinations at the DNA level to produce antibody diversity but employs the same principles to expand genetic possibilities at the RNA level as well.

Our most recent efforts, carried out in collaboration with Thomas Waldmann of the National Cancer Institute, have been devoted to the study of "non-T, non-B" cell leukemia, one of the major types of acute lymphocytic leukemia (ALL). Non-T, non-B cells are so designated because they have neither characteristic immunoglobulins nor T-cell antigens on their surfaces. There has been considerable controversy over the cellular origin of this class

of disease. We have known for a few years that many so-called non-T, non-B cells have in fact already committed themselves to B-cell development, as demonstrated by the presence of μ chain in the cytoplasm. More recently, we were able to show that many such cells have undergone the initial recombinational events of B-cell differentiation but were unable to form a functional immunoglobulin gene.

Our approach to this problem has a double intention. First, classification of these leukemias into B-cell or T-cell series provides a highly sensitive diagnostic marker with therapeutic implications. Second, clonal expansions of leukemic B cells that have been arrested at different stages of development represent a veritable cross section of B-cell differentiation suitable for investigating the accuracy of our predictions concerning developmental hierarchy in B cells.

Figure 6

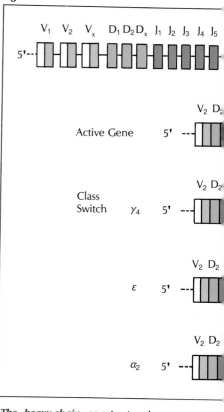

The heavy-chain constant-region genes are encoded on a single stretch of DNA. In the human genome, these heavy-chain genes have been localized to chromosome 14. Six strips of J sequences are lo-

We have found that the patterns of immunoglobulin gene rearrangement in leukemic pre-B cells are consistent with the postulated cascade of events in which μ-chain gene rearrangement precedes that of light-chain genes and in which κ-chain gene rearrangement generally precedes that of λ-chain genes. Of eight cases studied, we found one stem-cell type in which there were no immunoglobulin gene rearrangements. This set of cells reacted with a number of monoclonal antibodies to T-cell-associated antigens, suggesting that they may already have been committed to T-cell development.

The other seven cases could be classified as pre-B-cell leukemias and were placed in categories of gene arrangement reflecting a chronologic order of gene activation during B-cell differentiation. According to this scheme, a truly uncommitted B-cell or T-cell lym-phoid precursor would be expected to have all of its immunoglobulin genes in germ-line configuration (as was found in case 1). In cases 2 and 3, there was an attempt at μ-chain gene rearrangement associated with germ-line κ- and λ-gene configurations, a finding consistent with the proposed μ-chain/ light-chain hierarchy. Cases 4, 5, 6, and 7 displayed both aberrantly rearranged μ-chain genes and κ-chain gene rearrangement, a finding that appears to cancel out speculation that successful μ-chain gene rearrangement might be a necessary signal for light-chain gene rearrangement. Three of the cases (5, 6, and 7) had deleted κ-chain genes but had retained λ-chain genes in germ-line configuration. This supports our suggestion that human κ-chain gene rearrangements precede those of λ-chain genes. Case 8 showed μ-chain gene rearrangement and un-successful rearrangement of both κ-chain and λ-chain genes.

Our results suggest that immunoglobulin-gene rearrangements are surprisingly common among non-T, non-B lymphocytes. Previous studies based on the presence or absence of cytoplasmic μ chain categorized only 15% to 20% of these leukemias in the pre-B-cell stage of differentiation. However, the requirement for cytoplasmic μ chain may be too stringent a determinant, since there appears to be a potentially large population of lymphocytes that are already committed to B-cell differentiation but have failed to accomplish the V-D-J recombination needed for functional μ-chain synthesis.

Certain B-cell leukemias and lymphomas also have recently been found to be associated with another type of genetic rearrangement, i.e., translocations from a chromosome not normally related to im-

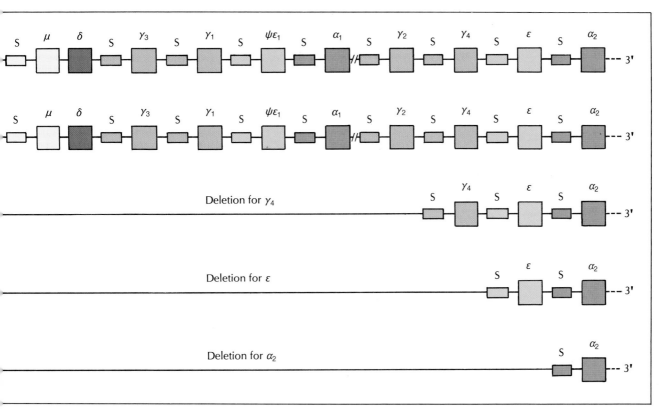

cated 2 kilobases to the 5' side of the μ sequence. The first step is a recombination event that associates one of approximately 100 V segments with one of about 50 diversity (D) segments and with a J segment to form active gene. Synthesis of μ chains is by transcription of the code up to the δ sequence.

Synthesis of δ chains is controlled by RNA splicing mechanism that deletes the μ sequence. Production of γ, ε, or α chains involves a recombination event that switches the V-D-J sequence to another site along the chromosome and deletes intervening sequences. Boxed S represents putative switch region.

munoglobulin synthesis (chromosome 8) to one of the immunoglobulin gene-bearing chromosomes (2, 14, and 22). It has been known for a few years that heavy-chain, κ-chain, and λ-chain genes are located, respectively, on chromosomes 14, 2, and 22. With recent advances in chromosomal hybridization techniques that make it possible to map genes more precisely to their chromosomal bands, Ilan Kirsch and his group have demonstrated that the human heavy-chain constant-region gene $\gamma 4$ is located on the same band to which a characteristic B-cell lymphoma or leukemia translocation occurs. It was also recently reported that the site of translocation onto chromosome 2 corresponds to the κ-light-chain gene band.

This phenomenon can be considered in the light of the George Klein–Janet Rowley version of the activated oncogene model, which suggests that translocation of genetic material that is normally "silent" to an active transcription site may be responsible for inducing and maintaining a malignant state. The best known example of this, of course, is the so-called Philadelphia chromosome in chronic myelogenous leukemia. In the case of immunoglobulin genes, it has been speculated that recombination of a heavy-chain or light-chain gene segment with an "incorrect" message from chromosome 8 might form an active gene capable of conducting large-scale production of an aberrant, oncogenic substance.

Studies of murine plasmacytoma and Burkitt's lymphoma cell lines by R. Taub and co-workers have provided good supportive evidence for this suggestion. They have been able to show that a somatically rearranged segment of mouse myeloma, which is joined to a DNA sequence that encodes the IgA constant and switch sequence, encodes the specific oncogene c-myc (the murine cellular analogue of the avian MC-29 viral transforming gene). This mouse c-myc sequence was used to show that human c-myc is located at the precise site on chromosome 8 from which the Burkitt's lymphoma translocation originates. Taub's group found that in many Burkitt's lymphoma lines, the c-myc gene region fragment has undergone a somatic rearrangement. In two of the lines studied, the c-myc and IgM region sequences were on the same DNA restriction fragments, suggesting that this segment included the crossover point for the translocation from chromosome 8 to 14.

The discovery of these translocations, which move a seemingly unrelated genetic message to a locus that normally undergoes a recombination event as a process of differentiation, has opened up a particularly provocative question: Might not the same diversity-generating mechanism that has proved so powerful for the expression of immunoglobulin genes be used in other genetic systems? As a hypothetical example, we might consider the events of cellular differentiation during embryogenesis, which require an enormous pool of information. One could postulate a recombination device used to "write addresses" on cells or endow them with the capacity for cell-type recognition. While such an example is pure conjecture, it does seem plausible that the immune system is not unique in its need for an expanded information bank.

The organization of the immunoglobulin genes demonstrates the concept that the genetic content of an organism represents a dynamic state in which rearrangements occur during the life of an individual as well as over evolutionary time.

It may be difficult to envision the immune system as both so consummately effective and consummately inefficient. In reality, that it is able to function at all appears to be a product of pure probability. A poker player who shuffled the cards and dealt them several million times could certainly come up with as many different combinations and as many winning hands.

Of course, the system also appears to be guilty of occasionally dealing out catastrophically bad hands. Although there is considerable controversy as to the precise implications of genetic recombination and translocation, few would deny that in our pursuit of the elusive factors that produce malignant transformations, further investigation of these phenomena is one of the best cards we have to play.

Structure and Biologic Activity Of Immunoglobulin E

KIMISHIGE ISHIZAKA *Johns Hopkins University*

Any discussion of the relationships between the structure of IgE and its biologic activity is rewarding in itself, particularly in the context of its established clinical role in the pathogenesis of atopic disease. But in addition, what has been learned of these relationships serves also to illustrate the ways in which the other immunoglobulin classes – IgA, IgG, IgM, and perhaps IgD – fulfill their antibody roles. Indeed, it is largely for this reason that this discussion of IgE was selected as the appropriate opening for this new series of articles on immunopathology.

It is an intriguing fact in this context that IgE is the most recent immunoglobulin class to be isolated, identified, and characterized. However, the studies that accomplished this are very much a part of a continuum that can be traced back to before the turn of the century, to the very beginnings of immunology. Early workers noted that patient sera had the ability to neutralize in vitro the activity of diphtheria and tetanus toxins. From these observations, immunology developed via experiments that demonstrated the ability of certain sera to agglutinate bacteria and to induce a precipitin reaction. Up to this point, these immunologic activities were generally considered to be properties of the serum rather than of any particular molecule or set of molecules. Following the discovery of the precipitin reaction, however, it was established that antibody activity involved proteins. Further studies characterized the molecule involved as a 6.5S or 7S gamma globulin. What evolved was essentially a unitary hypothesis that associated all antibody activity, that mentioned above as well as hemolysis, complement fixation, combination with bacterial, viral, and tissue antigens, etc., with a single type or class of immunoglobulin.

In the 1940s, some antibody activity was found not only in 7S but also in the 19S fraction of gamma globulin. However, it could not then be determined whether the larger protein was a single molecule or a polymer of 7S molecules, and the unitary concept persisted essentially intact until around 1960. Then another type of molecule – that is to say, a molecule with different antigenic properties from the classic gamma globulin – was identified; in present terminology this gamma globulin is IgA. At about the same time, it was determined that the 19S molecule was also antigenically differentiable; it is, of course, IgM. The original and major immunoglobulin class is IgG. All three of these molecules have a significant degree of antigenic cross-reactivity, so in this sense all the immunoglobulins have a familial relationship. At the same time they all have class-specific antigenic determinants. An additional unifying fact about immunoglobulins is their common morphologic derivation from plasma cells.

It may seem rather startling today that as recently as 1960 immunologists had still not defined so basic a concept as immunoglobulin class. In the intervening years, however, progress has accelerated phenomenally. Two additional Ig classes – IgD and IgE – have been identified, as have at least four IgG and two IgA subclasses. A great deal of this newer knowledge has come from the continuing check of myeloma proteins maintained by several investigators. This neoplastic disease is characterized by the production and secretion into the serum of large quantities of immunoglobulins of particular purity. It was through studies of the antigenic properties of these immunoglobulins – or so-called Bence Jones proteins – that IgD and the various IgG and IgA subclasses were identified.

The discovery of IgE, however, was made by another ap-

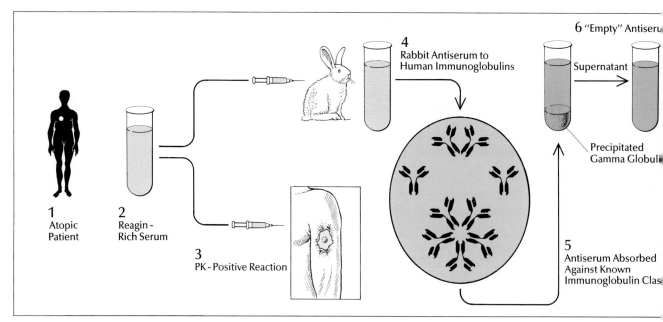

1
Atopic
Patient

2
Reagin-
Rich Serum

3
PK - Positive Reaction

4
Rabbit Antiserum to
Human Immunoglobulins

5
Antiserum Absorbed
Against Known
Immunoglobulin Class

6 "Empty" Antiseru

Supernatant

Precipitated
Gamma Globuli

Diagrammed above is the experiment that led to the conclusion that reaginic antibodies belong to a distinct immunoglobulin class – IgE. Patient with atopic allergy (1) serves as source of reagin-rich serum. Serum (2) is injected into nonatopic individual and evokes positive PK (passive transfer) reaction (3). An antiserum against human immunoglobulins is raised in rabbit (4).

This antiserum is then absorbed against previously known Ig classes (5), so that supernatant is devoid of antigamma globulin antibodies, or "empty" (6). Next, a small quantity of reagin-rich serum is added to "empty" antiserum (7) and another precipitate is produced by ultracentrifugation (8). This second supernatant is injected into nonatopic individual (9). The PK reaction is

proach. Back in the second decade of this century, Prausnitz and Küstner first identified reaginic antibody in the serum of persons with atopic disease. They showed that skin-sensitizing activity could be transferred with the serum of allergic individuals to normal individuals (the PK reaction). Over the years, as the various immunoglobulin classes were identified, first IgG and then IgA was suspected of being the offending atopic antibody. In fact, even IgM was tested extensively in the effort to identify reaginic antibody. It was work in our laboratories, then at the Children's Asthma Research Institute in Denver, that finally established that reaginic antibody belonged to a different immunoglobulin class - IgE. The critical experiment, summarized in the illustration above (Figure 1), involved removal of reagin from the serum of atopic individuals. At first, the reagin-rich fraction of the serum was injected into a rabbit to produce an antiserum, which in turn was absorbed with immunoglobulins of all classes then known, IgG, IgA, IgD, and IgM. With antibodies to these immunoglobulins absorbed out,

the antiserum did not produce precipitin bands against any of the known Ig classes. What was left, the so-called empty antiserum, should have been devoid of antibody. However, when a small quantity of reagin-rich fraction of serum from atopic patients was added back to the supernatant, an additional precipitate was observed and the supernatant was negative in terms of its ability to provoke a PK reaction in a nonatopic individual. This indicated that antireaginic antibody had been present in the antiserum and had combined with the reagin in the added serum.

To this evidence that reaginic antibody was not of any of the known immunoglobulin classes, we were able to add the demonstration, by radioimmunodiffusion and electrophoresis, that the immunoglobulin IgE developed a unique precipitin band and finally to correlate the "new" IgE with skin-sensitizing activity. Thus, we had met three basic criteria for an immunoglobulin class: ability to combine with specific antigen, unique antigenic determinants, and correlation with biologic activity.

It was noted earlier in this article that a major criterion in the differentiation of immunoglobulin class is antigenicity, i.e., each class has separable major antigenic specificities. It was also pointed out that all immunoglobulins cross-react with each other to some degree. Understanding of these relationships requires review of immunoglobulin structure, an appropriate starting point for which is the work of Rodney Porter in England.

Up until 1959, it had been generally believed that the antibody molecule consisted of a single polypeptide chain. In that year, Porter employed the proteolytic enzyme papain to split the molecule into three fragments. He found that two of the fragments were of essentially the same amino acid composition and that these two fragments contained the antibody activity, in the form of combining sites for antigen. To reflect their functional activity, these were designated the Fab fragments. The third fragment, in the rabbit gamma globulin preparation employed by Porter, was crystallizable; thus it became Fc.

The splitting of the molecule by pa-

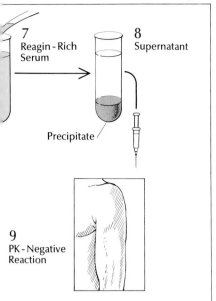

Figure 1

7 Reagin-Rich Serum

8 Supernatant

Precipitate

9 PK-Negative Reaction

negative, indicating that antibodies possessing reaginic activity have been removed. Reaginic antibody in the patient's serum was demonstrated by radioimmuno-diffusion, using the "empty" antiserum and ^{125}I-labeled allergen.

pain was an intrachain phenomenon, and at this stage Porter's concept of immunoglobulin was still of a single chain. However, during this same period, Gerald Edelman of Rockefeller University, then a graduate student, reduced the molecule with mercaptoethanol, a reagent capable of breaking disulfide bonds. His reasoning was that if the molecule were a single polypeptide chain, no fragmentation would occur via rupture of SS bonds. But if it were actually composed of multiple chains, reduction of the bonds would result in the separation of such chains. This work eventuated in the discovery that the immunoglobulin molecule is composed of four chains, two heavy and two light (see Figure 2, page 16). Further studies differentiated two light chain types, kappa and lambda. The heavy chains are the determinant of immunoglobulin class, so that the heavy chains of, for example, IgG molecules differ from those of IgA. Such class differences can be detected in amino acid sequences as illustrated in Figure 3 on page 17. The light chains are species-specific but not class-specific, and the proportion of κ and λ chains varies from species to species. In recent years, much information has been acquired on the genetic control of chain composition.

After the original studies of Porter and of Edelman, the obvious question was: How did the papain fragments relate to the polypeptide chains? Both of these scientists set out independently to answer the question. Their findings were in general agreement. Both found that the Fab fragments were composed of a complete light chain and the amino-terminal "half" of a heavy chain. The Fc consists of the carboxyl-terminal "halves" of the heavy chain.

It is interesting to note that early on in Porter's work, he described the Fab fragments as the "active fragments." Perhaps there was some bias here, since Porter's major interest was in determining how antibody combines with antigen. This is of course the activity that is in the exclusive domain of the Fab fragments with their structural variability providing the necessary specificity for this function (see Figure 4, page 18). Be that as it may, it is of more than historical interest that in the years when the structure of immunoglobulin was first being defined, there was general acceptance that the Fab fragments were more significant with respect to the activity of antibody molecules. Only more recently have studies permitted us to appreciate the many critical biologic functions subserved by the Fc.

One of the underlying reasons for the significance of Fc has already been mentioned, namely, that it is the determinant of immunoglobulin class. To put it another way, the specific antigenic determinant (or determinants) of the Ig molecule is in the Fc, while the antigens that account for Ig cross-reactivity between classes are on the Fab fragments. It should be stressed that immunoglobulin class is not simply a matter of nosologic convenience; rather it is an important factor in regulating the biologic behavior of the molecule with respect to such important considerations as complement-fixing ability, participation in phagocytosis, attachment to target cells, crossing of the placenta, and duration of antibody protection. All of these functional aspects will be discussed shortly. Before doing so, perhaps we can dispose of one further definition, that of immunoglobulin subclass. The subgroups within an Ig class have the same group-specific antigenic determinant as one another. However, in addition, each has within the heavy-chain polypeptide of the Fc fragment a subclass-specific antigenic determinant, which is identifiable immunologically and reflects differences of amino acid sequence among the various subclasses.

Let us turn now to some of the specific biologic phenomena that have been associated with the Fc fragment. To do this I would like to go back a few years and describe work done in our laboratories, although it should be stressed that parallel investigations were undertaken by other immunobiologists. Our interest was to clarify various biologic phenomena, such as complement fixation and anaphylaxis. We started from certain observations, namely, that these biologic events did not occur in vivo if antigen was present and antibody absent, nor did they proceed if antibody was present but antigen was not. Our hypothesis therefore was that the antigen-antibody complex somehow acquired biologic properties not possessed by either component alone.

We found that in the guinea pig the situation with respect to both complement fixation and the anaphylactic reaction was somewhat more complicated. It could be demonstrated that if one divalent antibody molecule combined with two antigen molecules, biologic activity was still lacking. On the other hand, complexes that included two or more antibody molecules were active. This suggested to us that perhaps the role of antigen was simply to bring the antibody molecules into proximity. The question that we then asked was whether antigen was necessary; what would happen if immunoglobulin was aggregated chemically, without antigenic participation?

Accordingly we prepared by chemical means nonspecific aggregates of IgG. And indeed these aggregates that lacked antigen possessed the same biologic capacities as antigen-antibody complexes. They could fix complement and they could induce the ana-

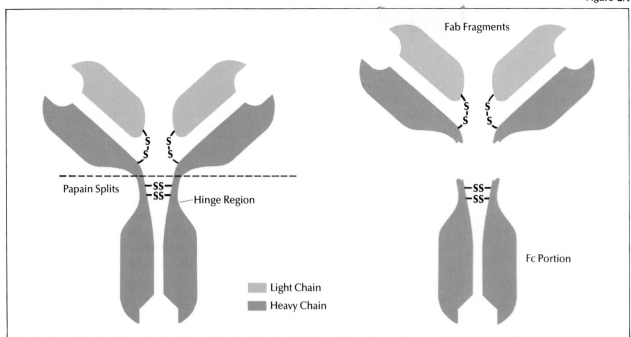

Diagrams synthesize structural conceptions of immunoglobulin molecules derived from work of Porter and of Edelman. Proteolytic action of papain splits molecule in hinge region to produce three fragments. Two, which are identical, have been labeled Fab and include combining sites for antigen; the remaining fragment – Fc – determines immunoglobulin class and subserves attachment of the immunoglobulin to target cells as well as a number of other immunobiologic functions. When a reducing agent is used to disrupt the disulfide bonds, the existence of four polypeptide chains – two heavy and two light – is demonstrable.

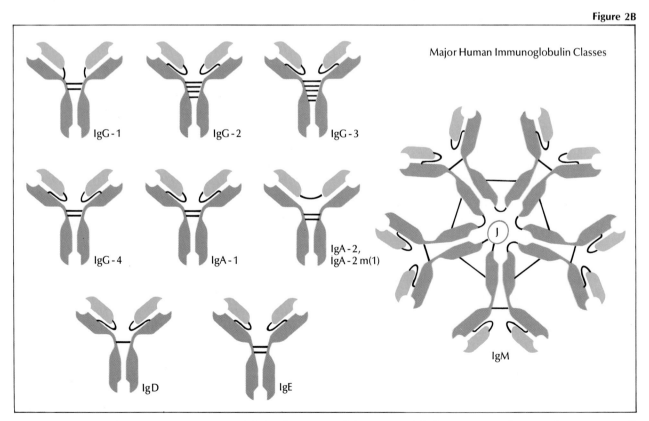

Schematic drawings depict the various immunoglobulin classes and subclasses with their varying interchain disulfide bonds. All of the immunoglobulins except IgM have a sedimentation coefficient of approximately 7S. Pentameric IgM is 19S.

phylactic reaction in guinea pigs. It was at this time that Porter described his work in preparing immunoglobulin fragments. We therefore prepared aggregates of both Fab and Fc fragments. The Fab preparations were inactive but the Fc fragments fixed complement and induced anaphylaxis. This and other experiments made clear that these biologic activities were associated with the Fc fragments (see Figure 5, page 19).

Since immunoglobulin class also could be correlated immunologically with the Fc, it seemed logical to hypothesize that different Ig classes would possess different biologic functions. A number of scientists initiated studies of class-function relationships, studies that eventuated in the delineation of a number of such differences, both qualitative and quantitative. Some of the differences are worth detailed description.

Both IgG and IgM antibodies are capable of fixing complement through the so-called classic pathway, that is, the pathway that begins with C_1 as the recognition unit, then proceeds through assembly of the so-called activation unit ($C_{4,2,3}$), and continues on to the membrane attack complex (C_{5-9}). Neither IgA nor IgE will fix complement through this pathway, although they appear to be able to do so through the more recently defined alternate pathway that starts with properdin and proceeds to the later complement components. With respect to the induction of the anaphylactic reaction in the guinea pig by human antibodies, only IgG antibody has this activity; neither IgA nor IgM does. IgM is extremely active in its ability to agglutinate red cells, while antibodies of the other classes are much lower in this capacity. And, of course, IgE antibodies are the only ones capable of skin sensitization as assayed by the PK reaction in humans and the analogous passive cutaneous anaphylaxis (PCA) in monkeys.

Although all of these reactions have major importance in immunologic protection and/or in immunopathology, perhaps even more interesting are the differences in cellular affinities that have been correlated with Ig class and subclass. For example, it has been found that two subclasses of IgG –

Figure 3

Human myeloma IgG γ chains		γ1	T	Q	K	S	L	S	L	S	P	G	COOH
		γ2	T	Q	K	S	L	S	L	S	P	G	
		γ3	T	Q	K	S	L	S	L	S	P	G	
		γ4	T	Q	K	S	L	S	L	S	L	G	
Animal IgG γ chains	Rabbit	γ	T	Q	K	S	I	S	R	S	P	G	
	Guinea Pig	γ2	T	Q	K	A	I	S	R	S	P	G	
	Horse	γ(T)	T	Q	K	N	V	S	H	S	P	G	
		γ(G)	T	Q	K	S	V	S	K	S	P	G	
	Dog	γ	T	D	L	S	L	S	H	S	P	G	
	Bovine	γ1	T	Q	K	S	T	S	K	S	A	G	
Human IgM		μ[Ou]	V	M	S	D	T	A	G	T	C	W	
Animal IgA		α1		M	A	Q	V	D	L	S	P	G	

The constancy of amino acid sequence in the carboxyl-terminal portions of IgG heavy chains is maintained not only from individual to individual but from species to species. Occasional variations are pinpointed above by absence of color background. In contrast, there is little homology between the COOH terminal residues of IgM and IgA (bottom two lines) and those of the IgG chains. Amino acid one-letter code used here is translated between the sequence diagrams on the next page.

IgG$_1$ and IgG$_3$ – have high affinity for many different types of phagocytic cells – neutrophils, monocytes, and macrophages (see Figure 6, page 20). This affinity exists whether the immunoglobulin is aggregated or in monomeric form. On the other hand, IgG$_2$ and IgG$_4$, as well as IgA, require aggregation in order to attach to phagocytes. This difference may be academic, since during in vivo participation in immunologic reactions immunoglobulin is aggregated by antigen.

From the point of view of biologic function, the significance of these cellular affinities is clear. In defending the host against bacteria and other microbial pathogens, antibody by itself is not destructive. The interaction in which it participates is antibody-antigen complexing, and this does not per se destroy or neutralize the pathogen. Such destruction, rather, is accomplished through the participation of chemical systems such as complement or comes about through phagocytosis, which is facilitated by the ability of the antibody Fc fragment to attach itself to the phagocytic cells.

There are, of course, other immunologic defense processes that do not require cellular participation. Among these is neutralization of toxins and of extracellular viruses. Both these processes take place in the circulation and are mediated by antibody.

Current evidence suggests that it is IgM and IgG antibody that functions mainly in the circulation, a view consistent with what is known of their biologic activities. IgM fixes complement and agglutinates red cells, but it does not have marked affinity for phagocytic cells. At least, such affinity is far less than that of IgG.

Immunoglobulin classes also differ significantly with respect to metabolism and ability to traverse the placenta. A major aspect of metabolism is duration of antibody viability. Again there is evidence that this is dependent on the Fc portion. Thus while the different classes of Ig molecules have very different half-lives, preparations consisting of isolated Fab fragments are all metabolized very rapidly – regardless of the Ig class from which the fragments are derived. On the other hand, when the whole immunoglobulin molecule is considered, IgG has a very much longer half-life than IgA, IgD, IgE, or IgM. This fact is of particular importance in passive immunization, in which new immunoglobulin synthesis does not take place. Passive immunization with IgG thus confers much more long-lived protection than that with antibodies of other Ig classes.

One type of passive immunization is a natural phenomenon: immunization of the fetus by maternal antibody.

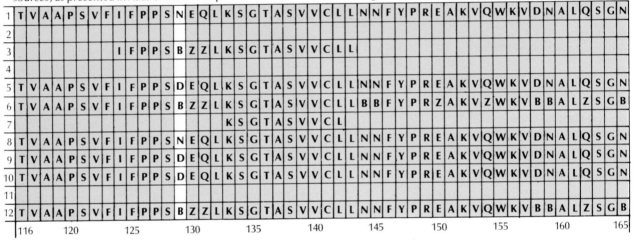

Amino acid one-letter notations: **A** – alanine, **B** – aspartic acid or asparagine, **C** – cysteine, **D** – aspartic acid, **E** – glutamic acid, **F** – phenylalanine, **G** – glycine, **H** – histidine, **I** – isoleucine, **K** – lysine, **L** – leucine, **M** – methionine, **N** – asparagine, **P** – proline, **Q** – glutamine, **R** – arginine, **S** – serine, **T** – threonine, **V** – valine, **W** – tryptophan, **X** – undetermined, **Y** – tyrosine, **Z** – glutamic acid or glutamine, **(-)** – gap in sequence. Note: Sequence data in these illustrations and the one on the preceding page are from many sources, as presented in Atlas of Protein Sequence and Structure, Vol. 5, Margaret O. Dayhoff, Ed., Georgetown University, 1972.

Variable regions of the immunoglobulin peptide chain are adjacent to the amino terminal. In kappa chain Bence Jones proteins from 12 human subjects (diagram at top), fewer than one quarter of the 115 residues (50 shown) are constant (color). In contrast, in the carboxyl half of the chains from same individuals (below), variation is seen in only three positions (e.g., in residue 129). It is widely believed that the portions of the chain that are folded into the antigenic combining sites of the antibody are the ones that manifest great variability of sequence, thus providing mechanism for specificity in immune recognition.

Since the infant is born without ability to respond to many different antigens, duration of maternal antibody persistence can have major survival significance. It is therefore interesting to note that only IgG crosses the placenta in considerable quantity, a fact that can be related teleologically to its longer half–life. There is evidence also that the capacity to synthesize IgM precedes that for IgG, and that IgA may be ingested with mother's milk.

To return now to the discussion of the affinity of various immunoglobulin classes for different homogeneous cell types, it can be noted that neither IgG nor IgA has any specific affinity for basophils or mast cells. These cells are of course the sources of histamine and slow-reacting substance of anaphylaxis (SRS-A) in hypersensitivity reactions. Indeed, it was our inability to designate these as target cells for any of the known immunoglobulin classes that led us to suspect reaginic antibody was derived from a previously undiscovered immunoglobulin.

Once we had identified IgE, work began in our laboratory and in other laboratories to characterize it physi-cally, chemically, and biologically. These efforts were greatly aided by the identification of a half dozen or so patients with IgE myeloma, which made available sources of IgE molecules in the purified form characteristic of myeloma proteins. One of the major thrusts of our investigations was the testing of the hypothesis that since reaginic antibodies are IgE, IgE molecules should have a specifically high affinity for the cell types with known pathologic roles in reaginic hypersensitivity, circulating basophils, and tissue–fixed mast cells.

We started with preparations of human leukocytes and of monkey lung fragments. (Lung tissue was chosen because of the obvious importance of the lungs in many atopic diseases such as ragweed allergy.) When the leukocyte preparation was incubated with antibody specific for IgE, histamine release resulted, indicating the presence of IgE in some portion of the leukocyte population. Similarly, the monkey lung fragments were incubated with E myeloma protein and then with anti–IgE; the result, again, was histamine release.

To achieve morphologic identification of the IgE-bearing cells, we then undertook autoradiographic studies. Specific anti-IgE antibody was labeled with ^{125}I and added to the isolated leukocytes in the presence of EDTA, an inhibitor of histamine release. Autoradiographs of the leukocytes demonstrated that the radioactive anti-IgE was attached to almost all cells containing metachromatic granules (basophils), but no combination occurred with any of the other leukocyte types: neutrophils, eosinophils, monocytes, or small lymphocytes.

When the same leukocytes were treated with iodine-labeled anti-IgG, most of the neutrophils and monocytes were labeled but none of the basophils, indicating the immunologic specificity of the IgE binding phenomenon. Completely parallel results were obtained with the tissue mast cells, although in these experiments the proximity of other cell types made it impossible to exclude the chance that some of the neighboring cells had IgE. Nevertheless, experiments over the years have made it abundantly clear that the major, if not the only, tissue cells sensitized by IgE are mast cells. We have also obtained firm evidence that the attachment to basophils and mast cells is a function of the IgE-Fc fragment. When preparations containing only the Fc fragment are used, binding takes place; it does not when the Fab fragment is employed.

Not only is the affinity of IgE molecules for basophils and mast cells highly specific but quantitatively it is extremely strong, far stronger, for example, than that of IgG molecules for macrophages or monocytes. There are a number of compelling biologic rea-

sons why this should be so.

In the experiments that sensitized the basophils and mast cells, the sequence of events included the direct attachment of IgE to its target cells. Implicit in this phenomenon is the presence on the target-cell membranes of specific IgE receptors. Only after the immunoglobulin or antibody attaches to the target cell does complexing with antigen, such as ragweed pollen, take place. The complex is then capable of transmitting the information that results in degranulation and release of histamine, SRS-A, eosinotactic factor, and perhaps other mediators of immediate hypersensitivity. The extremely high affinity between IgE and its target cells is most important in the context of two other pa-

rameters: extremely low concentration of IgE in the serum and the rapidity of catabolism of circulating immunoglobulin. Serum concentrations of IgE are generally in nanogram range, and rarely more than 1 μg/ml. (This is in contrast with IgG concentrations, which are in the range of 10 to 20 mg/ml, or some 10,000 to 20,000 times greater.) Unless the affinity of the molecule for its receptor is extremely high, a significant number of IgE molecules will not be bound; hence, there is a concentration of the immunoglobulin on its target cell that serves as a biologic compensation for the low concentration of IgE in serum and tissue fluids. This compensation has been quantified: the IgE affinity for basophils has been calculated at

Figure 5

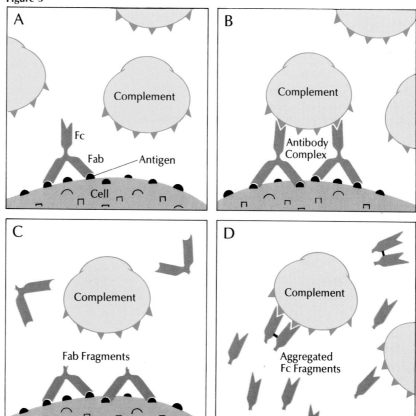

Summarized above are the findings of various experiments that have localized the ability to fix complement (via the classic pathway) to the Fc fragment of immunoglobulin. When intact IgG is used, a single immunoglobulin molecule, complexed with antigen, will not fix complement (A), but two or more IgG molecules, either complexed with antigen or nonspecifically aggregated, will do so (B). If IgG Fab fragments are substituted for whole immunoglobulin in the system, they can be complexed with antigen or otherwise aggregated, but complement fixation will not take place (C). However, aggregated Fc fragments alone will fix complement (D). Parallel observations have associated many other immunobiologic activities with the immunoglobulin Fc fragment.

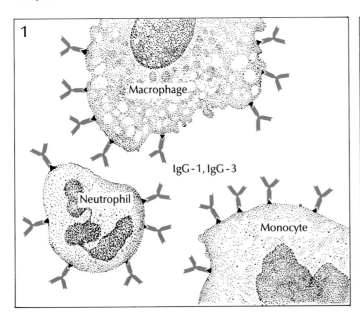

Different cellular affinities of the various immunoglobulin classes have important relationships to their biologic activities. Some of these affinities are represented above. IgG subclasses 1 and 3 have high affinity for phagocytic cells, such as macrophages, neutrophils, and monocytes, even without aggregation. IgA, IgG-2, and IgG-4 have similar cellular affinities, but re-

$10^9/M$, as compared with $10^5/M$ for IgG and monocytes, or a 10,000-fold difference.

The other factor, rapid catabolism, also provides a biologic rationale for high affinity. The half-life of IgE in the circulation is only two to three days. Yet we know that sensitization with reaginic antibody persists for a far longer time than that. One can get an allergic reaction by injecting antibody into the skin, waiting a week, and then injecting antigen. The explanation is that because of IgE's strong affinity for its target cells, dissociation is extremely gradual. Thus, high affinity does more than provide the IgE molecule with the capacity to concentrate on the cells it requires for functional expression. High affinity also maintains the association and permits persistence of biologic activity. Paradoxically, in the case of reaginic hypersensitivity this activity may be deleterious to the host. But from a teleologic point of view, one must assume that the hypersensitivity reaction has a still-to-be-discovered analogue that is, or has been, beneficial to the species in which it occurs.

Various facets of IgE–target-cell affinity have been extensively studied in an effort to determine whether they relate to susceptibility to atopic dis-ease. The question, of course, is whether there is a difference between atopic and nonatopic individuals in IgE–target-cell affinity. In most cases, such a difference has not been found. What has been observed is an enhanced level of serum IgE, which is related to elevated synthesis. As a result, the basophil receptors of atopic individuals are likely to be more highly saturated than those of normal individuals. A way of testing this in vitro is to incubate IgE with basophils. In such experiments, it has been found that nonatopic basophils are likely to bind more IgE molecules than cells from patients with atopic disease. Apparently, the former have more unoccupied receptors, since the IgE will complex only with such receptors.

There are some patients with atopic disease who have normal serum levels of IgE but whose basophils are as highly saturated as those of atopic patients with elevated serum IgE. In this minority, the basophils apparently do have an increased IgE avidity. The explanation probably relates to a genetic difference that causes an alteration in the receptor or cell surface structure. Perhaps these differences will be definable when investigators such as Metzger at NIH succeed in characterizing the IgE receptor.

In contrast to that of the receptor, the structure of the IgE molecule has been very well delineated. Let us turn now to this aspect of our discussion. As noted earlier, an IgE molecule consists of four polypeptide chains, two heavy chains (designated epsilon), and two light chains (κ) or (λ). Studies on myeloma proteins have yielded the information that IgE has a sedimentation coefficient of around 8.0S, that it is a glycoprotein, and that its carbohydrate moiety is about 12% of the total molecule. The molecular weight is close to 190,000. Each light chain has a molecular weight of about 22,500, each heavy chain of around 72,300. These last figures are derived from the findings of the Swedish investigators Bennich and Johansson. Others have calculated weights that are slightly, but not significantly, different.

Using papain digestion techniques, the native IgE molecule can be split into the Fc and Fab fragments. Further digestion will yield smaller fragments, permitting analysis of the content of the various fragments on the basis of antigenic determinants present on each. Figure 7 on page 22 provides a reference guide to the structure of the molecule.

The Fc fragments, made up exclusively of heavy-chain components, has

Figure 6

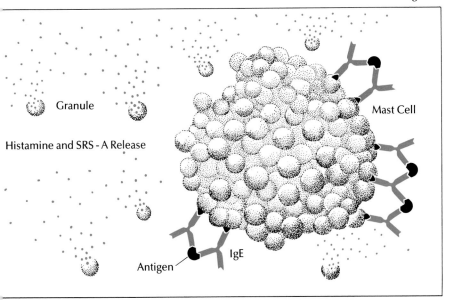

quire aggregation or complexing with antigen for attachment to phagocytes and for participation in opsonization. IgE molecules are unique in their affinity for basophils and mast cells and their ability to trigger histamine and SRS-A release.

been found to possess two antigenic determinants (ε_1 and ε_2) that are immunoglobulin class-specific. Each of the Fab fragments consists of a complete light chain and a portion of heavy chain designated as Fd. The Fd region possesses a third antigenic determinant (ε_0) that is idiotypic, that is, it is different for each E myeloma protein, depending on the individual patient from whom it was obtained.

Upon pepsin digestion, the carboxyl-terminal portion of the Fc fragment is split into small peptides, leaving a large fragment called $F(ab')_2$. This fragment consists of the two light chains, the Fd fragments of the heavy chains, and the Fc' regions, which consist of the amino-terminal third of the Fc. To exemplify the antigenic analysis that led to this "mapping," one can point out that it was found that the Fc' fragment shares the ε_1 with Fc. It was also determined that the $F(ab')_2$ shares antigenic ε_1 determinants with Fc and that the dimer includes the amino-terminal third of the heavy chain. Thus, it could be calculated that the Fc' is that amino-terminal third of heavy chain.

These structural data may seem esoteric. However, they have considerable bearing upon the biologic behavior of the IgE molecule. Before citing

some of the evidence that supports this statement, I should describe one other aspect of structure in some detail, the positioning of disulfide bonds. Studies both by Bennich and Johansson and by Kochwa and his colleagues yielded the information that each molecule of E myeloma protein contains 40 half cystine residues, which means that 20 disulfide bonds are present. Sixteen are intrachain bonds, 12 on the heavy chains and four on the light chains. Two more SS bonds connect the two heavy chains, both within the Fc' segment, one at the amino-terminal, the other at the carboxyl-terminal. The other two interchain bonds are at the hinges between the Fd segments of the heavy chains and the light chains. By consecutive increases in the concentration of such reducing agents as dithiothreitol (DTT) and alkylation, one can sequentially disrupt the disulfide bonds and determine the effects upon the biologic activity of IgE.

Among the properties that have been intensively studied in this way is the affinity between IgE and target mast cells and basophils. This affinity was measured by three parameters that have both clinical familiarity and pertinence: 1) the ability to sensitize primate skin in a reversed PK reaction;

2) the ability to sensitize human basophils as expressed by a reverse–type histamine release; and 3) the blockade of passive sensitization with reaginic antibody.

When a DTT concentration of 1 mM was used, the SS bonds between the heavy and light chains in the Fab fragment of the molecule were split; there was no diminution in the sensitizing potency of the reduced molecule as compared with the native protein. In a sense, this was expectable, since sensitization is dependent upon attachment of the immunoglobulin to cell receptors, a function we have already correlated with the Fc.

With an increased DTT concentration (2 mM), the bonds within the heavy chain lying between the hinge and the Fd were reduced. The resulting reduced-alkylated protein had a markedly reduced ability to attach to IgE target cells; what is more, the protein that did combine with basophils dissociated much more rapidly. Clearly the affinity had been diminished. It should be stressed that the bonds reduced at the 2 mM concentration lay entirely within the Fab fragment of the molecule; obviously the dogma that affinity of IgE for target cells is a function of the Fc required some qualification. A clue to the nature of this qualification resulted from a further experiment, with the protein reduced at the 2 mM concentration. The Fc portion of the reduced protein was separated from the Fab by papain digestion. When this was done, it was found that the affinity of the Fc was virtually equal to that of the untreated IgE. In other words, when the undisrupted Fc was attached to Fab protein that had been altered by SS bond reduction, it was unable to function with full biologic efficiency. When the undisrupted Fc was freed from the Fab, its affinity for target cells was fully restored. This finding strongly suggested that cleavage of disulfide bonds in the Fab portion of the molecule caused conformational changes impairing the ability of the Fc to attach to target cells.

To complete the picture, let me describe what happens if the reducing-agent concentration is increased to 10 mM. Now an additional fifth SS bond, one of the two inter-heavy

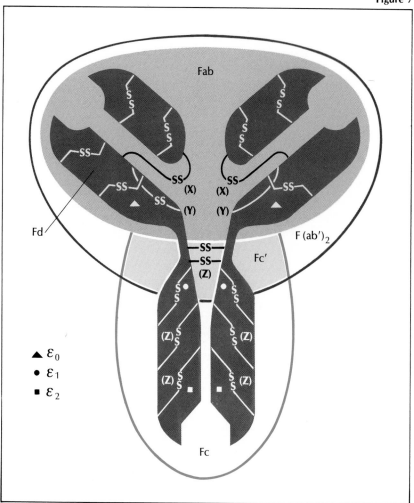

Some structural landmarks of IgE molecule are depicted above. The Fc fragments consist of heavy chain portions adjacent to carboxyl terminal and include class-specific antigenic determinants (ε_1 and ε_2). The Fab fragments include complete light chains and amino-terminal portions of heavy chain (Fd). Fd encompasses a third antigenic determinant that is idiotypic (ε_0). Presence of antigenic determinants has been critical to mapping of molecule. Other important areas of the molecule referred to in text are the F (ab')$_2$, consisting of the two light chains, the heavy chain Fd fragments, and the amino-terminal thirds of heavy chains (Fc'). Letters X, Y, and Z refer to the order in which SS bonds are disrupted in the reduction-alkylation experiments.

chain bonds in the Fc, is disrupted. However, neither of the heavy-chain antigenic determinants (ε_1 and ε) is degraded. This reduction-alkylation procedure results in the loss of both sensitizing and blocking activity. One can conclude that for the IgE to have

biologic activity – in this case target cell affinity – the Fc portion must be structurally intact. In other words, its tertiary structure or conformation cannot be altered to a degree that inhibits the capacity of the Fc to combine with receptors on the target cell

membrane. To some degree, the tertiary structure of the Fc is regulated by forces exerted from the Fab portion.

Such a relationship between conformation and biologic activity is not restricted to the IgE class of immunoglobulins. For example, Dorrington in Canada has shown that although the whole IgG-4 molecule does not fix complement by the classic pathway, the isolated Fc portion of the molecule will do so. Moreover, while this discussion has been largely restricted to the biologic activities related specifically to the Fc portion, tertiary structure appears equally important in relationship to Fab activity – which is mainly, of course, antigen-antibody combining capacity.

Also of considerable interest in this context is the concept of hypervariable regions of immunoglobulin, which has not been discussed here because it will be fully described in subsequent articles of this series. However, many readers will recall that amino acid sequence studies of Ig have shown that there are certain groups of amino acid residues in both light and heavy chains within the Fab portion that tend to vary from molecule to molecule much more frequently than do other sections of the chains. These hypervariable regions (see Figure 8, page 23) are believed to provide the mechanisms that permit the vast array of specificities required for immunologic function. If one looks at these hypervariable regions on a flat diagram in which the chains are simply presented linearly, they appear to be widely separated from one another. But x-ray diffraction studies have now shown that in actuality these regions are all found in close proximity, effectively surrounding holes in the tips of the molecules. They do in fact form the antibody's combining sites. So here we have another striking example of how conformational structure determines biologic function.

Figure 8

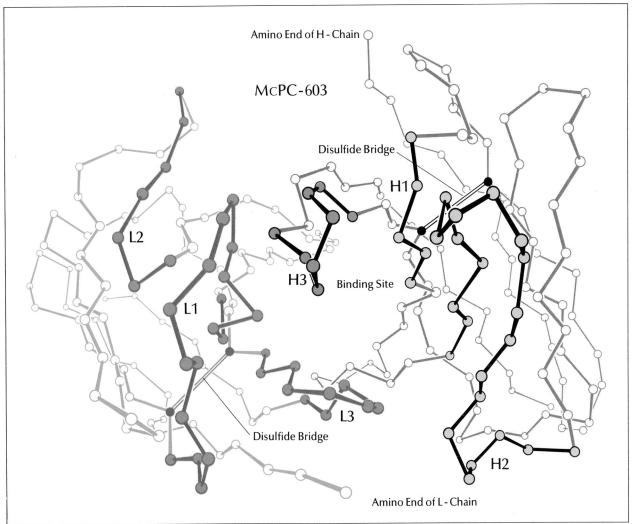

Amino End of H - Chain

McPC-603

Disulfide Bridge

H1

L2

H3

Binding Site

L1

L3

Disulfide Bridge

H2

Amino End of L - Chain

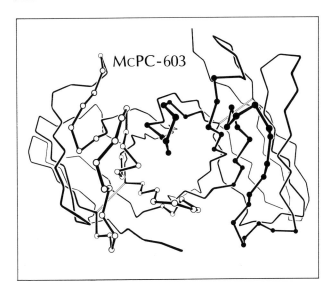

McPC-603

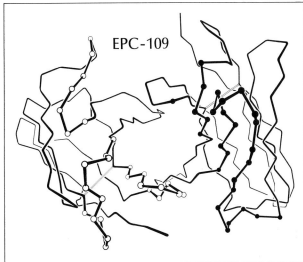

EPC-109

Three-dimensional model of mouse myeloma protein McPC-603, based on x-ray crystallographic data, calls out hypervariable "loops" of both heavy (H) and light (L) chains, showing their proximity to Fab binding site for the hapten phos- *phorylcholine. In smaller drawings, McPC-603 is compared with EPC-109. Conformation (and specificity) of binding site is changed by sequence differences corresponding to L1 and H3 loops (structural data from Davies and Padlan).*

Genetic Controls and Cellular Interactions in Antibody Formation

DAVID H. KATZ   *Medical Biology Institute, La Jolla*

That genes residing in the major histocompatibility complex (MHC) play an integral role in processes associated with immunologic recognition and cellular differentiation has become increasingly clear in recent years. Another major advance has been the delineation, in ever more complete detail, of the manner in which two major classes of lymphocytes, each having distinctive properties and functions, interact with one another in the development of effective immune responses. Taken together, these two groups of fundamental observations are enabling us to understand better how the immune defense system functions and regulates itself. They are also opening new avenues for research into methods of manipulating the immune system for therapeutic purposes when this is desirable. The scientific road that led to our present state of awareness has been complex and, in some instances, focused in seemingly different directions. To minimize the complexities as much as possible in this review, I will first discuss the major areas of investigation separately and then bring them together in an effort to delineate their close relationship.

Cell Interactions

It was clear to experimental immunologists during the 1950s and early 1960s that there were two distinct peripheral immune systems: one responsible for cell-mediated immunity, which was recognized very early to be associated primarily with the thymus and with cells originating in or influenced by the thymus; the other responsible primarily for humoral (antibody) immune responses. These two immunologic effector systems were originally regarded as distinct and discrete, having little or no apparent interrelationship. In 1966, however, first Henry Claman and his co-

workers in Denver and then, soon afterward, A.J.S. Davies in England and J.F.A.P. Miller and Graham Mitchell in Australia demonstrated that the development of antibody responses in mice required the concomitant presence of both thymus-derived and bone marrow–derived cells. This extremely important observation was based on experiments in which primary antibody responses to sheep erythrocytes were measured in irradiated recipients given either bone marrow cells alone, thymus cells alone, or a combination of the two cell types. Neither bone marrow cells nor thymus cells alone, they found, could reconstitute the capacity to develop antisheep erythrocyte antibody responses, but when both cell types were supplied exogenously, very good antibody production was obtained. Claman and his associates interpreted such results as indicating that antibody production required some form of interaction between the respective cell types. They held that only one of the cell types was the actual progenitor of the mature antibody-secreting cell, whereas the other (which they correctly guessed to be the thymus-derived cell) served some "auxiliary" function necessary for maturation of the bone marrow–derived cell into an antibody-secreting cell. Indeed, it was subsequently demonstrated by Miller and Mitchell that the bone marrow–derived cells, now designated as B lymphocytes, are exclusively the precursors of antibody-secreting plasma cells. The thymus-derived, or T lymphocytes, cannot differentiate into antibody-secreting cells but rather subserve a "helper" function that facilitates the differentiation of B lymphocytes into plasma cells.

Discovery of the phenomenon of "cell cooperation" prompted an intensive worldwide investigation into the bases and consequences of such cell interactions in the development of antibody responses. Subsequently similar studies were carried out on the occurrence of cell interactions in the development of cell-mediated immune responses.

Among the groups that embarked on these studies were N.A. Mitchison and coworkers in England, K. Rajewsky and his colleagues in Germany, and W.E. Paul, B. Benacerraf, and I at the National Institutes of Health. These studies had in common the use of hapten-protein conjugates, an approach that facilitated our understanding of recognition of distinct antigenic determinants by T and B lymphocytes. In general, it was found that recognition of haptenic determinants is primarily a property of hapten-specific B lymphocytes. T lymphocytes are primarily responsible for recognition of, and response to, the major determinants of the carrier portion of such conjugates. (It should be noted that there are also B lymphocytes specific for determinants on the carrier molecule, but under experimental conditions in which only antihapten antibodies are measured, such carrier-specific B lymphocytes are essentially ignored. In addition, it is also possible to find T lymphocytes with specific recognition capabilities for haptens, but under normal circumstances of immunization such hapten-specific T lymphocytes are relatively rare.)

The principle of experiments in which hapten-carrier conjugates are used to analyze cell cooperation in antibody responses is illustrated in Figure 2 on page 28. As shown in this diagram, if an animal is originally immunized with a hapten such as dinitrophenyl (DNP), coupled to a carrier such as ovalbumin (OVA), then the ability to obtain a secondary (or an anamnestic) anti-DNP antibody response ordinarily requires secondary immunization with DNP again coupled to OVA (group 1). If one attempts to immunize with DNP coupled to a second unrelated carrier, such as keyhole limpet hemocyanin (KLH), then little or no secondary anti-DNP antibody response would be observed (group 2). This inability to obtain a secondary antihapten antibody response unless the same carrier used for original immunization is also em-

ployed in the secondary challenge is a phenomenon known as the "carrier effect." It was originally described in 1963 by Z. Ovary and Benacerraf, then at New York University. Only several years later, as a result of the types of experiments discussed here, was it recognized that the carrier effect reflected a relative lack of sufficient numbers of carrier-specific T cells capable of helping the DNP-specific B lymphocytes to generate a secondary type antibody response. This conclusion followed from the fact that, as shown in Figure 2 (group 3), an animal immunized primarily with DNP-OVA can be stimulated to develop a secondary anti-DNP antibody response to DNP-KLH, provided this animal had been given a supplementary immunization with the carrier (KLH) alone at some time between the primary and secondary immunizations with the secondary carrier (KLH). Alternatively, in lieu of active immunization with the secondary carrier, such an animal can be stimulated to respond following the passive transfer of carrier-primed lymphocytes from a donor animal of identical histocompatibility genotype (i.e., from the same inbred strain). As shown in Figure 3, pages 30, 31, irradiated mice are used as recipients in the transfer of different cell populations obtained from donors immunized 1) with DNP-OVA (as a source of primed DNP-specific B cells); and 2) with KLH (as a source of KLH-specific helper T cells). As shown here, recipients of DNP-OVA-primed cells will respond to DNP-OVA (group 1) but not to DNP-KLH (group 2), unless a second cell population, primed to KLH, is co-transferred with the DNP-OVA-primed cells (group 3). It was this type of protocol that enabled M.C. Raff to demonstrate unequivocally that the KLH-primed cell type responsible for such helper activity is indeed of the T lymphocyte lineage.

Experimental approaches in both immunized animals and in cell transfer systems, such as those described above, have been used over the past eight years to analyze various parameters of T-cell function in cooperating with B cells in the development of antibody responses. As a result of these

studies, it is now clear that one of the main consequences of cell-cell interaction is to provide a regulatory force for controlling the magnitude and quality of such immune responses. With respect to the T lymphocytes, it has been well documented that their regulatory effects may either magnify or diminish antibody production. T cells responsible for enhancement are known as "helper" cells; T cells responsible for diminution are known as "suppressor" cells.

During the earlier years of investigation of cell cooperation phenomena and immune responses, emphasis was placed on the role of helper T cells. More recently, owing in large part to work by R.K. Gershon and his associates at Yale, the function of suppressor T lymphocytes has been intensively studied. In addition to the regulatory effects of T lymphocytes on magnitude of antibody production, it is clear that differentiation of subclasses of B lymphocytes responsible for producing different classes of antibodies requires the participation of T-cell regulation. Thus, T lymphocytes participate markedly in the effective development of antibody responses of the IgG, IgA, and IgE classes. In contrast, B lymphocytes capable of developing into mainly IgM-antibody-secreting cells appear to be somewhat less dependent for their differentiation upon participation of T lymphocytes.

At this point, it is pertinent to point out that the lymphocytes responsible for exerting these opposing regulatory effects, namely helper vs suppressor, actually constitute two distinct T-lymphocyte subpopulations. This conclusion has resulted from studies by H. Cantor at Harvard and E.A. Boyse at Memorial Sloan-Kettering Cancer Institute in New York ("Surface Characteristics of T-Lymphocyte Subpopulations"). To complicate matters further, Cantor, Gershon, and others have obtained evidence indicating that helper T lymphocytes regulate the development of suppressor T lymphocytes and vice versa, thereby indicating a rather closed circular network of cell-cell communication capable of self-regulating the immune system in apparently every imaginable direction.

Figure 1

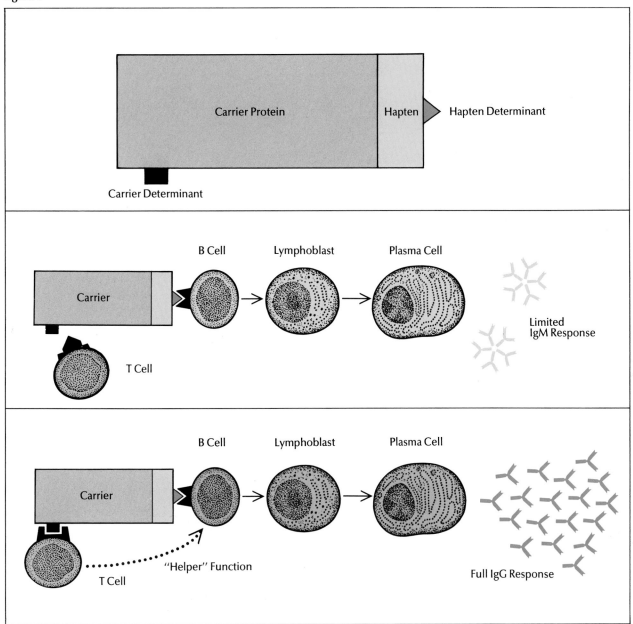

The concept that both T lymphocytes and B lymphocytes participate in an antibody response is diagrammed above. Shown in the top panel is a representation of antigen with both carrier and hapten components, each possessing discrete antigenic determinants. If the responding organism is competent to produce B cells able to recognize the hapten determinant but not to produce T cells for recognition of the carrier determinant, antibody to the hapten will be limited to IgM (middle). If the carrier determinant is also recognized by the animal's T cells, a full antihapten antibody response occurs (bottom).

Although the previous discussion has centered around the cell-cell interactions between lymphocyte classes and subclasses, it is also essential to acknowledge the very important role played by macrophages, both in immune responses in general and in the development and regulation of cell interactions in particular. The studies by E.R. Unanue and associates at Harvard have amply documented an important role for macrophages in the presentation of antigen to both T lymphocytes and B lymphocytes. Furthermore, Unanue and others have demonstrated the capacity of macrophages to secrete biologically active soluble mediators that themselves are capable of exerting a considerable influence on lymphocyte functions. In terms of their role in cell interactions, macrophages appear to be particularly important for the development of the helper type T lymphocyte, as indicated by the work of M. Feldmann and colleagues in London, and less important for the induction of suppressor function, although it should be noted that this point has not yet been definitively established.

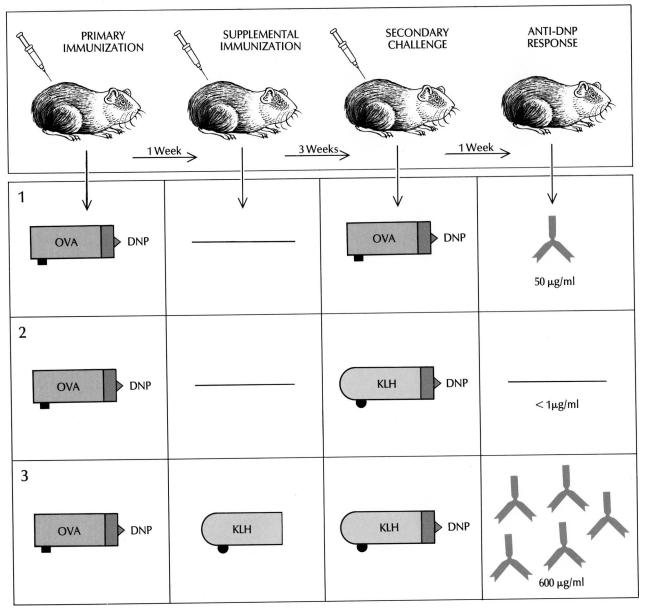

The generalized concept depicted in the previous figure is applied above in an actual experimental situation. The immunization schedule is shown at the top. If the animal is first immunized with the hapten DNP on an ovalbumin (OVA) carrier, and then challenged with the same hapten-carrier conjugate, an anamnestic anti-DNP antibody response is obtained. If the challenge is with a conjugate of DNP and a second carrier, KLH, the secondary response is almost nil. However, if, between the primary immunization and the challenge, the animal is presented with an immunizing dose of just the second carrier, then challenge with DNP-KLH will result in a full (and in these experiments actually heightened) antibody response to DNP.

Genetic Control of Immune Responses

In all mammalian species studied, including man, it has been found that the ability of an individual to respond to specific antigens is under the control of genes that reside in the chromosomal region known as the major histocompatibility gene complex; this has been well established by H.O. McDevitt. Additionally, in several species the particular chromosome on which this complex is located has been determined. In man, the MHC, known as *HLA*, is located on chromosome 15; in the mouse, it is known as *H-2* and is located on chromosome 17. The genes associated with the capacity to develop immune responses are designated *Ir*, for immune response.

Much has been learned in recent years concerning the characteristics of the responses controlled by *Ir* genes and thereby of their possible mechanisms of action. Among the most intriguing developments in this context are those that relate to cellular interactions in the immune response, specifically the interactions among the different classes of lymphocytes. As will be discussed further in the next section, considerable evidence has been obtained for the existence of genes in the MHC that specify products involved in cell differentiation – in either the process of antigen stimulation and/or in the interaction of cells belonging to different lymphocyte classes or subclasses. These latter genes have been designated as *CI,* for cell interaction, and may or may not be identical to *Ir* genes (as discussed below). There is evidence also to suggest that perhaps one or more of the gene products encoded in the MHC is associated in some manner with the receptor on cells of the T lymphocyte class. Finally, we have come to realize that just as there are genes controlling the immune response, so too are there genes governing the opposite phenomenon, immunosuppression.

The earliest work that led us to recognize that immune responses are indeed under genetic control began in the early 1960s, at the laboratories of Benacerraf at New York University. Experimenting with outbred guinea pigs, Benacerraf and his associates found that some individual guinea pigs were capable, others incapable, of developing immune responses to a synthetic polypeptide, poly-L-lysine (PLL), and to DNP hapten conjugates of PLL. Measuring both antibody formation and delayed hypersensitivity responses, Benacerraf and associates observed that the guinea pigs consistently proved to be either responders or nonresponders with regard to both criteria. It will be recalled that it was not until 1966 that antibody production was shown to depend on interactions between the two major lymphocyte classes, T and B. Therefore, the mechanism responsible for the parallel patterns of antibody formation and delayed hypersensitivity reactions in guinea pigs was inexplicable at the time these observations were made.

Subsequently McDevitt and his colleagues at Stanford carried out experiments with inbred mice in which certain strains were identified as responders and others as nonresponders to another synthetic polypeptide, (T,G)-A--L. Out of these studies came

the absolute documentation that the ability of inbred mice to respond to this and to other antigens with limited numbers of determinants was controlled by genes located within the *H-2* major histocompatibility gene complex of the mouse. This linkage was established by crossbreeding experiments using congenic strains of mice, i.e., strains genetically identical to those that were either responders or nonresponders *except* for the portion of the chromosome that contains the *H-2* complex. In this way it was possible to demonstrate that responsiveness and nonresponsiveness segregated genetically in an absolute linkage with the *H-2* complex.

It is pertinent to cite the fact that mapping *Ir* genes within the *H-2* complex was made possible largely as a result of previous genetic studies in mice over many years, initiated by P. Gorer and G.D. Snell and their associates. From this research, a vast array of recombinant mouse strains had emerged in which numerous chromosomal crossover events had occurred in the course of multiple matings. Such events can be defined and studied by serologic techniques so that the investigator working with recombinant inbred mice can know with reasonable certainty where the chromosomal breaks leading to a strain's particular genetic constituion are located. In this way, extensive analysis by D. Shreffler and J. Klein and their colleagues has resulted in the current map of the *H-2* complex of the mouse, shown in the diagram (Figure 4 on page 33).

As can be seen in this diagram, the complex is divided into nine regions and subregions. On its left and right ends are regions designated *K* and *D,* respectively. These regions were identified, in general, by the ability of one mouse strain to recognize another mouse strain immunologically, either by rejecting skin grafts or by making antibodies to alloantigens encoded by genes in each of these regions. The *S* region shown on the map was first defined by Shreffler, now at Washington University, St. Louis, and is known to code for certain components of the complement system. Between the *S* and *D* regions, there is the *G* re-

gion, which contains genes whose products constitute certain murine erythrocyte alloantigens. Between the *K* and the *S* regions lies the region designated as *I,* where the various *Ir* genes, among others, are located. In extensive studies, the *I* region has been further subdivided into five subregions; this subclassification is based on various findings relating either to the existence of *Ir* genes and/ or to specific, serologically definable antigens encoded by genes located within the specific subregions.

Having described the various genetic regions of the *H-2* complex, let us now return to the cellular side of the immune response in which *Ir* genes appear to be involved. As noted earlier, the first *Ir* gene or genes to be discovered controlled the ability of guinea pigs to respond to the synthetic polypeptide PLL. The definitive expression of that response was the elaboration of antibodies to PLL when animals were immunized either with the synthetic polypeptide alone or with conjugates in which PLL served as a carrier for DNP (or similar) haptens. In addition to controlling the ability of individual animals to produce antibody responses to PLL, the relevant *Ir* genes also determined the ability of such animals to make delayed hypersensitivity responses, a function known to be subserved by T cells. Similarly, genetic responder animals were found to be capable of exhibiting antigen-induced in vitro T-lymphocyte proliferative responses, whereas nonresponder animals were unable to do so. In other words, there was a precise correlation between the T-cell proliferative response and the capacity for delayed hypersensitivity (as shown by skin testing) and humoral antibody responsiveness.

At this time (the mid-1960s), Benacerraf and I. Green made an additional observation that proved highly significant: namely, that nonresponder animals unable to produce anti-DNP antibody in response to DNP-PLL could do so when the DNP-PLL was complexed to a second carrier molecule, bovine serum albumin (BSA). Guinea pigs so immunized now made anti-DNP antibody that was quantitatively and qualitatively indistinguishable from the antibody

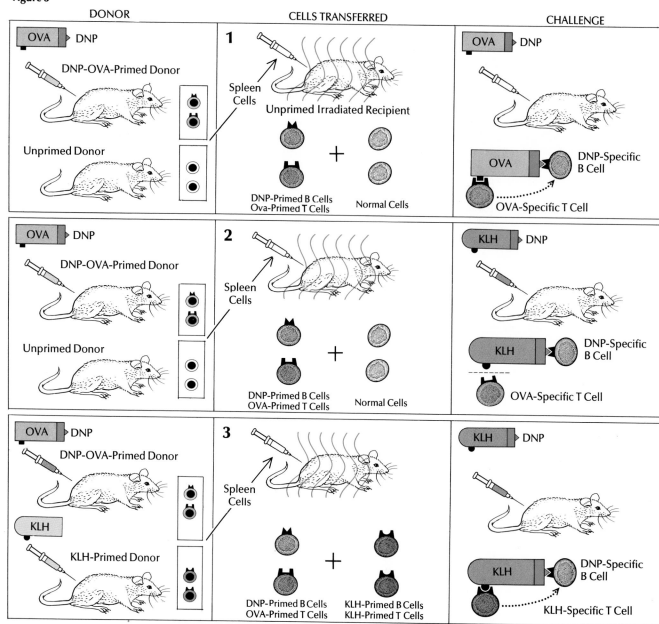

DONOR   CELLS TRANSFERRED   CHALLENGE

In place of active immunization experiments, the "carrier" effect can be demonstrated in cell transfer experiments. In all three of the experiments summarized here, lymphocytes are passively transferred from two donor animals to an irradiated recipient. In the top two schemes, the donors are an animal immunized with DNP-OVA and an unimmunized animal. In the third case, an animal immunized with just the KLH carrier is substituted for the unimmunized donor. Thus, in experiment 1, the transferred cells include DNP-primed B cells, OVA-primed T lymphocytes, and "normal" cells. Challenge with DNP-OVA

made by the genetic responder animals. Moreover, these animals were able to develop delayed hypersensitivity responses to BSA. They were still incapable of such responses to PLL, even though they could produce antibody directed against the DNP determinants linked to the PLL.

Once cooperative interactions between T and B lymphocytes were dis-covered, it was possible to interpret the above observations. To wit, an animal *lacking* the *Ir* gene required for antibody responses to DNP-PLL could produce antibody if it was provided with a molecule to which its T cells were capable of responding – namely, BSA. Thus, the expression of the particular *Ir* gene involved clearly appeared to be at the T-cell level. Or to put it another way, there was no defect in the capacity of the DNP-specific B cell to respond to the DNP determinant on PLL provided that the animal's T cells were stimulated by an antigen to which they could respond.

A number of observations now seem to indicate that the function of his-tocompatibility-linked *Ir* genes lies primarily at the T-cell level. For exam-

Figure 3

RESPONSE

Anti-DNP Response

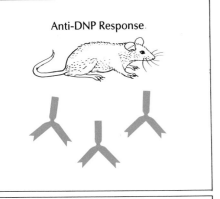

No Anti-DNP Antibody Response

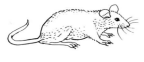

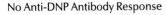

Anti-DNP Response

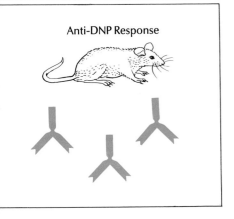

produces anti-DNP response. In 2, the same cells are transferred, but challenge is with DNP-KLH, and response is lacking. In 3, KLH-primed T cells are transferred. DNP-KLH elicits response.

ple, all immunologic responses in which histocompatibility-linked *Ir* genes have been identified are responses classified as thymus-dependent, i.e., in which the ability to obtain an antibody response to a thymus-dependent antigen requires the direct cooperative participation of T lymphocytes. There also exists a small class of thymus-independent antigens,

which are capable of inducing antibody responses of a limited nature in the *relative* absence of T-cell participation. Such responses are in general limited to the IgM antibody class, are of short duration, and usually manifest little or no capability for inducing anamnestic antibody response.

Mitchell and others, working at Stanford in the early 1970s, also contributed to the notion that *Ir* genes function primarily at the T-cell level. One of the group, C. Grumet, had found that nonresponder strains of mice to (T,G)-A--L, although unable to make a normal type of response to this antigen comparable to those of responder strains, were nevertheless capable of producing a limited antibody response, restricted to the IgM class, following appropriate immunization. Mitchell and associates simply took groups of responder and nonresponder mice to (T,G)-A--L and either subjected them to surgical thymectomy or performed sham thymectomies on control groups of both types of strains. When such animals were subsequently immunized with (T,G)-A--L, the sham-operated responder mice developed normal responses to (T,G)-A--L consisting of both IgM and IgG classes; sham-thymectomized nonresponder animals behaved in a fashion normal for them, namely, they produced limited IgM antibody responses.

The important observation, however, was that the thymectomized responder strain mice produced antibody responses to (T,G)-A--L that were indistinguishable from the nonresponder strains whether the latter had been thymectomized or not. Thus, thymectomized responder mice also were unable to produce anti-(T,G)-A--L antibody responses other than those of a limited IgM quality, with no switchover to IgG. Such observations certainly made a very strong argument in favor of the concept that *Ir* genes function primarily at the T-cell level.

The first hint that, at least in certain strains of mice, the *Ir* gene defect leading to nonresponse might exist at the B-cell rather than the T-cell level, came from G. Shearer, E. Mozes, and M. Sela in Israel, who used a complex cell transfer system with a limited

number of donor bone marrow cells. Very recently, M.J. Taussig, first with Mozes in Israel, and subsequently with A. Munro in England, provided corroborating evidence for the existence of *Ir* gene functional expressions at the B-cell level. These later studies employed considerably different methodology in which special techniques enabled these investigators to obtain soluble, and biologically active, mediators from tissue culture preparations of previously immunized T lymphocytes from (T,G)-A--L-primed donor mice.

In the context of our present discussion, the crucial findings concerning the issue of whether *Ir* genes function at the B-cell level and/or T-cell level have come from studies in which it proved possible to stimulate T lymphocytes of nonresponder animals to produce soluble mediators following stimulation with (T,G)-A--L, mediators that in turn were capable of providing some cooperative "help" for B cells obtained from responder strain donors. On the other hand, in certain instances, the (T,G)-A--L-specific soluble mediators have been found unable to stimulate B cells obtained from nonresponder strains. Conversely, in some nonresponder strains it has been found that the B cells are capable of responding to the biologically active factor derived from (T,G)-A--L-stimulated responder strain T lymphocytes, but their T lymphocytes are defective in their capacity to produce such factors. In other words, depending on the circumstances, a nonresponder individual may be a nonresponder either because of a defect in *Ir* gene function at the T-cell or B-cell level or, in some instances, at both. Such findings, and others made in somewhat different systems discussed below, are the basis of the current concept that the *Ir* genes are integrally concerned with cell-cell interactions in immune responses.

An interesting addition to the complexity surrounding the functions of *Ir* genes has been the recent finding that in certain immune responses genetic control involves the function of *two*, rather than one, *Ir* genes. The finding suggesting two-gene control of some responses has come from several sources, including Taussig and Munro in England and Rajewsky and associates in Germany. The most extensive studies of this type have been those performed by M. Dorf and Benacerraf and their associates at Harvard, in which the antigen used has been the synthetic polypeptide glutamic acid, lysine, phenylalanine (GLϕ). One can briefly summarize the case for two-gene involvement as follows: the earlier assumption that only a single gene determined whether a given inbred strain of animal would be a responder or nonresponder was based on the finding that in most instances, matings between nonresponder animals almost inevitably produced nonresponder offspring. However, in the case of GLϕ (as well as certain other antigens), it was found that in selected instances, matings between two nonresponder strains produced offspring capable of developing a response. Extensive genetic analyses led to the conclusion that in such instances both of the original nonresponder strains lack one of two genes necessary for response to GLϕ. The gene missing in one strain is different from the gene missing in the second strain. Therefore, when two such strains are mated, their offspring will inherit one of each of the two necessary genes for responsiveness from the opposite parents, and this process of genetic complementation results in reconstitution of the capacity of such offspring to respond to the antigen in question. There are many speculations as to what determines the requirement for two genes to control a given immune response, but firm conclusions on this point will not be reached until work now under way in several laboratories is completed.

Another variable that adds to the complexity of the entire subject is the heterogeneous range of T-cell functions, a range that led to the delineation of the functionally distinct subpopulations of T cells. As discussed earlier, helper T lymphocytes function to amplify or increase the magnitude of responses of B cells or other T cells, while suppressor T lymphocytes regulate, in a negative manner, a given immune response.

Awareness that there are suppressor T cells developed independently of the research in the genetic control of immune responsiveness. When it became clear that T-cell helper function is missing in some nonresponder animals, however, Gershon decided to explore whether one could detect the presence and activity of suppressor T lymphocytes in such nonresponders. Indeed, Gershon, together with P.H. Maurer and C. Merryman at Jefferson Medical School, observed that in one murine system under *Ir* gene control – namely, the response to the synthetic polymer GAT – nonresponder animals were able to express a T-cell response as measured by antigen-stimulated in vitro DNA synthesis. The authors suggested from these results that, although unable to produce a positive response to GAT, T lymphocytes of nonresponders may in fact be capable of developing suppressor T-cell function following GAT stimulation. Subsequently, Kapp, Pierce, and Benacerraf at Harvard confirmed this prediction by demonstrating that animals unresponsive to GAT nevertheless produced antigen-specific T cells, which, after stimulation with the antigen, functioned as suppressors of the GAT response. (This could be shown because under ordinary conditions, cell cultures of nonresponder lymphocytes are able to produce a GAT-antibody response when stimulated with a conjugate of GAT coupled to bovine serum albumin. But when cells from another animal stimulated with GAT alone are added to the culture, the antibody response to GAT coupled to BSA is abolished.)

More recently, P. Debré and Benacerraf have further explored the phenomenon of suppressor T cells in genetically controlled systems and have obtained evidence for a distinct gene system, known as *Is* (immune suppression) genes, that determines the capacity of a given individual to induce specific suppressor T lymphocytes following antigen stimulation. These experiments have raised the additional intriguing possibility that *Is* genes serve as a counterbalancing force to *Ir* genes in controlling immunologic responsiveness. Like the situation with *Ir* genes, however, it has yet to be established precisely what the molecular products of such genes may be in terms of their functional activities.

Genetic Restrictions on Cell-Cell Interactions

Since 1970, several laboratories have demonstrated an additional role for histocompatibility gene products in regulating immune responses. (The term, "histocompatibility gene products," in this context refers to those molecules involved in the recognition of foreign cells [e.g., transplanted tissue cells], rather than those molecules involved in recognition of and response to specific antigens, i.e., the *Ir* gene products.)

The studies to be described were concerned with the ability of lymphocyte classes and subclasses to interact with one another, as well as with macrophages, as a function of their histocompatibility genetic constitution. The first experiments that indicated a possible role of histocompatibility antigens in the mechanism by which cells interact in the immune system were performed by Paul, Benacerraf, and me at NIH. We found in guinea pigs that we could circumvent the need to prime helper T cells to a given carrier in order to facilitate the response of hapten-specific B lymphocytes to the relevant hapten-carrier conjugate (see Figure 3). Our method was to transfer unprimed allogeneic immunocompetent cells that were obtained from lymph node and spleen. As schematically illustrated in the diagram (Figure 5, page 35), transfer of allogeneic cells (cells of a genetically different histocompatibility antigen type) induced an enhanced secondary antibody response to DNP even though one changed from carrier A to carrier B between the first and second immunizations.

Experimentally, it was then established that this phenomenon, called the "allogeneic effect," arose from the fact that the donor lymphocytes recognized and reacted with the "foreign" histocompatibility antigens of the recipient animal. As a result of this "graft-versus-host" reaction, the recipient B cells differentiated to mature antibody-secreting cells; most important, this capacity of allogeneic unprimed T cells to stimulate differentiation of hapten-specific B cells was indistinguishable in its ultimate effects from the capacity of carrier-primed syngeneic T cells to mediate this function under physiologic circumstances (Figure 6, page 36).

These experiments provided fruitful early clues to our knowledge of genetic limitations upon interactions between the two lymphocyte classes. To understand the line of reasoning involved, one must keep in mind that recognition of and reaction to histocompatibility or transplantation antigens is for the most part a T-cell function and that differentiation to antibody-secreting cells is a capability restricted exclusively to B cells. The allogeneic effect suggested that, as a consequence of the reaction of immunocompetent donor T lymphocytes with B cells of the recipient, a strong stimulatory signal was somehow transmitted to the recipient cells – a signal that one could assume involved molecules on the cell surfaces of both donor and recipient lymphocytes. Such findings led us to ask what might be the physiologic counterpart of this interaction. In view of the ability of allogeneic cells to circumvent the need for specifically primed T-cell recognition of carrier molecules – and, more precisely, as a consequence of the ability of such allogeneic cells to interact with foreign surface histocompatibility molecules on the target recipient cells – we began to suspect that the histocompatibility molecules may represent the very surface structures that are normally involved in the mechanism of T-B-cell interaction within a given individual.

We set out to test these suspicions experimentally and at the same time to evaluate the role of genetic background on the control of these interactions. Briefly, T. Hamaoka, Benacerraf, and I sought to determine whether T-B-cell cooperation could occur between cells of the respective lymphocyte classes when such cells were obtained from donors that differed at genes in the major histocompatibility complex, and importantly, under conditions in which the allogeneic effect was prevented from occurring. In order to do this, appropriately primed T cells and B cells from mice of different inbred strains A and B were transferred to irradiated recipient mice in either syngeneic or allogeneic reciprocal mixtures and then

Figure 4

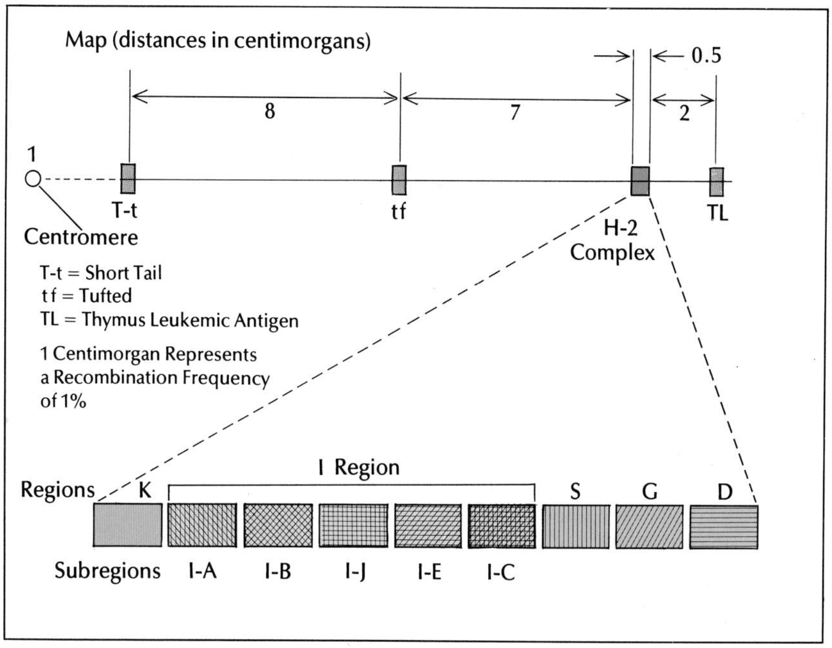

Map shows location of major histocompatibility complex (H-2) in the mouse, including the I region that contains immune response genes (Ir), as well as genes that code for molecules involved in cell interaction (CI), and immunosuppression (Is). In addition, several soluble factors involved in the immune response appear to contain antigens associated with genes located in the I region of the H-2 complex.

tested for their capacity to interact in response to an appropriate DNP-protein carrier conjugate.

The results of these studies demonstrated clearly that the ability of T and B cells to interact effectively in development of an immune response required that the respective cell types be genetically identical at the major histocompatibility gene complex. Mixtures of T and B lymphocytes, differing at certain critical genes in the MHC, either completely failed to interact or interacted weakly. Genetic mapping analysis localized the genes responsible for effective cell interactions to the I region of the complex that, by definition, is the same region in which the Ir genes reside. We could not at this stage of our research determine whether the genes responsible for controlling effective cell interactions were the same as or different from those known to govern immune responses. We designated the former genes as CI, for cell interaction.

An experiment was performed very early in these genetic studies that strongly suggested a close functional relationship between CI and Ir genes.

In the background of this experiment was the knowledge that under normal circumstances, carrier-primed T lymphocytes from an F_1 hybrid offspring of two different parental strains display an equal capacity for providing helper activity to hapten-specific B lymphocytes of either of the two respective parents – provided the carrier used for initial sensitization is one to which both parental strains are genetically capable of responding. We employed a carrier molecule to which one parent strain was a responder and the second parent strain a nonresponder (the F_1 hybrids of such matings are, of course, responders). Such carrier-primed F_1 T cells were found to be capable of providing helper activity for hapten-specific B cells of the responder, but *not* the nonresponder, parental type. This type of observation indicated either that the responsible Ir genes were capable of controlling the function of the B lymphocytes as well as T lymphocytes, and/or that the Ir genes concerned with this particular response were actually controlling the effectiveness of interactions between the T and B lymphocytes involved.

Studies from our laboratory concerning the role of MHC gene products in controlling cell-cell interactions between T and B lymphocytes were complemented by studies of interactions between macrophages and T lymphocytes at the NIH by A.S. Rosenthal and E.M. Shevach. They used T-cell–enriched populations of lymphocytes from two different guinea pig strains to study the response to sensitization by purified protein derivative (PPD). When the macrophages and lymphocytes employed were from the same strain, the macrophages proved capable of stimulating the T cells to high levels of DNA synthesis. However, when the histocompatibility barrier was interposed by using macrophages of one genetic strain and lymphocytes from another, the DNA synthetic response was abolished or greatly reduced. Further analysis, including reactions between lymphocytes and macrophages obtained from F_1 animals and from the two parental strains, added support to the investigators' conclusion that optimal macrophage-T-cell interactions are mediated in some way by histocompatibility molecules or closely related membrane structures. More recently, similar studies by Feldmann and colleagues in London have demonstrated that in the mouse the most effective macrophage-T-cell interactions in the development of helper T-cell function occur when the macrophages and T lymphocytes, respectively, are obtained from individuals genetically identical at the *I* region.

Further studies by Shevach and Rosenthal of response patterns in the guinea pig to antigens known to be under single *Ir* gene control demonstrated that lymphocytes of F_1 offspring of responder-nonresponder matings were poorly stimulated by nonresponder parental macrophages pulsed with such antigen. Similarly treated macrophages from the responder parent produced markedly higher stimulation of the F_1 lymphocytes. Such results imply that *Ir* gene products have a role governing effective macrophage-T-cell interactions.

The foregoing series of observations indicated that genetic compatibility at the *I* region is required for the most effective interactions not only between T and B lymphocytes but also between macrophages and T lymphocytes. In interpreting these genetic restrictions, we inferred that histocompatibility antigens are integrally involved in the mechanism by which such cell interactions take place. We proposed that such interactions either are mediated by identical *CI* gene products on the surface membranes of T and B lymphocytes, or, alternatively, that T lymphocytes of a given individual have the capacity to recognize and react with an appropriate *CI* gene product on the surface membranes of autologous B lymphocytes. This reasoning would suggest that failure of effective cooperation between T and B lymphocytes derived from genetically nonidentical individuals results either from dissimilarity of the genetically distinct *CI* gene products or from an inability of the T cells to recognize and react appropriately with *CI* gene products on the genetically distinct B-cell population.

An important series of observations made in a somewhat different system have provided additional insights into this question, particularly with respect to whether such interactions occur via identical molecules or through some form of self-recognition phenomenon. R.M. Zinkernagel and P.C. Doherty, working first in Australia and later in the United States, found that the capacity of cytotoxic T lymphocytes to lyse and thereby destroy virus-infected target cells depends on MHC gene identities between cytotoxic T-lymphocyte and target cell populations. In contrast to the situation with T-B-cell interactions and macrophage-T-cell interactions, the genes involved in determining effective cytotoxic T-lymphocyte target cell lysis were found to map in the *K* and/or *D* regions of the mouse *H-2* complex. Precisely identical observations were made independently by G.M. Shearer and associates at the National Institutes of Health using a slightly different cytotoxic T-lymphocyte system. Following extensive investigations of this phenomenon, the collective implications of the observations of Zinkernagel and Doherty and of Shearer and his associates have been that the genetic restrictions in cytotoxic T-lymphocyte function for effective target cell lysis most probably reflect some form of self-recognition. These observations, in turn, have been very important in influencing thinking about the probable mechanism of genetic restrictions in other types of cell interactions controlled by *I* region genes. One can easily envisage a similar form of self-recognition by T cells of the appropriate *CI* molecules on the surface of B cells and/or macrophages, as illustrated in Figure 6.

Adding to the complexity of such phenomena was another series of very important observations in which the requirement for MHC identity in T-B-cell interactions has been investigated using lymphocytes from chimeric individuals. A chimera is an individual artificially given relatively equal mixtures of hematopoietic and lymphoid cells derived from two genetically distinct sets of parents. Experiments using cells of this type by K. Bechtol and McDevitt at Stanford and by H. von Boehmer and J. Sprent in Basel showed that T and B cells, which had undergone their development in the same individual, so that they were mutually tolerant and would not undergo transplantation reactions against each other although they were derived from genetically distinct sets of parents, were indeed capable of undergoing effective T-B-cell interactions. Although such results were initially believed to be in direct contrast to observations from our laboratory indicating a requirement for genetic identity between T and B cells to obtain cooperative interactions, it now appears that we can make a reasonable explanation for these striking differences in results. The difference appears to stem from the fact that in one series of observations, T and B lymphocytes were obtained from fully mature donor animals that differed genetically and were then placed in contact with one another for a short period of time so that they might undergo cooperative interaction. In such instances cooperative interactions failed to take place whenever the respective lymphocyte classes came from donors differing at genes in the *I* region.

In contrast, in the case of the chimera experiments, the respective T- and B-cell classes had undergone de-

Figure 5

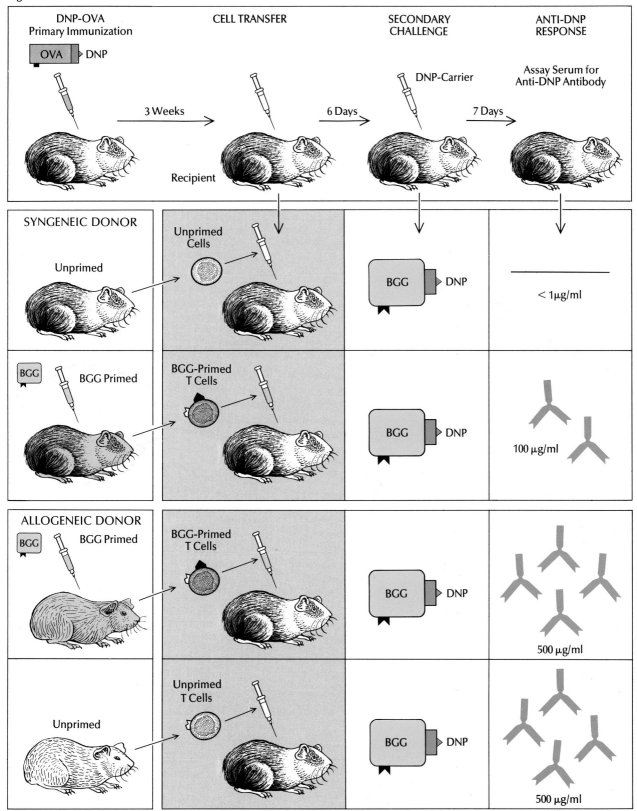

The phenomenon known as the allogeneic effect is schematized here. The upper panels, in which donor and recipient animals are of the same inbred strain, restates the point that to get an anamnestic response to a haptenic determinant, both donor cells and the recipient animal must be immune to carrier as well as hapten. But, when animals of different – or allogeneic – strains are used as cell donors, a response to the haptenic determinant will occur without carrier-primed T lymphocytes.

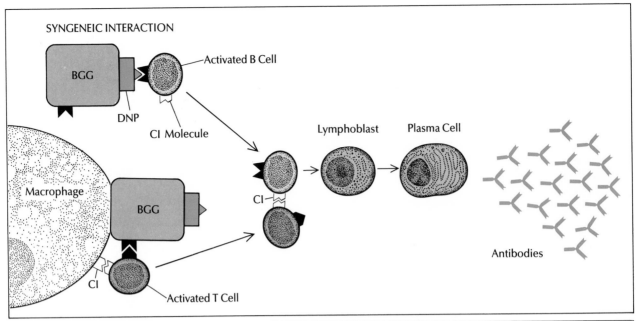

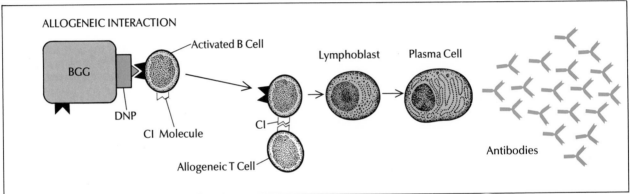

In syngeneic interaction (top), differentiation of B cells to produce antihapten antibody requires T-cell recognition of the carrier determinant, as well as B-cell recognition of the haptenic determinant. Specifically sensitized B and T cells will then interact with each other, with the cell interaction (CI) molecule of the B cell being engaged by the corresponding recognition site of the T cell. However, when two genetically different (allogeneic) donor animals are used, cell interaction will take place even when the T cells are not primed by exposure to the carrier determinant, and antihapten antibodies will be produced by differentiated B cells. It is believed that in both syngeneic and allogeneic situations; B-lymphocyte-T-lymphocyte interaction occurs as the result of recognition of cell surface molecules that are the products of cell interaction (CI) genes.

velopment from a very early stage within the same environment, or in other words had coexisted together through most of their lifespan. In this situation, the T and B lymphocytes derived from genetically different sets of parents were found to interact effectively despite differences in *I* region genes. This suggested to us that perhaps during the course of development, T and B lymphocytes "learn" to effectively interact in some way that has yet to be ascertained. This process, which we have called "adaptive differentiation," may involve a form of selection in which the ultimate result is the ability of T and B cells from genetically distinct backgrounds to effectively interact in order to maintain host integrity. Further investigation has documented the validity of the concept, as discussed below.

Adaptive Differentiation of Lymphocytes in Bone Marrow Chimeras

Adaptive differentiation describes the process by which differentiating stem cells adapt their functionally expressed self-recognition repertoire, and thus their ultimate cooperating phenotype, as a result of exposure to the MHC phenotype of the environment in which they differentiate. This has been substantiated largely by experimentation with irradiation bone marrow chimeras, most notably the results obtained with chimeric lymphocytes of $F_1 \rightarrow$ parent type (lethally irradiated parental hosts, of A or B type, repopulated with [A x B]F_1 bone marrow stem cells), which no longer display the indiscriminate interacting phenotype (i.e., for either parent) typical of conventional F_1 lymphocytes but rather interact preferentially with partner cells of host parental or F_1 type. Still to be determined are the ground rules of adaptive differentiation and the underlying mechanisms by which the self-recognition repertoire is sculpted by elements in the environment.

As an example of such studies, we tested the capacities of helper T lymphocytes and hapten-specific B lymphocytes primed in the environments of various combinations of bone marrow chimeras prepared between two parental strains (e.g., A/J and BALB/c) and their corresponding F_1 hybrid (CAF$_1$) to interact with primed B and T lymphocytes derived from conventional parent and F_1 donors as well as all of the corresponding bone marrow chimera combinations. Our results demonstrated clearly that 1) $F_1 \to$ F_1 chimeric lymphocytes displayed no restrictions in terms of cooperative activity with all of the various partner cell combinations; 2) parent$\to F_1$ chimeric lymphocytes manifested effective cooperative activity only for partner cells from F_1 or parental donors corresponding to the haplotype of the original bone marrow donor, thereby behaving phenotypically just like conventional parental lymphocytes; and 3) $F_1 \to$ parent chimeric lymphocytes displayed restricted haplotype preference in cooperating best with partner lymphocytes sharing the H-2 haplotype, either entirely or co-dominantly, of the parental chimeric host. Suitable control studies ruled out the existence of either nonspecific or specific suppression mechanisms as possible explanations for the restricted partner cell preference of $F_1 \to$ parent chimeric lymphocytes.

Another series of chimera studies was conducted to analyze further the sites of dominant influence on lymphocyte maturation with regard to the self-recognition capabilities normally displayed by regulatory helper T cells. This was accomplished by utilizing lymphocytes obtained from a variety of differentiating environments, including 1) $F_1 \to$ parent and 2) intact parental mice rendered tolerant as neonates to the MHC determinants of a second parental strain. Lymphocytes were removed from these environ-

ments and *adoptively primed* to KLH in irradiated, thymectomized F_1 recipients. The resulting helper T cells were then analyzed for their partner cell preferences when mixed with conventional DNP-primed B lymphocytes of either parental or F_1 origin in adoptive secondary responses in irradiated F_1 recipients. Irrespective of their initial environmental origins, T cells of such types could be adoptively primed to develop totally unrestricted helper cell activity for B lymphocytes of both parental types as well as of F_1 type. Such results indicate that the dominant influence on cooperative capabilities of helper T cells is exerted by the extrathymic microenvironment in which such cells undergo their early differentiation. Moreover, they demonstrate that the haplotype restriction displayed by helper T cells primed in, and taken directly from, $F_1 \to$ single parent chimeras is actually a *pseudo-restriction* since helper T cells with unrestricted cooperating phenotypes can be induced in such $F_1 \to$ single parent chimeric populations when adoptively primed in irradiated F_1 recipients. This pseudorestriction in cooperative capabilities was explained by a new concept termed *environmental restraint*.

Environmental restraint describes the process by which the environmental milieu can exert nonpermissive influences on the development of functional interacting partner cells corresponding to one of the possible (and actually existing) CI phenotypes inherent in a given lymphoid cell population. In other words, despite the fact that the F_1 lymphoid cells residing in an $F_1 \to$ parent chimera consist of self-recognizing subpopulations corresponding to each of the two inherited parental CI types, the parental host environment is permissive for expression (in that environment) of only that subpopulation corresponding to the CI phenotype of the parental host. For reasons that have yet to be delineated, that same environment is nonpermissive for emergence of the second parental type subpopulation.

Thus, our current working hypothesis is that adaptive differentiation is a dynamic rather than a static process and that the self-recognition repertoire within a given species enjoys a certain

degree of plasticity. Moreover, we feel that the plasticity of the self-recognition repertoire is determined by the occurrence of responses against self-specific receptors for CI molecules (i.e., αCI), and these, in turn, determine the immune response phenotype for a given individual.

Soluble Lymphocyte Factors, T-Cell Factors, and MHC Gene Controls

During the same period of time in which an important role for MHC genes in the development of cell interactions became established, a series of related observations had been made in somewhat different systems. In the last four or five years, a number of investigators have shown that under antigen stimulation, T lymphocytes can release biologically active soluble factors and that these factors in many instances encompass many of the effects of the whole T cell on either the B lymphocyte or other T cells. The bulk of such studies have employed in vitro systems. The first observations along these lines were by R. Dutton and his colleagues at the University of California at San Diego. These investigators used mixed leukocyte cultures (MLC), which provide an in vitro analogue of transplantation reactions, and found that molecules were released in the supernatant that could be substituted for intact T lymphocytes in facilitating an in vitro response to erythrocyte antigens by a suspension of B cells.

A number of investigators have confirmed these findings. In our own laboratory at Harvard, D. Armerding and I have extended the observations in studies that sought to determine whether such biologically active factors from the MLC (prepared as illustrated in Figure 7 on page 38) consisted of molecules that might include major histocompatibility gene products. In collaboration with David Sachs of the National Cancer Institute, we found that the soluble T-cell factor that we were studying did include antigenic determinants known to be coded by genes in the I region of the mouse H-2 complex. These antigens, known as Ia antigens because of their derivation from I region genes, were discovered and studied exten-

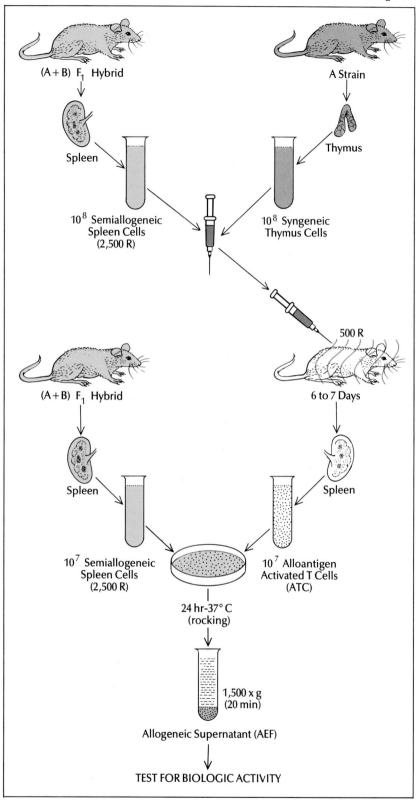

The method of preparing allogeneic effect factor (AEF) in a mixed leukocyte culture (MLC) system is schematized above. AEF, so prepared, has been shown to include antigenic determinants known to be coded for by genes in the I region of the mouse major histocompatibility (H-2) complex. These Ia antigens are most abundantly expressed on lymphocytes and also found on macrophage surfaces.

sively by Shreffler and C. S. David, now at Washington University, by Jan Klein and his colleagues at the University of Texas Southwestern Medical School, by G.J. Hammerling and McDevitt at Stanford, and by Sachs at the National Cancer Institute. Ia antigens have been found to be most abundantly expressed on cell surface membranes of lymphocytes and to a lesser extent on macrophages.

In our experiments we utilized antiserum directed against the Ia antigens to see whether such antiserum would react with the biologically active factor, allogeneic effect factor (AEF), in our MLC supernatants. Not only did such a reaction take place – but it was strong enough specifically to remove all biologic activity from our AEF preparations. Our initial conclusion was that the biologically active molecules present in AEF, which are capable of interacting in some way with B lymphocytes, possessed determinants coded for by genes in the *I* region of *H-2*.

Shortly after these observations were made, independent studies by Taussig, Munro, and Mozes both confirmed and expanded them. As discussed earlier, using the (T,G)-A--L system to study T cells from responder and nonresponder mice, they first showed that immunized T cells in culture released into the supernatant a factor specific for (T,G)-A--L; this factor was able to replace T cells in interactions with B cells. The specificity of the factor for (T,G)-A--L was demonstrated in several ways, perhaps most importantly by specific immunoabsorption, through which the factor's activity could be completely removed. It was of great interest that the factor in the initial studies could be obtained from either responder or, in some instances, nonresponder T cells but would only interact with B cells from responder animals. This is the evidence alluded to earlier that in some animals the defect of nonresponse may occur at the B-cell level. In further experiments with other strains, it was found that in some cases nonresponder B cells were stimulated by (T,G)-A--L-specific factors derived from T cells of responder animals, while in others there were nonresponders who could neither produce the factor nor yield B cells responsive to stimulation by the factor. Thus, in these experiments the defect of nonresponse was shown to be at the T-cell level in some individuals, in the B cells in others, and in both T and B in still others. In all cases, response or nonresponse was under the control of the *I* region within the major histocompatibility complex of the mouse. The specific factor capable of stimulating B cells to respond to (T,G)-A--L also was found to contain determinants coded by *I* region genes, as reflected by the ability specifically to remove the biologic activity of such factors with an appropriate anti-Ia antiserum.

In a somewhat different system, Tomio Tada and his colleagues in Japan have detected antigen-specific suppressive T-cell factors that also possess determinants associated with Ia antigens. Another such factor has been demonstrated by Kapp, Pierce, and Benacerraf at Harvard.

The discovery of these antigen-specific T-cell factors that appear to have Ia antigen determinants is not only of great importance with respect to supporting our understanding of the role of MHC gene products in cell-cell interactions, but is also pertinent to the question of the basis of specific antigen recognition by cells of the T-lymphocyte class. It should be pointed out that the molecular nature of the antigen-specific T-cell receptor has been a subject of considerable controversy over the past six or seven years. The difficulty in defining the molecular nature of the T-cell receptor has been in sharp contrast to the ease of identifying the receptors on B lymphocytes as immunoglobulins. It is relatively simple to find Ig molecules on the surface membranes of B cells using conventional techniques of immunohistochemistry, notably fluorescent antibody or immunoradioautography. By appropriate experimental approaches, it has been demonstrated unequivocally that readily detectable surface immunoglobulin molecules on B lymphocytes are synthesized by these cells, serve as antigen-specific receptors, and parallel quite closely, in the structural sense, the ultimate antibody secreted by mature plasma cells.

Similar attempts, using conventional techniques, to identify immunoglobulin molecules on the surface of T lymphocytes failed to reveal the presence of immunoglobulin molecules. Because of this difficulty in detecting surface immunoglobulin on T cells and because of the strong relationship between *Ir* gene function and T-cell responses, it was hypothesized that perhaps *Ir* genes code for the molecular entity that serves as the antigen receptor on T lymphocytes. This, of course, implied distinctly different genetic origins for antigen receptors on T and B cells. This, then, is the context for the studies in the past few years that suggest the existence of antigen-specific molecules, apparently produced by T lymphocytes and capable of exerting biologic regulatory effects on other lymphocytes, with *I* region–determined antigens (and, incidentally, no immunoglobulin determinants). These findings are consistent, in principle, with the hypothesis that histocompatibility-linked *Ir* genes may code for antigen-specific molecules serving as T-cell receptors.

However, also during the past few years, some very compelling data have been obtained in different experimental systems implying that at least part of the genetic information determining the specificity of the T-cell receptor is identical to that determining the specificity of the immunoglobulin receptors on B cells. Before we discuss these studies, it is important to understand that the control of immunoglobulin synthesis is genetically unique in that the immunoglobulin gene system is the only one known to involve the participation of two discrete structural genes in the synthesis of a single polypeptide chain. Thus, a structural gene for the variable, or *V*, region of the immunoglobulin molecule integrates somehow with another structural gene for the constant, or *C*, region to form a single chain composed of *V* and *C* regions. There are antigenic determinants associated with each region, and the ones most pertinent to this discussion are those determinants unique to the area of the *V* region–specific antigen combining site. Such determinants are known as idiotypes, and antibodies reacting with idiotypic determinants are known as anti-idiotypic antibodies.

Two similar experimental systems have been used by H. Binz and H. Wigzell in Sweden and by Rajewsky and K. Eichmann and associates in Germany. They have provided some very illuminating information with respect to the T-cell receptor. In essence, the investigators utilized anti-idiotypic antibodies prepared in such a way as to display specific reactivity with idiotypic determinants present on immunoglobulin molecules (and therefore encoded by *V* region genes of conventional immunoglobulin) as probes to analyze T-cell receptors for the presence or absence of identical idiotypic antigen determinants. The crucial observations from such studies have been that anti-idiotypic antibodies directed against *V* region determinants of conventional immunoglobulin molecules can, under appropriate experimental conditions, react with T lymphocytes whose receptor specificities correspond to the combining site specificities of the immunoglobulin molecules against which the anti-idiotypic antibodies are directed, and vice versa. Furthermore, by utilizing appropriate anti-idiotypic antibody preparations it has been possible specifically to isolate molecules from T lymphocytes that display antigen-binding capabilities. Thus it has been demonstrated that molecules isolated from T cells are very similar in size to one of the chains of conventional immunoglobulin; such T-cell-derived chains do not, however, possess any detectable antigenic determinants known to be present on conventional immunoglobulin. Nevertheless, inheritance of the relevant T-cell receptor idiotype is clearly linked to genes coding for one of the chains of conventional immunoglobulin *C* regions. Moreover, such T-cell molecules do not possess antigenic markers of the histocompatibility gene complex.

Therefore, at the present time such data strongly imply that the *V* region of the T-cell receptor is encoded by the same genes that encode *V* regions of conventional immunoglobulin; however, the structure and genetic origin of the remainder of the polypeptide chain are still a mystery. Furthermore, we are now in somewhat of a dilemma with respect to understanding the derivation and physiologic importance of the other nonimmunoglobulin antigen-specific molecules discussed above that are believed to come from T cells and that bear antigenic determinants encoded by histocompatibility genes.

Conclusion

We have reviewed the evidence for the existence of *I* region genes that are involved in regulation of immune responses *(Ir)*, that regulate cellular interactions between lymphocytes and macrophages *(CI)*, and that also appear to direct lymphocytes toward immunosuppression *(Is)*. The evidence is not yet conclusive with respect to the question of whether or not these genes are distinct from one another. Moreover, we have documented the case for the existence of biologically active soluble factors obtained from lymphocytes that appear to be derived from genes located in the *I* region of the MHC; these factors seem able to subserve the roles of positive response, suppression, and cell interaction, and the active molecules of these factors appear to bear antigenic determinants that are *I* region gene products. As stated above, the antigen receptor on T cells appears to be an entity quite independent of MHC gene products, but the origin of antigen specificity in certain MHC-encoded soluble factors has yet to be elucidated.

The unifying fact in all of these studies and their results, then, is the control exerted from the MHC genes. This fact begins to provide some perspective as to the functional relevance of the cell surface histocompatibility antigens, previously of interest largely because of their relevance to organ transplantation. It seems obvious that, in evolutionary terms, these antigens had to owe their existence to needs more integral to life than merely providing frustration for transplantation surgeons. We are just beginning to identify the myriad biologic functions related to this system.

Our present understanding makes it reasonable to speculate that organ differentiation even outside of the lymphoid system may be controlled by these and related cell surface molecules, namely the gene products of the MHC. From the physician's viewpoint, a less remote possibility is that understanding the histocompatibility genes and their products will afford some means to control those immunologic responses that cause not only transplant rejection but also autoimmune and atopic diseases and other immunopathologies – both those that are recognized and those still only suspected.

This train of events is in some respects already under way. A number of studies have statistically associated various arthritides with particular specific major histocompatibility *(HLA)* haplotypes. It is probable, therefore, that these relationships are determined by *HLA* genes. Absolute proof of this in humans is not yet available but is very strong in several animal systems. For example, experimental autoimmune encephalomyelitis in the rat, a disease that is regarded as a possible experimental model for multiple sclerosis in humans, has been definitely linked to the major histocompatibility complex of that species. This implies that susceptibility to certain diseases may result from the presence of an *Ir* gene that may cause the animal to respond deleteriously to the basic CNS protein that induces the disease. Alternatively, the etiology may involve the absence of an *Is* gene that may be required to prevent the animal from reacting aberrantly to the CNS protein.

It is also noteworthy that some association has been established between certain persons allergic to ragweed antigen E and *HLA* histocompatibility type. Again, one could argue as to whether it is the presence of an *Ir* gene or the absence of an *Is* gene that causes the response in these patients. It is, of course, also possible that in normal individuals both *Ir* and *Is* genes are present and that it is the disruption of normal homeostatic balance between the two that can lead or contribute to disease.

Our understanding of genetic control of lymphocyte recognition and differentiation processes has increased substantially over the past five years. Thus, concepts that were hardly imaginable a decade ago concerning the role of the MHC in controlling cell-cell communication and certain aspects of recognition in the immune system have enabled us to view normal cell differentiation and its control with a quite different perspective. From these new perspectives have also developed new ideas in terms of the mechanisms by which immunocompetent cells transact their necessary and usually unmistakable communication processes, which, we now know, determine the overall response pattern developed by the individual in both health and disease. It is probable that future studies will broaden our understanding of the genetic basis of self-recognition and of the cell-cell interactions that depend upon such self-recognition processes. Moreover, we should develop a clearer picture of the mechanisms underlying adaptive differentiation and the boundaries of the plasticity of phenotypic self-recognition. Finally, isolation and characterization of the *CI* molecules involved in such processes should clarify many of the existing ambiguities and questions that exist with respect to the general issue of MHC restrictions. In a broad sense, we might also expect that information obtained in studies such as these will further our basic knowledge of cell differentiation, receptor expression, self-recognition, and other developmental processes involved in multicellular organisms.

Be that as it may, there seems little doubt that we are on the verge of showing that the presence or absence of MHC genes and their products is of major consequence for health and for disease. Ability to manipulate the cell surface antigens specified by these genes clearly would constitute a powerful force for the prevention and treatment of disease.

Surface Characteristics Of T-Lymphocyte Subpopulations

EDWARD A. BOYSE *Memorial Sloan-Kettering Cancer Center and*
HARVEY CANTOR *Harvard Medical School*

The term "lymphocytes" refers to the class of cells that bear specific receptors for antigen, and therefore are directly responsible for all specific immune responses. They are of two sorts: 1) the T lymphocytes (or T cells), so called because their maturation requires processing in the thymus, and 2) the B lymphocytes (or B cells), which require processing in the bursa of Fabricius in birds or in a presumed homologous organ in mammals that has not yet been located.

This chapter is concerned with T cells and the various immune functions that they perform. As we shall see, despite their uniform morphology, the T cells are by no means a homogeneous population; they comprise subclasses, or sets, of lymphocytes with different and even seemingly opposing functions. It is common knowledge that a particular immune response may be beneficial under some circumstances and injurious in other circumstances. Ultimately, the key to therapeutic control over immune responses of patients may lie in improved understanding of the formation and operation of different T-cell sets.

In the immediately previous chapter in this volume, D.H. Katz dwelt on the fact that the production of specific antibody is an exclusive property of B cells, but that B cells generally require the cooperation of T cells in order to do so (see "Genetic Controls and Cellular Interactions in Antibody Formation"). Thus one property of T cells, "helper function," is to assist B cells to make antibody. A second well-known property of T cells is to bring about the rejection of foreign grafts, and of cells that have been rendered antigenically foreign, by infection with a virus for example, or by malignant transformation; this is associated with the "cytotoxic" or "killer" function of T cells.

Yet another function of T cells has been suspected from investigation of immunologic tolerance or unresponsiveness. Thus the "adoptive" transfer of lymphocytes from an unresponsive animal to a normal animal may render the recipient unresponsive, in the same way that immune resistance can be transferred adoptively from a specifically resistant donor to a normal recipient.

Experiments such as these led to the postulate of a "suppressor" function for T cells. At some risk of oversimplification, we may regard suppressor function as a necessary homeostatic control mechanism that keeps the complete immune capacity of individuals in trim.

A vital point arises: Can all T cells perform all the immune functions mentioned above; and are the responses of T cells governed entirely by extraneous conditions relating to encounters with antigen? Or, alternatively, are different sets of T cells, programmed to respond in different ways, generated by the organism as part of its normal developmental history? These questions resolve themselves into the practical problem of finding out whether it is possible to subdivide the T-cell population of unimmunized animals into different sets that, when confronted with antigen, are able to make only one or another of the possible T-cell responses.

We have a clear answer in the mouse: helper T cells are programmed for that function during development; killer and suppressor T cells are programmed and generated separately from helper T cells, although it is too early to say whether killer and suppressor cells are generated independently of one another during development. That is one of the key issues in current research on lymphocytes.

The following is a brief account of how it came to be

known that functionally different sets of T cells are generated during the normal physiologic process of differentiation. The information comes from immunogenetics. It may be helpful first to recall some familiar immunogenetic systems. In the ABO and other blood group systems, surface components of red cells, known as "A," "B," "Rh," etc, are recognized by antisera produced by individuals lacking one or another of these antigens. Tissue typing is similar to blood typing, i.e., histocompatibility antigens, which are surface components of nucleated cells, are recognized by antisera produced when an individual of one histocompatibility type is immunized against an individual of a different histocompatibility type. In the same way, antisera produced by immunizing mice with T cells of other mice identify systems of antigens expressed on T cells. Just as there are several different blood-group "systems," so there are several T-cell systems in the mouse. This itself is of no great interest, but the further investigation of these T-cell systems has led to some important findings.

First, it has been established that certain of these T-cell surface compo-nents (antigens) are found *only* on T cells; others are found on T cells and some other cell types, but not all cell types. Thus we see that these components of the T-cell surface have some special relation to the T cell per se, and are not simply building blocks required to make a functional plasma membrane. Those who like to think in terms of genetics envisage "gene programs," or sets of genes, that are selectively expressed in T cells. We can go further: we can enquire whether each of these special components of the T-cell surface is expressed on all mature functional T cells or only on certain sets with particular functions.

Table I (below left) lists the best known T-cell systems:

1) The first is G_{IX}. G_{IX} antigen has been identified as the hallmark of one of a class of molecules known as gp70 (glycoprotein of molecular weight around 70,000). As indicated in Figure 1 (at right), the notable feature of the G_{IX}-gp70 molecule is in addition to being a constituent of the thymocyte plasma membrane in various strains of mice, it also forms the major component of the envelope of certain leukemia viruses. This is not simply a case of the leukemia virus picking up this molecule to make its coat as it "buds" through the plasma membrane, because the molecule is thought to be coded by the viral genome. It will be recalled that the genome of such viruses is regarded as the RNA phase of a DNA viral genome that is integrated in the chromosomes of the cell. In its role as a component of the T-cell surface, G_{IX}-gp70 appears as a mendelian character obeying the usual rules of inheritance. It is only when T cells begin to produce virus, and most leukemias of mice originate from T cells, that we see G_{IX}-gp70 in its other role as a part of an oncogenic virus. It is an open question whether mendelian expression of the G_{IX}-gp70 T-cell surface molecule represents partial expression of a viral genome or a normal trait that assumes a pathologic connotation in the event of spontaneous virus production and leukemogenesis. This is the no-man's-land between mendelian genetics and viral infection. Many think viral genomes of the leukemia type are not just unwelcome intruders

Table 1

Alloantigen Systems Expressed Exclusively or Selectively* on Thymic Lymphocytes

System	Location of Genes
G_{IX}*	Two unlinked genes (location unknown) required for expression of G_{IX}
TL	Chromosome 17; *close to H-2D*
Thy-1*	Chromosome 9
Ly-1	Chromosome 19
Ly-2/Ly-3	Chromosome 6 (may be a single locus or two closely linked loci)
Ly-5	Unknown (not linked to any of the above)

*G_{IX} and Thy-1 participate in other differentiative programs

Figure 1

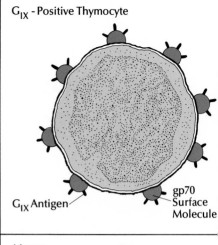

G_{IX} - Positive Thymocyte

G_{IX} Antigen

gp70 Surface Molecule

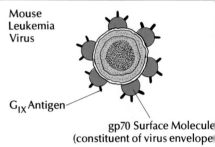

Mouse Leukemia Virus

G_{IX} Antigen

gp70 Surface Molecule (constituent of virus envelope)

A provocative relationship exists between G_{IX} surface antigen of thymocytes and an envelope component of mouse leukemia

but necessary parts of the genome.

2) The TL system, which is coded by genes on chromosome 17, will also be mentioned only briefly, because once again the T cells of some mice are TL-negative, just as blood group O individuals express no product referable to the ABO locus. Thus TL can scarcely play an essential role in immune responses, because the immune capacity of TL-negative mice is not obviously impaired. However, the TL surface component (TL antigen) has a key part to play in lymphocyte research, because its expression marks the early phase of T-cell differentiation in the thymus, which makes it a valuable marker.

3) The Thy1 surface component of T cells, coded by a gene on chromosome 9, is another element that is unlikely to have a use in discriminating T cells from one another, because it is expressed in the programs of other cell types, such as skin and brain. But it is not expressed on B cells. Thus Thy1 antiserum is useful for distinguishing

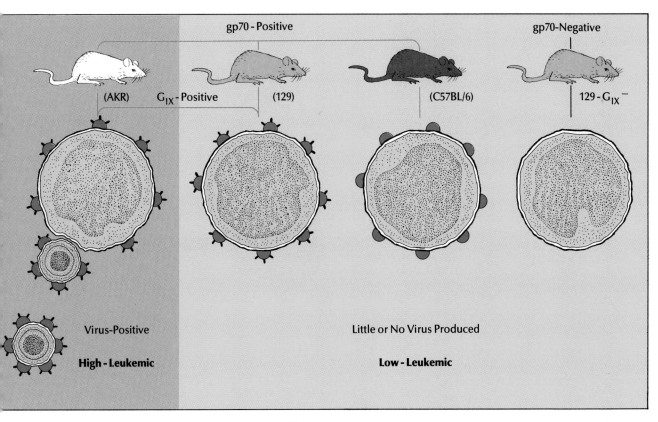

gp70 - Positive

gp70 - Negative

(AKR) G_{IX} - Positive   (129)   (C57BL/6) 129 - G_{IX}^-

Virus-Positive

Little or No Virus Produced

High - Leukemic

Low - Leukemic

virus. The glycoprotein (gp70), on which G_{IX} is expressed, is, in AKR and 129 mice, a constituent of the plasma membrane; similar glycoproteins, not expressing G_{IX}, are found on thymocytes in other mouse strains (e.g., C57BL/6). G_{IX}-gp70 also is the main constituent of leukemia virus envelopes. In high-leukemic mice, such as AKR, the dual roles of G_{IX}-gp70 are apparent.

T cells as a class from B cells as a class, for eliminating T cells from heterogeneous populations for experimental purposes, and for enumerating the total number of T lymphocytes present in a given preparation of cells.

4) The Ly1 component, coded by a gene on chromosome 19, is of more immediate importance to this discussion, because this component is expressed only on T cells, and all mice express it (in one or another of its alternative forms: Ly1.1 or Ly1.2).

5) The Ly2 and Ly3 components, both of which are coded by genes on chromosome 6, are of interest for the same reason as Ly1 (hence the similar notation "Ly"). These two are treated together tentatively because the two genes are tightly linked, and these two systems have not so far exhibited any differences other than the fact that genetically they are coded by distinguishable loci. It remains to be seen whether further immunogenetic analysis will identify discrete functions for these two genes, and this should be

borne in mind especially with regard to our present inability to distinguish separate identities for cytotoxic T cells and suppressor T cells.

6) It is now known that the Ly5 system is a complex one and not confined to T cells; rather it is expressed on all or most hematopoietic cells but on no other cells. Moreover, the Ly5 molecule has been shown to exist in at least three different forms, each having different molecular weights and each expressed independently of the other forms on cells of different hematopoietic lineages.

Although our knowledge of Ly5 is thus far quite limited, its inclusion here serves to emphasize that those Ly systems that have been investigated by no means exhaust the possibilities of this type of lymphocyte analysis. What is written in this brief review may represent only a beginning of the contemporary dissection of the immune apparatus.

Having described the six systems for the T-cell population listed in Table I,

we can use them to follow the life history of the T cell (Figure 2, page 44). All six systems are represented at the stage of development of the T cell, which is attained immediately the precursor cell, or "prothymocyte," reaches the thymus on its migration from the bone marrow (or spleen, in rodents). The prothymocyte, it will be noted, expresses only an *H-2* (major histocompatibility) surface component, an antigen found on the plasma membrane of almost all cell types and therefore of little relevance to this discussion. (The prothymocyte may, of course, have other surface components that have not so far been recognized.) In a convenient shorthand, the "surface phenotype" of the prothymocyte en route to the thymus is denoted G_{IX}^- TL^- $Thy1^-$ $Ly1^-$ $Ly23^-$ $Ly5^-$. On arrival, the prothymocyte is induced to become a thymocyte with the new surface phenotype G_{IX}^+ TL^+ $Thy1^+$ $Ly1^+$ $Ly23^+$ $Ly5^+$. The name thymocyte is given to the major population of thymic T cells that are not yet functionally mature. Later, something more will be said about the conversion of prothymocytes into thymocytes. For the moment it is sufficient to note that this takes place without cell division, that it can be monitored in vitro and so intimately analyzed, and that it involves the manifestation of a program in which the products of at least six genes become expressed as the characteristic surface phenotype.

First we can make a statement about changes in surface phenotype that accompany the differentiation of thymocytes into the functional T-cell population of the immune system as a whole. In so doing, we can imply corresponding changes in the gene programs that govern the expression of the six systems named. The main features of this maturation sequence are that G_{IX} and TL cease to be expressed, Thy1 continues to be expressed, but in considerably reduced amount, while the Ly systems are expressed differentially on selected sections of the T-cell population.

A word needs to be said at this point about the serologic methods on which this work is based. The basic technique is the cytotoxicity assay (as schematized in Figure 3, below right), which is the equivalent of the familiar complement-dependent hemolytic test used with red cells. As with hemolysis by antierythrocyte antibody and complement, lymphocytes exposed to, say, anti-Ly1 or anti-Ly2 sera, in the presence of complement, are lysed. This lysis can be monitored by the use of trypan blue, which stains lysed cells but not living cells, or by the release of a radioactive label from the lysed cells. This permits the proportion of lymphocytes lysed to be estimated, and it enables cells bearing a particular cell-surface component, say Ly1, to be eliminated from a T-cell population, leaving only the cells that do not bear that particular cell-surface component.

In this way it has been shown that the T-cell population of lymph nodes or spleen, for example, contains lymphocytes that are, say, Ly1$^+$Ly2$^-$, or Ly1$^-$Ly2$^+$. Analysis of this sort reveals that the T-cell pool contains three separate T-cell classes. We refer to them in shorthand as the Ly123 class, the Ly1 class, and the Ly23

Figure 2

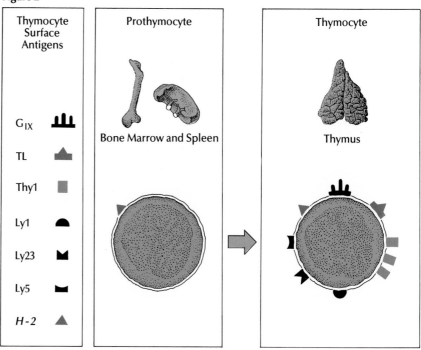

The surface changes that occur with differentiation of lymphocyte precursors to functional T cells are schematized. For reference, the symbols used to represent the various molecules that have been identified on thymus cell surfaces are catalogued in the left-hand panel. Before cells reach the thymus (prothymocytes), the only consistently present surface component expressed is the H-2 histocompatibility determinant. In the thymus one finds thymocytes displaying the full array of surface molecules (except that some

Figure 3

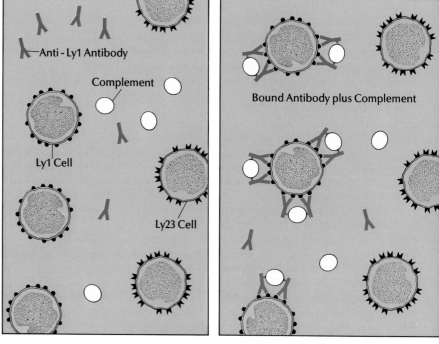

Diagrams summarize the cytotoxicity assay system that has been used in identifying surface components that are differentially expressed on T lymphocytes. Example here shows identification of cells expressing Ly1, and cells expressing Ly23, in a suspension of T lymphocytes. One adds antibody against one of the two cell types (anti-Ly1) and

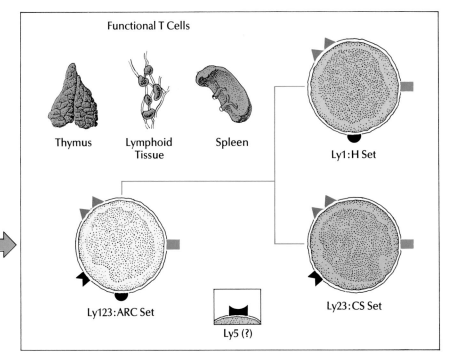

Functional T Cells

Thymus

Lymphoid Tissue

Spleen

Ly1:H Set

Ly123:ARC Set

Ly5 (?)

Ly23:CS Set

strains lack G_{IX} and/or TL). In the thymus and peripheral lymphoid sites, cells have undergone further differentiation, with reduction in the amount of Thy1 displayed, enrichment of H-2, and differential expression of Ly1 and Ly23. The Ly123 lymphocytes can be regarded as a pool of cells that have acquired antigen receptors (antigen-reactive cell =ARC) but are not yet functionally committed. Other antigens – G_{IX} and TL – have been lost. The fate of Ly5 remains to be elucidated.

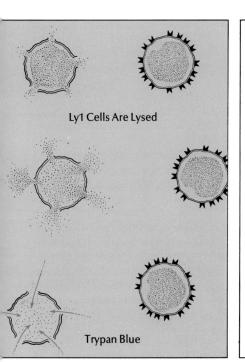

Ly1 Cells Are Lysed

Trypan Blue

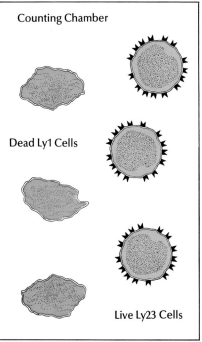

Counting Chamber

Dead Ly1 Cells

Live Ly23 Cells

complement. T cells with Ly1 surface components will complex with the antibody, and complement-mediated lysis will ensue. The lysed cells can be identified by labeling with trypan blue. The remaining intact cells can readily be counted, and they can be used in tests to correlate immune function with cell type.

class. (Again it should be emphasized that this may represent only a first and relatively gross categorization of the T-cell population and that the use of Ly5 and other new immunogenetic T-cell markers yet to be analyzed may add further refinements to the detailed classification of T cells.) Thus, speaking in genetic terms, we now have T cells expressing three programs that differ from each other and from that of the thymocyte.

Now we are in a position to examine the question whether these differentiative programs that we recognize by Ly surface components, the Ly phenotypes, include information that decides what the functions of each T-cell set shall be. We have already seen that three discrete T-cell functions have been inferred: 1) helper function, required for B cells to make antibody; 2) cytotoxic function, required for the destruction of antigenically foreign cells; 3) suppressor function, which sets a limit to the production of antibody by B cells and to immune responses mediated by other T cells.

It is a striking testimony to the advancement of immunologic technology during the last several years that these T-cell functions are all amenable to analysis by stringent tests in vitro. It has thus been possible to answer the question posed above, concerning the relation between the programming of surface composition and the programming of function, by examining in vitro the functional capacities of T-cell populations from which one or another of the three classes named has first been eliminated by exposure to the respective Ly antiserum and complement.

The picture that has emerged (see Figure 4, page 46) is that the surface phenotypes, represented by the Ly systems, are jointly programmed with function. Thus the Ly1 class is responsible for helper function and can conveniently be denoted the Ly1:H class. The Ly23 class is capable of cytotoxic (killer) and suppressor functions, and so can be denoted the Ly23:CS set; it remains to be seen whether this set will ultimately prove to be subdivisible. Our present view of the Ly123 set is that this is an intermediate pool of T cells that has acquired receptors for antigen but has not yet been com-

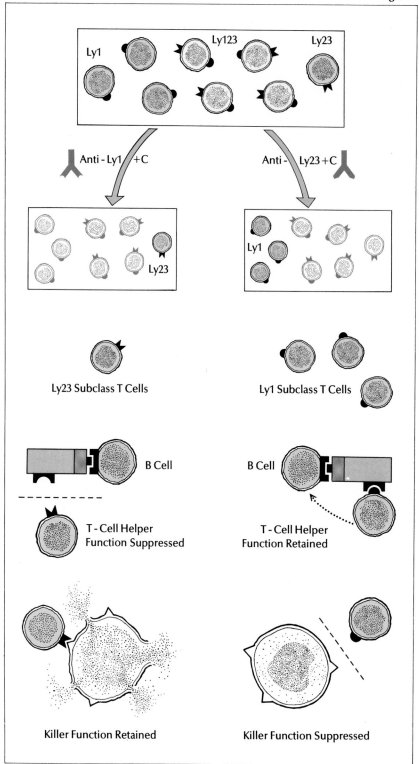

Correlation of Ly surface profile with functional precommitment of various T-cell subpopulations is done by the cytotoxicity method diagrammed above. If one starts with an unfractionated population of T cells (top rectangle) and adds Ly1 antiserum and complement, the result is lysis of Ly1 and Ly123 cells. The surviving T cells are then found to lack the capacity to act as helper cells, but to be competent in terms of their cytotoxic, or killer, function. If, on the other hand, one introduces an Ly23 antiserum into the system, it is helper function that is retained, and killer function that is lost.

mitted to H or CS functions (Figure 2).

So far, so good. But no self-respecting biologist cares to deal very long with models in vitro without periodically returning to check their validity in vivo. That is why the following confirmatory experiments are greatly reassuring:

A well-known method of obtaining mice that have no T cells is to thymectomize them, subject them to lethal irradiation, and restore them with bone marrow from which T cells have been eliminated. This is the so-called B mouse. If we are correct in presuming that Ly1:H cells and Ly23:CS cells are independently differentiated and self-sustaining populations, then the infusion of one of these populations into a B mouse should provide that mouse only with T cells of that particular surface phenotype, Ly1 or Ly23, and should confer on the recipient only the functions appropriate to that T-cell set. These experiments have been done, and the results were as predicted (and as indicated in Figure 5, facing page). The recipient B mouse acquires T cells whose Ly phenotype and function correspond only to the T-cell set originally infused.

There is a clear suggestion here that we should be on the lookout, not only in the mouse but also in man, for hereditary immunodeficiency syndromes that may be caused by mutation of genes that are programmed to be expressed only in T cells of the Ly1:H or Ly23:CS categories. Such mutant mice (or human subjects) would be expected to exhibit the same discrete defects in T-cell function that are observed in B mice that have been provided only with Ly1:H or Ly23:CS T-cell sets.

Parallel experiments with the Ly123 set, which in practice are more difficult, have not yet been accomplished, but this will be an important step in testing the conclusion that this is the store of receptor-positive intermediary cells that regulates the supply of functionally committed Ly1:H and Ly23:CS cells.

To summarize so far: T cells that have different immune functions, and that can be identified and isolated by the use of discriminating Ly antisera, are generated autonomously as an integral part of the mouse's program of development. Thus the physiology of T-cell development appears as follows:

The thymus receives a migrant population of prothymocytes, which ostensibly are indistinguishable from one another, converts these without cell division into thymocytes bearing the complete set of T-cell surface markers, and exports at least three sets of separately programmed functional T cells.

What view should we now take of thymic function? This can be viewed in two parts:

1) Induction of prothymocytes, which precedes mitosis.

2) The channeling of the thymocyte population into separate pathways of differentiation, which very probably involves cellular proliferation.

We know quite a lot about the former, but precious little about the latter. The reason that the first step, prothymocyte induction, is fairly well understood is that it can be studied in the test tube, as mentioned above. By extensive studies that will not be described in detail here, it seems clear that the conversion of prothymocytes to thymocytes is normally brought about by a thymic hormone, or inducer, called thymopoietin.

Thymopoietin has been isolated and fully sequenced; in fact an active fragment based on the structure of the parent molecule has been synthesized. It has further been established that induction can be brought about in vitro by a number of agents that react with the cell surface but are physiologically irrelevant, and also by the "second messenger" cyclic AMP. At first it may seem surprising that prothymocytes can be induced by such a variety of agents, as well as by the specific physiologic inducer, but in fact this is a familiar story to developmental biologists. The prothymocyte, they would say, is already "committed" or "determined" – perhaps "programmed" is the simplest term – to become a thymocyte. In the ordinary course of events, thymopoietin provides the right signal at the right time in the right place for the prescribed program to become manifest. The signal that thymopoietin conveys instructs the prothymocyte to express its predetermined gene set through the

Figure 5

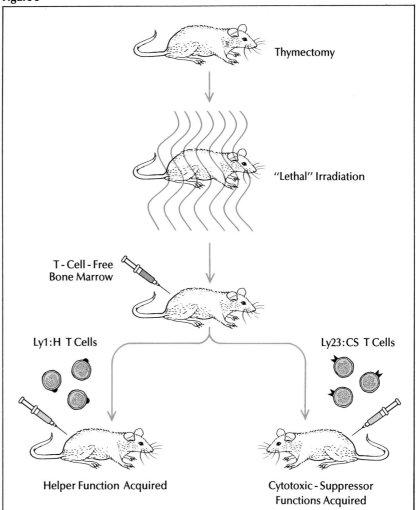

Thymectomy

"Lethal" Irradiation

T-Cell-Free Bone Marrow

Ly1:H T Cells

Ly23:CS T Cells

Helper Function Acquired

Cytotoxic-Suppressor Functions Acquired

Experiments in vivo confirm that surface Ly profiles are correlated with functional commitments of T cells. "B" mice are produced by thymectomy, followed by "lethal" irradiation, and then by inoculation of T-cell-free bone marrow. This reconstituted B mouse has B lymphocyte competence but no T cells. If B mice receive Ly1:H T cells, they acquire helper function (lower left). If B mice receive Ly23:CS T cells, they acquire cytotoxic-suppressor functions but not helper function (lower right).

medium of cAMP, as is the case with many examples of cellular function that are controlled by external molecular signals. It follows that from time to time prothymocytes may be induced to become thymocytes at inappropriate sites by exposure to nonspecific inducers released by infection, trauma, or necrosis. In fact this is the probable reason why mice in which the thymus is congenitally absent nevertheless commonly have cells that bear the T-cell surface markers discussed above; it would not be surprising if patients with thymic aplasia were also found to have some

lymphocytes expressing early T-cell markers. Moreover, this implies that if the induction of prothymocytes to immature thymocytes were the only function of the thymus, then this tissue would hardly be essential and individuals with congenital absence of the thymus would not be so immunologically crippled as in fact they are.

It is well to bear this in mind when considering the therapeutic use of agents that can induce prothymocyte differentiation. In this same vein it is at present unsafe to reason beyond the concept that these are calculated to

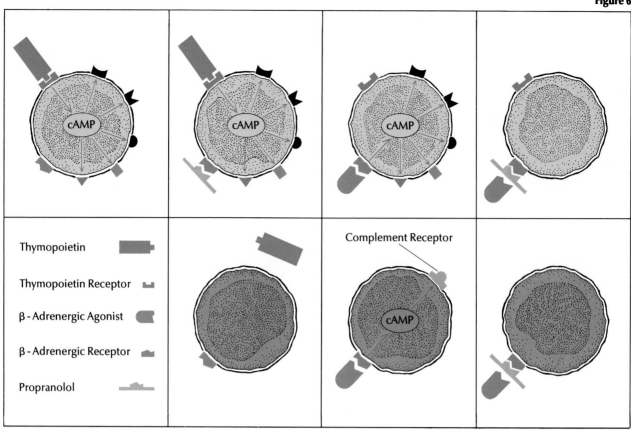

The specificity of thymopoietin as an inducer of thymocytes can be demonstrated with the dual induction assay. The upper row of diagrams shows the T-cell induction assay as described in the text. The lower row of diagrams shows a B-cell induction assay in which a B-cell marker, the complement receptor, becomes expressed. Thymopoietin induces only T cells. Agents that react with β-adrenergic receptors, for example, can induce both B and T precursor cells. The distinction of specific from nonspecific induction, in this case, is reinforced by the action of propranolol, which blocks induction of both cell types by β-adrenergic agonists, but the pharmacologic β-blocking agent does not interfere with induction of T cells by thymopoietin.

drive T-cell differentiation to a point represented by the thymocyte. It is useful, however, to make a distinction between nonspecific inducing agents, of which there are several, and the specific inducing agent thymopoietin and its synthetic derivatives. (Such a differentiation can be achieved by means of the so-called dual induction assay, depicted in Figure 6, above.) One must reckon with the probability that the former could indiscriminately induce differentiation in accessible committed cells of many types, whereas the inducing activity of the latter should at least be restricted to lymphocytes. It may well be, in view of the magnitude of the task of elucidating the post-thymocyte phases of T-

cell differentiation, that the therapeutic evaluation of specific and nonspecific inducers, and of thymic preparations generally, will depend for some time on empirical trials in vivo. Here it must be recorded that there is little concrete experimental therapeutic evidence in the mouse to guide us, despite the ample opportunities that laboratory mice provide for establishing such points beyond question. Therefore, while there is good cause for reasonable optimism in the matter of therapeutic trials of thymic products in man, there are also good reasons for forming a clear picture of what exactly has and has not been established experimentally in the mouse, and for being aware of the pos-

sibility of adverse results.

This brief review should suffice to indicate the truly remarkable advances that have been made in the understanding of T-cell differentiation and function in the last few years. But we do not have in our hands any agent that can dependably restore immune competence to an athymic mouse. Between the thymocyte and the functional T-cell pool lies unknown territory. Antisera capable of delineating the subcompartments of the human T-cell population that parallel those described in the mouse are just beginning to be defined. The precise identification of the human counterparts of the Ly systems must surely be ranked as a very important aim.

5

Suppressor T Cells
And Suppressor Factor

BARUJ BENACERRAF *Harvard Medical School*

Important insights into the mechanisms of immunity have been gained through the discovery of a suppressor system mediated by T (thymus-derived) lymphocytes. Among the regulatory functions of this system are the "turning off" of the immune response in certain circumstances and the maintenance of specific tolerance in others. This suppressor system has now been found to include not one but three different types of suppressor T lymphocytes and a soluble suppressor factor, and the genetic controls over the system have been defined. Allowing, of course, for the time lag of perhaps five to 10 years that normally separates the laboratory demonstration of a concept from its application clinically, one can readily foresee manipulation of the suppressor system in many areas of medicine: to prevent and treat autoimmune disease, to strengthen resistance to infections, and to tip the balance between host defense mechanisms and certain types of cancer in favor of the patient.

This article will seek to describe the steps that have brought us to our present knowledge of this T cell–mediated suppressor system and to outline the reasoning and some of the preliminary evidence of its potential clinical applications.

The first information concerning suppressor lymphocyte activity was provided by Gershon and Kondo of Yale in 1970. In a paper published in the British journal *Immunology*, these investigators described experiments in which adult mice were made tolerant to sheep erythrocytes by standard methods of inducing specific nonresponsiveness. Cells from these tolerant animals were then adoptively transferred to mice able to produce an antibody response to sheep RBCs, after which the recipients were found to have become tolerant to the sheep cell antigens. Subsequently, it was demonstrated that this specific nonresponsiveness was conferred by the transferred T lymphocytes. This was shown by subjecting the donor cells to antiserum to thy 1 (theta) antigen, a surface molecule found exclusively and universally on T cells, plus complement. When such selective functional destruction of T cells was accomplished prior to their inoculation into the recipient animals, the animals were no longer rendered nonresponsive by adoptive cell transfer (see Figure 1).

These findings at the beginning of the decade set in motion intensive research into the immunobiologic characteristics of suppressor T cells. Suppressor activity was subsequently identified in conjunction with thymus-dependent antibody responses involving many of the immunoglobulin classes, including IgG, IgA, and IgE, as well as with a variety of cellular immune responses, including contact reactivity, delayed hypersensitivity, and, most recently, cytolytic T-cell reactions, such as are seen in allograft rejection and host defenses against some kinds of tumors. It has become clear that suppressor T cells subserve a generalized homeostatic or regulatory function in the overall immunologic system. As suggested at the outset, these cells appear to provide a mechanism for turning off immune responses that otherwise might overwhelm the host. It is not yet clear whether the same subpopulation of T cells is involved in suppression of all of the immune responses cited above. However, as will be discussed later, it is known that at least three differ-

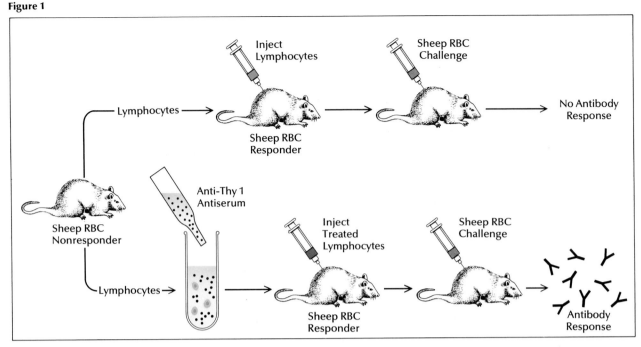

The first experimental evidence for the existence of suppressor T cells came from the laboratories of Gershon and Kondo. As schematized here, they made mice tolerant to sheep erythrocytes and transferred this specific nonresponsiveness to other mice by lymphocyte transfer (top). The fact that T cells were responsible for this adoptive transfer was shown when transferred lymphocytes were treated with anti-thy 1 antiserum prior to injection into recipient, thus destroying the T cells. When this was done, recipient no longer lost the ability to respond to sheep cells (bottom).

ent T-cell populations (Ts$_1$, Ts$_2$, Ts$_3$), functioning collaboratively, are involved in the suppressor system.

Another product of this intensive research has been identification of the genetically determined surface molecules—or antigens—on the suppressor T cells. As noted, they carry the thy 1 antigen, which establishes that they are T lymphocytes. They also carry surface Ly antigens, which are variable from subset to subset. However, one surface marker that appears to be uniquely characteristic of suppressor cells is a molecule coded for in the I-J subregion of the I region of the major histocompatibility (H-2) complex, known as the I-J antigen (see Figure 2).

At this point in the exposition, it is necessary to review briefly the evolution of our understanding of the genetic controls over the immune response. More than a decade ago, I discovered that if synthetic antigens of highly restricted heterogeneity were employed, some individuals within a species would react to immunization with an antibody response, others would not. When inbred mouse or guinea pig strains were used, response or nonresponse would be characteristic of the entire strain (see D. H. Katz, "Genetic Controls and Cellular Interactions in Antibody Formation"). Analysis of this phenomenon revealed that specific individual genes controlled responsiveness to thymus-dependent antigens, that the genes for response were dominant, and that they mapped in a discrete region within the major histocompatibility complex of all species tested (including humans). This region was designated as the I region, and the relevant genes were identified as Ir (for immune response). It is well to keep in mind that while the effector phenomenon eventually controlled by Ir genes is elaboration of antibody—a function subserved only by B lymphocytes—the actual control is always exerted over T-cell activity. Thus, the failure of an animal to elaborate antibodies to a particular antigen was first of all tracked to inhibition or functional deletion of helper T-cell activity.

The existence of Ir gene control in experimental systems was under intensive study when Gershon and Kondo discovered the existence of suppressor T cells. Their findings posed some obvious questions. Was the absence of antigenic response in any of the systems under study consequent to the generation of suppressor T cells? If so, was this a general phenomenon in all of the systems under Ir gene control?

In seeking to answer these questions, we chose a model system that we and other investigators had previously employed in studies of Ir genetic phenomena. We injected selected strains of mice with a synthetic terpolymer composed of L-glutamic acid, L-alanine, and L-tyrosine (GAT). The antigen is one of narrowly restricted antigenic specificity, with few enough determinants to permit analysis and to minimize responses to undefined antigenic components. Furthermore, we were able to take advantage of the previously established fact that one could stimulate a nonresponder mouse to make antibodies against synthetic antigens such as GAT by coupling the polymer to a carrier that the mouse recognizes as antigenic. The recognition is expressed by the generation of helper T cells and the production of antibody to the antigen (GAT). The immunogenic carrier selected for these experiments (which are summarized in Figure 3) was methylated bovine serum albumin (MBSA). Essentially, what these experiments demonstrate is that one can bypass the genetic defect (nonresponsiveness) with respect to the antigen GAT by employing a complex that includes an immunogenic carrier. Not incidentally, this experiment also pinpoints the Ir-controlled restriction to the stimulation of the T cell. Only after the helper T cells are induced does the animal have the B-cell population needed to produce specific anti-GAT antibody.

Simply stated, mice bearing three different H-2 haplotypes (H-2^p, H-2^q, and H-2^s) can be shown to be nonresponsive when injected with GAT antigen alone, but they produce anti-GAT antibody when the primary immunization is carried out with conjugates of GAT and MBSA. With this in mind, we were able to design what proved to be critical experiments in the development of our understanding of the suppressor phenomenon. These experiments involved primary immunization of the mice with GAT. Predictably, the animals did not produce an immunologic response to a GAT challenge. We then challenged them with GAT-MBSA; in this sequence, since the primary immunization had been with GAT alone, the animals again failed to produce antibody. What is more, this nonresponse was transferrable. When we took lymphocytes from nonresponder GAT-immunized animals and injected them into mice of the same strains, the recipient animals became nonresponsive to GAT-MBSA. Moreover, it could be shown that the cells responsible for the adoptive transfer of nonresponsivity were suppressor T cells, as follows:

If the cells drawn for transfer were incubated with anti-thy 1 or with anti-Ly 2,3 antisera before inoculation into the recipient animals, the recipients were able to make anti-GAT antibody when challenged with GAT-MBSA.

The fact that the ability of the animals to respond to GAT when it was coupled with a recognizable carrier was abolished if the conjugate immunization was preceded by GAT alone suggested that two different competitive pathways were being induced. In one, the generation of suppressor T cells appeared to be the dominant event; in the other, generation of helper T cells prevailed. The experiments described above had unmasked the fact that in this system the animals had developed a primary suppressive response to GAT and that this response was effected by suppres-

Figure 2

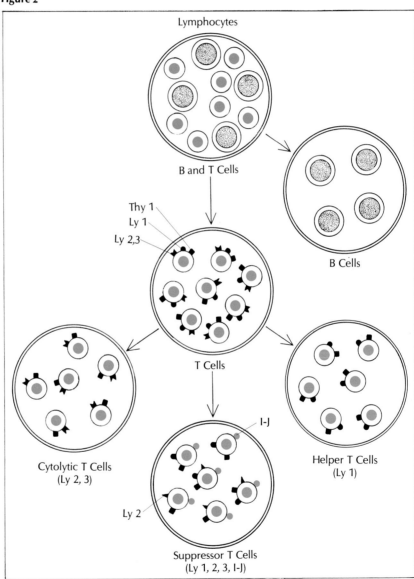

The differential pathway of suppressor T cells, as reflected in determinants on the surface, is diagrammed above. The presence of thy 1 antigen on all T-lymphocyte surfaces differentiates these cells from B lymphocytes. Ly-antigen differences are also distinctive; indeed each subset of suppressor T cells has different Ly markers—Ly $1^+,2^-$ for Ts_1, Ly (1^+), 2^+ for Ts_2, and Ly 2^+ for Ts_3. However, all suppressor T cells bear the unique H-2-coded I-J surface determinant.

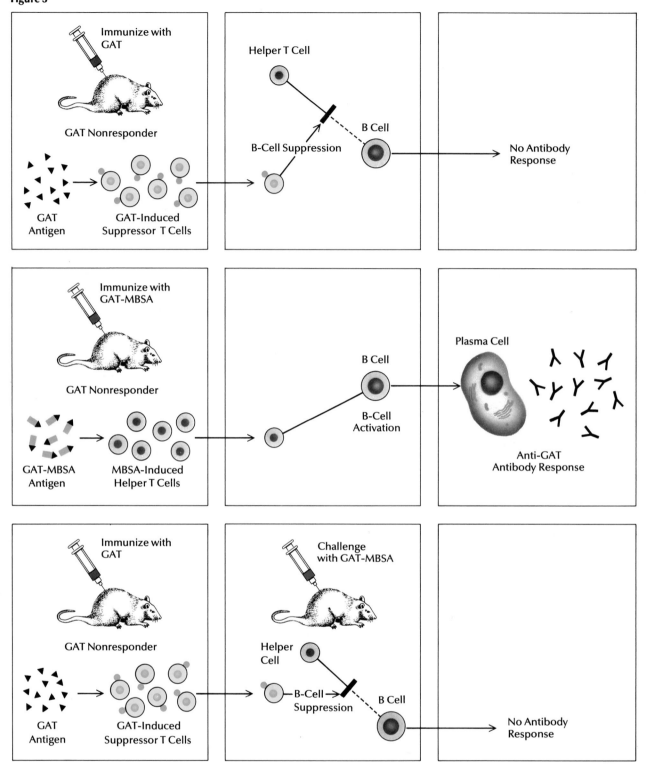

Use of synthetic polypeptide antigen GAT in defining basic characteristics of the suppressor T cell is depicted graphically. When a mouse of nonresponder strain is immunized with GAT, no specific antibody will be produced (top). The evidence suggests that the antigen induces a clone of specific suppressor T cells, and these lymphocytes interact with either helper T cells or B cells to turn off antibody-producing capacity. However, if GAT is presented to the animal on an MBSA carrier (middle),

helper T cells will be produced as a consequence of recognition of carrier. Thus the GAT T-cell–recognition defect will be bypassed, and specific anti-GAT antibody will be elaborated. However, when immunization with plain GAT precedes GAT-MBSA immunization (bottom), the primary immunization with GAT will induce specific GAT suppressor cells, and this pathway will dominate when GAT-MBSA challenge is made. As a result, no antibody will be produced.

sor T cells. What is more, the development of this suppressor cellular response was independent of the form in which the GAT antigen was presented to the nonresponder animal, as long as the GAT was not coupled in the primary immunization with a carrier that the animal was able to recognize. Subsequently, it was found that in responder animals, there were immunologic manipulations that resulted in the generation of suppressor T cells, but in such situations one effectively had to bypass the dominant helper pathway.

The next question posed was: Is the suppressor T-cell response related to the fact that these animal strains are nonresponders? In the model we have been discussing, involving GAT as the antigen and certain H-2 haplotypes, the answer is yes. This was shown by instituting certain procedures known to eliminate suppressor T cells prior to immunization with GAT. One such modality is pretreatment with cyclophosphamide. Suppressor T cells are considerably more sensitive to cyclophosphamide than helper cells. If after such treatment, one proceeds with the experiment exactly as described above—first immunization with GAT and then with GAT-MBSA—the animals will make not only antibody to the secondary immunization but even a small quantity of antibody to the primary immunization with GAT. There appears to be a minor helper pathway in these animals that is normally totally masked by the predominant suppressor pathway (see Figure 4).

However, it should be stressed that the preferential generation of suppressor T cells does not account for all Ir gene-controlled nonresponse phenomena. Only some strains of nonresponder animals can be demonstrated to produce suppressor T cells. In other strains, the nonresponse can be attributed to a failure to generate helper T cells. In such animals, neither helper nor suppressor T cells are produced. From the physician's point of view, this is an important fact to keep in mind when

Figure 4

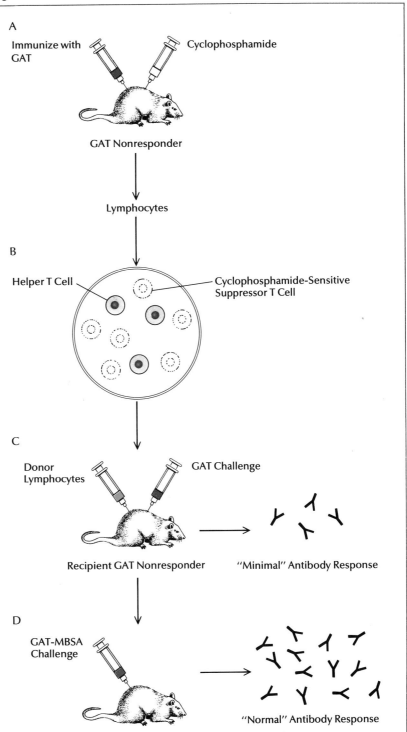

Ability of cyclophosphamide to abolish suppressor T-cell activity in the GAT system can be shown by injecting antimetabolite into nonresponder animal at the same time as one immunizes with GAT (A). This effectively eliminates cyclophosphamide-sensitive suppressor T cells but not helper T cells (B). When lymphocytes from an animal so treated are injected into syngeneic mouse and recipient is challenged with GAT, it produces a weak anti-GAT antibody response (C), indicating that minor helper T-cell pathway can be unmasked by eliminating suppressor T cells. In contrast to nonresponse seen in the absence of cyclophosphamide (cf Figure 3), recipient produces a "normal" antibody response to secondary challenge by GAT-MBSA (D).

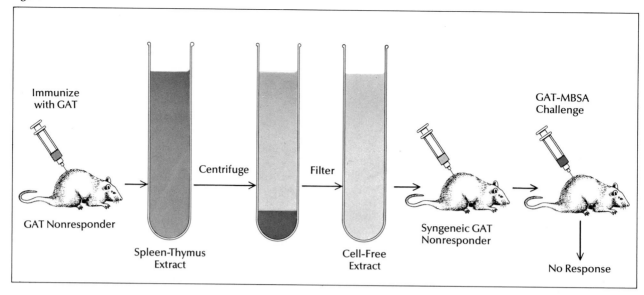

Existence of soluble suppressor factor generated by initial (cyclophosphamide-sensitive) suppressor T cells can be deduced if nonresponder animal is immunized with GAT and an ex- *tract is made from its spleen and thymus and treated to become cell-free. This extract, injected into syngeneic mouse, will make it nonresponsive to primary challenge with GAT-MBSA.*

we discuss the possibility of manipulating the suppressor systems to enhance antitumor host immunologic responses. Such manipulation is likely to offer promise only for those tumors that provoke a suppressor T-cell response.

In biologic terms, what has been shown is that both suppressor and helper responses are positive phenomena. From this follows the logical recognition that the suppressor pathway can be defective, even as the helper pathway can be defective. Both pathways are under control. Indeed, using techniques of genetic analysis, we have demonstrated the validity of this proposition. To do this, we resorted to another synthetic antigen, since with the GAT system, only three H-2 nonresponder haplotypes are known, an insufficient number to provide reasonable expectation of finding a defect. The antigen we chose is a copolymer closely related to GAT, polyglutamic tyrosine, or GT. With this synthetic antigen, responsiveness is confined to a few random-bred mice of the Swiss type, while all of the 20 inbred mouse strains tested are nonresponders.

We essentially repeated the sequence of experiments with GT that had been performed with GAT.

We showed that primary immunization with GT alone did not elicit antibody to GT; primary immunization with the hapten conjugate GT-MBSA did. But here the observations diverged. Preimmunization with GT did not alter the recipient's ability to respond to GT-MBSA in some of the strains studied. In others, it did. Analysis of the genetic defect in the suppressor pathway showed that control is located on an allele within the I region of the H-2 complex. In other words, the generation of specific suppressor cells (or the lack of such cells) and the generation of specific helper cells (or their lack) is genetically coded for within the same region of the genome.

Up to this point, we have been discussing suppressor T cells as if they were a single cell type. In fact, as already noted, three different populations of cells have been identified, one of which can be functionally characterized as initiating suppressor T cells, the others as effector suppressor T cells. Their functional differences have been delineated, as have certain differences in their properties.

However, before we get into detailed comparison of these cell types, it is necessary to bring into

the discussion the component that mediates between the inducer and effector cells: soluble suppressor factors.

The first description of antigen-specific suppressor factor was made by the Japanese investigator Tada. He was working in a nongenetically restricted system using a complex antigen, keyhole limpet hemocyanin (KLH), to which he produced suppressor T cells in mice. Tada then posed the question: Could something be extracted from the lymphoid tissue of these mice that would explain the suppressive action of these cells? He made an ultrasonicated extract from the thymus and spleen of mice that had been specifically suppressed in their responsiveness to KLH, and he produced a cell-free supernatant from this extract. Next, he injected this crude supernatant into normal (nonimmune) animals or introduced it into cultures of cells from such animals. In both models, the extract was found to be capable of suppressing responses to KLH.

Motivated by Tada's observation, we decided to apply his findings in our genetically restricted systems. Once again, we used the model predicated upon injection of the antigen GAT and the conjugate

GAT-MBSA into mice that were genetically nonresponsive to the former but able to make antibody when presented with the latter. As diagrammed in Figure 5, we immunized the mice with GAT, then made cell-free extracts from their thymuses, spleens, or both. These extracts were injected into syngeneic nonresponder animals, which were then challenged with GAT-MBSA. The animals failed to make antibody to the complex; parallel results were obtained in cell cultures in which the suppressor phenomenon was extremely sensitive, operating even when the extracts were diluted more than 1,000-fold. In short, the cell-free extracts appeared to induce suppressor activity similar to that induced by the antigen to which the animals were nonresponsive. Also noteworthy was the fact that the suppression of the response to GAT-MBSA could be achieved by injection of the cell-free extract either on the day of immunization with the complex or a week before such immunization. Moreover, the suppressive activity could be transferred to a second recipient. These experiments strongly suggested that here was a set of unusual molecules with highly promising biologic properties.

From our knowledge of the cellular kinetics of T lymphocytes, it seemed possible that the cell-free extract was inducing a population of suppressor cells. There was also reason to suspect that there might be two different sets of T cells. (At this stage of the experimentation, the existence of a third suppressor T-cell subpopulation was not suspected. As will be discussed subsequently, identification of what we now know as Ts$_3$ cells required use of another experimental system.)

As has already been pointed out, one could forestall the generation of suppressor activity with a primary GAT or GT immunization if one treated the animal with cyclophosphamide. This can be done with relatively small doses of the antimetabolite, on the order of 20 mg/kg. If this treatment is administered two or three days prior to immunization, the animal loses its nonresponsiveness and becomes a responder to the antigen. One can therefore conclude that the initial suppressor T cells normally responsible for the animal's tolerance are highly sensitive to cyclophosphamide. However, if during the course of treatment with cyclophosphamide, the same animal is also injected with the cell-free extract from another GAT- or GT-immunized mouse, it will develop suppressor T cells (see Figure 6).

We concluded from this finding that there must be two distinct suppressor T-cell populations, the first cyclophosphamide-sensitive, the second, cyclophosphamide-resistant. The observations also provided us with a clue as to the function of the cell-free extract, or, as we should now designate it, the suppressor factor. At this juncture in our studies, we had circumstantial evidence (later confirmed) that the suppressor factor was produced by the initial suppressor T-cell population. Similarly, we had shown that even in the absence of such initiating suppressor T cells, the factor could induce a second population of effector suppressor T cells. Additionally, the fact that the first population was cyclophosphamide-sensitive and the second was not was conceptually attractive, since it made biologic sense for precursor cells with a requirement for division and proliferation to be inhibited by

Figure 6

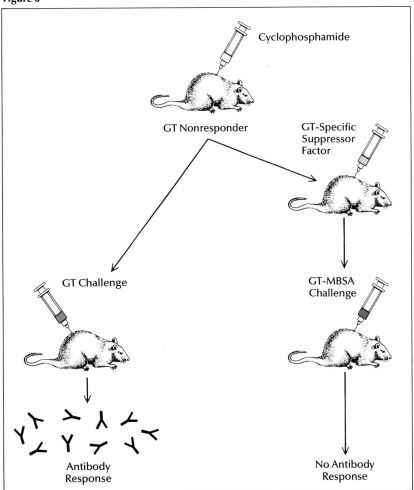

An additional demonstration of the role of specific suppressor factor is shown here. Mice used are GT nonresponders but can be induced to respond to GT by treatment with cyclophosphamide (left). However, if one introduces GT-specific suppressor factor, recipient animal will prove nonresponsive to GT-MBSA (right).

Figure 7

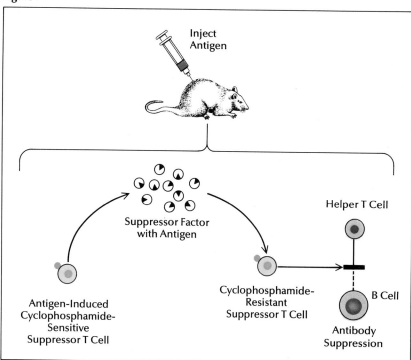

Inject Antigen

Suppressor Factor with Antigen

Helper T Cell

Antigen-Induced Cyclophosphamide-Sensitive Suppressor T Cell

Cyclophosphamide-Resistant Suppressor T Cell

B Cell

Antibody Suppression

Schematic summarizes the events that are believed to take place when an animal is exposed to antigen to which it is genetically nonresponsive. Antigen first induces a cyclophosphamide-sensitive population of suppressor T cells. These lymphocytes elaborate a soluble factor that combines with small quantities of antigen and induces a second—cyclophosphamide-resistant—suppressor T-cell clone. It is these effector cells that actually suppress the antibody-producing B cells. Also suggested is the likelihood that this system subserves the homeostatic role of turning off antibody response that threatens to overwhelm the host.

an antimetabolite and for an already differentiated subset of effector cells to be unaffected by such a chemical.

Serendipitously, we also had a genetic strain of mice in the GT system that provided us with an animal model for demonstrating these phenomena. The A/J mouse strain (haplotype H-2^a) does not develop suppressor cells when immunized with GT. It thus behaves as nonresponder strains do when treated with cyclophosphamide. But when this mouse is inoculated with cell-free extract from a suppressor strain immunized with GT, it becomes a nonresponder to GT-MBSA. In other words, it develops suppressor T cells that can be adoptively transferred.

Having summarized the basic evidence not only for the existence of two populations of suppressor T cells (still holding in abeyance dis-

cussion of the third subset) but also for the existence of a soluble suppressor factor that apparently induces the differentiation of the initial suppressor cells to effector cells, let us review the important properties of the suppressor factor.

First of all, it is clear that the factor is a T-cell product. We have shown that elimination of T cells from either intact animals or in vitro cultures will prevent production of suppressor factor. We have also specifically shown that neither B cells nor macrophages can elaborate the factor.

It has also been established that the suppressor factor is antigen-specific. When produced in response to GAT immunization, it will not alter responsivity to GT-MBSA, to red blood cells, or indeed to any other type of antigen. Its functional specificity is paralleled by equal specificity in its ca-

pability to bind the eliciting antigen. Thus, for example, if one passes GAT factor through several columns, one of which contains the specific GAT antigen while the others contain other antigens, all of the factor will be absorbed by the GAT column, and the material eluted from that column will be as active as, or even more active than, the factor prior to absorption.

We can also define some important physical characteristics of the suppressor factor molecule. Its molecular weight is about 50,000 daltons. This was demonstrated by passing the molecule on a column with different pore sizes. The maximum-size pore through which the factor passed was consistent with a molecular size corresponding to about 50,000 daltons.

More significantly, we have discovered that the factor molecule bears an antigenic determinant coded for in the I region of the H-2 complex. For those mouse strains for which appropriate antisera are available, we can establish that the antigenic determinants are coded for in the I-J subregion. I-J restriction has been demonstrated by immunizing the H-2^k mouse (a haplotype that produces suppressor T cells and suppressor factor against the GT antigen) with GT. When the resulting GT suppressor factor is treated with anti-I-J antiserum, the factor is specifically retained by the antiserum on a column.

An additional demonstration of the antigenic determinant comes from sequential absorption experiments. If the GT suppressor factor is placed on an antigen (GT) column, it will be absorbed by that column. Suppressor factor activity can then be eluted from the column. Furthermore, if the eluate is then absorbed into a column containing anti-I-J antibody, the antibody will retain the factor. Elution will once again permit recovery of the full suppressor factor activity. If one puts the results of these experiments together, one can delineate this sequence: initial suppressor T cells produce, and can have extracted from them, an I-J-determinant-bearing molecule that is antigen-specific and capable of inducing the formation of specific effector suppressor T cells.

In the course of these studies we also determined that the crudely extracted factor had some antigen bound to it. Apparently, the antigen originally injected in the animal to induce suppressor T cells persists long enough to bind to the suppressor molecules, in a very small but biologically highly significant quantity.

This brought the investigation to the point at which a critical question could be asked. Is the minute amount of antigen that is complexed to the factor molecule in the crude extract important in the sequence leading to generation of effector cells? One way to answer that question was to investigate whether suppressor T cells could be generated by purified factor with no antigen at all. It was found that this could not be done. On the other hand, the purified extract was extremely suppressive in culture when antigen was added back into the system. It should be stressed that in these systems the amount of antigen required was extremely small, as little as 10 or 15 ng. Such quantities are far below those that are needed to induce suppressor T cells initially.

With the information presented thus far, one can begin to bring into focus the homeostatic role of the four-stage suppressor system: 1) the induction by appropriate antigen of the initial cyclophosphamide-sensitive suppressor T cells; 2) elaboration by these lymphocytes of I-J-determined suppressor factors; 3) combination of factor molecules with small quantities of the immunizing antigen; 4) factor (plus antigen)-mediated induction of specific effector suppressor cells (see Figure 7). Clearly, this system provides a very sensitive means for augmenting a suppressor phenomenon in physiologic situations when an antibody response threatens to become an overreaction, since the effector phase can be induced with minimal amounts of antigen.

In the studies described to this point, we have largely confined the discussion to two suppressor-cell subtypes, Ts_1 and Ts_2, but have indicated that a third subtype with characteristic phenotypic surface markers also exists. Discovery of Ts_3 cells came about only after studies of suppressor phenomena in delayed hypersensitivity reactions were undertaken in our laboratories. In fact, two different groups of investigators were involved in the studies, each using a different sensitizing agent. One group headed by Mark Greene and involving Man-Sun Sy, Alfred Nisonoff, and Ronald Germain probed specific suppression of responses to azobenzenearsonate (ABA); the other group working with Martin Dorf employed the 4-hydroxy-3-nitrophenyl acetyl (NP) system. Since their findings were remarkably similar, we will confine our description to the ABA system experiments.

The ABA system was chosen for studies of contact sensitivity because it had been observed that ABA-specific antibodies produced

Figure 8

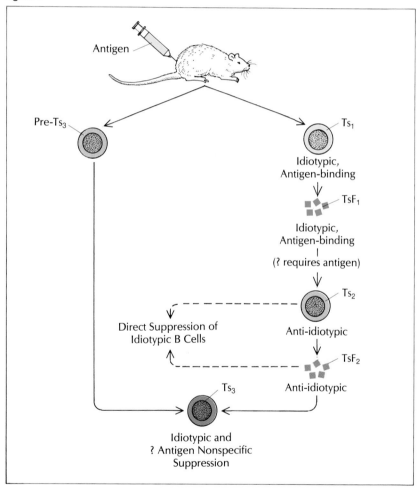

This summary diagram depicts the suppressor pathways starting with antigen encounter. At the same time as the antigen triggers the antigen-binding Ts_1 cells, it can cause differentiation of precursors to effector Ts_3 lymphocytes. The latter can also be activated by Ts_2 cells via idiotype-anti-idiotype interaction. The Ts_2s can also be induced either in the presence of antigen or by idiotypic receptor mechanisms involving the Ts_1 cells. The Ts_2 lymphocytes can function as immediate effectors by direct suppression of idiotypic B cells or via induction of the Ts_3 subset. In all cases the soluble suppressor factors (TsF) can subserve the functions of the lymphocytes that produce them.

in A-J strain mice share a unique idiotype. Perhaps, it was reasoned, T cells involved in the ABA response, including suppressors, would share the same idiotypic marker, thus facilitating analysis of the cellular response. This reasoning proved accurate.

The general scheme of the ABA experimentation can be summarized as follows: A-J strain mice when immunized with ABA-conjugated spleen cells will develop suppressor T cells (Ts$_1$) within four or five days. When these spleen cells are transferred to a normal mouse, they will inhibit the recipient animal from mounting a normal delayed hypersensitivity reaction to ABA. In other words, a mouse that has not received a suppressor-T-cell transfer and is sensitized either intradermally or subcutaneously to ABA will, on challenge between days five and seven, manifest a delayed hypersensitivity reaction. However, a recipient who receives suppressor cells from the first suppressed mouse concomitant with immunization will be anergic. It was discovered that the Ts$_1$ cells must be injected early in the immunization process because they are afferent inducer cells. That is, they are not suppressing directly

but only through initiation of the suppressor pathways that led to development of the second-order efferent suppressor cells (Ts$_2$). Up to this point, the results of the experimentation essentially paralleled the findings in the GAT system, and there was no reason to alter the concept that Ts$_2$ is the final effector cell in the pathway.

In fact, we discovered that this was not so. The discovery came from transfer of Ts$_2$ into immunized animals that had been treated with cyclophosphamide. It will be recalled that in the GAT system, cyclophosphamide treatment could prevent the induction of nonresponsiveness when administered at the level of the Ts$_1$ cell, which is cyclophosphamide-sensitive, but suppression could be achieved by circumventing the Ts$_1$ with injections of Ts$_2$ or its soluble factor, since Ts$_2$ is cyclophosphamide-resistant. In the ABA system, Ts$_2$-cell transfers will not suppress the immune response in a cyclophosphamide-treated animal. The implication was that a third lymphocyte subset was present. Like Ts$_1$, this subset is cyclophosphamide-sensitive, but unlike the first-order cell, the Ts$_3$ cell is functioning in the efferent effector mode rather

than as an inducer. Figure 8 summarizes the suppressor pathway, including all three subsets and their soluble factors, as it has been defined within the ABA (and NP) systems.

Once it was deduced that the Ts$_3$ cell existed, a systematic effort was made to identify it. This has been done. We now know that the Ts$_3$ is I-J-positive (along with all suppressor T cells) and Ly-2-positive and that it is induced during sensitization, with a functional commitment to turn off the immune response when it is activated in the normal pathway. The Ts$_3$ is idiotypic since it is the target of an anti-idiotypic Ts$_2$ cell. Finally, although the Ts$_3$ cell is triggered by specific antigen, its suppressive activity can be nonspecific because what it is suppressing is the inflammatory response that is common to all delayed hypersensitivity reactions.

In parallel with our studies of the Ts$_3$ cell, we have considerably enhanced our knowledge of the soluble factors. It can now be demonstrated that each of the subsets has a soluble factor that can subserve all of the functions of the cell that produces it. It is interesting to note that Ts$_3$ factor can function in a cyclophosphamide-treated animal simply because it no longer "needs" its cyclophosphamide-sensitive cell. Somewhat paradoxically, therefore, the Ts$_3$ cell is the only suppressor that has a soluble factor that doesn't need to interact with a cyclophosphamide-sensitive cell to effect a turnoff of the immune response system.

In the work described up to now the concentration has largely been on the operation of the suppressor system in subjects that are genetically nonresponders to specific antigens. Obviously, the system would have a more universal significance if it also functioned when the animal is responsive to the immunizing antigen. And indeed our investigations show that it does under certain circumstances. There are several ways in which the T-lymphocyte response can be deflected from a helper pathway to a suppressor pathway.

Figure 9

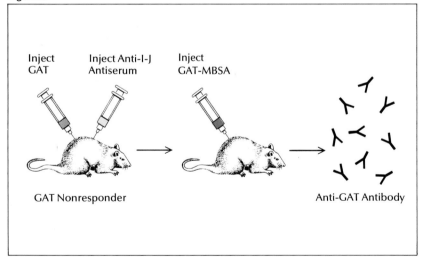

One can show that the generation of suppressor T cells is controlled by genes in the I-J subregion of the major histocompatibility (H-2) region of the mouse. If anti-I-J antiserum is injected into a nonresponder mouse along with antigen, that animal will subsequently make specific antibody when challenged with the tolerated antigen complexed with a recognizable carrier molecule.

If one takes animals that are responders to GAT and prepares cultures of their spleen cells, then adds antigen in quantities five to 10 times that which could be expected to induce an antibody response, suppressor T cells will be induced. This can be shown by injecting T lymphocytes from this culture into a recipient responder animal and going through the procedures previously described for demonstrating suppressor activity. Excess antigen, therefore, is one way in which a suppressor response can be incited in a responder animal.

If, in the same system, one depletes the culture of macrophages, suppressor activity can be obtained with normally immunogenic quantities of antigen. Keep in mind that a critical step in antibody formation is the presentation of antigen by the macrophage to the lymphocyte. It therefore appears that one way of converting an animal from the helper to the suppressor pathway is to bypass the macrophage.

The role of the macrophage was further confirmed in experiments involving F_1 hybrids between responder and nonresponder strains. The mouse strains selected for these experiments were Black-6 (Bl-6) and DBA-1. The Bl-6 is a responder to GAT, the DBA-1 a nonresponder. When the two strains are crossed and the offspring are immunized with GAT, they respond and make antibody to GAT. The ability of the hybrids to respond must of course be inherited from their Bl-6 parents. If one now takes the spleen cells from the F_1 hybrids and cultures them, secondary responses to antigen presentation can be tested. These responses vary with the macrophages used to present antigen to the cultured cells. If the Bl-6 macrophage is employed, an antibody response is achieved. If, on the other hand, the nonresponder DBA-1 macrophages are used for antigen presentation, no antibody is produced. Here then is convincing evidence that at least one of the defects leading to suppressor rather than helper activity is at the level of the macrophage.

Figure 10

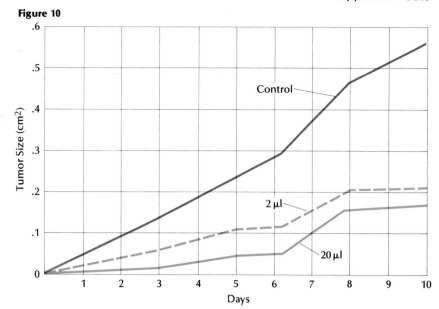

Graph shows effect of anti-I-J^k antiserum on growth of sarcoma 1509A in A/J mice. Curves represent tumor growth in controls, in animals treated with 2 µl/day of antiserum, and in mice treated with 20 µl/day of antiserum.

To return to the homeostatic raison d'être of suppressor cells, it can definitely be stated that they monitor and regulate antibody response to a variety of antigens. Not too many years ago, we thought of antibody as the elusive feedback mechanism through which the immune response was limited. That is to say, we regarded antibody itself as the sole mechanism for eliminating antigenic molecules from the circulation—by complexing with or denying antigen access to target cells by preempting binding sites. The whole relationship, it was assumed, depended on the affinity of antibody for antigen or for antigenic binding sites. Now it can be seen that with suppressor T cells there is a much more efficient feedback system. In practically all situations, an excess of antigen will stimulate the generation of suppressor cells. Recently, Gershon and Cantor have even shown that suppressor cells will be mobilized by an excess of helper T cells. There appears to be no doubt that the suppressor T cell serves teleologically as an "off-switch" for the immune response.

A second important biologic role that assuredly can be attributed to the suppressor system is to establish tolerance to self-antigens. The experiments described above demonstrate that suppressor T cells can replace response with nonresponse at very low levels of antigen. This is in contrast to B-cell tolerance, which requires large doses of antigen (see W. O. Weigle, "Immunologic Tolerance and Immunopathology"). The suppressor system provides a pathway through which T-cell tolerance can be established with minimal antigen bound to suppressor factor. This combination is capable of inducing a clone of effector suppressor lymphocytes. What remains to be clarified is the nature of the event that provides sufficient antigenic stimulation to initiate the differentiation of the first, factor-producing suppressor T cells.

On the immunopathologic side, it can readily be appreciated that any system as sensitive as the suppressor system can be triggered to function when such function is detrimental to the host. Indeed, there is now evidence that in many experimental tumor systems, the tumor-bearing animals produce suppressor T cells that turn off their antitumor immune responses. One of the most persuasive demonstrations of this phenomenon

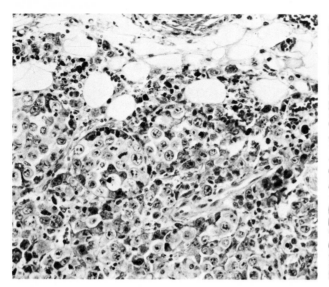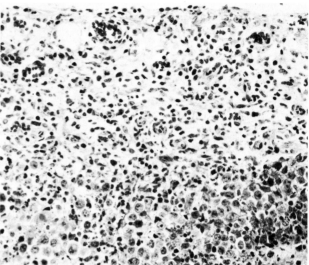

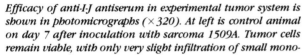

Efficacy of anti-I-J antiserum in experimental tumor system is shown in photomicrographs (×320). At left is control animal on day 7 after inoculation with sarcoma 1509A. Tumor cells remain viable, with only very slight infiltration of small mono- *nuclear cells at tumor's periphery. At right is comparable picture in mouse treated with anti-I-J^k antiserum. An intense leukocytic infiltrate can be seen adjacent to and within tumor cells, which are markedly necrotic.*

was made by Mark Greene at Harvard. He showed that in mice bearing tumors known to be antigenic but that cannot be rejected because of the size of the antigenic load, specific suppressor T cells can be identified in splenic and thymic tissue. When these cells are passively transferred to an immune animal bearing the same tumor, rejection of that tumor is prevented. The tumor-protective effect was found to be specific for the tumor growing in the animals from which the cells were obtained. Also, the suppressor T cells were found to be producing suppressor factor, which, in turn, was inducing clones of suppressor cells.

On the basis of such experiments, a question that looms large is: Can the suppressor system be manipulated either to enhance a positive immune response or to reverse a negative response?

Our first pilot experiments designed to answer this question did not involve tumor-bearing mice or tumor antigens but rather employed normal mice challenged with sheep red blood cells. Just preceding the injection of the RBC (in a very small dose), we treated the mice with minimal doses of syngeneic anti-I-J antiserum. The re-

sult was a two- to threefold increase in antibody to sheep RBC. It should be stressed that these experiments were done in animals that were not part of a genetically restricted system (not inbred, that is) and that normally are responders to the sheep RBC. Therefore, the most plausible explanation for our findings was that the anti-I-J antiserum interfered with the development of suppressor cells and suppressor factor. In addition, these experiments confirmed the previous observations suggesting that in both responders and nonresponders, thymus-dependent immune response includes both helper and suppressor T-cell activities. If one turns off the suppressor system, one leaves the field open to the helper T cells, with consequent amplification of the conventional immune response. We have obtained essentially the same or parallel results with other antigens, notably such complexes as GAT-MBSA.

With such experiments to guide us, we then turned to the genetically controlled or restricted systems, particularly those involving nonresponder strains. An experiment of this nature is diagrammed in Figure 9. In this, anti-I-J antiserum

was administered with GAT to SJL strain (H-2^s) nonresponder mice. On a subsequent secondary challenge with GAT-MBSA, the mouse responded to the complex and produced anti-GAT antibody. Similar results were seen when the H-2^k mouse was treated with anti-I-J and immunized with GT and GT-MBSA.

In addition, the anti-I-J antiserum turns these two strains of mice into minimal responders to GAT and GT, respectively—the responses, of course, occurring to the primary immunizations with these two synthetic antigens. Effectively, the anti-I-J antiserum mimics cyclophosphamide, immunologically eliminating the initial suppressor T population even as the antimetabolite does so chemically. Moreover, the antiserum does so at extremely small doses (on the order of 10 μl), a finding that has obviously important potential clinical significance.

Next we turned to tumor systems in which previous investigations had revealed the presence of suppressor T cells. A/J mice were injected with 10^5 or 10^6 sarcoma 1509A or sarcoma 1 cells. Normally, inoculations of these cells will produce extremely rapidly growing and inevitably lethal cancers. However, with these inoculations, we also injected the mice with 2.0 µl of anti-I-J antiserum daily for 10 days. The dramatic inhibition of tumor growth under this regimen is graphed in Figure 10. Histologic alteration of the tumors occurred in tandem, with the tumor tissue of the anti-I-J-treated animals showing extensive infiltration by mononuclear cells, as shown in Figure 11. Finally, when we looked for suppressor T cells specific for the tumor in these animals, we could not find any.

While this experimentation is still in its early stages, the evidence to date certainly justifies the conclusion that in tumor systems where the presence of suppressor cells is demonstrable, elimination of these cells with anti-I-J antiserum dramatically alters the balance of immunity in favor of the host. A cautionary statement must be appended: Not all tumor systems appear to stimulate suppressor cells.

In concluding this presentation, let me underscore that the ways we have been looking at the suppressor system will undoubtedly be considered highly primitive a few years hence. But already we have learned enough to project the possibility that a renaissance in immunology is approaching. An entirely new category of immensely powerful regulatory molecules is coming into scientific focus. The suppressor factor is perhaps the first; it is certainly not the only one. A number of laboratories in this country, in England, and in Israel have studied an analogous helper factor that also bears I region (but not I-J) determinants.

We can, I believe, be confident that we are learning the mechanisms of regulation at the T-cell level. This knowledge has immense potential for application once we have developed human counterparts of the antisera that are so active in mice. There is some evidence that these regulators are preferentially effective with respect to particular antibody classes, for example, the IgE-mediated responses that are of course so important in allergic syndromes. There is also considerable evidence that chronic bacterial and viral infections stimulate not only specific but also nonspecific suppressor cells. It is not unreasonable to speculate that these cells could explain the mechanism, or one of the mechanisms, of chronicity. In short, we are gaining new perceptions about many of the most perplexing problems of immunology. These perceptions permit us not only to be more realistic about the true nature of these problems but also to be more realistically hopeful about arriving at the solutions, in the laboratory and clinic.

Lymphoid Cells as Effectors Of Immunologic Cytolysis

JEAN-CHARLES CEROTTINI *Ludwig Institute for Cancer Research, Lausanne*

The term cell-mediated immunity has been employed for a long time, primarily to describe one of the two major domains of immunologic effector activity. In this usage, it is most often juxtaposed to and distinguished from antibody-mediated, or humoral, immunity. Until very recently, the two had been thought of and studied as two quite discrete sets of phenomena. But as our understanding of both immunopathology and immunobiology advanced in the 1970s, we have more and more recognized the interdependence of so-called humoral and so-called cellular immunity. On the one hand, for example, we have learned that, more often than not, an antibody response is facilitated by cooperation between thymically differentiated lymphocytes and bone marrow–derived lymphocytes (see D.H. Katz, "Genetic Controls and Cellular Interactions in Antibody Formation"; E.A. Boyse and H. Cantor, "Surface Characteristics of T-Lymphocyte Subpopulations"). On the other hand, it is now evident that effector immune mechanisms often involve the participation of both antibodies and cells. Thus, we have acquired evidence that there exists a cytotoxic lymphocyte population that depends for its effect upon ability to recognize and interact with antibody molecules that coat the surface of target cells.

It is this lymphocyte population, the K cells, that will be the subject of the latter portion of this presentation. The first part will describe and discuss the cytotoxic thymus-derived cells, or cytotoxic T lymphocytes (CTL).

A basic difference between CTL and K cells is that the former appear only after immunization, that is, they are a product of T-cell responses to surface membrane antigens, and perform their function in the absence of detectable antibody and complement activities. In contrast, K cells do not require such immunization but function by interaction with appropriate antibody that has coated the surface of the target cell. In biologic terms, there seems to be an analogy with the complement system, whose lytic sequence via the so-called classic pathway is initiated by attachment of its first component to appropriate antibody on a cell surface. When antibody is absent, however, the lytic sequence can proceed via the so-called alternate pathway (see H.J. Müller-Eberhard, "Chemistry and Function of the Complement System"). Clearly, the lysis of unwanted cells conveys sufficient survival advantage to require the persistence of an array of mechanisms designed to cope with all contingencies.

Historically, the concept of cellular immunity probably owes its birth to Metchnikoff, who early in this century postulated the role of phagocytes in host defenses against pathogens. However, the modern appreciation that lymphoid-cell populations could function as effectors of target-cell lysis came only after tumor and transplantation biologists demonstrated that the tissue reactions they were studying involved mobilization of lymphoid cells along with other cells such as macrophages, PMN leukocytes, and monocytes. Subsequent experiments demonstrated that the immune response to an antigen could be transferred from individual to individual by transfer of immune lymphocytes.

More detailed analysis of the observed phenomena has proved extremely difficult to achieve in vivo both because of the complexity of the events and because of the need to differentiate among the various cytolytic-cell populations involved. Progress became dependent on the development of appropriate in vitro analogues of the allograft reaction. Although a number of such procedures have been developed, not until less than a decade ago was the system perfected that has probably been most productive. Since a great deal of the information presented in this review is based on this technique – assay of the release of radioactive chromium-51 by lysed target cells – it is appropriate to describe it briefly.

As diagrammed in Figure 1 (facing page), the ^{51}Cr-release assay is simple in conception. The target cells (either fresh or cultured cells may be employed depending on the experiment) are prelabeled with ^{51}Cr in the form of sodium chromate. After diffusion through the cell membrane, the isotope is retained in the cytoplasm for a relatively prolonged period of time unless the target-cell membrane is sufficiently damaged to allow the efflux of intracellular molecules. The released isotope is no longer the chromate ion and is not reutilized. In the assay system commonly used, the radiolabeled target cells are incubated with immune lymphoid cells, and the amount of radioactivity released into the medium is measured after a few hours. Since the assay is independent of target-cell multiplication, the only parameter measured is direct cytolysis. The percentage of target cells lysed will, of course, depend on the concentration ratio of effector cells to target cells. Under optimal conditions, i.e., when highly susceptible target cells are incubated with a lymphoid population containing a high frequency of effector cells, cytolysis is detectable within a few minutes. Incubation for several hours may be required with less susceptible target cells and/or less active effector-cell populations.

The use of ^{51}Cr release also facilitates such procedures as the competitive inhibition assay (see Figure 2, facing page) to determine the specificity of CTL activity. In this procedure, a population of immune T cells (including CTL) is incubated with ^{51}Cr-labeled target cells bearing the immunizing surface antigens (target cells X). Next, these immunized T cells are mixed with equal aliquots of ^{51}Cr-labeled target cells X and of unlabeled target cells X. The amount of isotope

released into the extracellular medium will be reduced by about half as compared with a mixture in which all of the target cells are tagged. However, when the labeled target cells X are mixed with unlabeled cells (Y) bearing antigens to which the T cells have not been immunized, there is no reduction in lysis as expressed by extracellular ^{51}Cr. This demonstrates that the CTL killing is entirely specific.

The first description of cell-mediated cytotoxic reactions was made in 1960 by Govaerts, who reported that thoracic duct cells from dogs that had rejected kidney allografts were able to destroy donor kidney cells in vitro. This finding, which was confirmed in subsequent studies of allograft immunity in mice, suggested that immune lymphoid cells had a role in target-cell lysis in vitro, but it did not rule out the possibility that the actual effector of cytotoxicity was specific alloantibody. When several investigators demonstrated that this antibody actually diminished cell-mediated lysis, this seemed to militate against such a role for the immunoglobulin. However, it was then observed that the appearance of alloantibody after immunization temporally coincided with the formation of cytotoxic cells. The development of quantitative in vitro assays made it possible to settle this question and, in addition, to prove that the cytotoxic cells belonged to the T-cell lineage.

The critical experiments were performed by Brunner, Nordin, and the author, employing parallel in vitro techniques for the measurement of cell-mediated lysis and antibody response as these phenomena were expressed in the graft-vs-host reaction. This reaction, it will be recalled, occurs when grafted lymphoid cells attack and destroy the tissues and cells of the graft recipient. Our experimental design (see Figure 3 on page 66) involved giving a lethal radiation dose to recipient mice and then transplanting them with cells derived from allogeneic donors. We did this transplantation with lymphocyte-rich cell inoculates derived from either donor spleen, donor thymus, or donor bone marrow. The assumption was that the spleen cells would be a mixed B- and T-cell population, the thymic cells

would be predominantly T cells, and the bone marrow cells predominantly B cells.

Five days after inoculation of the recipient animals, examination of their spleens revealed that the cells therein were almost entirely of the donor genotype. These cells were then assayed in vitro by the ^{51}Cr method for cell-mediated cytolytic activity against recipient target cells and for the presence of alloantibody-forming cells by a plaque-forming–cell (PFC) method, using the same target cells. The results can be summarized as follows:

1) Cells of donor splenic origin were strongly positive for both cell-mediated cytotoxic and PFC activities.

2) Thymic cells were positive for cytotoxic lymphocytes but devoid of PFC.

3) Bone marrow cells showed no cell-mediated cytotoxicity.

These findings argued strongly for the existence of specifically cytolytic T cells. The argument was bolstered when spleen cells in this system were treated with anti-Thy 1 antiserum and complement prior to the testing of their activities. It will be recalled that

Opposite page: Figure 1 depicts the steps in the ^{51}Cr-release assay of cytolytic activity. The putative target cells are labeled with radioactive sodium chromate, the label being incorporated into the cytoplasm. Then lymphocytes specifically immunized to the target cells are added and the mixture is incubated. The cytolytic activity of the lymphocytes can be measured by assaying the ^{51}Cr that has been liberated into the medium upon cell lysis. This system can be adapted into a competitive inhibition assay that serves to define the specificity of lytic activity (Figure 2). Thus, when the specifically immunized lymphocytes are mixed with equal quantities of labeled and unlabeled target cells "X" (top), the unlabeled cells will compete on equal terms with the labeled ones, and the amount of ^{51}Cr detectable in the extracellular medium will be reduced by about 50%. On the other hand, if labeled target cells "X" are mixed with unlabeled cells "Y" (bottom) that do not possess surface antigens to which the lymphocytes have been immunized, there will be no inhibition of ^{51}Cr release.

Figure 1

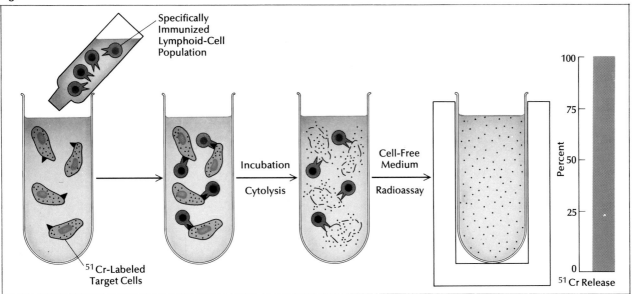

Specifically
Immunized
Lymphoid-Cell
Population

Incubation

Cytolysis

Cell-Free
Medium

Radioassay

^{51}Cr-Labeled
Target Cells

Percent

^{51}Cr Release

Figure 2

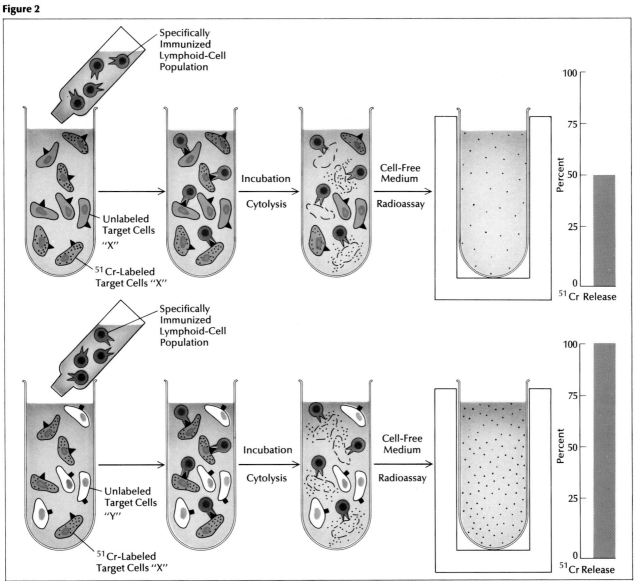

Specifically
Immunized
Lymphoid-Cell
Population

Unlabeled
Target Cells
"X"

^{51}Cr-Labeled
Target Cells "X"

Incubation

Cytolysis

Cell-Free
Medium

Radioassay

Percent

^{51}Cr Release

Specifically
Immunized
Lymphoid-Cell
Population

Unlabeled
Target Cells
"Y"

^{51}Cr-Labeled
Target Cells "X"

Incubation

Cytolysis

Cell-Free
Medium

Radioassay

Percent

^{51}Cr Release

Figure 3

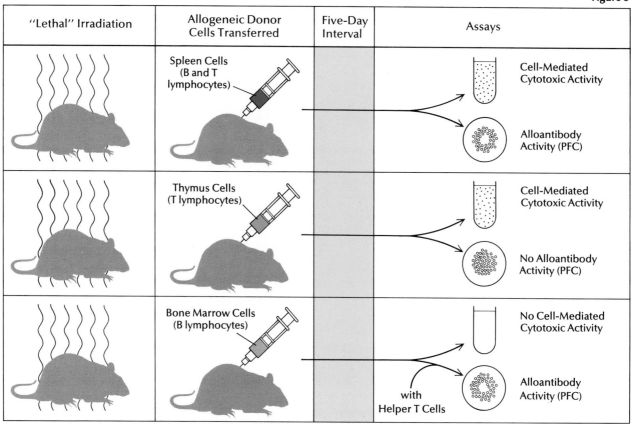

"Lethal" Irradiation	Allogeneic Donor Cells Transferred	Five-Day Interval	Assays
	Spleen Cells (B and T lymphocytes)		Cell-Mediated Cytotoxic Activity / Alloantibody Activity (PFC)
	Thymus Cells (T lymphocytes)		Cell-Mediated Cytotoxic Activity / No Alloantibody Activity (PFC)
	Bone Marrow Cells (B lymphocytes)		No Cell-Mediated Cytotoxic Activity / Alloantibody Activity (PFC) with Helper T Cells

Diagram summarizes critical experiments in localizing cytolytic activity to a T-cell subpopulation in a graft-vs-host system. Mice are first depleted of their own lymphoid cells by "lethal" irradiation, then injected with allogeneic spleen, thymus, or bone marrow cells. After five days, immunization of allogeneic donor cells against recipient histocompatibility antigens has taken place, and lymphocytes are withdrawn and assayed for cytotoxic activity by ^{51}Cr assay and for alloantibody-forming activity by plaque-forming cell (PFC) method, using recipient target cells. Cytotoxic activity clearly correlated with immunization of donor T cells, antibody activity with B cells (with a requirement for helper T cells).

the Thy 1 surface alloantigen is a marker for T cells (see Boyse and Cantor) and that treatment of a mixed lymphoid-cell population with anti-Thy 1 antiserum and complement specifically eliminates T cells. Indeed, it was found that treatment of spleen cells with anti-Thy 1 and complement abrogated cell-mediated cytotoxicity without affecting alloantibody PFC. As similar findings were obtained with spleen cells from mice immunized with allogeneic cells, it became clear that the in vitro cell-mediated cytotoxic reactions observed in allograft systems and in graft-vs-host reactions were caused by effector T cells.

More recently, it has become clear that CTL belong to a subpopulation of T cells that is distinct from the T cells that function as helpers of B cells in the antibody response. As discussed in detail by Boyse and Cantor in their

article, at least two T-cell subsets can be identified and isolated by the use of antisera directed against Ly surface components. Thus, CTL express the Ly 123 phenotype, whereas helper T cells are Ly 1.

In vitro assays have also permitted study of the kinetics of CTL responses. It was found, for example, that when allogeneic living tumor cells were injected into the peritoneal cavity of a mouse, T cells removed from the animal spleen showed lytic activity within three or four days. The activity increased continuously until it reached maximum levels at 10 to 11 days postinoculation. It remained detectable for 60 to 90 days. At the peak of the response, the heaviest concentration of CTL was found at the rejection site, the peritoneal cavity in this instance, with descending concentra-

tions (in order) in the blood, the thoracic duct, the spleen, and the lymph nodes. Evidence with respect to the development of memory cells during the response is not as direct as in the case of B-cell responses, but circumstantial evidence strongly favors such development. For example, accelerated rejection of second allografts occurs in a time frame consistent with anamnestic CTL responses. One also can observe in the accelerated "second-set" response a marked increase in the number of CTL generated.

It is likely, however, that anamnestic CTL responses are not only quantitatively different from primary responses but also include some qualitative difference.

Other investigations have delved into the cellular events involved in the generation of CTL. Initial studies

Figure 4

have concentrated on CTL responses in intact animals, but, because of the obvious difficulties encountered with in vivo systems, more recent approaches have involved in vitro models, in particular that of the mixed leukocyte culture (MLC). This is the system best known for its application in the matching of donors to allograft recipients in human transplantation situations. The basis of MLC is that if lymphoid cells from one individual are mixed with those of another, differences in antigens coded for within the major histocompatibility locus will lead the two different cell types to stimulate each other, causing a proliferative response. By pretreatment of one of the two individuals' lymphocytes with either x-irradiation or mitomycin C (to prevent their proliferation), MLC can be made unidirectional. In such an MLC system, not only do lymphocytes proliferate but also effector T cells such as CTL are generated.

With the development of appropriate culture conditions, it has been possible to keep the reactive lymphoid-cell population alive for several weeks and, hence, to determine the differentiation pathway and the fate of the effector T cells completely in vitro. Based on the results of several recent studies, the following picture (see Figure 4, this page) has emerged The immediate precursors of CTL are small, dense lymphocytes that express the Ly 123 phenotype. Before antigenic stimulation, they lack cytotoxic activity, although they are presumably equipped with specific receptors. Upon stimulation with appropriate cell-bound antigens, for example surface constituents coded for by the major histocompatibility complex, the CTL progenitors bearing the relevant receptors are triggered to proliferate and differentiate into medium- to large-sized cytotoxic cells directed against target cells that display on their surfaces the immunizing antigens. The question then arises whether the generation of CTL requires a cooperation between various cell types, even as the formation of antibody-producing cells may require a collaboration between their progenitors and helper T cells. While CTL formation is independent of the presence of B cells, there is some uncer-

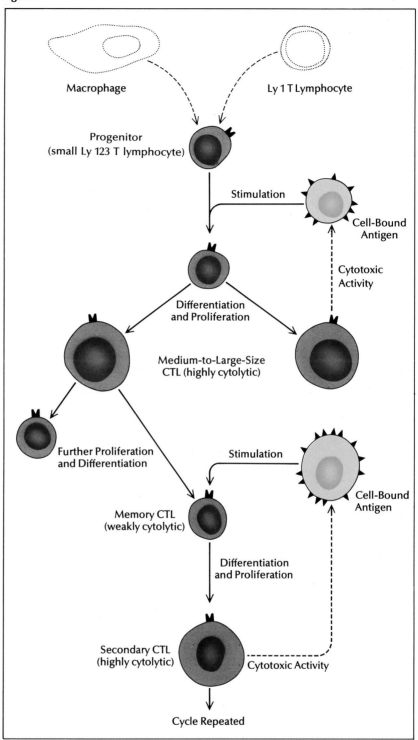

Currently held concepts of CTL induction and differentiation are presented graphically. It is believed the immediate precursors are small, dense T cells that express Ly 123 surface molecules. On stimulation with appropriate cell-bound antigens (with a possible requirement of cooperation from macrophages and/or Ly 1 T lymphocytes), the progenitors are triggered to proliferate into large, less dense cytolytic lymphocytes active against cells bearing the immunizing surface antigens. Further differentiation and proliferation take place, yielding both cytolytic cells and memory cells. The latter are weakly cytolytic but upon further antigenic stimulation will differentiate to a population of cytolytically highly active secondary CTL.

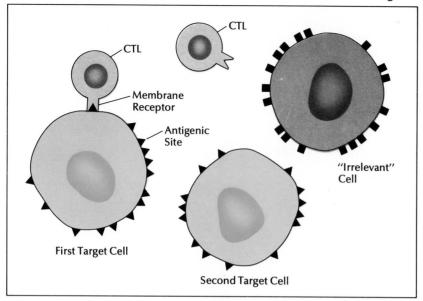

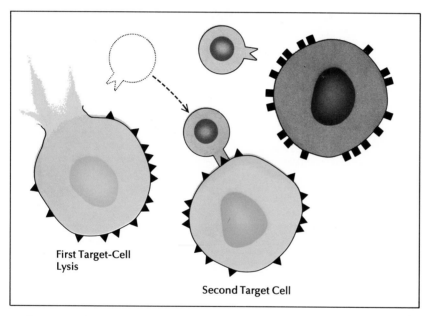

As demonstrated in vitro, the events of CTL cell lysis involve direct contact between the immunized lymphocyte and the surface of a target cell bearing the immunizing surface antigen. As symbolized in upper panel, no interaction will take place between CTL and cells not bearing specific immunizing antigenic determinants. Once CTL has lysed one specific target cell, it will dissociate from that cell and subsequently go on to attack another cell bearing the same antigenic surface components.

fraction thereof, are not end cells, but may further differentiate and undergo several cycles of proliferation and/or differentiation. The progeny of the large-sized CTL is a population of small lymphocytes, the lytic activity of which decreases as a function of time. However, when these are reexposed to the original stimulating antigen, they rapidly regain the ability to kill and undergo extensive proliferation.

Let us turn now to what actually happens in CTL-mediated lysis, or at least what happens when such a reaction is brought about in vitro. It has been shown that actual contact must be made between the effector lymphocyte and the target cell (see Figure 5, this page), and that this contact depends initially on the presence of membrane receptors on the T cell that interact with the corresponding antigenic determinants on the surface of the target cell.

The biochemical nature of the CTL receptors is not yet known, but there is clear evidence that they are not immunoglobulins of the classes found in serum. Earlier, it was mentioned that by using ^{51}Cr in a competitive inhibitory assay, one could establish the specificity of CTL activity. It is now evident that the basis of such specificity is related to the establishment of effective adhesions between CTL and the relevant target cells. In early studies, this was documented by adsorption of CTL on target-cell monolayers. In particular, such adsorption experiments have been used to demonstrate that concomitant immunization of an animal against two different sets of histocompatibility antigens results in the formation of CTL, which, at the single-cell level, are specific for either one or the other antigenic specificities, but not for both (see Figure 6, facing page). In the first step, a lymphocyte population obtained from mice immunized against allogeneic cells of two different genotypes (H-2^x and H-2^y) are incubated with monolayer cultures of fibroblasts from each of the donor strains. When the lymphocytes that do not adhere to the monolayers are then assayed for CTL activity against H-2^x and H-2^y target cells, the results are as follows: The lymphocyte population, after adsorp-

tainty as to the obligatory role of accessory cells such as macrophages and/or other antigen-reactive T cells (see E.R. Unanue, "The Macrophage as a Regulator of Lymphocyte Function"). Recently, it has been proposed that optimal induction of CTL, at least in vitro, involves participation of Ly 1 cells that cooperate, directly or via soluble factors, with CTL precursors. In-

deed, soluble growth-promoting factors active on CTL (and other antigen-activated T cells) have been identified. One of these factors, designated T-cell growth factor or interleukin 2, appears to be produced by some antigen- or mitogen-activated Ly 1 cells.

What is the fate of the effector cells, once formed? Recent studies have demonstrated that CTL, or at least a tion on H-2^x monolayers, has little activity against H-2^x target cells, but is fully active against H-2^y target cells. Conversely, the activity of the nonadherent lymphocytes recovered after adsorption on H-2^y monolayers is unimpaired against H-2^x target cells, but strongly diminished against H-2^y target cells.

More recently, the process of cell-to-cell contact required for CTL-mediated lysis has been investigated, using target cells in suspension instead of monolayers. Thus, it has been shown that the effector T cells, or at least a fraction thereof, strongly adhere to the relevant target cells within a few minutes. Usually, binding occurs between one CTL and one target cell, leading to the formation of rela-

tively stable "doublets." By using a technique that allows the separation of cells according to their size, it has been possible to isolate these doublets for further examination by transmission and scanning electron microscopy (see Figure 7 on pages 70, 71). The formation of firm adhesions is an energy-dependent process, since the effector cells must be alive and metabolically active. Binding is inhibited by cytochalasin B, a chemical known to interfere with the lymphocyte contractile microfilaments. Moreover, there is reason to believe that the cyclic nucleotides have an important role in regulating the effectiveness of cell-to-cell contact.

Operationally, binding of CTL to target cells is followed by a second

phase whereby the target-cell membrane is damaged. This phase, which depends on the presence of calcium, takes place within a few minutes and leads to the actual disintegration of the target cell thereafter. The exact nature of the primary lesion is not yet known, although there is suggestive evidence that an increase in membrane permeability may be involved. In this respect, the mechanism of CTL-mediated lysis would be analogous to that postulated for complement-dependent lysis (see Müller-Eberhard). It should be noted, however, that there is no evidence that complement may play a role in target-cell killing by CTL. Similarly, secretion by the effector cells of toxic factors has yet to be demonstrated.

Figure 6

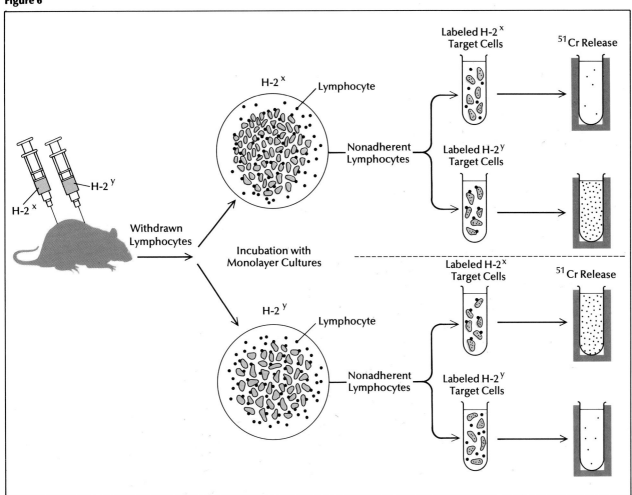

Dual immunization of animals against antigens of different major histocompatibility (H-2 in mice) specificities will result in CTL cells having one or the other, but not both, cytolytic specificities. This can be shown by adsorption of lymphocytes *from such an animal on monolayers of cells of each allotype. The nonadherent lymphocytes will then manifest cytolytic activity only against target cells of the "opposite" genotype, that is, H-2^x-adsorbed against H-2^y and vice versa.*

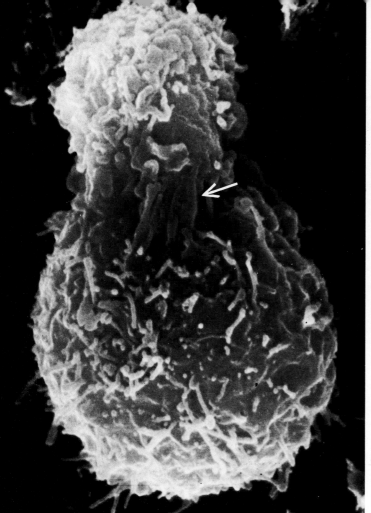

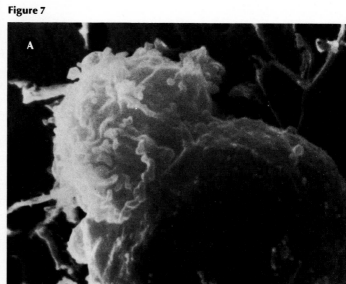

Figure 7

The scanning electron micrograph above (x7,200) shows conjugate of CTL with a large target cell after incubation. Note many microvilli on target-cell surface and closely apposed surface projections in zone of contact between cells (arrow). SEMs at right show a cytolytic sequence. First (A) conjugate is seen after 20 minutes of incubation with smooth-surfaced target cell (x7,400). After 40 minutes (B) target cell has developed polymorphous projections (arrow), and additional T cells and another target cell can be seen (x4,500). At the same time (C), closeup of target-cell surface shows numerous blebs (x11,800). Also at 40 minutes, another SEM view (D) of the target-cell surface shows membrane defects through which apparently granular submembranous areas can be seen (x10,200).

Scanning electron micrographs are from Ryser, J.E., Sordat, B., Cerottini, J.-C., and Brunner, K.T., Eur J Immunol 7:115-116, l977. Magnifications are those originally published in this report.

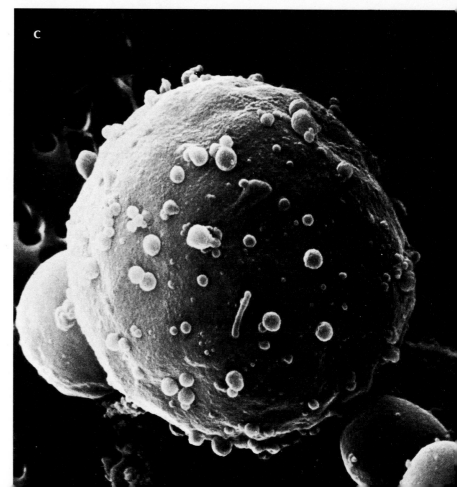

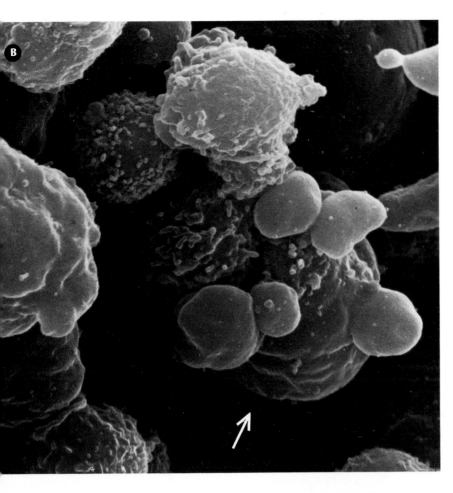

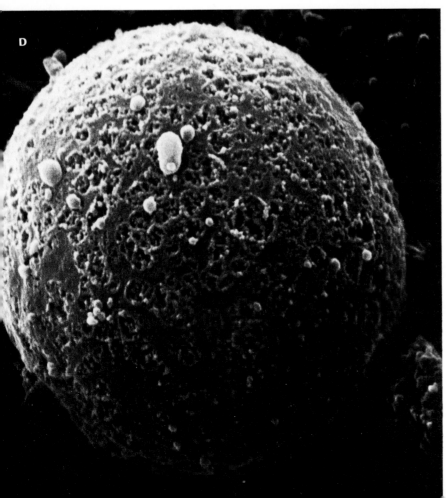

Whatever the mechanism may be, it is evident that the lysis process is unidirectional, i.e., target-cell killing has no effect on the viability of the effector cells. In fact, it has been demonstrated that one CTL, after destroying one target cell, does dissociate from the dying cell and proceeds to its next contact with an intact target cell.

It will be noted that most experiments that have demonstrated the cytolytic capacity of T lymphocytes have employed allogeneic systems, either allograft (or its in vitro counterparts) or allogeneic tumors. CTL activity has also been detected in systems based on syngeneic tumor cells, but in general it has been much weaker. From the biologist's point of view, this has been interpreted as indicating the dominant role of the transplantation antigens in invoking the CTL response. From the clinician's point of view, the biologist's interpretation may help explain some of the disappointments to date in the effort to direct immunologic phenomena against human cancer. Since cancers are derived from autologous tissues and cells, the experimental evidence appears quite consistent with the thesis that (even assuming the emergence of new or altered antigens) the concentration of cytolytic T lymphocytes would not be sufficient to mount an effective attack against a large mass of tumor cells.

It should be pointed out that CTL not only may play a role in promoting graft rejection or in inhibiting tumor growth but may participate in the defense mechanisms as well as in the immunopathologic reactions operative in some infections. Along this line, it is now evident, at least in the mouse, that effector T cells are formed after infection with certain viruses and that they can kill in vitro target cells infected with the relevant virus. While the mechanism of CTL-mediated lysis of virus-infected cells is similar to that reported for allogeneic target cells, a major finding has been the demonstration of a genetic restriction in these CTL activities (see R. M. Zinkernagel, "Major Transplantation Antigens in Host Responses to Infection"). This suggests that an important function of the effector T-cell system in animals is to recognize infection-induced anti-

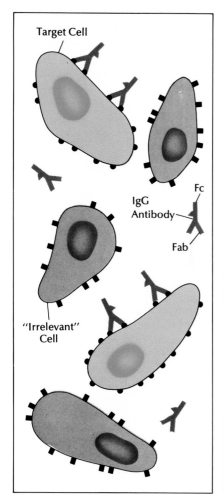

Target Cell

Fc

IgG
Antibody

Fab

"Irrelevant"
Cell

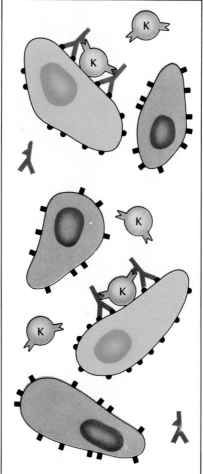

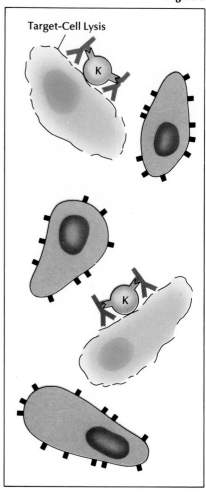

Target-Cell Lysis

Antibody-dependent K-cell cytolysis achieves specificity only through specificity of IgG antibody. IgG first coats target cell (left); K cell then attaches to antibody by means of an Fc receptor (middle); the ensuing lysis (right) requires surface contact between K and target cells. Gray cells are unaffected because there is no antibody against them.

gens on its own cells and to eliminate such cells.

Antibody-Dependent Cytolysis: The K Cells

As pointed out above, antibody may inhibit CTL-mediated lysis, presumably by covering up antigenic determinants on the target-cell membrane that are identical to, or closely associated with, the structures recognized by the effector-cell receptors. In contrast, there are lymphoid cells that function as killer cells only when target cells are coated with antibody.

The existence of antibody-dependent (AD) cytotoxic lymphoid cells – or K cells – was first demonstrated by Perlmann and his colleagues in man, and by MacLennan in the rat. Further

studies, using the ^{51}Cr-release assay described before, have shown that human K cells are small-sized mononuclear cells that are mainly found in peripheral blood and in the spleen. They are poorly represented in lymph nodes and do not belong to the pool of recirculating lymphocytes (they are absent from thoracic-duct lymph). As already noted, K cells are formed independently of any immunization and thus are found in peripheral blood of any healthy blood-cell donor.

The main surface characteristic of K cells is the presence of receptors specific for the Fc portion of IgG molecules (Fc receptors). Until recently, there was no evidence that AD cytotoxic lymphocytes interact with antibodies other than IgG. There is now some indication that IgM anti-

body-dependent effector cells may also exist, but these lymphocytes appear to be distinct from IgG-dependent K cells.

The finding that the complementary determinant for the K-cell receptor was in the Ig Fc made it necessary to consider the relationships between these cells and various nonlymphoid cells that also have Fc receptors – monocytes, macrophages, and PMN leukocytes. In fact, studies aiming at the characterization of the cells operative in AD cell-mediated cytotoxicity have revealed considerable heterogeneity in the type of effector cells according to the nature of the target cells used for their detection. This heterogeneity is best illustrated by the results obtained in man when peripheral blood is used as the source of effector

Figure 9

cells. When chicken red cells are used as target cells, PMN leukocytes, monocytes, and K cells are all found to kill in the presence of anti-chicken red cell IgG antibody. IgG antibody-coated *human* red cells, however, are lysed in the presence of monocytes and PMN but are unaffected by purified lymphoid preparations. In contrast, target cells such as lymphocytes or cell lines of lymphoid or nonlymphoid origin usually are not killed by monocytes and PMN in the presence of antibody, while the same sensitized target cells are readily lysed by K cells.

If one dismisses the nonlymphoid cytotoxic cells as the source of AD cytolysis, one is still left with a question: How do we know that AD cytolysis is not mediated by CTL functioning in a different context from that of immune cytotoxic T cells? This is perhaps the most likely source of doubt as to whether K cells do indeed form a discrete cytolytic cell population.

To answer the question, let us go back to the earliest evidence for a separate population of antibody-dependent cytolytic lymphocytes: distribution studies performed by MacLennan and Harding with rat lymphocytes. In these experiments, the highest concentrations of AD cytolytic cells were found in peritoneal exudates, the next highest in the spleen, followed in order by the blood lymphocytes and the lymph nodes. K-cell activity was essentially nil in the thymus and the thoracic duct. Additional studies involved rats that had been thymectomized, irradiated, and reconstituted with bone marrow cells. Antibody-dependent cytotoxicity was not diminished in spleens of such T-cell depleted rats.

In man, it appears that most peripheral blood T cells are not involved in K-cell activity. However, the possibility exists that a subpopulation of T cells equipped with Fc receptors may participate in the overall AD cell-mediated cytotoxicity. What about the possibility that K cells are identical to B cells? The evidence here seems to weigh heavily toward the negative. For instance, it has been found repeatedly that blood lymphocyte populations from patients with severe hypogammaglobulinemia, while devoid of cells with surface immunoglobulin (a characteristic of B cells), possess nor-

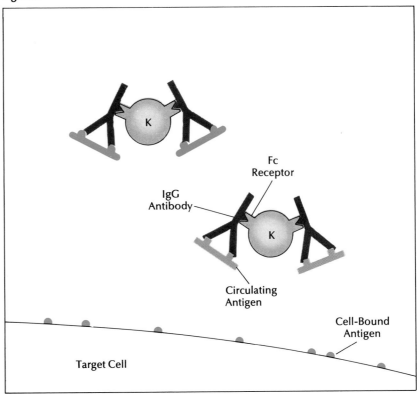

Circulating antigen-antibody complexes may inhibit antibody-dependent cytolysis by combining with K-cell Fc receptors and thus preventing K-cell attachment to antibody-coated target cell (above). However, if complexes have excess antibody against same antigenic determinants as those in target-cell surface they may promote K-cell activity by bringing K cells, attached to complex, to the target-cell surface (below).

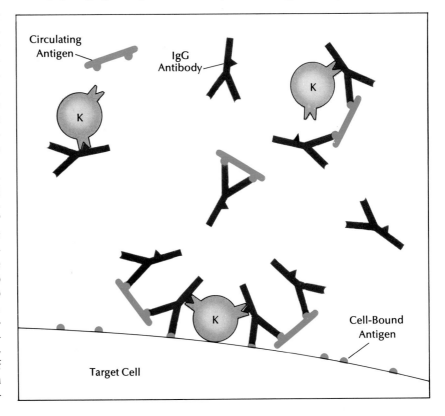

mal AD cytotoxic activity even after depletion of contaminating monocytes and PMN leukocytes. More recently, surface marker analysis of individual K cells has clearly indicated that they lack detectable amounts of surface immunoglobulin.

A good portion of the discussion on K cells to this point has been focused on the fact that they cannot easily be classified as belonging to the majority of immunocompetent B or T cells. Perhaps it is now time to start defining what they are, or at least what at the present time we believe they are. K cells appear to be a heterogeneous population of lymphoid cells that carry on their surfaces Fc receptors (although, to make one more negative point, all lymphocytes with Fc receptors are not K cells).

There is evidence suggesting that K cells in human peripheral blood represent a small fraction (not more than 5%) of the total lymphocytes and are comprised within a population with Fc receptors of high avidity. It is the Fc receptor that endows the K cell with relatively nonspecific reactivity; this sharply differentiates the K cell from the immune T cytotoxic lymphocyte, the specificity of which is antigen-directed. Since the specificity of K cells is entirely secondary to the specificity of the antibody with which it reacts, it is in effect the antibody that selects the target cell for the K cell (see Figure 8 on page 72).

Since K-cell–mediated lysis depends on the association between the K-cell Fc receptor and antibody on the target-cell surface, it is not surprising that this phenomenon can be inhibited by soluble antigen-antibody complexes, probably as a function of the ability of the soluble complexed immunoglobulin moieties to compete for the Fc receptor with the target cell–bound immunoglobulin (see Figure 9, page 73). Complexes of any specificity may be inhibitory, the only requirement being the accessibility of Fc de-

terminants to the K-cell Fc receptors. The situation might be different with soluble complexes containing anti-target-cell antibodies. If such soluble complexes are in antibody excess, one could envisage that they are first bound (via the antibody Fc portion) to K cells, which are now able to react with the target cell through binding of the complex via the Fab (antigen-binding site) portion of the antibody. In such cases, target-cell lysis might be markedly enhanced. This type of complexity, arising out of the relative nonspecificity of K cells, as well as the lack of specific markers for these cells, has made it extremely difficult to study the effector role of K cells in vivo. However, in theory at least, it might provide the basis for significant clinical use of K-cell cytolysis, i.e., against cancers. Obviously, it would be easier to produce large amounts of antitumor cell IgG than high numbers of specific cytolytic T cells. Conceivably, one could raise such an IgG-containing antiserum and use it therapeutically as a bridge to bring K cells into contact with tumor cells. Let me emphasize that this is highly speculative; indeed, attempts to do this have been completely unsuccessful to date in any in vivo system.

It appears that the actual events occurring during K-cell–mediated cytolysis are very analogous to those described for target lysis by CTL. We do know that direct contact between the K cell and the antibody IgG-coated target cell is required and that the process is energy-dependent. Under optimal conditions, target-cell lysis is detectable within a few minutes and it increases linearly as a function of time. Several of the inhibitors effective in CTL-mediated lysis (such as cytochalasin B or EDTA, a chelating agent) are also active in K-cell–mediated lysis. However, a recent study of divalent cation requirements indicates that K-cell activity can develop in the presence of calcium alone, while both

magnesium and calcium are required for CTL activity.

While evidence that one K cell may kill several target cells has been provided, it also appears true that the lytic activity of these effector cells decreases after interaction with antibody-coated target cells. Whether this is due to a blockade of Fc receptors or to an inactivation of the lytic machinery is unknown.

Throughout this review, I have tried to emphasize that most of the information with respect to K cells, and indeed with respect to CTL, must be derived from in vitro studies. Before concluding, let me mention the belief that we are probably approaching the time when we will be able to follow and analyze these effector cells in vivo. It is now possible to distinguish CTL from other T-lymphocyte populations by surface antigenic markers. This should be a powerful tool for the study of such phenomena as the actual role of CTL in transplant rejection or tumor immunity. It should also facilitate efforts to separate CTL effects from nonlymphoid cytolytic cell effects as well as from K-cell lysis. We should also be better equipped to confirm or refute the long-held suspicion that cytolytic T cells directed against virally induced antigens on cell surfaces may be responsible for various forms of viral pathology.

The day is probably not far off when we will have analogous markers for the K cell so that some of the in vivo studies that have proved so difficult to perform will be brought within the realm of realization. For the moment, what is clear is that in the past we have been too absolute in our dissociation of humoral and cell-mediated cytotoxic functions. The recognition of antibody-dependent, cell-mediated cytolysis, even if the demonstrations have had to be in cell mixes and cultures rather than in intact animals, should move us toward a more holistic attitude with respect to this important aspect of immune responsivity.

Natural Killer Cells

RONALD B. HERBERMAN   *National Cancer Institute*

Since its discovery 10 years ago, natural killer (NK) activity has been one of the more mysterious immune functions. Recently, we have gained some insight into the cellular basis of this function and its range of effects. NK activity was originally identified purely as an immediate cytotoxic response to tumor cells. Indeed, it has since become likely that NK cells, along with macrophages, provide the body's first line of defense against malignant growth. But now we can also hypothesize a role for NK activity in the rejection of bone marrow transplants, in graft-versus-host disease, as a regulator of cellular development, as a major producer of interferon and an effector of its action, and as a barrier to microbial infections. Our understanding of NK activity has even progressed far enough for us to consider its direct exploitation as an anticancer therapy.

NK activity was first recognized when immunologists studied cell-mediated responses against tumor cells in cancer patients and in healthy individuals. To their surprise, lymphoid cells from entirely normal subjects had the same properties. In addition, the targets of NK activity were not restricted to a particular histologic tumor type. The name "natural killer" was given to this property because it mediated a cytotoxic reaction and appeared "naturally"—i.e., without the need for sensitization.

These properties distinguish NK activity from other known cytotoxic, cell-mediated functions of the immune system, cytotoxic T lymphocytes (CTLs), and killer (K) cells (see J.-C. Cerottini, "Lymphoid Cells as Effectors of Immunologic Cytolysis"). Table 1, which appears on page 76, summarizes the characteristics of the major cells with well-defined immune activity. Most significantly, CTLs must first be exposed to the antigenic determinants of the target cell and then progress through a seven- to 14-day maturation period before they can function. They are part of the T-lymphocyte class of cells, sharing their morphology and their need to mature in the thymus gland. NK activity continues to be expressed in athymic or neonatally thymectomized mice or rats and, in fact, is at supernormal levels in such animals.

K cells are responsible for antibody-dependent cell-mediated cytotoxicity (ADCC). The effector cells for this function have a surface receptor that recognizes and binds to the Fc portion of IgG molecules. Thus, when a cell is coated with IgG, it becomes a target for K activity. Recent work by Tuomo Timonen in my laboratory resulted in the purification of the cells responsible for NK activity, large granular lymphocytes. It turns out that these cells do possess Fc receptors on their outer surface and also exhibit all the other properties of K effector cells. NK and K activities therefore appear to be two manifestations of the same cell, and it is only circumstance that determines which function is expressed (see Figure 1 on page 77). Since they were discovered independently, however, and since these functions are so easily distinguished, I will refer to the two activities as separate entities.

The targets of human NK cells in vitro are primarily human tumor cells, either established cell lines or, to a lesser extent, primary tumor cells. Some normal cells also can be killed by NK cells, particularly poorly differentiated cells, such as fetal fibroblasts, immature thymocytes, and colony-forming cells in bone marrow. In vitro killing is usually assayed visually or by insertion of chromium-51 into cells and evaluation of lysis by release of the radioisotope.

Human NK cells have been found to consist of a few clonal subpopulations, each with a somewhat different target specificity. One way this has been shown is by

Table 1. Characteristics of NK and Other Immunologic Effector Cells

	NK Cells	T Cells	Monocytes or Macrophages	Polymorphonuclear Leukocytes
Morphology				
Size	Medium (12–15 μ)	Small (9–12 μ)	Large (16–20 μ)	Medium-large (12–18 μ)
Cytoplasmic/ nuclear ratio	High	Low	High	High
Nucleus	Slightly indented	Round	Markedly indented	Multilobed
General features				
Adherence to plastic surfaces	No	No	Yes	Yes
Phagocytosis	No	No	Yes	Yes
Cell surface markers				
Receptors for sheep erythro- cytes (human cells)	Yes, on about 50% (low affinity)	Yes (high affinity)	No	No
Receptors for IgG	Yes	< 10% of cells	Yes	Yes
Antigens				
Human	Most or all cells: HNK-1, OKM1, asialo GM1, OKT10 Subsets: 9.6, Ia	Most or all cells: 9.6, OKT3 Subsets: OKT4, OKT8	Most or all cells: OKM1, asialo GM1 Subset: Ia	Most or all cells: OKM1, asialo GM1
Mouse	Most or all cells: NK1, NK2, asialo GM1, Ly 11, Ly 5, Qa 5, ?Mph 1	All cells: Thy 1, Lyt 1	Most or all cells: Mac 1, asialo GM1, Mph 1	
Functional charac- teristics				
Spontaneous reactivity	Yes	No	Yes	Yes
Period for de- velopment or augmentation of cytotoxic reactivity	In vivo: within 4 hr; in vitro: within 1 hr	Primary response: > 5–7 days; memory re- sponse: 2–5 days	In vivo: 5–10 days; in vitro: < 18 hr for most stimuli	In vitro: within minutes
Nature of target	At least several widely distributed antigenic specificities	Wide array of specific antigens; im- portant role of MHC- restricted antigens	Specificity not clearly defined; selectivity for tumor targets	Apparently nonspecific but some selectiv- ity for tumor targets
Cytotoxic reac- tivity against IgG antibody-coated targets	Yes	No	Yes	Yes
Activating factors	Interferon, TCGF, lectins, antibodies, retinoic acid, PGE	Specific antigens, lectins, LAF, TCGF, interferon, T-cell helper factors	MAF, interferon, wide variety of foreign materials (e.g., bacterial endotoxin, phor- bol esters)	Contact, lectins, cytochalasin E, phorbol esters
Inhibition of reactivity	PGE, nonspecific macrophages and other suppressor cells, phorbol es- ters, cyclic AMP	Specific and non- specific T sup- pressor cells and factors, macro- phage suppressor cells, interferon, PGE, cyclic AMP	PGE, phorbol esters	Inhibitors of serine esterases
Growth factors	TCGF	TCGF	Colony-stimu- lating factor	Colony-stimulat- ing factor
Possible mech- anisms of cyto- toxic effects	Protease, phospho- lipase, cytotoxin	Protease, osmotic	Reactive oxygen species, protease, lysozyme, phago- cytosis, PGE, in- terferon	Reactive oxygen species, protease, lysozyme, phago- cytosis
Production of soluble medi- ators	Interferon, TCGF	Wide array of lymphokines	LAF, colony-stim- ulating factor, PGE, many en- zymes, interferon	Many enzymes

monolayer adsorption experiments, performed by John Ortaldo. NK cell populations are incubated on monolayers of target cell lines. The cells that do not bind are removed and tested for their cytotoxic activity against both the adsorbing cell and other targets. We have shown that essentially all of the activity against one target can be removed from an NK population without significantly depleting all NK activity against some other targets. By this means, we have arrived at a minimum estimate of five or six human NK subpopulations.

A complementary experiment has involved the isolation of clonal NK cell lines. This is feasible because NK cells grow and divide in culture for at least a month when they are provided with T-cell growth factor (TCGF, or interleukin-2). Three human NK-cell clones, isolated from three different subjects, have been grown in my laboratory. One is cytotoxic against carcinoma cells in vitro but has very low activity against leukemia target cells. The other two clones kill both these targets to about the same extent. We have also been able to generate about 25 different clones of mouse NK cells, and they display a similar mixed target pattern.

This specificity does not appear to be due to major histocompatibility (MHC) antigens on the surface of target cells. In fact, some of the most susceptible targets are human cells that lack HLA determinants and mouse cells that are missing H-2 determinants. This is in contrast to cytotoxic T lymphocytes, which appear principally to recog-

Cytolytic T lymphocytes must differentiate under antigenic influence before they are able to kill a target cell. Natural killer/killer cells respond to a target immediately. The activity expressed by an NK/K cell depends on the type of target it encounters. Cells coated with IgG are vulnerable to antibody-dependent cell-mediated cytotoxicity. Certain transformed, microbially infected or other cells are susceptible to NK attack in the absence of antibody. Subpopulations of NK cells with different target specificities have been identified.

Figure 1

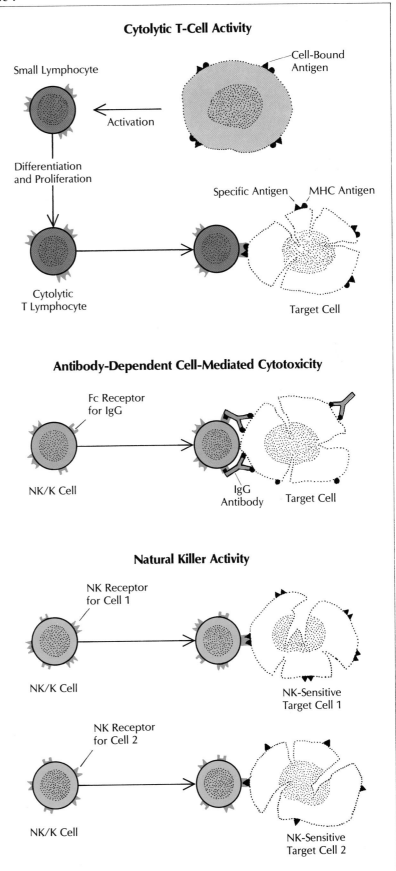

Figure 2

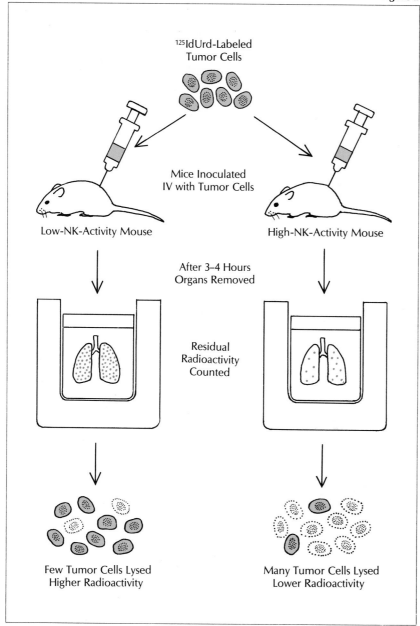

¹²⁵IdUrd-Labeled
Tumor Cells

Mice Inoculated
IV with Tumor Cells

Low-NK-Activity Mouse

High-NK-Activity Mouse

After 3–4 Hours
Organs Removed

Residual
Radioactivity
Counted

Few Tumor Cells Lysed
Higher Radioactivity

Many Tumor Cells Lysed
Lower Radioactivity

An in vivo assay for NK activity has been devised in which labled tumor cells are injected into mice. Time is allowed for localization of these cells in various organs (e.g., lungs) and radioactivity in these organs is measured. It is deduced that high NK activity will result in fewer surviving tumor cells and therefore less radioactivity.

nize their specific antigens in close association with MHC antigens.

NK cells were first discovered during the search for an antitumor CTL, and even now, when one is trying to develop a specific cell-mediated activity, the question arises of how much activity is actually attributable to NK cells. This is a particular concern because a number of the methods used to generate CTLs will also generate NK activity. For example, the usual way to induce cellular cytotoxicity in vitro is through a mixed lymphocyte culture. In this process lymphocytes are incubated with stimulating, allogeneic cells, typically for five to seven days. A number of laboratories have consistently found that this creates NK in addition to CTL activity. This overlap can frequently go unnoticed since the usual target cells for cellular cytotoxicity, phytohemagglutinin-induced blasts (metabolically active, DNA-synthesizing T cells that are induced in a lymphocyte population after its exposure to PHA), are highly resistant to NK activity. But when other targets, particularly tumor cells, are used, the combination of CTL and NK activity can become very confusing.

Another confusion results from the now common practice of expanding a population of CTLs by growing them in culture. It has been assumed that if TCGF is used in the medium, the only cells that would grow out would be CTLs. Instead, both NK and K activities are also found in these cultures.

Determining the in vivo activity of NK cells is even more difficult than assaying in vitro activity. About all that can be done is to correlate the level of NK activity in mice with the resistance of those mice to the growth of a transplanted tumor. Many studies, in a number of laboratories, have shown that the greater the NK activity, the greater the resistance. This type of experiment presents a problem, however, because of the long time required to evaluate in vivo tumor growth. And any presumed correlation might involve an indirect effect of NK cells in tumor rejection, such as their release of a factor like interferon, which could produce the same tumor-inhibiting result as a direct, cytotoxic action.

C. Riccardi, of Perugia, Italy, has developed an in vivo assay that evaluates more directly the role of NK cells (see Figure 2 on this page). He injects mice with ¹²⁵I-iododeoxyuridine (IdUrd)-labeled tumor cells and determines the distribution of these cells in the mice over the course of a few hours. He has found an excellent correlation between NK activity and the speed of clearance of radioactivity, particularly from their lungs. Mice with spontaneously low NK activity or mice that have have been given NK-suppressive treatments, such as x-irradiation, cyclophosphamide, or hydrocortisone, show poorer clearance.

The role of NK cells in controlling primary tumors is still more difficult to determine. The only evidence that we can apply is suggestive, not definitive. This includes the low incidence of spontaneous or carcinogen-induced tumors in animals with high NK activity, the high incidence of lymphoproliferative disease in humans and animals with low NK activity, the enhancement of NK activity by retinoic acid, an agent that retards tumor development, and the strong inhibition of NK activity by some carcinogens or tumor-promoting agents.

Tumor cells that are at first highly susceptible to NK activity can develop into progressively growing tumors. The ways in which tumor cells escape NK elimination are not clear, but they may involve resistance to lysis. Lytic resistance in a cell can be induced by interferon and be reversed in some cases by treating it with RNA or protein synthesis inhibitors. Loss of NK

activity in intact animals may be at least partially due to suppressor T cells, macrophages, or other lymphoid cells. Prostaglandins may also depress NK activity, since treatment with prostaglandin-synthesis inhibitors, such as aspirin or indomethacin, can restore NK activity.

NK cytotoxic activity requires direct binding between the NK cell and its target. Neither the binding receptors on NK cells nor their recognition sites on target cells have been characterized. The nature of the actual killing event, which results in target-cell lysis, is also unknown. Lysis is blocked by low temperature or other conditions that interfere with NK-cell metabolism. However, protein and RNA synthesis and cell division are not required. There is no evidence that any accessory cell type or factor is needed for NK cytotoxicity.

Although the mechanism of target-cell lysis by NK cells is unknown, there is evidence of at least two different processes. Workers in several laboratories, including my

own, have found that a series of specific protease inhibitors interfere with NK cytotoxicity. Experiments also have shown that inhibitors of phospholipase A2, which depress production of lysolecithin, will lower NK activity. Whether proteases or lysolecithin, or both, are directly responsible for the lysis of target cells is still not clear. We now believe a sequence of events may be needed for target-cell lysis. If any of the steps in this sequence are interfered with, cytotoxicity is affected.

When an NK cell lyses a target, it can dissociate from that cell and, after about two hours, bind and kill another target cell. This "recycling" capability has been directly demonstrated by Timonen (see Figure 3 on this page). If the NK cells are treated with interferon, they recycle more rapidly.

There is increasing evidence that NK cells play a role in resistance to microbial infections. Most studies, which involved viruses, have indicated that infected cells are considerably more sensitive to NK-cell

Figure 3

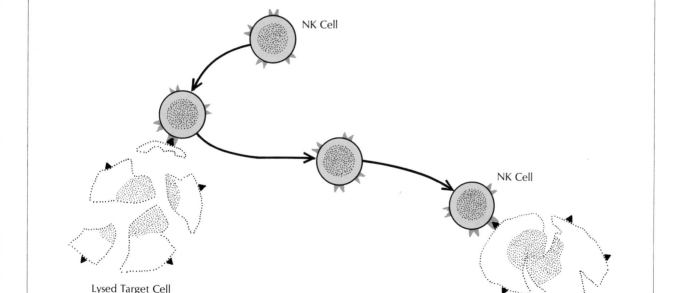

NK Cell

NK Cell

Lysed Target Cell

Second Target Cell

NK cells recycle. After an NK cell has bound to a target cell and lysed it, it will dissociate from the dead target and be able to bind to and lyse a new cell. This phenomenon was demonstrated experimentally by microscopic observation of isolated NK–target cell complexes. A two-hour recovery period is usually required, but interferon makes recycling go faster.

lysis. In vivo resistance to several types of viruses (e.g., herpes simplex type 1 and mouse cytomegalovirus) has correlated with NK activity. Resistance of mice to the malarial parasite *Babesia microti*, to fungi, and to the bacterium *Listeria monocytogenes* has also been found to be greatest in animals with high NK activity.

Until about three years ago, any work with NK cells involved the use of a mixed population of cells that were largely composed of T cells, B cells, and macrophages. About 5% of the cells contained NK activity. Then E. Saksela and Timonen, in Helsinki, observed a correlation between NK activity in their cell preparations and a characteristic cell morphology that appeared with Giemsa staining. These cells are called large granular lymphocytes (LGLs). They are about 50% larger than a typical lymphocyte with a higher proportion of cytoplasm that contains azurophilic granules and a kidney-shaped nucleus (see Figure 4 on the opposite page).

Shortly after the LGL–NK correlation was made, Timonen and I decided that it was important to determine what fraction of NK activity could be accounted for by this cell type as well as what fraction of LGLs could be shown to have NK activity. Our approach was to prepare as pure a population of LGLs as could be obtained and then analyze the cellular properties. The isolation protocol was based on Timonen's observation that LGLs could be separated from other lymphoid cells by the use of density centrifugation gradients prepared with Percoll, an inert silica polymer. Since LGLs have a relatively low density, due to their large cytoplasmic content, they migrate to a discrete region of the gradient.

When the isolation procedure became technically refined, it was possible to go from the starting population, with about 5% NK cells, to a preparation that was about 80% NK cells. We were then able to further increase the purity by applying an earlier observation of the behavior of NK cells with respect to binding to sheep erythrocytes. Typi-

cal T cells rosette very well with sheep erythrocytes, even at high temperatures. NK cells are about equally divided into an absolutely nonrosetting fraction and cells that will rosette but only under optimal conditions, i.e., at low temperatures. Thus, by performing a rosetting protocol at a high temperature, most of the remaining T cells could be removed while leaving behind virtually all NK activity. In this manner 90% to 95% purity has been routinely achieved.

The relationship of LGLs to NK activity turned out to be very straightforward. All of the NK activity is found in the highly enriched LGL population. Fractions depleted of LGLs have no NK activity, even though they have most of the T cells from peripheral blood and have virtually all other functions intact. As noted earlier, the ADCC activity also segregates in the LGL fraction, suggesting that these cells have K activity as well.

This purification protocol does not involve the "creation" of NK activity, as measured by total lytic units. We often end up with about 120% to 150% of the starting activity in the purified LGL preparation, but this is probably due to the removal of certain inhibitory cells. This hypothesis is supported by experiments that mix pure LGLs with non-LGL fractions, with a resultant loss of some NK activity, suggesting inhibitory-cell participation.

High NK activity is not inevitably associated with a high number of LGLs. This probably reflects the presence or absence of factors that regulate LGL activity, particularly interferon. For example, age-related differences in NK activity in the mouse are believed to reflect the degree of activation of their pool of NK cells rather than any change in the number of cells. In humans, the highest proportion of LGLs is in peripheral blood (7% of all nucleated cells) and in suspensions of cells from the lungs (7%), followed by the spleen (4%), peritoneal exudates (3%), and lymph nodes (1%). Few, if any, LGLs are detectable in the thymus or bone marrow.

The concept that NK and K activities are attributable to distinct cell populations is based on an error. Early studies indicated that mouse and rat NK cells lacked Fc receptors, giving rise to the concept that these were spontaneously appearing lytic effector cells that did not have Fc receptors and so could not be responsible for ADCC. Only later, after a more careful examination, was it realized that both human and rodent NK cells have Fc receptors.

In the past few years it has become evident that in most cases, if NK activity is interfered with, ADCC activity is also affected, and vice versa. In addition, enrichment or depletion of one activity enriches or depletes the other as well. This recognition culminated with our purification of LGLs, when it became apparent that essentially 100% of LGLs have Fc receptors. It now appears that almost all, if not all, of the NK and K cytotoxic activities in humans arise from the same cells. It is, therefore, the milieu in which these cells appear that determines how they act. If they confront tumor or other sensitive cells, they exhibit NK activity. If they meet cells coated with an appropriate antibody, they show ADCC activity.

Craig Reynolds, in my laboratory, has arrived at the same conclusions concerning the properties of rat LGLs. We have found LGLs with similar properties in just about every species we have looked at except, until recently, mice. Now we have found similar cells there as well. The problem seems to have been that in mice these cells are smaller and their granules are very labile once the cells are isolated.

It has been more difficult to determine whether the NK and K activities are contained in only a certain fraction of LGLs. To investigate this question, we have mixed purified LGLs with various populations of target cells and visually determined what fraction of the LGLs attach. Only about 10% to 50% of the LGLs bind to a given target, but if different targets are mixed with an LGL preparation, the proportion of bound cells rises by about an-

Figure 4

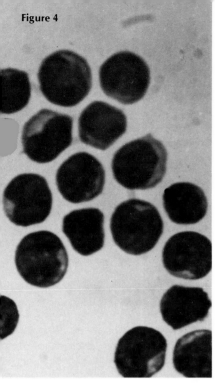 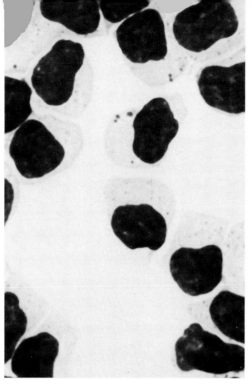 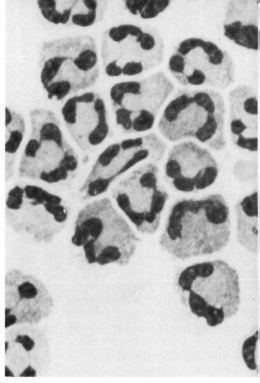

Micrographs compare morphology of small lymphocytes, or T cells (left), large granular lymphocytes, or NK cells (center), and polymorphonuclear leukocytes (right). LGLs are distin- *guished from other lymphocytes by their large size (about the same as PMNs), greater amount of cytoplasm, which is filled with azurophilic granules, and kidney-shaped nuclei.*

other 10% to 15%. This indicates that while many of the LGLs can recognize a target, they vary in their binding specificities, and the specificities overlap. It appears that LGLs are divided into subpopulations that can recognize different targets.

We can also measure cytotoxic activity using a method developed by E. Grimm, working with B. Bonavida at the University of California in Los Angeles. Mixed LGLs and target cells are suspended in a dilute agarose solution that prevents recycling by immobilizing the cells. This preparation is incubated for various periods of time and then trypan blue dye is added, which selectively stains dead cells. We find that the most sensitive target cells are almost all killed by 12 to 24 hours after their exposure and binding to LGLs, compared with only 5% to 10% of unbound target cells that take up the dye in control suspensions. Certain target cells are not killed by LGLs as efficiently. Only 25% to 30% of certain carcinoma targets will die after they have been bound by LGLs. This experiment also revealed that if non-LGL lymphoid cells are used, they bind to the targets but they do not cause lysis.

Because LGLs contain both NK and K activities, we must be very careful if we wish to measure only one of these functions. When we are assaying human cells for ADCC activity, we use a mouse target cell that is completely resistant to NK cytotoxicity. Thus, if the cell is not coated with antibody, virtually no target killing occurs. We are able to rule out K activity in our NK assays by performing the experiments with immunoglobulin inhibitors or by using purified LGL preparations that do not contain immunoglobulins or B cells.

We have evaluated the phenotype of pure LGLs by other parameters. Ortaldo assembled a panel of monoclonal antibodies that he has used, along with a fluorescence-activated cell sorter, to determine the pattern of surface antigens' appearance among these cells. This pattern does not coincide with what is found on typical T cells, B cells, or monocytes. For example, the most commonly used anti–T cell monoclonal antibody is OKT3, which does not appear to recognize LGLs. But two or three other monoclonal

antibodies, which react with about the same percentage of T cells as OKT3, recognize at least half of an LGL population. For example, one monoclonal antibody that is believed to recognize the sheep cell receptor on T cells reacts with about half of the LGLs. This makes sense since, as I have stated, about half of the NK cells are known to totally lack the ability to rosette sheep erythrocytes.

We have also analyzed LGLs with monoclonal antibodies that react with other leukocytes. One of these, OKM1, reacts primarily with monocytes and granulocytes, but it also recognizes 80% to 90% of LGLs.

The reason for such sharing of cell-surface markers is unknown. However, it seems likely that LGLs have diverged from the T stem-cell lineage. When LGLs are put into a culture with TCGF, they retain their morphology and NK activity. But after about seven days their surface markers change, shifting to the pattern seen in typical mature T cells. I suspect that LGLs are ordinarily in a state of differentiation that does not fit into any well-defined leukocyte category. If their differentiation is given a

81

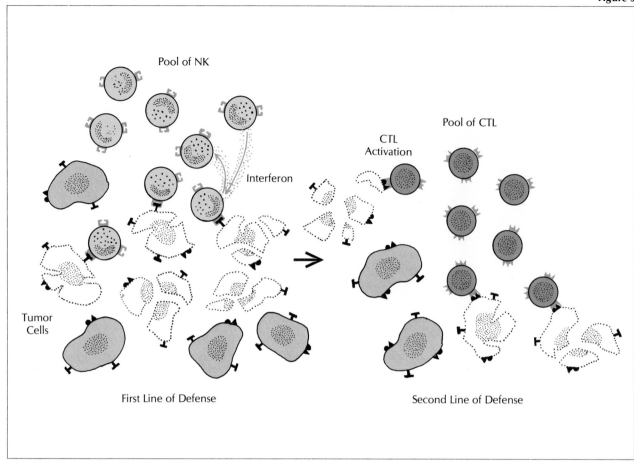

The identification of several different cell cohorts capable of cytolytic function suggests a sequence of defensive responses to, e.g., tumor cells. NK cells, perhaps functionally enhanced by interferon, would immediately kill many, perhaps all, of these cells. If any should escape NK destruction, immunized cytotoxic T lymphocytes would mount a second attack.

push, so to speak, in a culture medium with TCGF, they will then replicate and begin to resemble a typical T cell. The fact that LGLs react to TCGF also suggests that they somehow fit into the T-cell lineage, since this factor does not appear to affect any other type of leukocytes.

The only other structural characteristics of human LGLs that have been examined are their granules. C. E. Grossi and M. Ferrarini, in Italy, have isolated lymphoid cells that we believe to be LGLs, based on their morphology and their surface receptors for the Fc portion of IgG. Various histochemical stains have indicated that granules in these cells are primarily lysosomes. However, Mariana Henkart, an electron microscopist at NIH with whom we have collaborated, suggests instead that the granules contain actin

bundles. It is possible that these bundles allow the cells to move around and attach, and they may have a role in cytotoxicity. But Henkart has had great difficulty seeing the actin in rat LGLs, even though these cells have very prominent granules. At this point, I believe that the granules are lysosomal and that the actin and the characteristic granules are probably separate phenomena.

Interferon has a central role in the function of NK cells. Not only does it enhance NK activity, but it is also released by NK cells, thus apparently acting as a positive self-regulator. These properties of interferon were first discovered when researchers tried to see whether NK cells exhibited a CTL-like anamnestic response. When CTLs are first exposed to an antigen, it takes seven to 14 days for them to re-

spond, but when there is a second exposure to the same antigen, peak CTL activity appears in three to five days.

It seemed likely that NK cells also have an anamnestic response, based on their behavior in mice and rats. In these animals, NK activity is not present at birth and only begins to appear at the age of three to four weeks. Peak NK activity occurs at six to eight weeks of age, and then it declines to an almost undetectable level when the mice are three months old. If tumor cells are injected into the adult animal, however, a spike of NK activity appears within three days, an observation that is reminiscent of the anamnestic response. But further investigations have suggested that immunologic memory has nothing to do with this behavior. We have found that NK activity can be induced by interferon as well as by viruses, bacterial adjuvants, and poly I:C (small, synthetic segments of double-stranded RNA). Since many of these agents induce interferon, we believe it plays a major role in stimulating NK activity.

Comprehensive in vivo and in vitro experiments with interferon have shown that it acts only in a species-specific manner—mouse interferon, for example, induces NK activity only in mouse lymphoid cells. Interferon also boosts K activity, suggesting that although LGLs express these two activities separately, their regulation can overlap. In contrast, interferon does not appear to affect CTL activity.

The current experimental use of interferon in cancer patients has been reported to be accompanied by a rise in NK and K activities within a few days following treatment. Indeed, the basis for any antitumor effects of interferon may be its ability to enhance NK and K activities. If this is the case, it may provide ways to improve interferon-therapy protocols by, for example, allowing clinicians to use doses that sustain optimal levels of NK and K activities. The amount of interferon required may be significantly less than the nearly toxic doses now frequently used—and which are usually determined by purely empiric criteria.

Interferon has recently been subdivided into more than 15 different types, which fall into roughly three broad categories—alpha, or leukocyte; beta, or fibroblast; and gamma, or immune. Every type that has been tested induces NK activity, but the potency of each varies. Both beta and gamma types produce a uniformly high level of induction. When 10 different alpha types were tested, they ranged from a similar high level of induction down to a 50-fold weaker level of potency. By using very pure interferon, or by using interferon made by bacteria with a recombinant interferon gene, we have shown that the induction activity is attributable to interferon itself and not a contaminant.

In vitro exposure to interferon for as little as 10 minutes is sufficient to increase NK activity within one to two hours. If interferon is injected into mice, they exhibit increased NK activity in two to three hours. When interferon inducers are used, the NK response appears more slowly, depending on how long it takes for the inducer to raise interferon levels. It may take 12 to 24 hours, or even two to three days.

NK cells appear to be affected by certain other agents as well. As noted, they will proliferate in response to TCGF, which also augments their cytotoxic activity. LGLs have recently been shown to produce TCGF after stimulation with a mitogen and a potent tumor-promoting agent, phorbol myristate acetate.

The interferon- and TCGF-releasing abilities of LGLs indicate that these cells are important immunoregulatory agents. These properties also show that LGLs can react to foreign materials in a variety of ways. It should be cautioned, however, that it is not known whether those cells that release interferon, TCGF, or any other substance also have cytotoxic activity. It is possible that a nonlytic LGL subpopulation is responsible for the release of these substances.

The question of whether other substances induce NK activity has not been easily answered, since many putative agents have turned out to work via interferon. Retinoic acid, a vitamin A analogue, increases NK activity, in both mice and humans, and it does not seem to be an interferon inducer. If anything, in fact, retinoic acid may interfere with interferon production. Certain plant lectins and antibodies directed against NK cells also appear to be effective inducers. The antibodies must be added in the absence of complement so there is no killing of the NK cells. Antibody directed against the H-2 antigens of mouse NK cells, for example, will increase their cytotoxic activity. This is not a result of enhanced binding of the NK cells to their targets due to the antibody, since human target cells can be used and the same cytotoxic enhancement is seen. Antibodies do not seem to affect K activity.

Based on our knowledge of NK activity and other immune effector cells, we can now construct a likely scenario for the process of immune surveillance (see Figure 5 on page 82). The immune system seems to be composed of two levels, one a natural or nonspecific line of defense and the other an induced specific immunity. The natural line is present constitutively or can be rapidly induced. Thus, when a microorganism, a cancer cell, or some other agent appears, NK cells and, probably, macrophages as well deal with the agent very quickly. In many instances these mechanisms alone may be sufficient to deal with the problem.

Although the NK system is not as

Table 2. Possible Functions of NK Cells

Natural killer activity and destruction of tumor cells

Natural killer activity against microbial agents (virus-infected targets, parasites, fungi, or bacteria)

Destruction and/or control of growth and development of some normal hematopoietic and thymus cells

Antibody-dependent cell-mediated cytotoxicity against antibody-coated tumor or other target cells.

Contribution to graft-versus-host disease or autoimmunity (e.g., aplastic anemia, multiple sclerosis)

Secretion of interferon and TCGF and consequent immunoregulatory activity

Figure 6

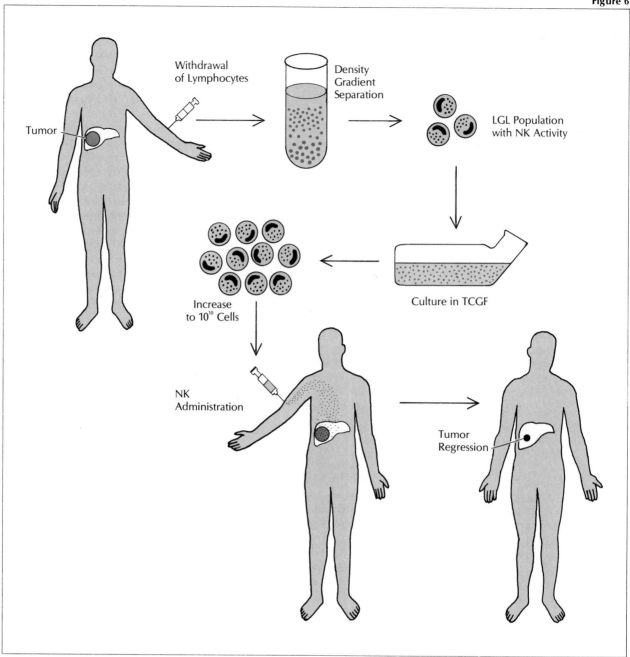

The possibility of NK-cell therapy of tumor patients is under active investigation. An approach hypothetically would involve withdrawing lymphocytes from the patient, then isolating the

NK cells and growing them in vitro by the use of T-cell growth factor. These cells would be infused back into the patient, where they might lead to the elimination of tumor.

sophisticated nor, most likely, as potent as the induced immune response that involves T and B cells, it does demonstrate a certain degree of discrimination. Most normal cells are extremely resistant to NK activity, whereas most tumor cells are sensitive. A normal, adult fibroblast is usually resistant, but if it is infected by a virus, it be-

comes sensitive. NK cells, as well as CTLs and K cells, can kill their targets very rapidly, beginning within about an hour and lysing a large fraction within four hours. Macrophages are much slower, usually requiring at least 18 hours to kill their targets.

NK cells may not be involved exclusively in immune surveillance

and protection (see Table 2 on page 83). There is evidence that they also have a role in regulating the response to bone marrow transplants and the development of certain cells. Mice given lethal doses of radiation are no longer able to reject skin grafts, but they can still reject bone marrow grafts from entirely unrelated strains. Nude, athymic mice have the same ability, so the bone marrow response cannot be a thymus-dependent property as are skin graft rejections. On the other hand, beige mice—C57 black mice with genetic defects that affect coat color and cause lower NK activity, while leaving typical T-cell activity nearly normal—tend to accept bone marrow transplants more readily than mice with higher NK activity. Riccardi, using a variation of the IdUrd technique described earlier, has shown that normal bone marrow cells are cleared from a new mouse host most rapidly when NK activity is high and slowly if it is low.

The genetics of bone marrow graft rejection also indicate that something other than T cells is involved. Certain experimental mouse F_1 hybrid offspring will reject bone marrow from both parents. Skin grafts from either parent are not rejected by these offspring because they recognize antigens in the graft as self. Additionally, a number of treatments that affect NK activity also seem to affect natural bone marrow resistance. It now appears very likely that NK cells are the principal effectors of natural resistance to bone marrow grafts.

NK activity against syngeneic bone marrow cells has been observed in addition to the stronger reactivity against allogeneic parental cells. This indicates that NK cells are at least somewhat autoreactive. It will be of interest to see whether the same cell can discriminate between homozygous and heterozygous cells, or whether separate NK subpopulations mediate these specificities.

NK cells may also be involved in some way in the graft-versus-host (GVH) response. The mechanism involved in this process has never been clear, but there appears to be a correlation between the incidence of GVH disease and the level of NK activity in a patient prior to a marrow transplant. When patients are given immunosuppressive treatments to allow a bone graft to take, their typical T cell–mediated functions do not reappear for three months or longer. NK activity, however, begins to return—sometimes within days and certainly within one month—so when GVH disease appears, usually about seven days after the graft, it is accompanying the resumption of NK activity.

While these correlations suggest that NK cells may cause GVH disease, there are alternative explanations. GVH may, for example, result in elevated production of interferon, and this causes enhanced NK activity. We will soon examine the role of NK cells in GVH disease experimentally. One test will be to inject LGLs into irradiated mice to see whether these cells do induce GVH disease.

A group in Sweden has recently shown that the stem cells from bone marrow are quite susceptible to NK killing in vitro. Thus, another function of NK cells may be to regulate the normal differentiation of certain cells, such as hematopoietic stem cells. There may be a certain point in the differentiation pathway when stem cells are most susceptible to this control, and it may involve something other than cell killing—NK cells may simply inhibit stem-cell growth. There is, however, no clearly recognized role for NK cells in stem-cell regulation. It seems difficult even to design experiments to examine this question.

Another population of normal cells that are sensitive to NK activity are undifferentiated thymocytes. NK cells may be involved in regulating the number of T cells that eventually mature. A California group has evidence that of the thymocytes developing in the thymus, only one in 10,000 ever leaves. The others die within a few days of maturation. This may not be an expression of the cells' limited life span but the result of down-regulation that is similar to what may happen to bone marrow stem cells.

In addition to the possible pathologic involvement of NK cells in GVH disease, some patients with aplastic anemia may have very active cytotoxic cells that seem to fit the characteristics of NK cells. Depressed NK activity in mice and humans has been associated with the proliferation of various types of tumors, particularly when the tumor burden is large. Chédiak-Higashi syndrome is a specific deficiency of NK activity that is associated with a high incidence of lymphomas. Kidney allograft recipients on immunosuppressive therapy have severely depressed NK activity and also have a high risk of developing lymphoproliferative and other types of tumors. Other diseases associated with depressed NK activity are active multiple sclerosis and systemic lupus erythematosus. The role of low NK activity in the pathogenesis of autoimmunity is unclear.

Efforts to boost NK activity for therapeutic purposes have usually involved interferon, either giving it directly or giving an interferon inducer. Soon, however, we will explore the alternative of directly administering NK cells (see Figure 6 on the opposite page). LGLs would be isolated from a cancer patient, grown to large numbers in vitro, and then infused back into the cell donor. As a prelude to this effort, we will first determine how well these cells are accepted by the patient and how they distribute in the body. The laboratory study of LGLs and NK activity has brought us to a level of knowledge that places us on the verge of direct clinical exploitation.

Macrophages as Regulators Of Lymphocyte Function

EMIL R. UNANUE   *Harvard Medical School*

Mononuclear phagocytes, represented by monocytes and macrophages, have close interactions with lymphocytes and play a critical role in immunity. During the induction of an immune response, the handling of the antigen by the phagocyte is an essential step for the lymphocyte to become activated. Subsequently, the activated lymphocyte regulates the microbicidal and cytocidal function of the macrophage.

The classic definition of the macrophage is "a phagocyte," but macrophages are also highly secretory cells. In fact, the secretory function of the macrophage may be as important as phagocytosis. Certainly, both functions are closely related, since phagocytosis is the major stimulus for secretory activity. In its role in immunology and inflammation, the macrophage not only acts as a scavenger of foreign material but also secretes a multitude of substances involved in tissue repair and reorganization, antigen recognition, and lymphocyte differentiation and proliferation.

These functions represent a phylogenetic elaboration of the role of the primitive phagocytic cells that eliminate foreign material in invertebrate species. In the course of evolution, the lymphocyte "learned" to make a critical distinction: Those antigens taken up by the phagocytic macrophages are pathogenic, and they should be recognized as foreign and destroyed; but antigens encountered in the extracellular environment that are not associated with macrophages do not require elimination. Expansion of macrophage function to include regulation of lymphocyte response to antigens provided a mechanism to insure lack of immunity to self.

The lymphocyte-regulatory functions of the macro-

phage are influenced by a number of variables, including the state of differentiation and maturation of the macrophage, the structure and quantity of antigen present, and whether the antigen is under genetic control. Since macrophages belong to the reticulo-endothelial system (a term used in Aschoff's classification to include cells that are capable of taking up a number of vital dyes), they originate from the promonocytes, a bone-marrow stem cell line. The promonocytes, it should be noted, have differentiated at an earlier step from the stem line that is committed to the lymphoid cells (see Figure 1, page 88) and can be characterized by the presence of certain surface markers that are found preferentially in the mature macrophage. The most easily identified of these markers is the Fc receptor, a structure on the cell membrane that binds the Fc portion of the heavy chain of IgG.

Another surface marker, the complement (C3) receptor, binds the cleaved product of the third component of complement. The cell membrane also has many other receptors, known to be involved in phagocytosis but yet to be biochemically characterized. After several cell divisions, the promonocytes enter the circulation as the blood monocytes; eventually they seed in different tissues, where they differentiate into tissue macrophages. Thus, the Kupffer cell of the liver, the alveolar macrophage of the lung, the microglia of the central nervous system, and the peritoneal macrophage are all mononuclear phagocytes. As the macrophage matures, its phagocytic capacity increases. It acquires more receptors, more lysosomes, and more endocytic capacity than the promonocyte or the monocyte.

Current understanding of the interrelation between

macrophage and lymphocyte functions began in the early 1960s with the observation by immunologists that phagocytosis is an important event in the induction of immunogenicity. As a basis for understanding the relationship between phagocytosis and immune responsiveness, it is important to keep in mind the sequence of events involved in the former.

Phagocytosis consists of two phases (see Figure 2, page 89): 1) an attachment phase, in which the macrophage, through its cell membrane receptors, binds the antigen (bacteria, viruses, protein molecules, and cellular components), and 2) an interiorization phase, in which the antigen is taken into the cell and lysed. Interiorization consists of invagination of the cell membrane to form an endocytic vesicle around the antigenic particle. The endocytic ves-

Figure 1

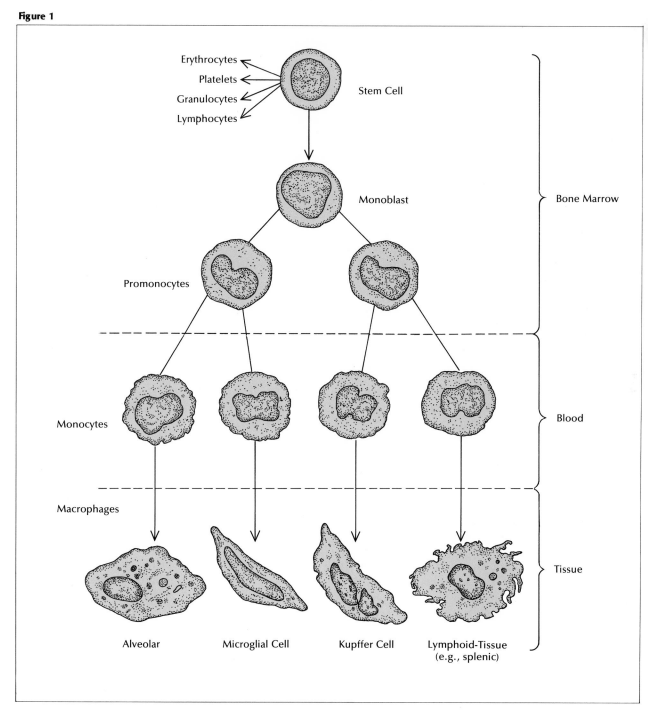

Macrophages are differentiated from bone marrow stem cells that are also the progenitors of many of the other cellular elements of the blood. In the marrow compartment, differentiation goes forward to the promonocyte stage. Promonocytes further differentiate to blood monocytes and then to macrophages that seed as specialized cells in various tissues, exemplified above.

Figure 2

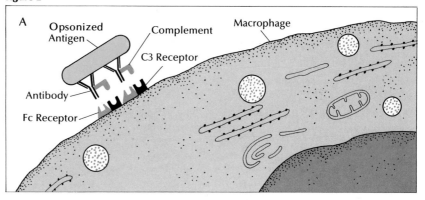

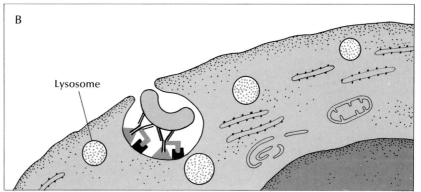

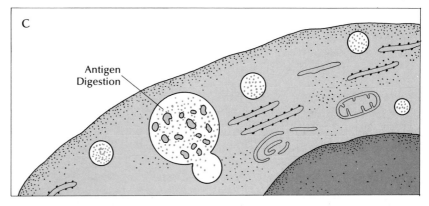

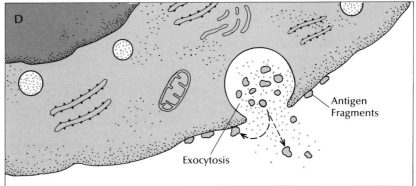

icle flows into the cell and attaches to a lysosome containing proteolytic enzymes that digest the antigen.

Phagocytosis is greatly facilitated if the antigen has been opsonized, that is, coated with antibody and complement, because the macrophage is then capable of binding it through its Fc and C3 receptors. Complex structures with many binding sites, such as foreign red cells, bacteria, and viruses, are strong antigens. One factor responsible for their strong immunogenicity is their extensive uptake by the macrophages. Proteins, on the other hand, are generally weak antigens. Albumin injected into a rabbit circulates with a half-life that is more or less equal to the half-life of the rabbit's native albumin. Although the foreign albumin is taken up by the macrophages, it binds weakly to the cell membrane and rapidly dissociates from it. However, if the albumin is polymerized the number of binding sites is increased, and the macrophages take up the protein polymers avidly.

The enhanced immunogenicity of antigens taken up by the macrophages was first demonstrated by B. Benacerraf and associates in a "biological filtration" experiment that compared the immune responses to protein polymers and to monomers (see Figure 3, page 90). When a mixture of protein polymers and monomers was injected into a rabbit, the polymers were rapidly taken up by the various tissue macrophages, whereas the monomers remained in the circulation. If the protein monomers were extracted from the plasma of the first rabbit and injected into a second rabbit, no antibody response occurred, and a state of tolerance was induced. Other experiments indicated that the purified polymers resulted in a very strong immune response, much higher than that found by injection of the mixtures of polymers and monomers. The experiment demonstrated that the capacity of an antigen to interact with the macrophage determined if it was a weak or strong antigen.

The first in vitro experiments on immune induction by macrophages were done in the early 1960s by M. Fishman, F. L. Adler, and asso-

Phagocytosis of antigen is greatly facilitated by opsonization, because antigen complexed with antibody and complement can attach to the macrophage surface through receptors specific for these immunoreactants (A). Interiorization begins with invagination of the macrophage membrane (B) and proceeds to the formation of a vacuole that merges with a lysosome (C). Lysosomal enzymes digest the antigen. Fragments are then released back into the circulation (D), with some adhering to the cell membrane.

Figure 3

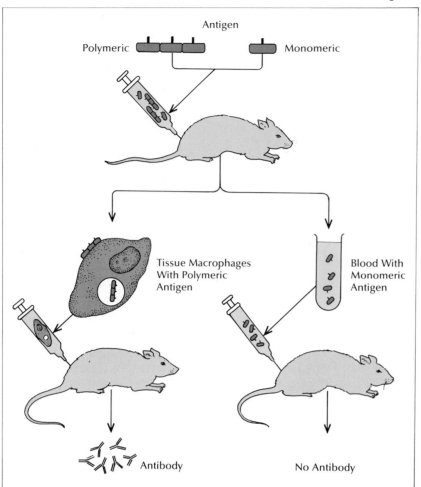

This diagram combines the "biological filtration" experiments of Benacerraf et al and a number of macrophage transfer experiments. An antigenic mixture of polymers and monomers is injected into a mouse. Both isolated tissue macrophages and blood are taken from the mouse and injected separately into two animals. The macrophage recipient responds with specific antibody, and the blood recipient does not, which indicates that the polymers were taken up by the macrophages and were immunogenic, while the monomers remained in the circulation and were nonimmunogenic.

phage-bound antigens were clearly more immunogenic than soluble antigens. This was especially evident with weak antigens, such as serum albumins, which were found to be 1,000- to 10,000-fold more immunogenic when macrophage-bound than when they were injected in soluble form. Later, the enhanced immunogenicity of macrophage-bound antigen was shown in vitro utilizing a haptenated protein, dinitrophenylated keyhole-limpet hemocyanin (DNP-KLH), as the antigen (Figure 4, page 91). DNP-KLH-primed spleen cells were incubated for four days with the antigen in one of three forms: macrophage-bound, free, or adherent to a culture dish. The cells were then assayed by the plaque method for the number of antibody-forming cells. Once again the immunogenic response to the macrophage-bound antigen was greatest. Moreover, antigenicity was virtually abolished by the elimination of T cells. The latter finding, when considered together with an earlier observation that thymectomized mice were unable to respond to a challenge with macrophage-associated antigen, indicated that an immune response required recognition of both hapten and carrier determinants by B and T cells, respectively. Subsequently, we showed that both hapten and carrier determinants had to be present in the same molecule of macrophage-bound antigen if an antibody response was to occur. This finding is in keeping with the classic observation that immunogenicity requires two foreign determinants in the same molecule.

It is now well established that in order for the T cell to become a helper cell or an effector cell for delayed sensitivity, it must recognize antigen in the context of a macrophage. The interaction between macrophage and T cell is essential; without it, the T cell will not proliferate. The essential role of a macrophage in its interaction with the lymphocyte results from two processes: 1) presentation of antigen and 2) secretion of biologically active molecules. Furthermore, genetic control of the immune response is exerted at the level of the macro-

ciates at New York University. The antigenic stimulus used in these experiments was a bacteriophage. The virus was presented to macrophages first, and then an extract of the macrophages was prepared. Lymphocytes were then presented with either a cell-free extract of the macrophages or the bacteriophage directly. Because an antibody response was produced only to the macrophage extract and not to the bacteriophage alone, these investigators postulated that the macrophage was in some way instructing the lymphocytes to make a response. Their suggestion that an information transfer between macrophage

and lymphocyte took place via the macrophage RNA has never been definitely established. Nevertheless, these experiments were the first in which attention was called to the crucial role of macrophage-extracted antigen in lymphocyte recognition.

In our studies of the antigen-presenting function of the macrophage, we have assayed for antibody responses that require T- and B-lymphocyte collaboration and T-cell differentiation and proliferation. We used live macrophages that were incubated with radioactive antigens and then assayed for their immunogenicity. The results of our early in vivo studies showed that macrophage presenting the antigen.

Genetic mapping analyses have localized the genes responsible for effective cell interactions to the I region of the major histocompatibility complex (MHC), H-2 in the mouse and HLA in the human.

The MHC has been analyzed extensively in the mouse, and several regions have been identified. Genetic control of the interaction between the T cell and the macrophage has been localized to the I region. Genes in the I region code for a product, Ia, found not only on the macrophage membrane but also on the B cell and on some subsets of activated T cells. The I-region-coded molecules found on the cell surface are Ia antigens.

The Ia antigens have been identified biochemically as two polypeptide molecules of 33,000 and 25,000 molecular weights. It has been shown that only about one third of macrophages isolated from the peritoneal cavity and spleen bear Ia antigen. Furthermore, only the Ia-positive macrophages appear to be involved in the antigen-presenting function (see Figure 5, page 92).

Recent studies in our laboratory indicate that Ia antigens can be synthesized by all macrophages. However, synthesis takes place only during a brief period in the life history of the phagocyte, particularly during the monocyte-to-early-macrophage stage. Expression of Ia antigens is increased in the activated macrophage.

The key observation leading to the hypothesis that Ir genes function at the macrophage level was made by E. M. Shevach and A. S. Rosenthal at the NIH in 1973. In the course of in vitro experiments on T-cell proliferation in response to macrophage-associated antigens, they made the discovery that in order for T-cell proliferation to occur, the T cell had to be syngeneic with the macrophages. The expected interaction with antigen did not occur when T cells from one strain of guinea pig were mixed with macrophages from another strain, one with a different MHC genotype. These results pointed to the genetic restriction on T-cell-macrophage interactions, with the controlling genes located in the I region of the MHC.

Further evidence that the macrophage participates in the expression of genetic control of the immune response comes from other experiments by A. S. Rosenthal and associates at the NIH. They used insulin as the antigen in the hybrid offspring of two strains of guinea pigs: strain 2, which reacted to only the determinants in the A chain of insulin, and strain 13, which reacted to only the determinants in the B chain. The F_1 hybrids were immunized with insulin, the T cells were isolated and mixed in culture with macrophages from either parent strain, and it was found that the T cells responded to only the A chain in cultures containing strain 2 macrophages and to only the B chain in cultures containing strain 13 macrophages. These results suggested that the macrophage selectively determined the specificity of the immune response. Since immunologic responsiveness is under Ir gene control, the manner in which macrophage presents antigen to T cell may be relevant to immune response to many determinants.

In its role as an antigen-presenting cell as well as an antigen-processing cell, the functions of the macrophage seem to be somewhat contradictory: How is the same cell able to remove antigen from the extracellular milieu, degrade it, and still present it to the lymphocyte? We have done a number of experiments addressed to this question. These confirm that the bulk of macrophage-bound antigens are indeed phagocytized and undergo extensive lysosomal digestion. But we can postulate two possible ways in which antigenic molecules could escape degradation, at least temporarily, and become available to lymphocytes.

One pathway involves antigen bound to the macrophage membrane. In experiments using hemocyanin as the antigen, we found that a small number of antigen molecules remain on the membrane for a finite period of time, despite the interiorization of a majority of the membrane-bound molecules. Removal of the surface-bound molecules by treatment with trypsin or by antibody greatly reduces the immunogenicity of the macrophage-associated hemocyanin.

Figure 4

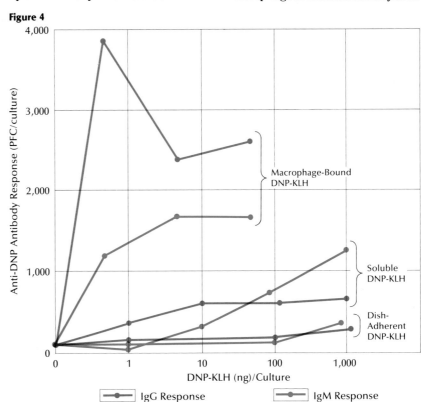

Experiments with the haptenated protein antigen DNP-KLH documented the amplification of immunogenicity resulting from macrophage binding.

Figure 5

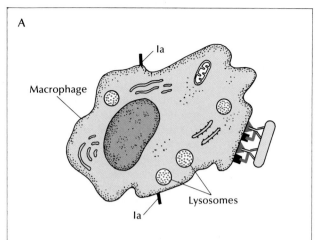

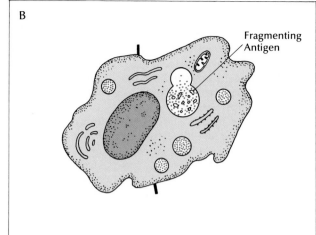

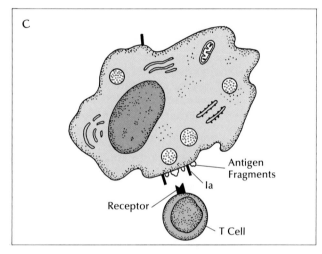

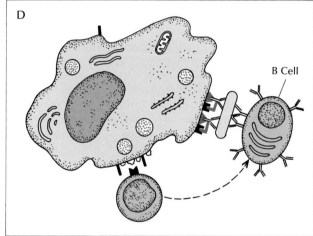

Schematically represented is the role that Ia-positive macrophages may play in antigen presentation and in initiating an immune response. Panels A and B encompass phagocytosis and digestion of opsonized antigen. T lymphocytes are mobilized and react to the macrophage-processed antigenic fragments, with the Ia determinate apparently regulating the interaction (C). At the same time, B cells recognize whole opsonized antigen, also on the macrophage membrane, providing a stage for B-T interaction (D).

The second pathway involves molecules of antigen that are phagocytized but escape complete digestion by lysosomal enzymes and are returned to the extracellular milieu by the process of exocytosis. Our studies have shown that macrophages release partially fragmented molecules of antigen continuously and for long periods of time, although in small amounts, and that these fragments are capable of binding antibody. Since concomitant release of cytoplasmic enzymes, such as lactic dehydrogenase, could not be demonstrated, lysed macrophages did not appear to be the source of the extracellular antigen. That the released antigen had been derived from intracellular sources was demonstrated by exposing macrophages to antigen and permitting phagocytosis of most of the antigen molecules. Any remaining surface-bound antigen was then removed by trypsin. This treatment did not halt the release of antigen into the medium, however. Furthermore, when antigen was recovered from the medium, it was clearly as immunogenic as the native molecule. It appears that phagocytosis of membrane-bound soluble antigens by the macrophage is not 100% complete: The few molecules that remain surface-bound and/or are slowly interiorized may serve an antigen-presenting function.

On the basis of these findings, we have proposed alternative mechanisms for macrophage presentation of antigen to the lymphocytes. One involves the macrophage membrane-bound antigen molecule that remains accessible for some period of time and that is probably recognized by the B cell. It is known, from the experiments of M. Sela et al more than a decade ago, that the antigen molecule recognized by the B cell is the native molecule in its tertiary configuration. The other way is through the fragmented molecules that escape complete digestion. It has been shown repeatedly by a number of investigators that the T cell does not discriminate between native and denatured antigen. Perhaps the T cell recognizes the fragmented antigen, which may have some association with Ia molecules.

Some support for this concept has been provided by experiments of P. Erb and M. Feldmann in London. The available evidence, therefore, suggests that the macrophage presents antigen through a membrane-bound molecule recognized by the B cell and also through a molecule that has been processed through an MHC-controlled step recognized by the T cell. The T cell then responds, proliferates, and/or secretes mediators that influence other T cells, macrophages, or B cells.

How is the Ir gene control exerted at the level of the macrophage? There are no clear answers yet. The Ir gene codes for the Ia antigens, molecules that are definitely crucial for the interaction, perhaps because they associate with or link to the fragmented antigen discussed earlier or because they are crucial as cell-to-cell interaction molecules. Not mutually exclusive with the above is the possibility that the Ir genes could code for enzymes that are critical for the handling of the antigen molecule.

It now appears that the interactions between macrophages and lymphocytes take place in two stages. In the first (immune-inductive) stage, the Ia-positive macrophages bind the antigen and present it to the T cells. The T cells are then able to secrete lymphocyte mediators, such as chemoattractants, which summon fresh macrophages from the bone marrow, and macrophage-activating factor, which induces microbicidal activity. The macrophages become highly activated and kill any pathogen that interacts with them, including tumor cells. This is the stage of cellular resistance or delayed hypersensitivity essential for resistance to intracellular pathogens. In the second stage, the T-cell-activated macrophages can be either Ia positive or Ia negative, but first, only Ia-positive macrophages can recruit T cells.

These two interactions can be reproduced readily and studied in culture. The experimental system developed in our laboratory involves infecting mice with an intracellular facultative bacterium, *Listeria monocytogenes* (see Figure 6, page 94). It is known that resistance to Listeria infection involves interaction of specific anti-Listeria T lymphocytes with macrophages. In our experiments, a few days after infection, the T cells are isolated from the peritoneal exudate and cultured with normal macrophages and dead Listeria organisms. Within a few minutes, the T cells adhere firmly to the Ia-positive macrophages containing the bacteria. In a few hours, a number of mediators are produced, including a 15,000-dalton mitogenic protein (MP) secreted by the macrophages and a macrophage-activating factor secreted by the T cell. (The amount of MP produced is determined by adding the culture fluid to ^{3}H-labeled thymocytes and measuring thymocyte proliferation. The macrophage-activating factor is assayed by adding the fluid to normal macrophages and assaying their cytocidal function, which is stimulated by the factor.) By 24 hours, the macrophages in the T-cell-macrophage mixtures, including the Ia-negative macrophages, are activated and exhibit microbicidal and tumoricidal properties, and the T cells undergo extensive proliferation. All biologic effects – secretion of mediators, activation of macrophages, and T-cell proliferation – require that the T cell interact with Ia-bearing macrophages and that genetically both come from strains of mice sharing the same I region (see Figure 7, page 95). In contrast, MP and macrophage-activating factor, once synthesized, show no genetic restriction.

The interaction between T cell and macrophage that results in production of lymphocyte mediators is important in infections involving intracellular pathogens such as tubercle bacilli, *L. monocytogenes*, salmonellae, and brucellae. Unlike the pyogenic bacteria, which after phagocytosis are rapidly digested by the macrophage, these organisms survive inside the macrophage. Activation of the macrophage requires the two-stage interaction with the T cell described above.

As noted at the beginning of this article, the macrophage is a highly secretory cell. Its secretory products include complement proteins, lysosomal enzymes, neutral proteases, interferon, lysozyme, plasminogen activators, antigen fragments, and a number of less well-defined factors that appear to be involved in lymphocyte regulation. Secretory activity is determined to a large extent by the state of maturation of the macrophage and its function at a particular time. Some factors are secreted continuously, but most are secreted in response to antigen uptake and phagocytosis.

Our interest has been in the lymphoregulatory factors, four of which have been identified. The best characterized of these is the MP described previously. It was isolated from macrophage culture fluid in this laboratory and is very similar to a factor discovered by I. Gery and B. H. Waksman at Yale, who termed it "lymphocyte-activating factor." It is a powerful mitogen that stimulates cell division in both thymocytes and T and B cells. Some MP is secreted by macrophages under basal conditions, but secretion is greatly enhanced by phagocytic stimuli, exposure to endotoxin, the addition of activated lymphocytes or their products, or inhibitors of protein synthesis. Highly activated macrophages are poor secretors, whereas nonstimulated macrophages exposed to immune T cells and antigen generate large amounts of MP.

Two other lymphostimulatory factors have been found in macrophage culture fluid: one that causes differentiation of immune B cells into plasma cells in the absence of antigen and T cells and another that increases or decreases antibody production by T and B cells in the presence of antigen.

The first of these factors was detected in experiments using spleen cells from mice immunized to a haptenated protein, fluorescein on KLH. The immune spleen cells were incubated in different amounts of macrophage culture fluid for four days and assayed for antibody response by measuring the number of plaque-forming cells. The antibody response to the addition of the specific hapten-carrier combination was not further enhanced by the addition of an unrelated carrier protein (fluorescein on rabbit gammaglobulin). Furthermore, it occurred in the absence of antigen and in cultures depleted of T

Figure 6

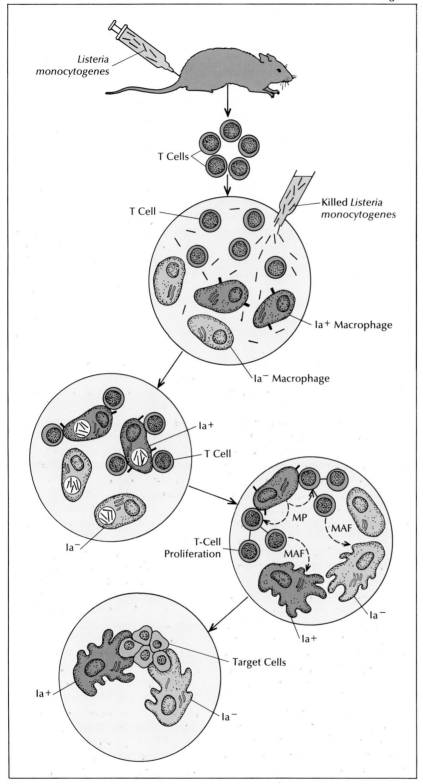

When T cells are taken from an animal that has been injected with live Listeria organisms and incubated with both Ia⁺ and Ia⁻ macrophages as well as with dead bacteria, the immunized lymphocytes will adhere only to the Ia⁺ macrophages. Mitogenic protein (MP) will be secreted by the macrophages and, in turn, stimulate T-cell proliferation. The T cells will secrete macrophage-activating factor (MAF). The T cell–macrophage interaction that results in these secretory activities is genetically restricted by the I region of the MHC. MAF activates both Ia⁺ and Ia⁻ macrophages, shown by ability to kill bacteria or tumor cells.

cells. These results indicate B cells, at a certain stage of maturation, differentiate into plasma cells upon interaction with the macrophage factor.

The fourth factor noted in macrophage culture fluid enhances or suppresses antibody production by primed spleen cells in response to the addition of antigen to the culture. Enhancement requires challenge with the same hapten-carrier conjugate used to prime the spleen cells. The antibody response is far greater than that seen without adding antigen and probably represents expansion of the T-cell helper function.

The evidence cited thus far supports the view that the macrophage participates in the antigen-driven differentiation of the lymphocytes through its antigen-processing and secretory functions during phagocytosis. The lymphocyte-proliferating effect of the macrophage secretory products – MP, B-cell-differentiating factor, and T-cell-activating factor – explain, at least in part, the enhanced lymphocyte response to antigen in the context of the macrophage.

In addition to regulating antigen-specific recognition, there is evidence that the macrophage participates in the antigen-*independent* differentiation of the lymphoid cell line through the secretion of still another lymphostimulatory factor. The results of recent experiments by D. I. Beller in this laboratory have shown that immature thymocytes can be induced to mature in macrophage culture fluid. The experiments were undertaken originally to determine whether MP, in addition to stimulating thymocyte proliferation, could induce differentiation into mature thymocytes. The experiments led to the discovery of thymocyte-differentiating factor (TDF).

It will be recalled that the T-cell stem line originates in the bone marrow as the prothymocyte. The prothymocyte migrates into the thymus, where it differentiates into the thymocyte. Monocytes and macrophages also are found in the thymus, and curiously, they are located strategically at the junction between the medulla and the cortex. Thymocyte maturation occurs as the thymocyte migrates from the cortex to the medulla, before it exits into the circulation. The T cell, in the course of differentiation from the thymocyte, acquires more H-2 antigen than its progenitor and then loses thymic-lymphocyte (TL) antigen. TL antigen is thus a valuable marker of T-cell maturation. The change from thymocyte to mature T cell may take place without cell division and involves a change in the cell surface phenotype.

In Beller's experiments, immature thymocytes were isolated and grown in macrophage culture fluid. After 48 to 72 hours, they were found to have changed their membrane properties, acquiring more H-2 antigen, losing TL, and becoming responsive in mixed leukocyte cultures. The impressive degree of maturation achieved was not due to contamination of the cultures with mature thymocytes. The change in H-2, for example, occurred in immature thymocytes that had been treated with mitomycin C and were not dividing. The phenotype change remained stable: The cells continued to respond to allogenic stimulation after removal of the macrophage culture fluid. The active factor in the medium has been identified as a 40,000-dalton molecule, which we have called thymocyte-differentiating factor (TDF). It can be distinguished from both MP and interferon. Thymocyte differentiation has also been induced by culturing thymocytes in the presence of macrophages isolated from the thymus. These macrophages are less mature than macrophages isolated from the spleen and serous cavities but are highly active in causing differentiation of the thymocyte.

Several other substances isolated from the thymus have been proposed for the role of TDF. In tissue culture these putative thymic hormones can induce conversion of the prothymocyte to a thymocyte. In view of the strategic location of the monocytes and macrophages in the thymus, it seems highly probable that the maturation step regulated by TDF follows the action of the thymic hormone(s) and converts the immature thymocyte to a mature T cell. In support of this notion is Beller's finding that the thymic hormones convert stem cells to prothymocytes

in vitro but do not produce the phenotype changes that signal T-cell maturation.

These observations are consonant with the hypothesis of multisignal regulation of T-cell maturation (see Figure 8, page 96). In the early phase of thymic differentiation, the commitment of the stem cell line to a thymocyte is regulated by thymic hormone(s). In the next phase, the maturation of the immature thymocyte to a mature T cell during its transit from the thymic cortex to the medulla is regulated by the macrophage factor secreted by cells in the corticomedullary junction. A question that remains to be explored is whether TDF influences the differentiation of T-cell subsets.

The role of macrophages in T-cell differentiation may extend beyond the secretion of TDF. Recent studies, particularly by R. Zinkernagel and M. Bevan, based on an early hypothesis of Niels Jerne, have implicated a role for the nonlymphoid thymic cells in the generation of the repertory of receptors of both cytolytic T cells and

helper T cells. The development of the specificity of receptors follows the interaction of the thymocytes with stromal cells bearing MHC determinants. David Beller and I have just found that the major nonlymphoid cell in the thymus bearing Ia is the macrophage, which suggests that this cell may well be controlling development of the receptor repertory.

Another factor identified in macrophage culture fluid influences neovascularization. In inflammatory conditions in which new blood vessel formation occurs, it has long been known that the endothelial cells in the new vessels that are surrounded by macrophages are in mitosis. The observation suggested a cause-effect relationship – that is, the macrophages secreted a product that triggered the replication of the endothelial cells, which led to formation of new blood vessels. In joint studies with R. Cotran's laboratory, such a substance, in fact, has been detected in macrophage culture fluid. For the assay, phagocytosis was induced in macrophages grown in tissue culture. Angiogenesis was tested in assays

Figure 7

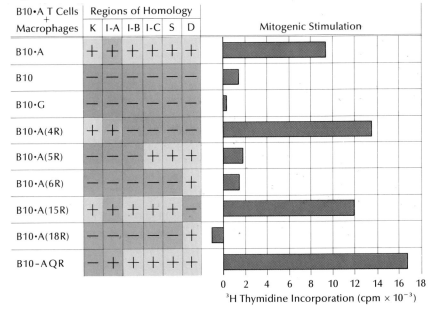

B10·A T Cells + Macrophages	Regions of Homology						Mitogenic Stimulation
	K	I-A	I-B	I-C	S	D	
B10·A	+	+	+	+	+	+	
B10	−	−	−	−	−	−	
B10·G	−	−	−	−	−	−	
B10·A(4R)	+	+	−	−	−	−	
B10·A(5R)	−	−	−	+	+	+	
B10·A(6R)	−	−	−	−	−	+	
B10·A(15R)	+	+	+	+	+	−	
B10·A(18R)	−	−	−	−	−	+	
B10-AQR	−	+	+	+	+	+	

0   2   4   6   8   10   12   14   16   18
³H Thymidine Incorporation (cpm × 10⁻³)

The need for I-A congeneity for cooperation between macrophages and T cells was demonstrated by assaying for mitogenic stimulatory activity with combinations of the two cell types. T cells from B10·A mice immune to Listeria were cultured with macrophages and killed Listeria organisms. The macrophages were derived from different mouse strains. Part of the H-2 map is shown, with regions shared between T cells and macrophages indicated. Essentially, significant stimulation occurred when cells were derived from animals with homology at the I-A locus of the major histocompatibility complex (H-2).

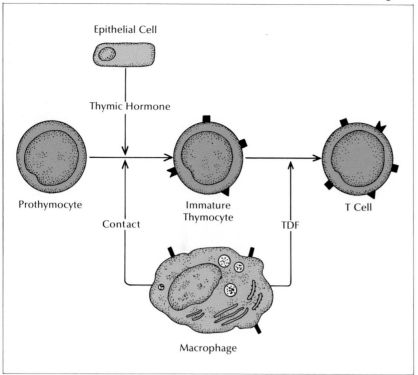

Epithelial Cell

Thymic Hormone

Prothymocyte

Contact

Immature
Thymocyte

TDF

T Cell

Macrophage

A scheme is presented for multisignal regulation of T-cell maturation. On entering the thymus, a prothymocyte is exposed to thymic hormone and establishes contact with Ia⁺ macrophages, with resultant differentiation into an immature thymocyte. Between the thymic cortex and medulla, a second signal is provided by the macrophage-secreted thymocyte-differentiating factor (TDF), which causes maturation to the functional T cell.

developed by J. Folkman and associates, who were the first to find an angiogenesis factor – in their case, derived from tumor cells. The conditioned culture medium was embedded in tiny plastic matrices, which were implanted in the corneas of live guinea pigs. After several days, stereomicroscopic examination of the eyes revealed new limbic vessels growing into the implantation site, which indicated the presence of an angiogenesis factor in the macrophage culture medium.

The finding suggests that the macrophage secretes a material that produces new vessel growth and may be relevant to the reorganization of connective tissue in inflammation. In damaged tissue, the growth of new connective tissue elements, such as blood vessels, is a reparative process. However, in certain inflammatory conditions in which there is a persistent influx of macrophages secreting angiogenesis factor, these cells may condition a pathologic reaction. For example, in immune complex glomerular nephritis, proliferation of endothelial cells is a prominent feature that correlates with infiltration of the glomeruli by macrophages.

This discussion of macrophage functions has implied that one cell performs phagocytic, antigen-processing and antigen-presenting, and secretory functions. Actually, it is not known whether the macrophage population consists of heterogenous or homogenous cells. It has been suggested by some that the macrophage passes through stages of differentiation and that each function may become more or less prominent at a given stage. It seems equally plausible that the macrophage, like the T cell, differentiates into subsets. At the present time, it is only possible to divide macrophages into two sets on the basis of the presence or absence of Ia antigen on the cell membrane. Whether the Ia antigen marks a stage in the differentiation of the macrophage is not clear. More Ia-bearing macrophages are found in the spleen than in the peritoneal cavity – which may indicate that as the macrophage matures, it loses Ia, but this point has not been established. One fact that has been determined experimentally is that the Ia-negative macrophages do not convert to Ia-positive macrophages. One can kill all of the Ia-positive peritoneal macrophages in a culture by the addition of anti-Ia antibody and complement, and this does not lead to conversion of the Ia-negative macrophages remaining in the culture.

Because the Ia antigen-presenting function of the macrophage is crucial to the development of an appropriate T-cell response to intracellular pathogens, some immunodeficiency diseases could involve a genetic defect at the level of the Ia-positive macrophage. It might be worthwhile to search among the T-cell and combined immunodeficiency diseases for abnormalities in macrophage-lymphocyte interactions.

Major Transplantation Antigens In Host Responses to Infection

ROLF M. ZINKERNAGEL   *University of Zurich*

Current studies of host defenses against intracellular parasites such as viruses or bacteria bring together two major fields of immunologic study: rejection of organ transplants and immune responses to infection in general. In the field of transplant rejection, relevant work with experimental animals originated perhaps half a century ago with tumor biologists who were seeking to transplant neoplastic cells and found it necessary for their purposes to develop inbred or syngeneic mouse strains. In terms of our understanding of immune responses and their genetic controls, the results of this contribution, particularly the work of P. Gorer and G. Snell, have been as dramatic as the clinical consequences of transplantation. The second field, the immune response to infection, dates back two centuries. This review will discuss aspects of the relationship between the two fields, specifically exploring what has been learned of the role of major histocompatibility antigens in immunologic protection against intracellular infectious agents.

Major Transplantation Antigens and Cellular Immunity

Until relatively recently, there were no clear, experimentally established data that defined the relationship between immune phenomena in infectious diseases and transplantation rejection. However, starting in the 1950s, a number of speculations pointed the way toward unraveling this relationship. One of the earliest suggestions was that cell-mediated delayed hypersensitivity against both chemical allergens and tuberculosis bacilli (BCG) was possibly not directed against either type of antigen per se, but rather against the antigens *and* the cells onto whose membranes they attached. In this sense, N. A. Mitchison pro-posed a commonality between transplantation reactions and responses to chemical allergens and at least one group of exogenous pathogens, exemplified by BCG.

A whole chain of speculation was inspired by Lewis Thomas's immunosurveillance hypothesis, namely, that certain immune responses had evolved to cope with continuous somatic mutation and that cancer could be regarded as a breakdown of these defenses. From this, H. S. Lawrence concluded that cell-mediated immunity in one sense may always be autoaggressive, in that it is directed not only against foreign antigenic determinants but at the same time against the "self" surface expressing those antigens.

In the 1960s, facts related to these hypotheses and connecting transplantation and infectious disease immunology were generated in both laboratory and clinical settings. F. Lilly demonstrated that susceptibility to disease could in some cases be linked to the major histocompatibility gene complex, which codes for major transplantation antigens. Then B. Benacerraf and H. McDevitt discovered that immune responses to many non-self antigens were genetically controlled by immune response (Ir) genes. They also established that these genes mapped within the major histocompatibility complex (MHC), which earlier had been defined on the basis of its function in coding for molecules involved in recognition of transplantation antigens.

On the clinical side, a *possible* relationship between transplantation and microbial immunology may be inferred from the associations discovered between certain diseases and major histocompatibility complex types (HLA) in humans. Such associations have been demonstrated for a number of disorders, virtually all of which are usually considered to have an autoimmune component. These include connective tissue diseases such as ankylos-

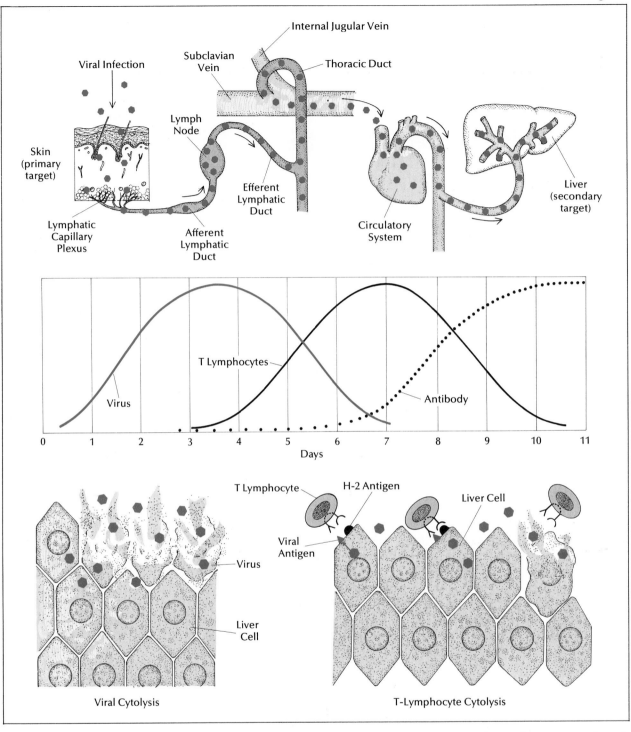

The illustrations above depict, in order, a typical route of viral infection, the kinetics of viral infection and response, and two different modes of viral pathogenesis. The viral route (top) is represented by a viral infection whose primary target is the skin, which serves as an entry portal to local or regional lymphatics. In the so-called hematogenous stage, the virus enters the blood circulation, and then travels to a secondary target organ, here typified by the liver. The middle panel contains standardized curves representing the kinetics of viral multiplication and of immune responses to the virus. Note that T-cell response only becomes measurable at the time the circulating virus peaks and, in turn, it peaks about when the virus has disappeared from the circulation (six to eight days). Humoral antibodies are detectable even later. Finally, the bottom panel suggests two ways in which viruses precipitate target-cell destruction. Highly cytopathic viruses (left) can lyse cells directly. With less destructive viruses, infection will result in translocation of viral antigens to the cell surface. Cytolytic T cells, with dual specificity for virus and self (H-2) antigens, both now expressed on the surface, will attack the infected cell and induce the lysis sequence.

ing spondylitis and rheumatoid arthritis. Obviously, none of these diseases has been shown to have an acute infectious etiology, so one must be equivocal about these associations as evidence of a relationship between transplantation antigens and immunologic phenomena in infectious diseases. The possibility that these diseases are related to infection by, or immunity against, slow or chronic viral infection is intriguing, perhaps even likely, but unproved.

Contemporaneously with the finding of such associations, several lines of direct evidence emerged that hint at an intimate relationship between the transplantation reaction and T-cell immunity against intracellular parasites. One was the experiments reported by G. J. Svett-Moldavsky, which demonstrated that if skin from a mouse that had been infected with a noncytopathic virus was transplanted into an uninfected syngeneic mouse the recipient would reject the skin graft. Without such infection, syngeneic animals – being essentially identical – accept each other's skin grafts. Clearly, then, to the recipient animal the virally infected skin graft represented a "self-plus-X" complex.

In the early 1970s, B. Kindred and D. Shreffler in Basel first described the concept that thymus-processed T lymphocytes and bone marrow–derived B lymphocytes cooperate in producing an immune response only when helper T cells are H-2 (the murine MHC) compatible with antibody-forming precursor B cells. Subsequently, this observation and that of the so-called allogeneic effect were thoroughly analyzed by D. H. Katz and Benacerraf at Harvard (see D. H. Katz, "Genetic Controls and Cellular Interactions in Antibody Formation"). Briefly, these studies established that B cells could be helped to produce antibodies either by H-2 I-restricted helper T cells or by allogeneic T cells recognizing the foreign H-2 determinants on B cells. A similar involvement of H-2 structures in T-cell interactions was established for proliferative T-cell responses when T cells were exposed to antigen on macrophages by E. Shevach and A. Rosenthal at NIH.

This became clear only when P. C.

Doherty and I, working in Canberra, discovered that virus-specific cytotoxic T cells were H-2 restricted. Cytotoxic T cells, specific for trinitrophenyl coupled to cell surfaces, similarly are under H-2 control, as shown by G. Shearer at the NIH. Finally, J.F.A.P. Miller in Melbourne demonstrated that still another T-cell function—induction of delayed-type hypersensitivity—was H-2 restricted. Thus, experiments of the last six years have shown that all known T-cell functions have dual specificity—for a foreign antigen and for a self-MHC structure—and that all T cells are MHC restricted. It has also become clear that this MHC restriction is probably a universal characteristic of T cells, since it has been documented in mice, rats, humans, and chickens. Teleologically, these findings, particularly for T-cell-mediated immunity against intracellular parasites, are intriguing, since they suggest that at least one important biologic function of transplantation antigens is in host defense against nonself antigens expressed on cell surfaces.

Immunity to Virus

Virus infection and immunity to virus follow general kinds of interrelated kinetics (see Figure 1 on page 98). Usually, virus infects a primary organ and spreads systemically, via lymph nodes during a hematogenous phase, to secondary target organs such as liver or spleen. *Most* viruses cause pathology by destroying host cells. Immunity then prevents further spread of virus and thereby prevents pathology. However, some viruses do not readily cause death of host cells and may be harmless in themselves. Instead, it is actually the humoral or cellular immune response to infection that, in functioning to prevent viral spread, causes disease by attacking infected cells; this will be discussed more fully later. After the induction of immunity, viral titers in blood and/or in tissues fall. In analyzing the phenomena, one must also keep in mind that during systemic infection of mice, virus often is no longer detectable six or seven days after initiation of infection. Virus-immune lymphocytes become detectable just as viral titers begin to fall, and they peak as the virus disap-

pears. In contrast, humoral immunity (antibodies) usually reaches detectable titers and peaks somewhat later.

Cell-mediated immunity against viruses can be evaluated by 1) measuring delayed-type hypersensitivity in vivo; 2) assessing specific release of macrophage inhibition factor (MIF) in vitro; or, most easily, 3) measuring in vitro the cytotoxic activity of virus-immune lymphocytes against virus-infected target cells labeled with a radioactive marker, such as ^{51}Cr. Release of ^{51}Cr is proportional to cell death caused by immune T cells (see J.-C. Cerottini, "Lymphoid Cells as Effectors of Immunologic Cytolysis.)" The effector cells in this assay have been defined as T cells by various criteria: 1) sensitivity to anti-T-cell sera plus complement; 2) necessity of direct T-cell to target-cell contact for lysis; 3) absence of antibody involvement; and, as will be discussed, 4) H-2 restriction of the effector mechanism.

For the present discussion, the immune response and immune pathology observed in lymphocytic choriomeningitis (LCM) virus and pox virus infections are of particular interest. When mice are infected systemically, the resulting severe infection has quite distinct characteristics. Mouse pox virus, as studied by R. V. Blanden in Canberra, is a cytolytic virus that causes massive cell destruction. This virus is comparable to pox (e.g., vaccinia) or influenza virus in humans. Immune reactions to such viruses are mainly protective, since they prevent cell destruction by virus.

LCM virus, in contrast, is poorly cytolytic and is not particularly damaging by itself. In fact, W. Rowe and G. Cole found that acute LCM disease in mice is not produced by the virus itself but rather by the immune response to the pathogen, thus establishing this disease as a model for certain kinds of predominantly cell-mediated autoimmune diseases in man. Subsequent work by M. B. A. Oldstone, F. J. Dixon, G. Mitchell, and McDevitt showed that there were some strain differences in susceptibility to this virus, which suggests that there may be a component of H-2 gene control in the pathologic process.

In our own experiments, Doherty

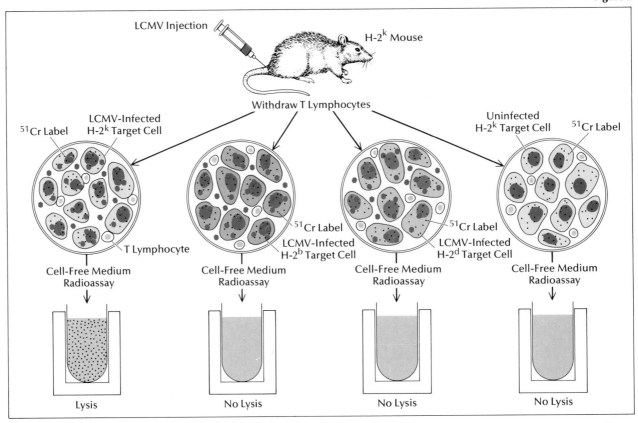

This diagram summarizes experimental evidence for both the H-2 restriction and the dual specificity of cytolytic T-cell responses to viral infection. If a mouse with an H-2^k haplotype is infected with lymphochoriomeningitis virus (LCMV), T cells from that animal will lyse target cells infected with the same vi- *rus, but only if the target cells carry the same H-2 haplotype. Thus, infected H-2^b and H-2^d cells will not be lysed nor will uninfected H-2^k target cells. When an F_1 hybrid mouse is used as the lymphocyte donor, target cells of either parental haplotype will be lysed but not cells of a third H-2 specificity.*

and I were able to demonstrate that if one taps cerebrospinal fluid at the time when LCM virus-infected mice are very sick, one finds large numbers of cytotoxic T lymphocytes. Therefore our speculation was that the differences in strain susceptibility to LCM virus infection might be accounted for by a difference in the number or activity of the cytolytic effector T cells that the animals could mobilize in response to the virus. To test this hypothesis we selected inbred mice of different strains and injected them intracerebrally with LCM virus. After seven days, when the animals were clinically acutely ill and when, from earlier studies on the kinetics of immunoresponsive cells, we knew that the cytolytic T-cell response should be maximal, we sacrificed the animals, removed their spleens, and tested the splenic virus-specific cytotoxic activity. For these experiments, we used a

^{51}Cr release assay on virus-infected fibroblasts taken from H-2^k mice.

We found that immune T cells from C3H mice (H-2^k), which were syngeneic with the target cells, and from all other mice having the H-2^k haplotype, could kill the infected H-2^k target cells (see Figure 2 above). On the other hand, LCM virus–immune T cells from H-2^d or H-2^b mice could not lyse the infected H-2^k target cells. Moreover, LCM virus–immune lymphocytes from H-2^d mice lysed infected H-2^d targets but not H-2^k or H-2^b targets. F_1 hybrids between H-2^k mice and H-2^b mice lysed infected target cells of both parental types but not cells of the unrelated H-2^d type. Further analysis demonstrated that these virus-specific cytotoxic T cells were usually restricted in the respect that they could lyse only infected target cells that expressed the serologically defined major transplantation anti-

gens present in the donor animal.

These experiments clearly indicated that the cytotoxic T lymphocyte has a dual specificity: first, for the virus against which it has been immunized and whose antigens it can recognize on the target-cell surface, and second, for the self component coded for in the H-2 major histocompatibility complex and similarly represented on the target-cell membrane.

The more precise mapping of the genes involved in this system required use of genetically defined strains of mice that differ from one another with respect only to small segments of the genome, specifically in the MHC (see map, Figure 3 on page 101). These experiments confirmed that the restriction is indeed imposed by structures coded for by H-2 genes. More precisely, virus-specific cytotoxic T cells are restricted by the K and D regions of H-2, which also code for the serologically defined major transplantation antigens.

From what has been described so far, one can stress several observations: MHC restrictedness appears to be a very prominent characteristic of T-cell function. Whenever T cells are involved in immunologic activity they express a dual specificity for a foreign antigen and – differentially dependent on the T-effector function – for a cell-surface self component coded for in the major histocompatibility complex. In contrast, all antibody-mediated immune phenomena – including opsonization, antibody-plus-complement-mediated lysis, and antibody-dependent cytolytic cell activity – are unrestricted genetically, and are uniquely responsive to foreign antigenic determinants.

T-Cell Recognition and the Thymus

Before turning to the immunopathologic implications of the role of cytolytic T cells as attackers of virus-infected cells, we should briefly discuss an area that remains a significant and unresolved controversy – the nature of the recognition structures on the T lymphocyte that provide for this dual specificity. Two basic models have been proposed, the dual recognition model and the single recognition, or altered self, model (see Figure 4 on page 102). The dual recognition concept suggests that so far as cytolytic T cells are concerned, the MHC determinants are coded for in the K and D regions, while for the nonlytic T cells, including helper and macrophage-activating lymphocytes, the determinants are products of I-region genes. On the basis of work by H. R. Ramseier, J. Lindenmann, H. Binz, and H. Wigzell and studies by K. Rajewsky and K. Eichmann, it is generally hypothesized that foreign antigen probably is recognized by a classic type of receptor with a variable region (like that of immunoglobulin) to afford the necessary array of specificities required to recognize the almost infinite variety of antigenic determinants. The nature of the cytolytic T cell's receptor for self, which is directed toward the K and D gene products, is unknown.

The single recognition model proposes that T cells have only a single receptor site, which serves either to recognize a complex formed between the self determinant and the foreign-antigen determinant or, alternatively, to recognize the self marker only after it is "altered" by viral infection.

Despite the fact that the T-cell receptor(s) still lacks biochemical characterization, we know some important aspects of the biology of T cells and of their interactions with other cells, particularly infected target cells. Recently, we have obtained experimental evidence that without exposure to antigen, T cells in the thymus acquire the restricted specificity for the MHC that is expressed in the thymus. Thus, T cells are destined a priori to recognize self-MHC structures as expressed by thymic epithelial cells. The evidence for this concept derives from the following experiment done in collaboration with G. Callahan, A. Althage, S. Cooper, and Jan Klein here at Scripps. One can construct hybrid $(H\text{-}2^b \times H\text{-}2^k)$ F_1 mice that lack functional T cells, because their thymuses are removed surgically before mature T cells appear. These mice are incapable of generating virus-specific cytotoxic T cells during a virus infection and often die of it. What happens if one gives one of these mice that has no T cells or thymus a new thymus of $(H\text{-}2^b \times H\text{-}2^k)F_1$ origin, or substitutes a new thymus of either $H\text{-}2^b$ or $H\text{-}2^k$ parental origin? Is the restricted specificity dictated by the H-2 of the thymus? In fact, when thymuses of $H\text{-}2^k$ origin were transplanted into $(H\text{-}2^b \times H\text{-}2^k)$ mice without thymuses or mature T cells, they

eventually became capable of generating virus-specific cytotoxic T cells restricted to $H\text{-}2^k$ only but not to $H\text{-}2^b$ – and vice versa (see Figure 5 on page 103). Thus, the restricted specificity of T cells is selected during the T-cell maturation in the thymus.

The implications of this finding, theoretical and practical, are far-reaching. While for the most part they lie outside the scope of this review, there are two that merit brief mention. First, although both models of T-cell recognition are explainable in terms of this finding, a dual recognition model may fit it better. Second, the practical implications are compelling enough to warrant their consideration in efforts to treat immunodeficient patients by reconstitution with stem cells or with thymus grafts.

The latter point can be better appreciated by keeping in mind what happens if a lethally irradiated mouse of $H\text{-}2^k$ type is reconstituted with bone marrow stem cells of incompatible $H\text{-}2^b$ origin. The animal will survive, but it will not be able to generate virus-specific cytotoxic T cells or to make a useful antibody response. The same holds true if an $H\text{-}2^b$ mouse that lacks both thymus and T cells is transplanted with a thymus graft of incompatible $H\text{-}2^k$ origin. One possible explanation is that in both examples stem cells of $H\text{-}2^b$ type mature in an $H\text{-}2^k$ thymus to recognize $H\text{-}2^k$ as self. Since B cells, macrophages, and T cells are of donor origin, and themselves express $H\text{-}2^b$ self markers, the T cells recognize a self that is not really self. Therefore, interactions between T cells and other

Figure 3

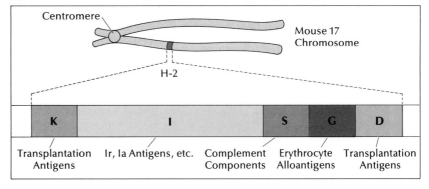

The map locates the mouse major histocompatibility (H-2) complex and indicates the regions in that complex involved in immune response activity. Some of the known products of genes of these H-2 regions are indicated.

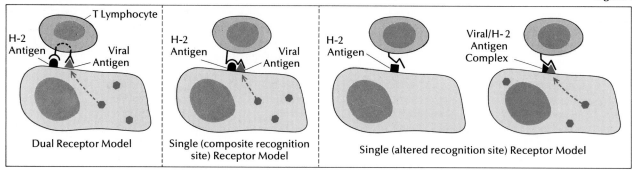

The nature of the T-lymphocyte–receptor structure is still a matter of disagreement. Drawn here (and described in the text) are several of the hypothesized models, each of which could provide for the dual specificity common to immune T cells.

cells – B lymphocytes, macrophages, or infected liver cells – cannot occur. Immunoincompetence results.

Major Transplantation Antigens and CTL

Do the self H-2 cell surface structure determinants play a direct role in the killing of target cells? Building upon the studies of others, we together with Oldstone used the F-9 teratocarcinoma cell line, originally derived from a mouse with an H-2^b haplotype. This cell line does not express major transplantation antigens, i.e., it lacks K and D determinants. Both normal H-2^b and F-9 cells are readily infectable with viruses (see Figure 6 on page 104). Virus-specific killer T cells from H-2^b mice were assayed either on infected macrophages from H-2^b mice or on infected F-9 cells. Although both types of target cells were virus infected, lysis was observed only with the H-2^b cells, not with the F-9. In other words, cells *not* expressing K or D determinants were not lysed by virus immune cytolytic lymphocytes. These results were at least consistent with the interpretation that K- and D-coded determinants, which are normally detected by serologic means, are directly or indirectly involved in killing by virus-specific T cells. They also argued in favor of the proposition that the K and D determinants are either the receptors or a necessary part of the receptors for the lytic message.

Additional evidence that K and D structures are involved in cytolytic interactions stems from work with mutant mice bred by I. K. Egorv in the USSR and by D. W. Bailey and J. J. Kohn at the Jackson Memorial Laboratory and at Harvard. These mutant mice differ from their wild-type ancestors, having undergone mutations in the K or D regions of their H-2 complexes. The results of these experiments indicated that the stronger the skin-rejection reactions between mutant and wild-type animals, the less able were virus-immune T cells from mutant mice to lyse infected target cells of wild-type origin, and vice versa. This suggests the ability to recognize a K or D structure as self and the ability to see it as foreign and destroy it are inversely related.

What is the biologic relevance of the in vitro phenomena we have been describing? That is, what are their roles in immunologic responses to viruses?

Cytolytic T-cell phenomena have been studied for many years (see J.-C. Cerottini), and the role of these lymphocytes in transplant rejection has been well studied. However, the relevance of the reaction except in transplant surgery is unclear.

In experiments done by Blanden in Canberra, and here with R. M. Welsh, the antiviral protective potential in vivo of cytotoxic T cells was tested using a pox virus or lymphocytic choriomeningitis virus. Mice were infected with virus and then, six to eight days later, when killer T-cell levels were at their maximum, spleen cells from these immunized animals were transferred to normal animals that had been infected with the same virus some 20 hours previously, (to allow for expression of viral antigens), as shown in Figure 7 on page 105. These recipient mice were sacrificed 24 hours later in order to assess the number of infectious virus particles in their spleens. A reduction in infectious plaque-forming virus particles indicates that the transferred immune T cells are protecting the virally infected recipient animal. The controls for these experiments were transfers of spleen cells from nonimmune animals or animals immunized with an unrelated virus.

The immune spleen cells caused specific reduction of infectious plaque-forming virus particles in spleens by a factor of about 10,000 as compared with controls. Blanden had demonstrated earlier that the cells involved in this protection were predominantly T lymphocytes, and our experiments now revealed that the protection so afforded required H-2 compatibility at the K and D loci between immune T cells and recipient mice. Lack of such compatibility or compatibility at the I region alone obviated a protective effect. Furthermore, the kinetics of generation of cytotoxic activity in vitro and of the T cells' protective capacity in vivo were virtually identical. Thus, identity of cellular characteristics, kinetics, and H-2 restriction specificities all suggest that the cytotoxic effector T cell assessed in vitro and the antiviral effector T cell tested in vivo are probably the same. These findings, together with results from acute lymphocytic choriomeningitis virus infection of mice, which will be discussed later, are important for understanding the concepts of viral immunity and immunopathology: T-cell–mediated responses to viruses may effect lysis of infected host cells; therefore protection is mediated by host cell destruction.

How Can Virus-Immune Cytolytic T Cells Act Antivirally?

It is worthwhile to recapitulate the stages involved in viral infection of a cell: after virus absorbs and penetrates, its genetic information is integrated into the host cell's genetic replication machinery. Eventually, virus components reassemble, and mature virus is released by budding or by cell decay. Considering these events, it becomes clear that for immune cytolysis to be protective, it must take place reasonably quickly after infection. Indeed, maximum protection can be expected if the target cell is killed and lysed during the "eclipse" phase of the virus, i.e., after the viral antigens are expressed on the cell surface but before new viral progeny assemble. Some protection would still be provided once assembly of new viral progeny was in progress but would steadily diminish. With all new viruses assembled, the cytolytic T cell would cease to be protective.

Thus, virus-immune cytolytic T cells can be regarded as a first line of antiviral defense. The T cell that reaches the infected cell during the virus's eclipse phase can effectively abort the viral infection. However, it is important to emphasize that cytotoxic T cells are certainly not the sole such defense mechanism. Simultaneously, various humoral and cellular mechanisms, such as antibody and complement, lymphotoxins and lymphokines, interferon, and activated macrophages, enter the fray.

Since the foregoing postulates that for cytotoxic T cells to protect a host from viral activity, viral antigens must be expressed on the infected cell's surface before new viral progeny assemble. The question is this: Can such a point in time exist? There is experimental evidence that it does exist. Experiments with vaccinia virus have demonstrated that one can detect viral antigens by fluorescence on almost all target-cell surfaces within three hours after infection. Other experiments show that most new viral progeny assemble between four and eight hours after infection. The dependence of antiviral activity by T cells on the viral

Figure 5

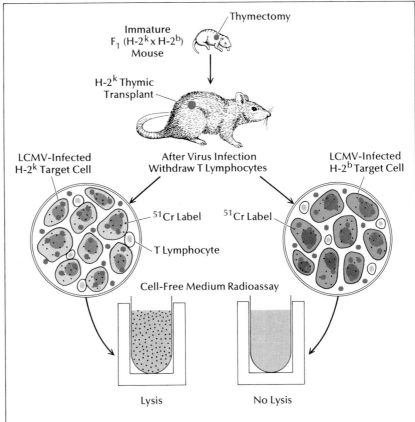

Key experiments supporting the concept that T cells acquire their restricted MHC specificity during differentiation in the thymus are schematized. In these experiments newborn F_1 ($H\text{-}2^k \times H\text{-}2^b$) mice were thymectomized. Subsequently, they were given thymic transplants from mice of the $H\text{-}2^k$ parental strain. When these mice were infected with virus, their lymphocytes were then able to lyse infected $H\text{-}2^k$ but not $H\text{-}2^b$ target cells.

infectious cycle was illustrated by the following experiment (graphed in Figure 8 on page 106). Addition of virus-immune cytotoxic T cells to target cells one hour after infection resulted in a nearly 100% reduction in infectious viral particles produced by these target cells along with almost complete (more than 90%) lysis of the target cells. If the addition of the immune T cells to the acutely infected target cells was postponed until four hours after initiation of target-cell infection, the decrease in virus titer was minimal, although target-cell killing was as great as if cells were added shortly after infection.

There is good evidence that for some viruses, the viral antigen may not even need to be "processed" through the cell's synthetic machinery to be a target for T cells. Several groups (J. Schrader, G. Edelman, and

U. Koszinowski) have shown that Sendai virus particles fuse with the cell membrane and make the cell a recognizable target that is lysed by virus-specific cytotoxic T cells without actual viral replication taking place. It should be noted Sendai virus is a classic fusion virus, and the phenomenon demonstrated in these experiments may be restricted to such viruses.

T-Cell–Mediated Immunopathology of Virus Infections

From the immunopathologic point of view, the rapidity of viral spread and the extent of viral infection at the time when virus-specific cytotoxic T cells arise are of great importance for the clinical outcome of the infection. As already mentioned, cytolytic viruses destroy host cells, and immunity stops

Figure 6

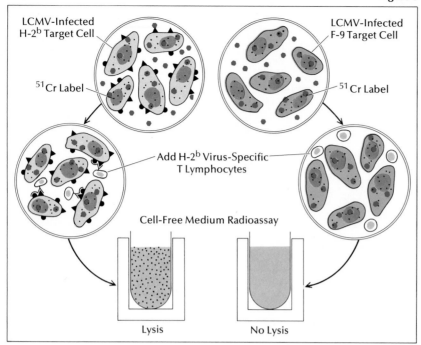

LCMV-Infected H-2^b Target Cell

LCMV-Infected F-9 Target Cell

^{51}Cr Label

^{51}Cr Label

Add H-2^b Virus-Specific T Lymphocytes

Cell-Free Medium Radioassay

Lysis

No Lysis

The probability that the biologic function of transplantation antigens is to provide a mechanism for immune T cells to kill infected target cells is supported by observations involving H-2^b target cells and F-9 target cells. The F-9 are a teratocarcinoma cell line derived from H-2^b mice and are comparable to normal H-2^b cell lines, except that they do not express major transplantation antigen determinants. Virus-specific H-2^b T cells will lyse infected H-2^b target cells but not F-9 cells.

further virus-mediated cell destruction and pathology; the sooner immunity is effective, the less pathology the virus causes. Even when viruses themselves do not harm the cells (e.g., LCM virus), the immune T cells can cause cell destruction and pathology; however, again, the sooner immunity arises, the less the virus spreads and the less pathology is caused by immune "autoaggression."

Early in this article, it was noted that intracerebral LCM virus infection of mice is a particularly interesting model, because the resulting disease appears to be caused by the responding T cells rather than by the virus. Therefore, acute LCM infection may serve as an example for the fact that antiviral cytotoxic T-cell activity is mediated by cell destruction that not only eliminates virus but also produces pathology and disease. It seems obvious that if cytolytic T cells can reach target cells very early in the infection and destroy them before the assembly of viral progeny, the damage will be localized and minimal. If, how-

ever, virus spreads extensively or in a physiologically critical organ, T cells may destroy vital cells. For example, after intracerebral infection, LCM virus spreads preferentially in the choriomeninges. Their destruction results in a breakdown of the blood-brain barrier and a lethal brain edema.

There is reason to believe that this LCM model may resemble human autoimmune hepatitis. If enough of the liver has been invaded by the hepatitis virus, the onslaught of cytolytic lymphocytes could be sufficient to reduce functional live tissue below the threshold required to sustain minimal liver functions. These relationships can be summarized as follows: First, with a highly cytopathic virus, the killer lymphocyte is beneficial, since, from the host's point of view, there is little alternative. Either the T cells will destroy the virus-infected cells or the virus will destroy the functional capacity of the virotropic organ or tissue. Second, under conditions of low viral cytopathogenicity and/or extensive spread of

some viruses in critical organs, the immune response may have a greater capacity to cause tissue damage than the infectious agent itself. It is perhaps no accident that many diseases presumptively classified as autoimmune appear to be associated with such viruses. This relationship suggests that sometimes what we call autoimmunity may in reality be a normal response to autologous cells that have been modified by foreign antigens on their surfaces.

MHC and Disease Susceptibility

These two aspects of T-cell–mediated immunity to viral infection may well be a key to understanding why susceptibility to many diseases seems to be associated with particular major histocompatibility allotypes. The more immunogenic cytopathic viruses are, with respect to inducing H-2 restricted cytotoxic T cells, the better protected is the host. In contrast, if generation of strong T-cell immunity (e.g., because of an H-2 coded defect in immune response regulation) is deficient, susceptibility is increased. As discussed above, for less cytopathic viruses where the T-cell immune response causes immunopathology, the relationship between T-cell immune response and survival is reversed. Here the more immunogenic viruses would *increase* the risk of immunopathologic damage, whereas weak (or defective) immune responses would decrease susceptibility to autoimmune types of virally induced immunopathologic diseases. In fact, most human diseases actually associated with the major transplantation (HLA) antigens are probably of the latter, autoimmune type (rather than examples of decreased responsiveness to acute infection). From a teleologic point of view, this relationship seems reasonable. Evolutionary pressures would be much greater against the survival of low responders to acute or fulminant viral diseases, because many members of a species would die before they could reproduce, whereas with slower, chronic, virally induced immunopathology, the hosts would not succumb until after reproduction.

These arguments can be extended to explain why major transplantation antigens are highly polymorphic and are coded by more than one locus. If only one MHC self marker existed it would be easy for viruses to mimic this antigen in order to escape immune surveillance under the protection of tolerance. However, the polymorphism of the MHC self markers means that only a few members of a species will be in danger of succumbing to a particular virus. This danger is further decreased by gene duplication in the MHC; i.e., there are two genes – HLA-A and B in humans or H-2K and H-2D in mice – that code for lytic cell-surface self markers. In a polymorphic system with gene duplication, heterozygosity for the MHC will be the rule and therefore each individual will possess an array of two to four different self markers coded in the various MHC regions. Thus, polymorphism, together with gene duplication and heterozygosity, will also maximize the immune responsiveness of the individual and optimize its survival.

Intracellular Bacteria

At the outset, we stated that this article would deal with immune responses to intracellular bacteria as well as to viruses. This portion of the discussion will be, of necessity, less extensive, since the relevant knowledge is considerably less developed. As was noted earlier, however, it can be demonstrated that the dual specificity that has been described with respect to self-plus-viral antigens applies also to intracellular bacteria. *Listeria monocytogenes* infection in mice is a relevant model here. The H-2 restriction in this experimental infection parallels that observed in the virus models, in the sense that, on adoptive transfer,

Figure 7

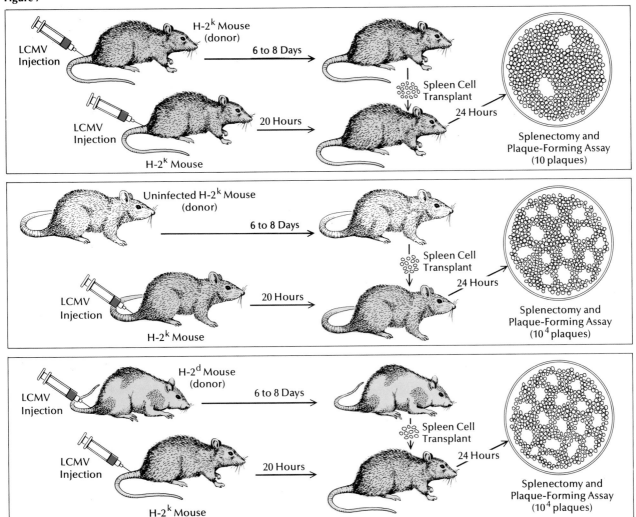

In vivo protection by specifically immune T cells can be shown by adoptive transfer experiments using spleen cells as a source of T cells. The number of viral particles in an infected recipient is determined by a plaque-formation assay in which multiplying virus destroys cells in monolayers, making "holes." An H-2^k mouse is infected with virus. Six to eight days later, its spleen cells are transferred to a syngeneic mouse infected 20 hours earlier; 24 hours later, the recipient is splenectomized. Plaque-forming units in the spleen are reduced by a factor of 10^4 compared with control tests, in which the donor mice are of the same H-2 haplotype, either uninfected or infected with a different virus, or virus-infected mice of a different H-2 type.

The relationship between the infectious cycle of virus and the protection afforded by immune T cells is shown by experiments graphed at the right. When the immune lymphocytes were added one hour after infection of target cells (before measurable increase in virus titers), there was a nearly 100% reduction in the number of virus particles released into the medium as measured by plaque-formation units (PFU). When immune T cells were assayed on the same target cells after four hours, T-cell protection was minimal. At the same time, immune lysis of the target cells exceeded the 90% level both when the immune T lymphocytes were added at one hour postinfection and at four hours postinfection.

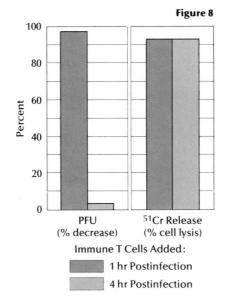

Figure 8

Immune T Cells Added:
█ 1 hr Postinfection
▒ 4 hr Postinfection

listeria-immune T cells can only protect mice that are H-2 compatible with the donor. This has been shown in experiments done cooperatively at Scripps, in Canberra, and at Washington University in St. Louis. However, there is an interesting divergence in responses to virus and intracellular bacteria. Rather than mapping to the K or D regions, the MHC-coded structures involved for effective bacterial response are coded by the I region.

The fact that protection against two of the most significant types of intracellular infection – viral and bacterial – is MHC restricted and mediated through T cells then poses the question: Why should one be controlled by K and D determinants, the other by I determinants? One possible answer is that the cell surface structures coded for by the K and D genes are the receptors, or are linked to the predominant receptors, for the lytic signals that promote T-cell–mediated cell destruction. In viral infections, cell lysis makes teleologic sense as a protective mechanism, because its occurrence during the eclipse phase of the infecting virus provides a means for aborting the infection. On the oth-

er hand, bacteria have no such eclipse phase; therefore, lysis of the infected cells by itself cannot kill intracellular bacteria nor subserve any protective function. Furthermore, viruses can associate with and infect many different types of cells, phagocytic and nonphagocytic, including liver, kidney, or skin cells. But intracellular bacteria can only be taken up by and infect phagocytic cells, such as monocytes or macrophages. Therefore, for antiviral protection, which can function for any type of cell and recognize alteration in any type of cell surface, a T-cell–mediated effector mechanism is needed that can be exerted against all infected cells. The fact that K or D MHC products are expressed universally and ubiquitously on all cells, both phagocytic and nonphagocytic, including T cells, liver, kidney, and skin cells, fits this requirement. In contrast, for intracellular bacteria the restricting MHC-cell surface markers need only be expressed on phagocytic cells. Again, the selective expression of I-region markers on macrophages and certain lymphocytes but not on most other somatic cells is compatible with this requirement. If the T cells

involved in protection against intracellular bacteria are not cytolytic and are not associated with antibody or antibody-producing B lymphocytes, what is their role in protection? A plausible answer is the one suggested by G. Mackaness and coworkers: that T cells probably function through soluble mediators or direct contact, activating macrophages and enhancing digestion of infective bacteria.

From this perspective – which reflects the findings of a great many immunobiologists – one can set forth, at least tentatively, a concept of the biologic functions of major histocompatibility antigens as follows: K- and D-coded structures are themselves receptors or are linked to receptors for lytic signals and permit cytolytic T cells to disrupt target-cell membranes; I-coded structures provide a broad array of cell-specific surface determinants that are receptors for differentiation signals. The latter differentiation signals may trigger antibody production in B cells, suppress activation of T cells, shift production of IgM to IgG in B lymphocytes, turn on or enhance production of proteolytic enzymes in the macrophage, and so on.

In conclusion, this review has sought to summarize the many relationships between T-cell immune phenomena and diseases caused by intracellular parasites, both viral and bacterial. We are only beginning to comprehend some of the underlying mechanisms, and we are still far from understanding either T-cell recognition or such complex phenomena as association of disease susceptibilities with the MHC. But a few more pieces have been added to the puzzle over the last few years. These have not only widened knowledge of basic immunology and the physiology of T cells but also improved our understanding of the pathogenesis and immunopathology of viral disease.

Immunologic Tolerance And Immunopathology

WILLIAM O. WEIGLE   *Research Institute of the Scripps Clinic*

In the framework of most immunologic discussion, normality is defined as a state in which an organism reacts to antigenic stimulation by the elaboration of circulating antibodies and/or by the activation of cells able to attack and destroy foreign tissues or microbial agents. One variation or another of these processes constitutes, in the usual sense, an immune response.

We know, however, that in nature there is a vital necessity for the organism to be immunologically unresponsive to molecules that in other circumstances are antigenic. This necessity is sometimes described as tolerance to "self" and, of course, the breakdown of such self-tolerance is generally considered to be the underlying pathogenetic mechanism in those diseases classified as autoimmune.

The systematic study of immunologic tolerance probably can be traced back more than a quarter of a century to the prediction by Burnet that specific unresponsiveness would result from the injection of antigenic material early in life. It remained for Billingham, Brent, and Medawar in their classic experiments to begin to delineate the conditions for such specific induction of tolerance. In the intervening years, there has been a progressive augmentation of the sophistication with which we can analyze the phenomena of immunologic tolerance. Thus, the recognition of the two discrete populations of immunocompetent lymphocytes – thymus-derived T cells and bone marrow-derived B cells – has made possible analysis of the significance of each in the induction and maintenance of tolerance. Further delineation of functionally different subpopulations of T cells has now made possible the postulation of a specific role for one of those subpopulations – the suppressor T cells – in certain models of tolerance. And because immunologists have shown that different immuno-globulin classes subserve different immunobiologic functions, we are now able to suggest that perhaps one of the factors determining whether the response to antigen will be immunocompetence or tolerance is the class of immunoglobulin on the surface of the responding cell.

All of these facets will be reviewed in this article. However, before doing so let us define further what is meant by immune tolerance. For purposes of arriving at a general definition, I will begin by pointing out that immunologic tolerance is as specific as immunologic responsiveness. It is a state of refractoriness to a particular antigen in some way induced by previous contact with that antigen. Specific unresponsive states that do not require antigen contact but rather are under genetic control have been well documented (see D. H. Katz, "Genetic Controls and Cellular Interactions in Antibody Formation"). The remainder of this review will deal only with specific unresponsive states resulting from contact with the antigen.

In addition, we now recognize two broad types of antigen-directed tolerance: central unresponsiveness, in which there is a functional deletion of cells competent to respond to a specific antigen, and peripheral inhibition, in which competent cells appear to be present but suppressed. Such suppression may be produced by suppressor T cells, by antigen, or by antibody-antigen complexes.

It will be recalled by readers of previous articles in this series that in most immune responses in which the effector phenomenon is the production by B cells of specific humoral antibodies, there must be an interaction between these B cells and T lymphocytes. In these so-called thymus-dependent reactions, tolerance can be achieved by rendering either B cells, T cells, or both, nonresponsive. In most situations, it is the T cell that is tolerant. If one is

Figure 1

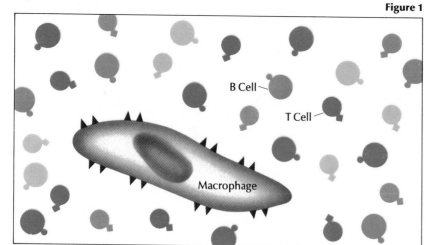

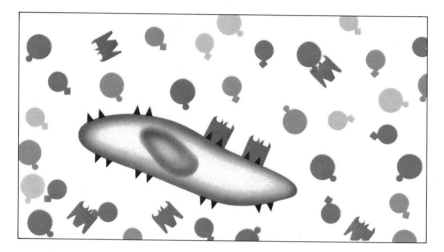

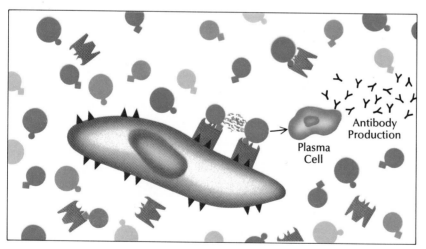

The role of the macrophage may be important in immunologic tolerance because of evidence that macrophages will not fix monomeric (tolerogenic) antigen. Thus, a critical step leading to antibody response may be deleted when competent lymphocytes encounter monomeric antigen. That step is diagrammed sequentially. In the top panel, T lymphocytes and B lymphocytes are depicted surrounding a macrophage, on the surface of which are antigenic receptor sites. When antigen is introduced (middle), both B and T cells are capable of reacting to complementary antigenic determinants. However, the B-T cell interaction necessary for antibody production may require the proximity provided by the macrophage through antigen fixation (bottom).

dealing with B cells derived directly from the bone marrow (and here, as will be seen later, it is important to differentiate between bone marrow cells and peripheral B cells, such as those from the spleen), it has been found that tolerance in such bone marrow cells requires much larger doses of tolerance-inducing antigen (tolerogen), is slower to develop, requires the persistent presence of the specific antigen, and is less durable – all as compared with the T cell. Since this is a critical concept both in understanding tolerance and in the etiology and pathogenesis of autoimmune diseases, let me describe some of the experimentation that helped us to define the relevant cellular kinetics.

The experimental system used to define these kinetic relationships employed as tolerogen, monomeric, or deaggregated, human gamma globulin (DHGG). Monomeric antigen of this type is as fully capable of reacting with host B and T cells as is the usual polymeric, or aggregated, form of HGG. However, the interaction with a monomer will be tolerogenic rather than immunogenic, as in the case of a polymer. It is still not completely understood why this difference exists, but our suspicion on this point, quite strongly supported by experimental evidence, is that the macrophage is implicated. It has been shown that macrophages are involved in the "handling" of antigen and its presentation to both B and T lymphocytes in a way that sterically optimizes the chance for interaction and antibody production, as depicted in Figure 1 on this page. It has been shown by several investigators that macrophages will not fix monomeric antigen. Therefore, it is hypothesized that, in the absence of such fixation, the deaggregated antigen is unable to bridge the gaps between B and T cells, and the exchange of information between helper T cells and B lymphocytes necessary to initiate antibody synthesis does not take place. Instead, the monomeric antigen selects out those lymphocytes capable of reacting with it from the pool of immunoresponsive cells and renders them unresponsive. As a result, subsequent exposure to this antigen, even in its aggregated, or immunogenic, form, will fail to elicit antibody.

At any rate, injection into mice of DHGG will induce tolerance, as shown graphically in Figure 2 on this page. An injection of 2.5 mg of DHGG will result in tolerance to human gamma globulin lasting for 130 to 150 days. The kinetics can now be examined by cell-transfer studies, in which the thymocytes and the marrow cells from the animal injected with tolerogen can be injected into an irradiated recipient animal of the same inbred strain along with cells of the "opposite" lymphocyte class from a third syngeneic animal. I will exemplify the typical findings in such experiments by describing the results that could be expected from such cell transfers conducted at time intervals after tolerogen injection of 10 days, 20 days, 40 to 50 days, and 130 to 150 days.

At 10 days, if the irradiated recipient animal receives thymocytes from the tolerized animal and bone marrow cells from a nonimmunized ("normal") animal, challenge with aggregated (polymeric) HGG will not result in an antibody response. If, on the other hand, the bone marrow cells are derived from the previously tolerized mouse and the thymocytes from a normal mouse, anti-HGG antibody will be produced by the recipient. If one keeps in mind the premise that tolerance in either of the two cell populations will inhibit antibody response, the conclusion from these experiments is that at 10 days after administration of a tolerogen, the bone marrow cells remain responsive, while the thymocytes are already tolerant.

These experiments, repeated at 20 days, will now show that if either the bone marrow cell or the thymocytes transferred into the irradiated recipient are derived from a donor exposed to tolerogenic HGG, the recipient will be unable to make antibody to immunogenic HGG. Apparently, both lymphocyte populations have become tolerant. This bilateral tolerance will persist until 40 or 50 days after the original injection of tolerogen, at which time the situation existing at 10 days will be restored, i.e., tolerance will be exhibited only if the thymus cell transfer is from the tolerized mouse; bone marrow cells from the same animal will be once again re-

Figure 2

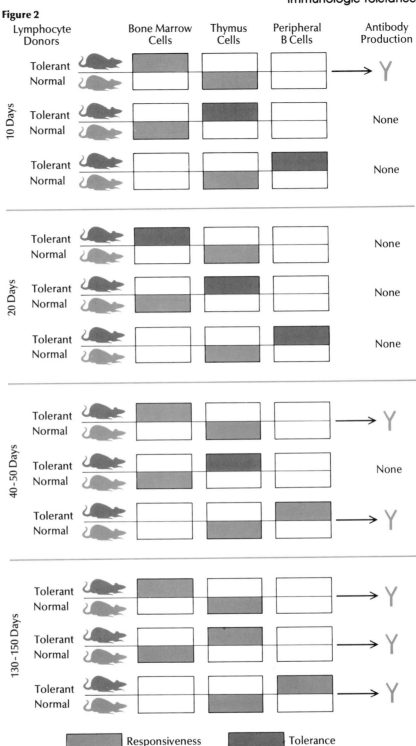

The results of cellular kinetic studies related to tolerance are summarized graphically. Ten days after injection of a tolerogen into donor mice, bone marrow cells from such a donor, injected into an irradiated recipient animal, will interact with normal thymus cells, and antibody will be produced. Both thymus cells and peripheral B cells will have already acquired tolerance. At 20 days, all three lymphocyte populations appear to be tolerant. By 40 to 50 days, both bone marrow and peripheral B cells have regained specific responsiveness to the tolerizing antigen. At 130 to 150 days, T-cell tolerance is lost and the animal will produce antibody to the antigen. No kinetic differences between thymus and peripheral T cells are discernible in these studies.

Table 1

Temporal Patterns of Immunologic Unresponsiveness to HGG in A/J Mice*

Site	Days of	
	Induction	Maintenance
Thymus	<1	120-135
Bone Marrow	8-15	40-50
Spleen: T Cells	<1	100-150
B Cells	2-4	50-60
Whole Animal	<1	130-150

*Injected with 2.5 mg DHGG on day 0

sponsive. And at 130 to 150 days, the immunocompetence of the thymocytes will return.

Within the same experimental design, one could also determine the relationship of dose to tolerance in bone marrow cells and thymocytes. Thus, if one employed three different doses of HGG – 0.1, 0.5, and 2.5 mg – in deaggregated, or tolerogenic, form for immunization of three different mice, and then waited 11 days to check on the immune responsivity of the animals' bone marrow and thymus cells to immunogenic challenge, a sharp difference would be observed in the proportion of bone marrow cells and of thymocytes that had been rendered nonresponsive. For thymocytes, the smallest dose induces tolerance in 96%, and each of the two larger doses achieves tolerance in 99% or more. On the bone marrow side, 0.1 mg induces only 9% of lymphocytes to be tolerant; 0.5 mg, 56%; 2.5 mg, 70%.

Having described these results for cell combinations in which the B-cell populations are contributed by bone marrow and T cells by the thymus – and historically speaking this was the system in which the B and T cellular kinetic differences for tolerance were first defined – let us return to the point made earlier, i.e., that peripheral B cells behave somewhat differently than do bone marrow cells (at the same time, it should be pointed out that the kinetics described for thymocytes have been found to be unchanged for peripheral cells).

In experiments carried out subsequent to the cellular kinetic studies described above, it was found that B lymphocytes from the spleen became specifically unresponsive to antigen within 72 hours after exposure to that antigen in tolerogenic form. Thus, the addition of normal thymocytes (T cells) to the system at this time did not "break" the tolerance to DHGG. From this and other experiments it was concluded that while bone marrow cells were "more resistant" to the induction of tolerance than thymocytes, peripheral B cells developed unresponsiveness in much the same time frame as did thymocytes. The differences between the two B-cell populations could be interpreted as reflective of varying stages of B-cell differentiation in which the functional ability to bind tolerogen is increased with maturation.

Clearly, had these experiments showing that peripheral B cells behaved more like T cells than like bone marrow cells with respect to induction of tolerance been paralleled with respect to duration of tolerance, then the concept of tolerance to thymus-dependent antigens being maintained essentially by T cells would have been refuted. However, fortunately for the integrity of this concept, it was found that the duration of unresponsiveness was similar in peripheral B cells and in bone marrow cells – 40 to 50 days. Thus the premise remained intact.

Taken together, the kinetic parameter of duration, as related to lym-

Figure 3

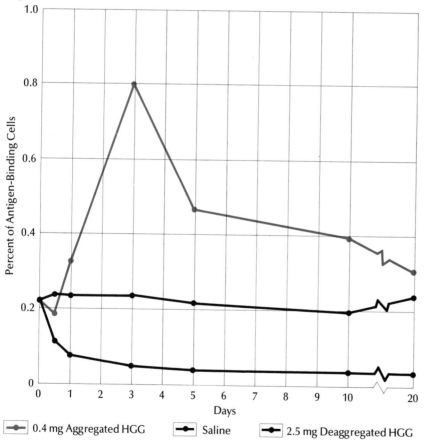

0.4 mg Aggregated HGG | **Saline** | **2.5 mg Deaggregated HGG**

Graph shows the effects of two different physical forms of antigen on the reactivity of mouse spleen cells. Aggregated (immunogenic) human gamma globulin causes immediate rise in specific antigen-binding cells, with a fourfold increase by day three. With deaggregated (tolerogenic) HGG, reactive cells are virtually eliminated.

Figure 4

Immunologic Tolerance

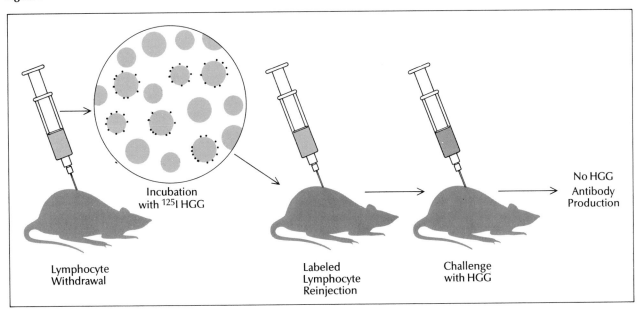

Incubation with ^{125}I HGG

Lymphocyte Withdrawal

Labeled Lymphocyte Reinjection

Challenge with HGG

No HGG Antibody Production

Cell "suicide" experiments have been used in studying tolerance. By incubating lymphocytes with labeled antigen (HGG), one can induce all lymphocytes with receptors to that antigen to self-destruction by surface concentration of radioactivity.

phocyte class (summarized in Table 1 and Figure 3 on page 110), appears to go a long way toward providing a reasonable working hypothesis for the cellular pathology underlying autoimmune disease. It will be recalled that Burnet first proposed that lack of immunity (or tolerance) to endogenous antigens was induced during embryonic or (in species born relatively immature) early postnatal life by exposure of these antigens in the circulation to those cell populations that are destined to differentiate to immunocompetence. An important fact is that this exposure must take place before immunocompetence has been developed. However, there are a number of tissue antigens that are only minimally diffused into the circulation and therefore will only be exposed to lymphocytes in minute quantities. It is reasoned then that for some tissues the antigen dose in immature or embryonic animals may be sufficient to render T cells tolerant but insufficient to do the same with respect to B cells. Or if B-cell tolerance is induced, it will be terminated unless a continuing antigenic stimulus is present in the circulation. Now we have an animal that is living precariously with respect to recognition of the self-nature of tissue components. Only the tolerant T cell stands in the way of autoimmunity.

And significantly, in the experiments described above, even T-cell tolerance eventually breaks down unless it is continuously maintained by repeated or chronic exposure to antigen.

Let us now look at this construction with respect to known autoimmune pathology. A frequently used and highly instructive example is thyroiditis, a disease that of course has well-established autoimmune pathogenesis both in man and in a number of species of experimental animals.

Theoretically, the suggested model of autoimmunity – in which one starts with T-cell tolerance and B-cell responsiveness to an antigen, and then some event or events intervene to circumvent the T-cell tolerance – makes a good deal of sense for thyroiditis. The antigen involved is thyroglobulin, which normally circulates in minute quantities. Experiments have shown that the immune response is thymus-dependent, so that the presence of both competent T cells and competent B cells is required for immune reaction. It seems perfectly plausible to postulate that the amount of thyroglobulin in contact with lymphoid tissues is sufficient to tolerize the T cells prior to their differentiation to immunologic competence but not adequate to do the same for B cells. Or, alternatively, perhaps originally both

T and B cells are made tolerant, but subsequently there is not enough circulating thyroglobulin to sustain tolerance in the B lymphocytes.

There is a good deal of hard experimental evidence to support the reality of this postulation. In mice with thyroiditis, it was shown that the animals have B cells capable of reacting with endogenous thyroglobulin and that these B cells have antigen-specific receptors for the thyroid protein.

An experimental approach that has been used to demonstrate that vulnerability to thyroiditis involves having only T-cell tolerance, along with B-cell responsiveness, is use of the so-called cell suicide technique (see Figure 4, above).

The underlying concept is that one can take a population of immunocompetent lymphocytes and induce self-destruction in all cells precommitted to reaction with a specific antigen by presenting to the population a large dose of antigen heavily labeled with a radioisotope. The precommitted cells will concentrate the antigen on their surfaces, and the resultant radiation exposure will destroy them. Thereafter, that lymphocyte population will be devoid of cells with receptors for the antigen and will be unable to interact immunologically with it, al-

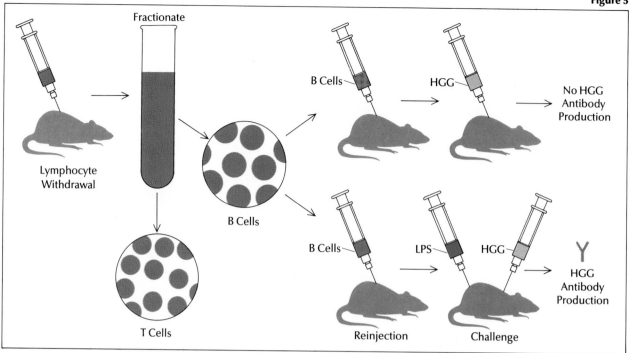

Schematized above are experiments in which all lymphocytes are extracted from an animal. When B cells alone are reinjected, there will be no response to challenge with HGG. When B cells plus lipopolysaccharide (LPS) are injected, antibody is produced, even though the animal still lacks T cells. The concept is that LPS provides mitogenic signal in lieu of T cells.

though as competent as ever to respond to other antigens. In Figure 4, this technique is first exemplified in a system employing HGG labeled with iodine-125.

In the application of this method to thyroiditis, mouse lymphocytes were employed. We separated and purified the B and T cells and successively incubated the two lymphocyte components with ^{125}I-labeled thyroglobulin. The question being posed by these experiments was: Do the mice have either T or B cells capable of interacting with endogenous or syngeneic thyroglobulin?

First the B-cell population was incubated with the labeled antigen, and these B cells were injected into an irradiated mouse along with normal T cells. Upon appropriate challenge with immunogenic thyroglobulin the mouse did not elaborate any circulating antithyroglobulin antibody, nor did it manifest thyroiditis. However, when the T cells were treated with ^{125}I thyroglobulin and injected into the irradiated animal with normal B cells, both an antibody response and thyroid disease ensued. This result emphasized the lack of the need of specific T cells and is further evidence that the T-cell population is tolerant to autologous thyroglobulin.

When those B cells that are competent to respond to antigenic thyroglobulin are destroyed by the suicide technique, autoimmune responsiveness to thyroglobulin is terminated because the capacity to make specific antibody is terminated. On the other hand, incubation with radioactive thyroglobulin leaves the T-cell population essentially unaffected because these cells, being tolerant to thyroglobulin, lack functioning receptors for the thyroglobulin antigens; they are therefore unable to concentrate these antigens on their surfaces and are spared exposure to lethal levels of radioisotope irradiation. This, then, bolsters the hypothesis that tolerance to thyroglobulin is maintained by T cells alone, and is consequently more easily disrupted than tolerance to those self-antigens sustained by both major lymphocyte populations.

In order to complete the picture of tolerance as it is expressed at the cellular level, at least with respect to thymus-dependent immune responses, some additional information with respect to macrophages is needed. In 1968, experiments were performed in our laboratory that showed that it was easier to induce tolerance in some inbred mouse strains than in others. Such strain differences strongly pointed to genetic controls over these differences. By using cell-transfer studies, Leskowitz and his coworkers showed that the facility to develop unresponsiveness was a function of macrophages. The generally accepted belief now is that the more efficient the macrophages are in handling antigen, the less likely is development of tolerance. It is felt that even in a deaggregated, or monomeric, antigenic preparation, there will be some "contamination" by aggregated antigen. If the macrophages are efficient enough, they will select out these trace amounts of immunogen and present them to the T cell, thus preventing tolerogen-induced unresponsiveness.

It was established early in the study of immune tolerance that the physical form of antigen presented to lymphocytes was critical with respect to whether the antigen would act as an immunogen or as a tolerogen. However, only recently has there begun to be an understanding of some of the mechanisms that govern the ability of monomers to turn off the immune responses, whereas polymers of the same antigen turn them on.

Central to these studies has been investigation of the relevancy of lymphocyte receptors, particularly those of B cells. It has long been known that B-cell receptors are immunoglobulin, and that it is the interaction between these surface immunoglobulin molecules and antigen that provides the specificity and the signal for B-cell differentiation to produce antibody. In 1971, Vitetta and Uhr reported that the B cells of adult mice had surface immunoglobulins of two classes, one of which was characterized by μ chains. Subsequently, parallel findings were made in man, with the μ chain molecules identified as IgM, and a second class, with δ chain molecules, as IgD. Although IgD has not been specifically identified in mice, one of the Ig receptors in this species has been characterized as either IgD or IgD-like. The finding that first linked these studies with tolerance phenomena was that in newborn mice the dominant immunoglobulin-receptor class is IgM, with the "IgD" developing later. This observation was then associated with the knowledge that it is much easier to induce tolerance in newborn than in adult mice, so it could be reasoned that this difference might be the result of the class differences in immunoglobulin receptors, with the Fc fragment of the IgM inducing tolerance, and the Fc of the IgD inducing responsiveness.

There are a number of ways in which this could come about. Perhaps the most plausible in terms of the still incomplete evidence on hand is that the IgM on the surface of a B lymphocyte lacks the ability to modulate (perhaps by aggregation) antigen, and that if such a receptor encounters monomeric antigen in the absence of IgD surface receptors, the signal transmitted to the lymphocyte will be tolerogenic. However, if the cell surface also has IgD receptors, the antigen will be aggregated by them and the effect will

Figure 6

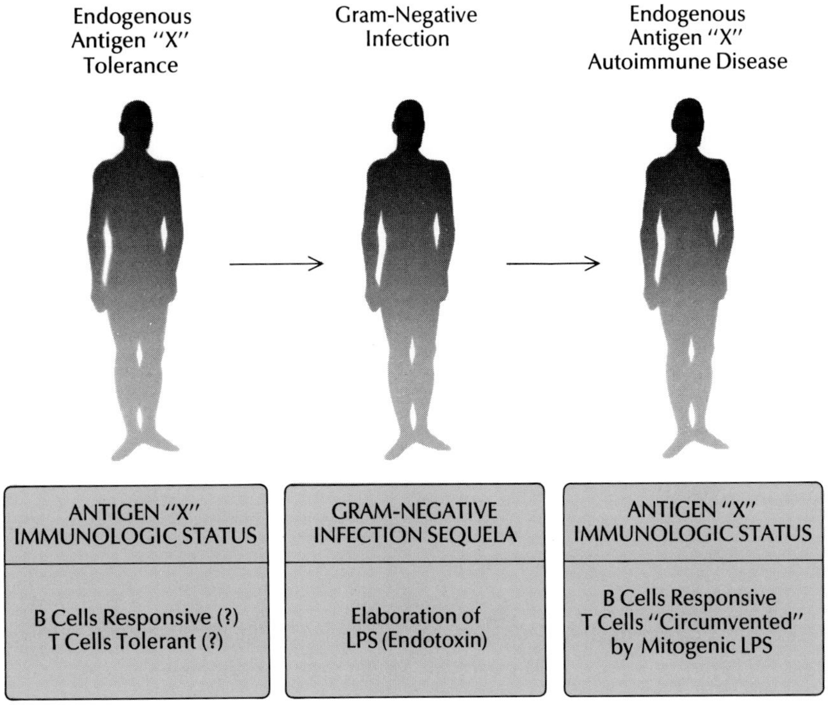

The diagram summarizes a theoretical mechanism for the breaking of autotolerance by endotoxin elaborated in the wake of a gram-negative septicemia. The assumption is that self-tolerance to endogenous antigen "X" is maintained by T cells alone. LPS (endotoxin) would interact with B cells, obviating the need for responsive T cells, and, as a result, autoantibody to antigen "X" would be produced.

be immunogenic. Thus, it is not the interaction with IgM that causes tolerance; rather it is the interaction with IgD that prevents it.

In a sense, then, the natural counterpart of the contrived experiment in which one presents the lymphocyte with polymeric antigen and gets an antibody response, while the presentation of monomeric antigen produces tolerogenicity, may be found in the differential roles of the IgD and IgM receptors. This, of course, still doesn't speak to the problem of why these two opposite reactions occur when two different physical forms of antigen are employed. For a hypothetical approach to this question, one has to look at current thinking on the nature of the signal or signals that turn B cells on to produce antibody.

We know that the cellular phenomena involve the interaction between antigen and B-lymphocyte receptor, with subsequent differentiation of the lymphocyte to plasma cells, and thence to a clonal population of mature antibody-producing B cells.

Since one starts with a single stimulated cell and proceeds to a multitude of specifically induced cells, obviously mitotic events must be interposed. A number of investigators have shown experimentally that antibody production by B cells requires a specific mitogenic stimulus. However, the steps leading up to this ultimate mitogenic stimulus are matters of considerable contention.

In a sense, the areas of dispute, although unquestionably of great importance to eventual understanding of both immune responsiveness and immune tolerance, remain somewhat esoteric. The debates focus on whether one or two signals are required to produce antibody response, or whether the signals originate directly in the activated T cell, or whether the T cell functions through receptors on the macrophage, or whether – if one accepts a two-signal model – tolerance results from the first signal being given without a subsequent second signal ever being given, etc.

Without delving too deeply into this

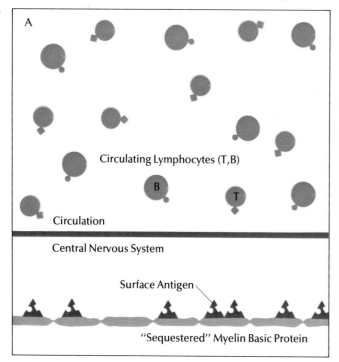

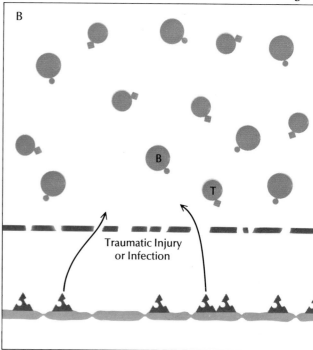

Another possible mechanism for autoimmune disease depends on sensitization of cytotoxic T cells. As exemplified by experimental autoimmune encephalomyelitis in rats, one starts with the antigen – myelin basic protein – sequestered from the circulation by the blood-brain barrier (A). Trauma or infection renders this barrier permeable, and small quantities of basic pro-

network of unsettled questions, it can be noted that most theories, and the evidence supporting them, are compatible with the notion that the final signal for B-lymphocyte differentiation and antibody production is delivered by mitogen. In some way, the mitogen has to be concentrated in proximity to or on the B-cell surface in sufficient quantity to induce the cell to produce antibody. In many situations, the mitogen may be produced by T cells or derived from plant or microbial sources, but in the case of polymerized antigen the need for such mitogens is obviated, and in a sense the antigen itself acts as a mitogen. Monomeric antigen, however, does not possess a repeating structure and therefore will not meet the quantitative needs of the B lymphocyte in differentiating to a dividing and antibody-producing cell population without participation of the helper T cell.

This line of reasoning suggests that for thymus-dependent antigens, T cells, after recognizing appropriate determinants on the antigen, are activated, allowing soluble factors to act mitogenically on the B lymphocyte; in this way the mitogenic requirements for antibody production can be met. As for so-called thymus-independent antigens, it is suggested by some investigators that this class is restricted to naturally polymeric molecules that do not require the participation of T cells or macrophages. The signal of mitogenic stimulation of the B cells comes directly from the interaction between those cells and the antigen.

A major portion of the experimental basis for these hypotheses has been developed in work with lipopolysaccharides (LPS) such as the gram-negative bacterial endotoxins. One of the characteristics of LPS not usually thought about in connection with their role in infectious diseases and their sequelae is that they are powerful B-cell mitogens. It is this property that has made them a significant tool for studying immunologic phenomena.

As depicted in Figure 5 on page 112, one can induce B cells to produce antibodies to thymus-dependent antigens in T-cell-depleted animals by injecting the antigen with LPS. In terms of the signal models alluded to above, this has been interpreted by different investigators in various ways:

1) If a two-signal system is accepted, then the antigen provides one signal, and the LPS, *substituting for the T cell,* provides the other by stimulating the B lymphocyte to undergo mitotic division.

2) If one adheres to the concept of a one-signal model, then the antigen can be viewed as necessary only for binding the T and B cells together, so that the mitogenic signal received by the B cell in this experimental system is the only one needed for the B cell to be stimulated to produce antibody. Obviously, however, such a signal would be nonspecific, and antigen would still be required in a natural situation to interact with those B lymphocytes that are capable of elaborating specific antibody.

At any rate, we have used the mitogenicity of LPS to study tolerance. What we did was to employ the cellular kinetic timing parameters discussed earlier to select animals that were unable to respond to an antigen because, although their B cells had regained competence, their T cells were

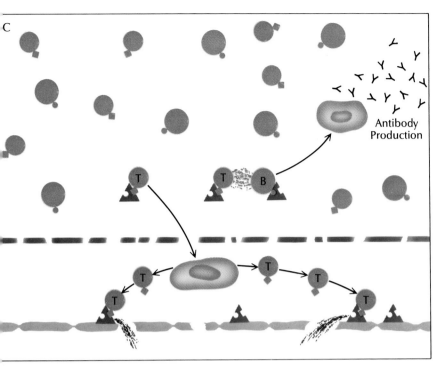

C

Antibody
Production

tein leak into the circulation (B). Both B and T cells are sensitized. While antibody is produced, this is not thought to be the mechanism for disease. Rather, the attack on myelin by activated specific cytotoxic T cells is believed responsible (C).

still in a tolerant phase. If antigen alone was injected into these animals, no antibody was detectable; but if antigen plus LPS was used, specific antibody was produced. In other words, the LPS circumvented the T-cell defect, effectively substituting for the T cells in the immune response. However, if tolerant animals were selected at a time when both B and T lymphocytes maintained tolerance (and this, of course, could be confirmed by cell-transfer experiments), the LPS did not restore specific responsiveness to the injected antigen. Apparently, whatever it is, the signal transmitted by the T cell can also be transmitted by the strongly mitogenic endotoxin molecule.

Is there an in vivo correlate of this laboratory demonstration of the ability of endotoxin to terminate an antigen-specific unresponsive state? Although the question remains unanswered, the possibilities are both intriguing and potentially of great significance with respect to immunopathology. It will be recalled that we have mentioned that some antigens circulate in extremely small quantities. Thyro-

globulin was cited; growth hormone and alpha fetoprotein are two other examples. There is good evidence that self-tolerance for these proteins is maintained entirely by the T cells, with B-cell immunocompetence. The precariousness of this state of immunologic affairs, implied earlier, can be all the more readily appreciated if we now add to the picture realization that bacterial lipopolysaccharides – endotoxin – can replace T cells in an immune response. One can now see how an infection, particularly one caused by gram-negative organisms (although viral products too have been shown to be mitogenic), could set off a train of events leading to, for example, antithyroglobulin antibody formation and "autoimmune" thyroiditis. This postulated sequence is illustrated in Figure 6 on page 113.

Another mechanism by which tolerance to T cells only could be circumvented in nature involves cross-reactivity between endogenous surface antigens and bacterial or viral antigens. Such a mechanism has been postulated with respect to cardiac M protein and the streptococcus. As with the tis-

sue antigens mentioned previously, M protein circulates in extremely minute amounts. It is a likely candidate as an antigen for which tolerance is maintained only by T cells. However, a streptococcal infection will elicit a T-cell response to a number of antigens, including those that cross-react with the myocardial protein. In effect, one can visualize a situation in which the bacterial infection contributes the necessary T-cell component against an antigen to which B-cell competence already exists. Now the host has all of the necessary reactive cells to mount an autoimmune attack on cardiac tissue. It is not known, however, whether this mechanism is directly involved in the pathogenesis of rheumatic heart disease.

All these examples so far have involved low-dose antigenic phenomena favoring B competence and T tolerance, and it is likely that this is a critical area in the pathogenesis of autoimmune diseases. However, it should be pointed out that there are experimental situations in which one can show the development of autoimmune phenomena resulting from the presence of competent lymphocytes in both B and T classes. Such a case is experimental allergic encephalomyelitis in rats. This disease can be produced by injecting syngeneic myelin basic protein into the footpad of the animal (see Figure 7 above). Now one sees both B-cell and T-cell responses eventuating in cerebral damage. The difference here is that the myelin protein is normally completely sequestered, with not even enough circulating to tolerize the T cells. What would be required naturally to incite autoimmunity would be some traumatic or infectious injury that caused the uncovering of sequestered antigens and their exposure to the circulation. Interestingly, the findings in these studies are that the actual organic damage results from the activation of cytotoxic T cells, which leads to an increase of vascular permeability and inflammation.

At the outset of this presentation, two distinctive types of tolerance were specified: central unresponsiveness, resulting from the functional deletion or paralysis of antigen-reactive cells, and peripheral inhibition. To this point, our discussion has been entirely on the various aspects of the first, "true" tolerance, if you will. Let us turn now to some of the phenomena that can be classified as forms of peripheral inhibition.

To introduce this section, I will summarize some experiments that have been done with New Zealand (NZB × W) F_1 mice. With age, these inbred animals frequently develop an autoimmune disease not unlike lupus nephritis in humans. Young New Zealand animals do not manifest the nephritic syndrome. Investigators have shown that as an older mouse begins to have the signs and symptoms of lupus, an injection of T lymphocytes from young animals of the same strain will halt the disease process. It has become clear that some cells or cellular factors, present in the young but lost with age, are protective.

In their presentation, E.A. Boyse and H. Cantor ("Surface Characteristics of T-Lymphocyte Subpopulations") point out that T cells differentiate into at least three functionally and morphologically separable subclasses, or sets, and that one of these is capable of inhibiting or turning off the B-cell response to an antigen. It has been claimed that suppressor T cells are central to the interpretation of the resistance that young New Zealand mice seem to possess against a disease that is apparently genetically determined in their strain. It is suggested that the young animals are endowed with such cells along with immunocompetent T cells and B cells that are capable of reacting to nuclear components. Although a loss of suppressor activity has been reported with increase in age, it has also been well documented that aged mice with autoimmune disease have an increased number of suppressor cells. It may be that during early life there is a transient loss of suppressor cells associated with initiation of an autoimmune process. However, the status of suppressor cells in the autoimmune phenomena in New Zealand mice is not yet resolved.

It is still too early to attribute any human diseases to failure of this form of peripheral inhibition, although there has been some suggestive evidence from several laboratories that such a phenomenon could be involved in lupus pathology.

There are several other forms of immunologic unresponsiveness that do not relate to the incompetence per se of antigen-reactive cells. One is the so-called enhancing or blocking antibody phenomenon that has been widely studied in relationship to tumor and transplant immunology. The concept one is dealing with is actually immunologic competition in which the foreign or antigenically altered tissue (the allograft or the tumor) evokes both a humoral antibody response and a cytotoxic T-cell response. In both situations it is the cell-mediated component that is capable of attacking the activating antigenic determinants; and in both it has been postulated that humoral antibody may be able to preempt the antigenic receptors and abort the cytotoxic response by such blockage. In the case of allografts, the result would be protection and toleration of the transplanted organ; in the case of the tumor, it would be protection against effective, i.e., tumor-destructive, immunologic responses, and therefore enhancement of tumor growth would result.

Finally, let me mention briefly one other form of transient tolerance that has been the subject of a great deal of study, i.e., the unresponsiveness that has been associated with so-called exhaustive differentiation. The theoretical basis of this is that it may be possible for an antigen to be introduced into a host in a dose so massive that it will engage, in a short time span, all of the functional lymphocyte lines genetically capable of specific response. All of these lines, including the appropriate precursor cells, will differentiate into antibody-producing cells. Additional antigen will then be tolerated simply because there are no further lymphocyte precursors able to respond, at least during the period required for regeneration. It should be added that it is extremely difficult to demonstrate this phenomenon in any experimental system, although it quite possibly does occur in nature and could even account for occurrence of overwhelming infections.

At the beginning of this presentation, it was noted that the systematic study of immunologic tolerance is now about a quarter of a century old. It was also pointed out that the last few years have been particularly fruitful because those of us working in the field have been able to transfer to it the great advances in sophistication resulting from increased understanding of genetic mechanisms and of the molecular interactions and complex cellular components and events that make up our immune defenses. In closing, it must be conceded that these advances have not yet brought us to the point at which we can prophesy the directions that will bring us to a full understanding of that remarkable homeostatic complex that is immune tolerance.

Lymphocyte Maldistribution And Immunodeficiency

MARIA DE SOUSA   *Sloan–Kettering Institute for Cancer Research*

The quantitative and morphologic evaluation of the lymphoid component of the peripheral blood traditionally has been the clinical measure of an individual's immunologic status. Blood studies are an important aspect of clinical studies, but the peripheral blood is only one compartment through which the lymphocytes circulate, and recent studies have made it clear that any attempt to investigate a disease of the lymphoid system is incomplete if only that compartment is analyzed. Lymphocyte depletion in the blood may mean that lymphocytes are accumulating elsewhere. Similarly, lymphocytosis may mean that cells are failing to circulate normally. In either case, lymphocyte maldistribution will have functional consequences, and indeed may be relevant to the pathogenesis of the immunodeficiency in certain apparently unrelated diseases, including lepromatous leprosy, Hodgkin's and Crohn's diseases, mycosis fungoides, systemic lupus erythematosus (SLE), alcoholic hepatitis, and a number of other chronic liver diseases (see Figure 1 on page 119).

Before considering those states in which lymphocyte maldistribution has been shown to occur, it is worthwhile to review normal lymphocyte circulation. Much has been learned since J. L. Gowans's demonstration that lymphocytes are long-lived cells whose rapid turnover in the blood is explained by their continuous circulation into the lymph through the peripheral lymphoid organs (see Figure 2 on page 120).

Both T and B lymphocytes circulate from blood to lymph, using common routes of entry and exit from the spleen, lymph nodes, and Peyer's patches in the gut. Within the lymphoid organs, however, they migrate and arrange themselves discretely and territorially (see Figure 3 on page 121).

On the basis of the specificity of lymphocytic territorial distribution, we have called the transit of these cells "ecotaxis." Studies using radiolabeled mouse thoracic duct or lymph-node lymphocytes have shown that within 24 hours after intravenous injection into genetically identical, syngeneic hosts, 70% to 80% of labeled cells have migrated to distinct T-cell and B-cell areas of the peripheral lymphoid organs. In the spleen, the outer regions of the white pulp, or malpighian bodies, where the germinal centers develop, consist mostly of B cells. T cells that enter the perifollicular and red-pulp areas of the spleen localize in the periarteriolar sheath, which is a thymus-dependent area. In the lymph nodes, the medulla, which consists of the sinuses and cords, is occupied mostly by maturing B cells, plasma cells, and macrophages. The outer cortical area of primary nodules where germinal centers develop also consists mostly of B cells. T cells that enter the postcapillary venules in the midcortex of the lymph nodes localize around these vessels. In Peyer's patches, the lymphoid tissue of the gut, B cells are found in the germinal centers and cortical areas and T cells in the dome and interfollicular areas.

Thus, unlike the heart, the liver, and the kidney, the peripheral lymphoid organs consist of nomadic cell populations of small lymphocytes that are in constant transit between the blood and the lymph. The molecular basis for lymphocyte ecotaxis is not known, but several recent findings may be relevant to the lodging of T and B lymphocytes in specific microenvironments within the lymphoid organs. Ultrastructural studies by J. E. Veldman of the reticulum framework in the stroma of the spleen and lymph nodes have revealed features peculiar to the T- and B-cell areas. In the thymus and thymus-dependent areas of the spleen and lymph nodes, the reticulum framework surrounds interdigitating cells with dendritic processes (IDC) and has an "open" structural pattern (see Figure 4 on page 122). The medulla in the lymph nodes, the equivalent medullary region in Peyer's patches, and the peritrabecular areas in the splenic red pulp contain most of the antibody-producing (B-cell) lymphocyte populations. The reticulum framework in these areas has a characteristic "closed" pattern containing single cells. The nodular peripheral areas in splenic follicles and in the outer cortex of the lymph nodes and Peyer's patches contain little reticulum and have a different type of dendritic cell, designated dendritic reticulum cell (DRC).

Another finding, from this laboratory, concerns the role of T-cell phenotype in the ecotaxis of lymphocytes to specific anatomic compartments within lymphoid organs and the influence exerted by the presence of selected T-cell subsets on the morphology of peripheral lymphoid organs. As is well known, T lymphocytes may function as helpers of B cells in the antibody response, as B-lymphocyte suppressors, and as cytotoxic or killer cells. Although these T-cell subpopulations are morphologically indistinguishable, E. A. Boyse and H. Cantor showed that they can be identified by certain cell-surface components. One surface component, known as Ly1, identifies helper T cells, and another, known as Ly23, identifies cytotoxic or killer cells (see E. A. Boyse and H. Cantor, "Surface Characteristics of T-Lymphocyte Subpopulations").

Our study of the fate of labeled Ly1 and Ly23 mouse lymphocytes injected into syngeneic hosts demonstrated Ly1 cells and Ly23 cells differ not only in immunologic function but in their pattern of distribution within lymphoid tissues. In addition, a much higher inci-

dence of germinal centers was found in the spleen and lymph nodes of B mice reconstituted with T-helper cells than in B mice reconstituted with unselected T cells or Ly23 cells. These findings indicate that the positioning of lymphocytes within the lymphoid organs is a function of cell phenotype and that ultimately one can read this contribution of individual cellular components in the morphology of the peripheral lymphoid organs.

In mammals, the tempo of circulation from blood to lymph is different for T and B lymphocytes. Labeled thoracic-duct and lymph-node B lymphocytes from mice and rats have been shown to have a slower tempo of circulation than thoracic-duct T lymphocytes (see Figure 5 on page 123). At one hour after intravenous injection into syngeneic recipients, 47% of labeled T cells are found in the spleen and lymph nodes and only 22% in the lungs and liver, whereas only 17% of B cells have reached the spleen and lymph nodes at one hour and 58% are still in the lungs and liver. This difference has been interpreted as reflecting a relatively longer sojourn of B cells in the major capillary networks and may be due to intrinsic differences in lymphocyte subpopulations, as well as to the functional need of B cells to be available in the circulation for antigen encounter.

The tempo of lymphocyte circulation is influenced by interactions between circulating cells and interactions with the territory crossed by the cells. One factor probably involved in controlling the tempo of lymphocyte circulation in vivo is a low molecular weight substance secreted by lymphocytes that we have called interaction modulation factor (IMF). T and B lymphocytes secrete different IMFs that modulate the adhesive interactions between lymphocytes in vitro. These interactions may also occur within lymphoid organs. The rate at which a lymphocyte travels in a given environment also may be influenced by factors produced by other cells in that environment.

As might be expected, alterations

in the lymphocytes or in the territory they cross change the normal pattern of circulation. Any modification of the lymphocyte surface results in reduced entry into lymph nodes and a concomitant increase in the number of cells that enter other compartments, particularly the spleen, lungs, and liver. For example, treatment of lymphocytes with neuraminidase causes a temporary sequestration of the treated cells in the liver. Treatment with trypsin causes an accumulation of lymphocytes in the blood. Concanavalin A, which binds to lymphocyte cell surfaces, causes an initial delay in the lungs and, later, an accumulation in the splenic white pulp. Treatment with lipopolysaccharides and phospholipases also alters lymphocyte circulation and delays entry into lymph nodes. Lipopolysaccharides cause an accumulation of lymphocytes in the spleen, and phospholipase A treatment results in a considerable holdup in the lungs. Changes in the territory through which the lymphocytes circulate also alter the normal pattern of circulation. Experimental modification of the lymphoid organs by irradiation, stress, or the injection of antigens or adjuvants can result in transient sequestration of lymphocytes in various compartments of the circulation. Subcutaneous injection of an antigen causes a temporary accumulation of lymphocytes in the lymph node that drains the site of injection. If the antigen is injected intravenously or intraperitoneally, the sequestration occurs in the spleen. Administration of the adjuvant dextran sulfate causes trapping of lymphocytes in the marginal zone of the spleen.

Most experimental models of abnormal lymphocyte circulation have a transient duration. In the experiments just described, the lymphocyte maldistribution resulting from enzyme, antigen, or adjuvant treatment lasted for less than 48 hours. The value of an experimental model, however, is to prove that a certain event can happen. That it can happen experimentally should alert us to the possibility that it can also occur in nature. In several disease

Figure 1

Lymphocyte Maldistribution in Selected Diseases

Hodgkin's Disease

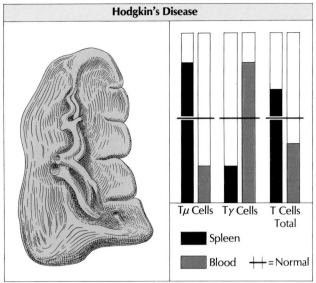

Tμ Cells   Tγ Cells   T Cells Total

■ Spleen
▧ Blood   ╫ = Normal

Crohn's Disease

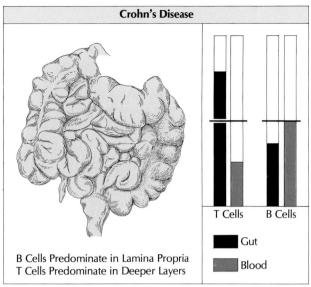

T Cells   B Cells

■ Gut
▧ Blood

B Cells Predominate in Lamina Propria
T Cells Predominate in Deeper Layers

Alcoholic Hepatitis; Chronic Active Hepatitis

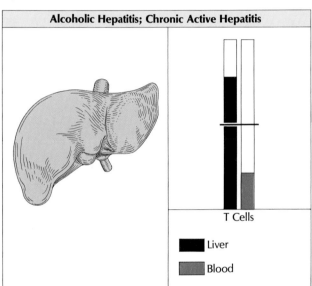

T Cells

■ Liver
▧ Blood

Rheumatoid Arthritis

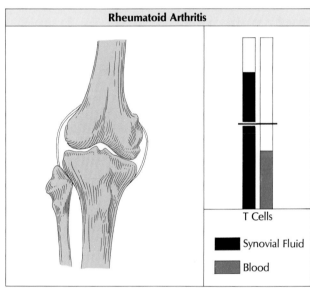

T Cells

■ Synovial Fluid
▧ Blood

Multiple Sclerosis; Aseptic Meningitis

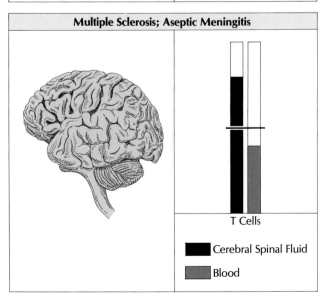

T Cells

■ Cerebral Spinal Fluid
▧ Blood

Tuberculosis

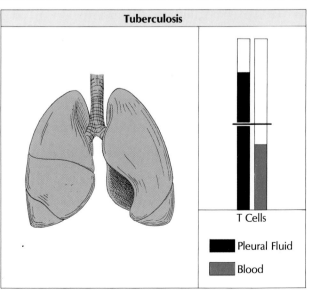

T Cells

■ Pleural Fluid
▧ Blood

states associated with immune deficiency, there is evidence that lymphocyte maldistribution rather than an absolute lymphocyte deficit occurs (see Figure 1).

Hodgkin's disease is associated with a well-recognized depression of the T cell–mediated immunity. This impairment in cell-mediated immunity is associated with anergy and increased susceptibility to certain types of infection, and the degree of lymphocytopenia correlates with the clinical stage of disease.

With the adoption of surgical staging of Hodgkin's disease by laparotomy with splenectomy and lymph-node biopsy, it became possible to examine not only the blood but other compartments of the circulation for evidence of selective T-cell depletion in patients with Hodgkin's disease. From studies in this laboratory as well as others, it has become apparent that large numbers of T cells are present in the spleens of patients with Hodgkin's disease, coincident in some cases with depletion of T cells in the peripheral blood.

Furthermore, differences in immunologic function of the lymphocytes in the peripheral blood and spleen have been detected. Peripheral blood lymphocytes from patients with Hodgkin's disease generally fail to respond in vitro to the mitogen phytohemagglutinin (PHA), whereas spleen cells from the same patients respond normally. We suspected that the dichotomy in mitogenic response between peripheral blood and spleen lymphocytes represented the absence of a specific T-cell subpopulation in the peripheral blood. Recent studies by S. Gupta and C. Tan at this institution have shown that the majority of T cells in the spleens of children with Hodgkin's disease belong to the subset defined by the cell-surface Fc IgM receptor. These are known as Tμ cells, and they are believed to be helper cells in interactions between T cells and B cells. Depletion of the Tμ subset was found in the peripheral blood of the same patients.

Normally, both Tμ and Tγ cells (which are identified by the pres-

Figure 2

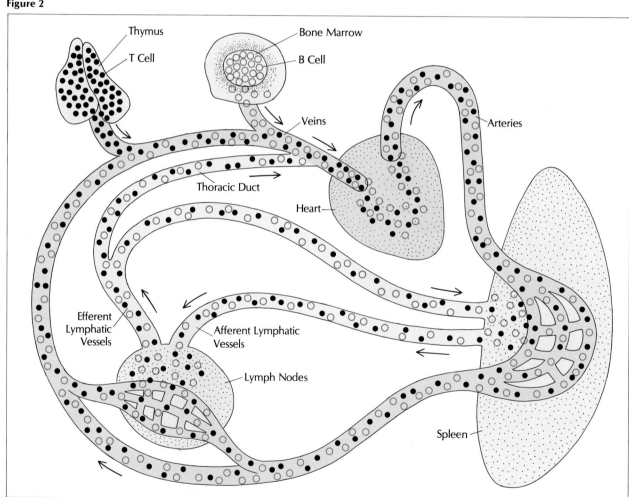

Lymphocytes move constantly in a dual circuit. From their sites of origin in the thymus (T cells) or bone marrow (B cells), they enter the blood, pass through the capillary networks, and enter the lymphatic circulation in the lymphoid organs, such as the spleen and lymph nodes. From the lymph circulation they pass back into the blood via such routes as the thoracic duct.

ence of cell membrane Fc IgG rather than the IgM receptor) are present in both the peripheral blood and the spleen. Tγ cells are believed to function as suppressor cells of B-cell differentiation to antibody-secreting cells. In the children with Hodgkin's disease studied by Gupta and Tan, Tγ cells were increased in the peripheral blood and depleted in the spleen. Thus, Hodgkin's disease appears to be associated with a maldistribution of subsets of T cells, with helper T cells increased in the spleen and depleted from the peripheral blood and suppressor T cells increased in the peripheral blood and depleted from the spleen.

From this finding, several functional consequences can be predicted. One is that the imbalance of T-cell populations in the periphery relates to the deficient cell-mediated immunity observed in these patients. Another is an effect on humoral immune function and immunoglobulin production. The increase in helper T lymphocytes in the spleen should be accompanied by changes in B-cell function and immunoglobulin production. Indeed, increased levels of serum IgG and IgA are frequently found in patients with Hodgkin's disease. Synthesis of these classes of immunoglobulin is known to be thymus-dependent.

Our interpretation of these findings is that in Hodgkin's disease, large numbers of T cells are sequestered in the spleen, where they function normally. The presence of unusually large numbers of T cells in the spleens of patients with Hodgkin's disease, at all stages of the disease, also has been reported by other investigators. The finding that the splenic lymphocytes in patients with Hodgkin's disease are normally responsive to PHA stimulation but the peripheral blood lymphocytes of the same patients are not suggests that sequestration of normally responsive T lymphocytes in the spleen occurs concomitantly with the appearance in the peripheral blood of a nonresponsive thymus-derived lymphocyte population. Therefore, the known anomalies of lymphocyte number and

Figure 3

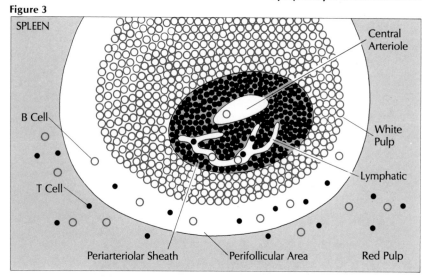

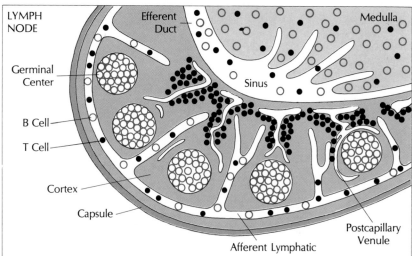

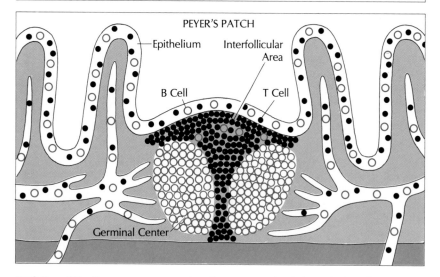

Both B and T cells use common routes of entry to and exit from the lymphoid organs, but within the organs they occupy separate territories. T cells localize around the periarteriolar sheath in the spleen, around the postcapillary venules in the cortex of the lymph nodes, and in the dome and interfollicular areas of Peyer's patches. B cells are found in the white pulp of the spleen, in both the germinal centers of the cortex and the medulla of the lymph nodes, and in the germinal centers of Peyer's patches.

Figure 4

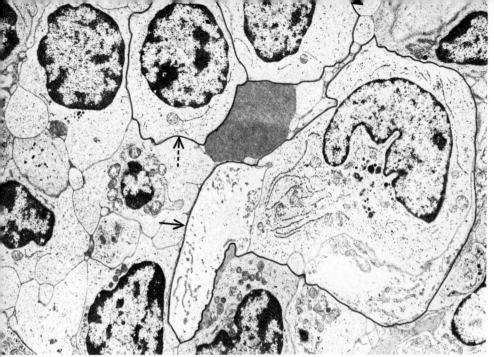

Ultrastructure studies have revealed different patterns in T- and B-cell areas of lymphoid organs. In human lymph node, T-cell areas have "open" reticulum and interdigitating cells (solid arrow) that interact with small lymphocytes (dashed arrows). EM courtesy of E. Kaiserling and K. Lennert, Kiel, West Germany. Their work has clarified the significance of environmental cell interactions in lymphomas.

function in the peripheral blood in Hodgkin's disease appear to reflect a maldistribution of T lymphocytes in the body rather than an absolute T-cell deficit.

Further evidence of lymphocyte sequestration in the spleen in Hodgkin's disease is seen in the effect of splenectomy on lymphocyte circulation and function. If T lymphocytes are sequestered in the spleen, an improvement in T-lymphocyte function would be expected to follow splenectomy. We examined the question in two children with Hodgkin's disease who were of the same sex and age, who were diagnosed clinically as stage 1-A, and who received the same treatment—irradiation of the involved lymph node—but one was splenectomized and the other was not. The peripheral blood lymphocyte response to PHA was used as the indicator of T-cell function and was tested before and at several intervals after splenectomy. Recovery of the response to values within the control range occurred more rapidly in the splenectomized patient than in the nonsplenectomized patient. In general, patients at all stages of Hodgkin's disease who are doing well

clinically show a return of the PHA response toward normal, and patients who are doing poorly or who relapse show persistently low responses to PHA.

Abnormalities of immune function (specifically, lack of cutaneous delayed hypersensitivity and weak lymphocyte response to PHA) similar to those seen in Hodgkin's disease have also been reported in patients with Crohn's disease. R. G. Strickland et al found evidence of T-cell sequestration in the involved colon and ileum of two patients with Crohn's disease. Examination of the resected tissues revealed lymphocytic infiltration in all layers of the bowel wall except within the superficial epithelium. In the mucosal lamina propria from either colon or ileum, the predominant cells were B cells, but in the deeper layers, 60% to 70% of the lymphocytic infiltrate were T cells. At the time of surgery, proportions and absolute numbers of peripheral blood T cells were decreased in both patients, whereas the proportions and numbers of B cells were normal. Two to six months after surgery, T-cell proportions and numbers had returned to normal, and

B-cell values remained normal. These findings indicate a clear-cut T-cell maldistribution in Crohn's disease.

Imbalances between peripheral blood and liver lymphocyte distribution were demonstrated by J. Sanchez-Tapias, H. C. Thomas, and S. Sherlock in a number of patients with chronic liver disease in whom lymphocytes were isolated from both sources. The percentages of lymphocytes identified as T cells in liver biopsy specimens were significantly higher than in peripheral blood in patients with alcoholic hepatitis or chronic active hepatitis, whether HB_sAg positive or negative, and not significantly different in patients with fatty liver, inactive alcoholic cirrhosis, or chronic persistent hepatitis.

The accumulation of mononuclear cells and plasma cells in non-lymphoid organs is one of the pathologic and diagnostic features of the connective tissue diseases. Studies of the proportions of T and B lymphocytes in the peripheral blood and synovial fluid of patients with rheumatoid arthritis have been carried out by a number of investigators. In the majority of cases studied, the proportion of T cells found in synovial fluid has been higher than the proportion in the **peripheral blood. Recent reports of success in treatment of rheumatoid arthritis with total lymph node irradiation represent a further indication, albeit indirect, of the importance of controlling lymphocyte migration to the joints in the management of the disease.**

The occurrence of lymphocyte maldistribution in patients with SLE is largely speculative, but P. D. Utsinger found that the lymphopenia always present in the disease is associated with decreases in peripheral blood T and B lymphocytes, and the more severe lymphopenia observed during active stages of the disease is attributable largely to further decreases in T-cell numbers. There is evidence that "autoimmune" formation of immune complexes in SLE is the result of a failure or dearth of suppressor T cells. Therefore, the question of whether

T-cell depletion occurs is even more specific.

In two central nervous system diseases, evidence has been found of T-cell accumulation in the cerebrospinal fluid. Several investigators have found patients with multiple sclerosis or aseptic meningitis to have significantly higher percentages of T cells in the CSF than in the peripheral blood.

The distribution of T and B lymphocytes in peripheral blood and pleural fluid in patients with pleurisy of various etiologies was recently examined by T. Petterson and associates. There were no significant differences in the percentages of T cells between pleural fluid and peripheral blood, except in pulmonary tuberculosis. In these patients, both the percentages and absolute numbers of T cells were higher in pleural fluid. The percentages of B lymphocytes, on the other hand, were lower in peripheral blood in all patients except those with congestive cardiac failure and were significantly lower in patients with tuberculosis, pulmonary malignancies, and nonspecific effusions.

A significant reduction in peripheral blood T-cell numbers is known to occur in a proportion of patients with solid primary or metastatic cancer, but the decrease has not been related either to the extent of local tumor infiltration by T cells or to the presence of disseminated disease. Direct studies of the fate of labeled lymphocytes in patients with chronic lymphatic (B-cell) leukemia done by K. Bremer and associates, and more recently by J. Wagstaff and coworkers, have revealed an impairment in the circulation of B leukemia cells from blood to central (thoracic-duct) lymph.

The basis of lymphocyte maldistribution in the examples cited above is not known, but an association between lymphocyte sequestration and pathology has been demonstrated in mycosis fungoides and in murine leprosy. Mycosis fungoides is characterized by an accumulation of lymphoid cells in the skin. One consequence of this maldistribution of circulating cells is their depletion from other circu-

latory compartments, as was dramatically illustrated in a case reported by R. Edelson's group now at Columbia University. In one patient, they demonstrated that episodes of cutaneous infiltration coincided with sharp decreases in the peripheral blood lymphocyte count (see Figure 6 on this page).

In human lepromatous leprosy, a depression of T-cell function is also well documented. After successful treatment, T-cell function returns to normal. Experiments by W. E. Bullock Jr. at the University of Kentucky in murine leprosy, the model for human lepromatous leprosy, demonstrated that a sequestration of circulating lymphocytes occurs in the spleen of infected rats. Murine leprosy is a slowly progressive disease that attacks lymphoid organs with a high degree of specificity. Six to 10 weeks after infection, the paracortical areas of lymph nodes are invaded by granulomatous infiltrates composed of histiocytes that displace the small lymphocytes normally present. At the same time, the splenic white pulp is infiltrated by granulomas containing *Mycobacterium lepraemurium*, which displace the lymphocytes from the periarteriolar lymphocyte sheaths. Bullock measured

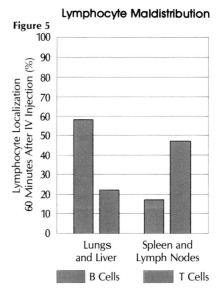

Figure 5

B cells circulate more slowly than T cells. In mice, the lungs and liver have 58% of the B cells and 22% of the T cells by one hour after injection. At the same time, only 17% of B cells, but 47% of T cells, are in the spleen and lymph nodes.

the output of radiolabeled thoracic-duct lymphocytes in both infected and control rats at intervals after intravenous infusion of the labeled cells from syngeneic donors. In the infected rats, the infused lymphocytes failed to circulate, as indicated by a low thoracic-duct output of labeled cells, compared with a definite increase in output in the non-

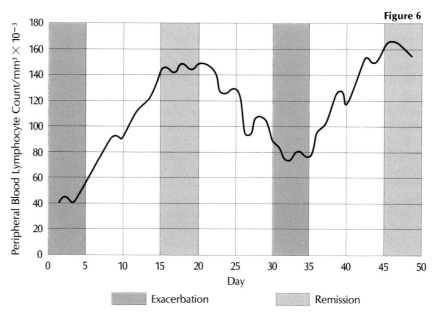

Figure 6

In periods of active disease, patient with mycosis fungoides exhibited cutaneous lymphocyte infiltration and lymphocyte depletion in peripheral blood. In remissions, peripheral blood lymphocytes increased (data of M. Lutzner, R. Edelson, et al).

infected controls. In subsequent experiments, the labeled lymphocytes were found in the spleens and, to a lesser extent, in the lymph nodes and livers of the infected rats. Splenectomy prior to infusion of labeled lymphocytes greatly increased the number recovered from the thoracic duct, although the amount did not return to normal. In contrast, induction of massive splenomegaly in control rats by intraperitoneal injection of methyl cellulose did not significantly disturb lymphocyte circulation. Bullock concluded that the disturbance of lymphocyte circulation in the infected rats was secondary to pathology in the splenic white pulp and paracortical areas of the lymph nodes and that the infected spleen became a major sequestering site for recirculating thoracic-duct lymphocytes in the infected animals.

Experiments with murine leprosy in this laboratory confirmed Bullock's finding that lymphocytes become trapped in the spleen. In the early stages of infection following intravenous injection, *M. lepraemurium* organisms are present in macrophages in the marginal zone, or thymus-dependent areas, of the spleen. As the organism proliferates, it spreads into the red pulp, but it does not invade the B-cell areas of the white pulp until the terminal stages of infection. In the lymph nodes, the mycobacteria are found primarily in the endothelium of the postcapillary venules in the outer section of the thymus-dependent area. The environmental predilection of the organism for T-cell areas and red pulp of the spleen is apparent within three months after infection, but in the terminal stages,

Figure 7

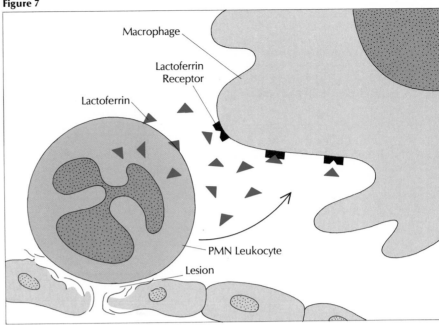

Iron may participate in abnormal distribution of lymphocytes. According to this hypothesis, lactoferrin secreted by PMN leukocytes may attract macrophages, which have receptors for the iron-binding protein (left). Macrophages secrete transferrin and ferri-

the general architecture of the spleen is replaced by macrophages containing *M. lepraemurium.*

It should be noted that the sequestration of lymphocytes in murine leprosy differs from the so-called lymphocyte trapping that occurs after antigen administration. "Trapping" can be detected in the lymphoid organ, draining the site of injection within a matter of hours, but it is transient, disappearing within hours, whereas sequestration does not develop until two to six weeks after infection, is more marked, and persists throughout the course of infection, and the circulating cells accumulate within the wrong compartment in the spleen itself (red vs white pulp).

Thus, two types of lymphocyte maldistribution (ecotaxopathies) can be envisaged: 1) a "gross" maldistribution between anatomic compartments, in which whole lymphocyte populations or, more likely, particular lymphocyte sets are reduced in the blood but have accumulated elsewhere in the recirculatory pathway; 2) a "fine" maldistribution between microenvironments within the lymphoid organs themselves, e.g., T lymphocytes that normally migrate readily to the center of the white pulp nodules in the spleen are retained in the marginal zone or red pulp. Common clinical immunology findings associated with a gross maldistribution are summarized in Table 1 and include depressed T cell–mediated immunity in peripheral blood, normal or increased levels of circulating thymus-dependent immunoglobulins (IgG and IgA), and imbalances of monocyte and T-cell sets in peripheral blood; frequently, identifiable (e.g., prostaglandins) or still unidentified "suppressor" factors are also detected. The tools to diagnose possible fine T-cell maldistributions within lymphoid organs only now are becom-

---

Table 1

Laboratory Findings To Be Expected* in Lymphocyte Maldistribution Syndromes

1. Depressed T cell–mediated immunity
2. Normal or increased levels of circulating thymus-dependent immunoglobulins (IgG, IgA)
3. Imbalances of monocyte and T-cell sets
4. Frequently identifiable (e.g., prostaglandins) or still unidentified "suppressor factors," detected in in vitro tests of immunologic function

*In peripheral blood tests

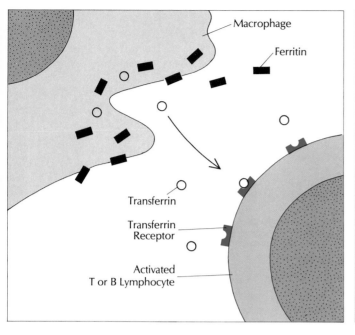

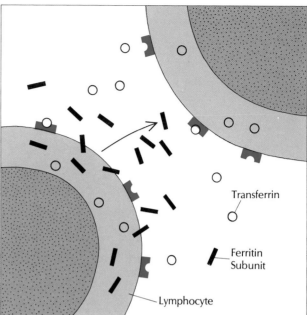

tin and attract activated lymphocytes, which have receptors for transferrin (center). Some lymphocytes also secrete transferrin and ferritin, and this may serve to further enhance lymphocyte

migration to the site (right). Thus, it is possible that the presence of iron in an organ or tissue could attract circulating lymphocytes with receptors for iron-binding proteins.

ing available with the production of monoclonal antibodies against selected T-cell sets.

Finally, why should T lymphocytes leave the normal recirculatory pathway and accumulate at such disparate sites as the mammary gland during lactation, the synovial fluid in rheumatoid arthritis, or the spleen in Hodgkin's disease?

Following earlier findings by C. P. Bieber and M. M. Bieber of unusually high amounts of ferritin in the spleen and other involved tissues of the Hodgkin's disease patients, the identification by Z. Eshhar and coworkers of ferritin as a suspected tumor-associated antigen in Hodgkin's disease, and more recent reports of siderosis in lymph nodes of Hodgkin's disease patients, we have been exploring the hypothesis that iron and iron-binding proteins (and probably other metals) contribute to the attraction of circulating lymphocytes to nonlymphoid sites (see Figure 7, above). The association of

T-lymphocyte migration to sites of iron deposition occurs in a number of physiologic and pathologic situations. The two best-known physiologic situations are lactation and iron absorption, but the presence of stainable iron is a well-known pathologic feature of rheumatoid arthritis, as discussed recently by D. Blake and colleagues. Although early biochemical studies of cells in the immune system had shown that iron-binding proteins were present in neutrophils, lymphocytes, and monocytes, only recently did compelling evidence become available indicating that such associations have significant functional implications. In addition, it has been shown that all cells of the immune system synthesize a ferritin with a subunit composition different from that of liver ferritin. By applying a recently developed reverse hemolytic plaque assay to the analysis of secretion of ferritin by mononuclear cells, Martins da Silva

in my laboratory has shown that after activation by mitogens in the presence of increasing concentrations of iron, cells of the immune system release increasing amounts of ferritin. In collaboration with M. S. Pollack and B. Dupont we have shown that this process is associated with HLA-A phenotype.

In conclusion, the possibility that cells of the immune system can have a primary role in protection from the potentially toxic accumulation of iron resulting from breakdown products of the red cell circulation, and that they can be "directed" to and accumulate at some abnormal sites through the synthesis and secretion of iron-binding proteins and expression of receptors for transferrin in activated lymphocytes, is no longer speculative. Moreover, it provides a unifying framework for many of the contradictions presently recognized in the theory of immune surveillance.

Section II
IMMUNOLOGICALLY RELATED EFFECTOR SYSTEMS

Chemistry and Function Of the Complement System

HANS J. MÜLLER–EBERHARD   *Research Institute of the Scripps Clinic*

Just about a century ago, it was recognized that serum contained soluble and heat-labile proteins that could lyse bacterial cells in the wake of an antibody response to those cells. At least 11 discrete proteins are involved in this lytic system, the classic complement pathway. Their mobilization from the serum occurs in a sequence that not only produces lysis of antigen-bearing cells but also contributes to another host defense mechanism, inflammation. About a quarter century ago—in 1954, to be precise—Louis Pillemer postulated the existence of a serum protein that is *not* antibody-dependent and that is active in early host defenses against bacteria and viruses. We now know that this protein, properdin, is a component of the so-called alternate pathway of complement activation.

The existence of these two pathways makes one appreciate—not for the first time!—that while evolution often results in biologic complexity and even apparent redundancy, such complexity is hardly pointless or inefficient. Our present evidence wholly supports the concept that the classic complement pathway operates when the target cells are able to evoke a complement-fixing (IgG or IgM) antibody response to initiate it. In contrast, the properdin pathway subserves the humoral cytolytic function when lytic activity is required before an antibody response has been expressed. The last role is, of course, that originally suggested by Pillemer's insight that properdin was involved in the very earliest host responses to bacterial or viral infections.

A diversity that can "cover" all eventualities underscores the evolutionary and biologic importance of cy-tolytic mechanisms to host defenses. In this context, it is interesting to note that a similar set of phenomena seems to be emerging with respect to cell-mediated immunologic responses. As was described in Chapter 6, at least two different classes of cytolytic lymphocytes, one antibody-dependent, the other antibody-independent, have now been identified.

As has already been noted, the first observations of the complement system, made 100 years ago, related it to cell lysis, specifically to bactericidal activity. From this starting point, the activities of complement were very soon extended by Bordet into the hemolytic system. This shift was largely a matter of convenience in the framework of late nineteenth century laboratory technology. It was a good deal easier to detect and quantify the egress of intracellular components of a red blood cell than to recognize the disruption of a bacterial cell. Unfortunately, this change in focus, however convenient, was to set back analysis of the bactericidal functions of complement by more than a half century. Yet, of course, the role of complement in the immunologic response to bacteria and viruses has far more biologic significance than does complement-mediated hemolysis. The immunologic functions, very possibly including a parallel role with respect to cancer cells, certainly account for the persistence of this complicated system in phylogeny. However, lest I appear to be blaming the erythrocyte too much for the long lag period between the discovery of complement and the appreciation of its immunologic significance, let me point out that until the 1950s the methodology of protein chemistry necessary for analysis of complement's significant functions had not been developed.

When modern protein chemistry techniques began to be applied, starting in the late fifties, both the complexity and the inherent beauty of the complement system were revealed. Today, we can correlate complement activities with discrete protein molecules with great precision. We can start with the initiation of the reaction and follow the eventual involvement of the 11 separate proteins in the classic pathway and the additional four in the properdin pathway. All of these molecules are present—often in precursor form—in the serum. The biologic denouement of their sequential array is the destruction of a target cell. En route, substances are produced that play major roles in inflammation.

Let us examine complement then as a sequence, starting with the classic pathway and turning later to the properdin, or alternate, pathway. We will begin appropriately with the so-called recognition unit of the classic pathway, C1, continue with discussion of the activation unit—C4, C2, and C3 (in that unorthodox arithmetical order)—and conclude with the membrane attack unit—C5 through C9.

The Recognition Unit

The recognition unit, C1, is a trimolecular complex, one molecule of which possesses the ability to recognize certain classes of antibody that have aggregated on the surface of an antigen-bearing cell. All three components of C1 are discrete proteins; they have been designated C1q, C1r, and C1s (see Figure 1, above). It is C1q that is capable of recognizing the antibody and fixing to a combining site in the Fc portion of the immunoglobulin. For this highly selective function of complement fixation to be carried out, the Fc portion of the immunoglobulin must be characteristic of either IgG or IgM antibody.

Physically and chemically, C1q is an unusual molecule. A glycoprotein, it is structurally very much like collagen in terms of both its

Figure 1

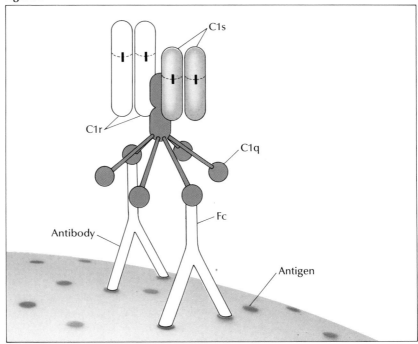

The drawing represents the recognition unit—C1—of the complement system. Shown is the fixation of two IgG molecules to a bacterial cell surface. C1q, a glycoprotein, recognizes and attaches to the Fc portions of the immunoglobulins, the first step required for activation of the other C1 complex molecules, C1r and C1s.

Figure 2

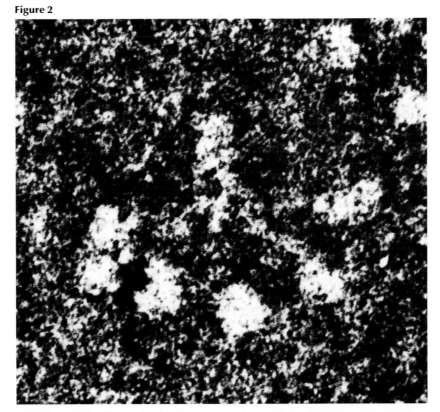

EM shows flower-like structure of C1q molecule. Molecular diameter is about 200 A. (Reprinted from E. Shelton, K. Yonemasu, and R. M. Stroud: Ultrastructure of the human complement component C1q. Proc Natl Acad Sci USA 69:65, 1972)

Figure 3

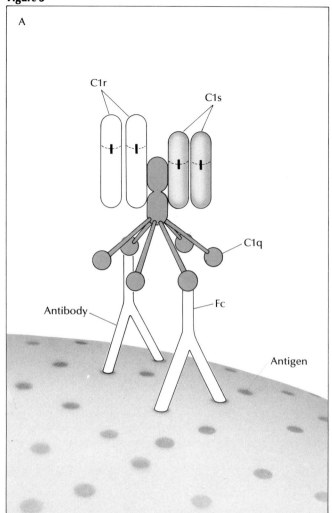

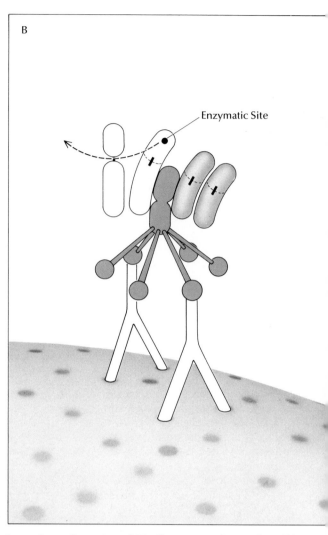

Attachment of the C1 trimolecular complex to fixed antibody initiates complement activation (A). It is postulated that a

change in configuration of C1q distorts one of two polypeptide chains of C1r, exposing an enzymatic site and resulting in the

protein and carbohydrate moieties. Even its primary structure—that is to say, its amino acid sequence—is very close to that of collagen. Figure 2, on page 129, provides an electron microscopic view of the C1q molecule. It looks very much like a bouquet of flowers, with blossom-like globular subunits appended to six stalks that meet in a common center. The "flowers" are in fact the binding sites for immunoglobulin Fc. These sites are dependent on the three-dimensional structure for their generation and availability for binding, and the Ig Fc's in turn must have several binding sites arranged in spatially appropriate orientations for the linkup to be made. Two IgG Fc fragments are

required for activation of C1q. Only one IgM molecule is needed, but since it is pentameric, the IgM molecule can provide up to five Fc binding sites for C1q.

When C1q attaches to the antigen-antibody complex, an internal activation of the whole C1 complex results. The explanation for this activation is far from complete, particularly as it relates to the rather unusual ability of C1q, a nonenzymatic protein, to alter C1r from its inactive proenzyme form to an enzymatically active molecule. Nonetheless, we have postulated a sequence of events that seems plausible on the basis of the pre- and postactivation structural char-

acteristics of C1r (see Figure 3, above).

The C1r molecule has two non-covalently linked polypeptide chains. After attachment of the entire C1 complex to the antigen-antibody complex, each of the original C1r chains is cleaved into two unequal chains held together by a single disulfide bond; there are now four chains, two with enzymatically active sites. This, of course, would be readily explicable if C1q were a proteolytic enzyme. However, we know that it is nonenzymatic, and what we have postulated is that C1q, on attachment to the immunoglobulin Fc, acquires a slightly different conformation. This change in shape, in turn, is believed to dis-

C

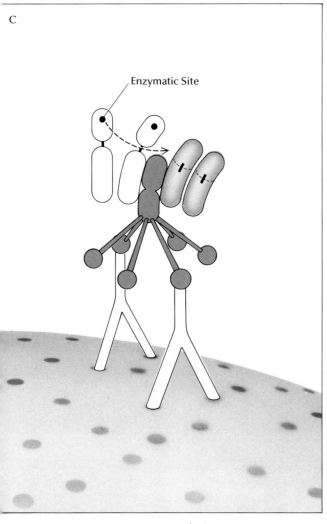

Enzymatic Site

D

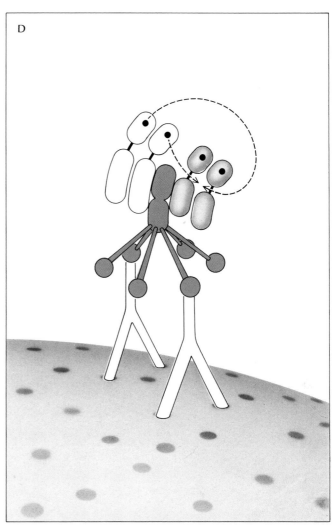

cleavage of the second chain (B). This cleavage opens a new enzymatic site, leading to cleavage of the previously distorted

polypeptide (C). The activated C1r fragments in turn cleave the C1s chains, generating two active fragments (D).

tort one chain of the C1r dimer. Without cleavage, this chain now becomes enzymatically active; its substrate is the neighboring chain of the dimer, which is cleaved. Following this first enzymatic cleavage in the complement sequence, the activated half of the dimer now acts enzymatically on the first chain, the one that had previously been only distorted by C1q, and cleaves it.

Whether or not this sequence proves to be the actual series of biochemical events involved in activation of C1r, what is clear is that, with this activation, enzymatically active molecular fragments are generated, and they act on C1s. This complement component starts

as a calcium-dependent dimer— consisting of two polypeptide chains that are cleaved by the action of C1r. The result is four fragments, two each with molecular weights of about 30,000 and 50,000 daltons, respectively. Like the C1r fragments, the two newly created chains are held together by a single disulfide bond. Indeed, the r and s components in their activated form are extremely similar in size, conformation, and amino acid composition, which suggests a common evolutionary ancestry. Perhaps more relevant in this context, the result of the activation of C1s by C1r is to provide a supply of enzymatically active C1s fragments sufficient to catalyze the reactions

required by the next unit of the classic complement pathway—the so-called activation unit. We are now ready for the conversion of three more inactive serum proteins into two active enzyme complexes.

The Activation Unit— C4, C2, and C3

With the activation of C1s, the conditions exist for the assembly of arguably the most important enzyme in complement's cytolytic activity (see Figure 4 on page 132). At this point, in addition to active C1s, the serum contains three complement components in their inactive precursor forms: C4, C2, and C3. In succession, C4 and C2 are activated by C1s to form a bimolecular complex, C4-C2, with two important functional characteristics. The transformation of both C4 and C2 from inactive precursor to active form is achieved when C1s cleaves away low-molecular-weight activation peptides, exposing receptors that permit C4 and C2 to fuse. Also exposed is a labile combining site on the C4 molecule that permits the complex transiently to attach itself to a cell surface. As will be made clear later, this attachment plays an important role in the development of a configuration on the cell membrane favorable to cytolytic attack.

Enzymatically, the C4-C2 complex has only one substrate, and that substrate is the next component of complement to be activated, C3. Because of this functional specificity, the bimolecular complex is also known as C3 convertase. Its action on C3 is to dissociate that molecule into two fragments, the smaller of which is designated C3a, the larger, C3b. In this dissociation, the C3a effectively moves out of the complement sequence and functions biochemically as an anaphylatoxin, becoming one of the two complement-derived anaphylatoxins that play a significant role in inflammation. (The other, to be discussed in sequence, is C5a.) C3a has its own biologic functions, including the ability to cause degranulation and histamine release

from mast cells, smooth muscle contraction, and release of hydrolytic enzymes from PMN leukocytes. In short, C3a manifests functional parameters not unlike those of IgE antibodies in hypersensitivity reactions, inducing many of the basic vascular phenomena characteristic of inflammation.

The larger fragment, C3b, subserves a dual function in the complement sequence itself. First of all, it associates with its own activating enzyme, C3 convertase, to form a trimolecular complex (C4-C2-C3b). And it modulates its activating enzyme so that it can now act on C5. As far as can be determined, the enzymatic site of C4-C2 is the same when it is functioning as C3

Figure 4

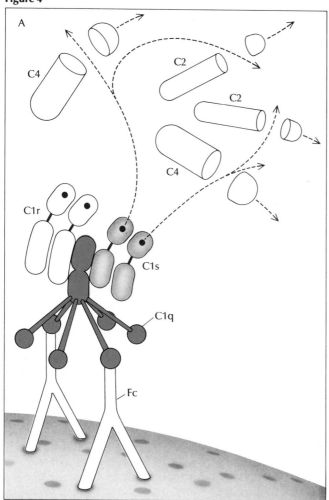

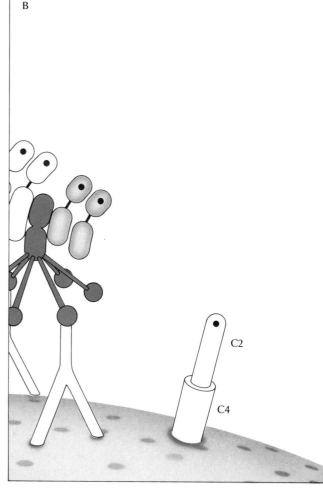

The assembly of the complement activation unit is diagrammed sequentially. Activated C1s attacks C4 and C2 in that order, cleaving off small activation peptides from each (A). This cleavage permits formation of a bimolecular C4-C2 complex and opens up a labile combining site on C4, permitting the complex to attach itself to the cell surface (B). Enzymatically,

convertase as it is when it functions with C5 as the substrate; however, the action on the latter will only take place after C3b is joined with it in a trimolecular complex. The modulation is apparently achieved by an effect on the substrate (C5) binding site. For reasons analogous to the designation of C4–C2 as C3 convertase, the trimolecular complex is enzymologically termed C5 convertase.

The second very important role for C3b is the generation of numerous monomeric C3b sites on the surface of the target cell. These sites are intrinsic to the so-called immune adherence phenomenon. A C3b-coated target cell presents specific receptors for lymphocytes, PMN leukocytes, monocytes, macrophages, and various other effector cells. The significance of the labile attachment of C4–C2 to the cell surface can now be placed in context. If one looks at the cell surface at this stage, one notes that the C4–C2 site is a center, and the C3b molecules are grouped in radial proximity to this center. Apparently, the C4–C2 molecule is responsible for attaching the C3b molecules in proximity to it on the cell surface.

Before proceeding with the classic complement sequence, let me note for future reference the fact that the attachment of C3b to cell surface represents the generation of the first condensation point, or juncture, between the classic and alternate pathways. As will be discussed, the C5 convertase of the alternate pathway uses surface-bound C3b molecules to attain its enzymatic functional integrity.

In terms of the classic pathway, the establishment of the trimolecular C5 convertase results in an attack on the C5 component, the final enzymatic reaction of the entire cytolytic sequence. C5 is cleaved in much the same way as C3. Once again, one smaller fragment, C5a, is produced, which exits from the complement sequence to function as a second anaphylatoxin. A larger fragment, C5b, in its nascent state becomes the focal point for the membrane attack unit.

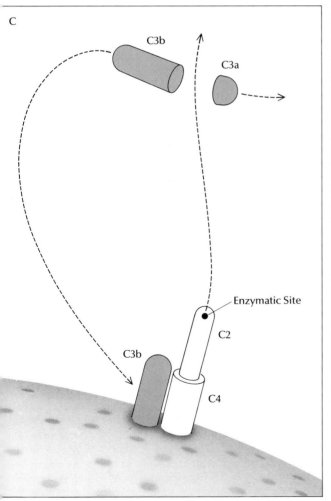
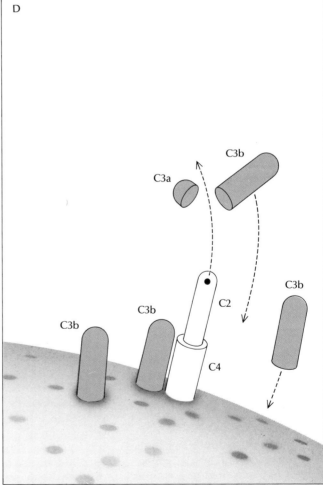

C4-C2 acts on C3 in the serum, splitting off the anaphylatoxin C3a, which functions in inflammatory processes. C3b has a dual role, forming a trimolecular complex with C4-C2 (C) and generating monomeric sites on the surface of the target cell (D). These C3b sites provide receptors for immune adherence of various effector cells (monocytes, PMN leukocytes, macrophages).

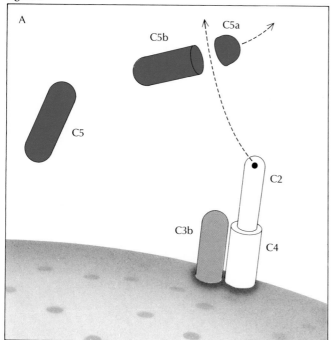

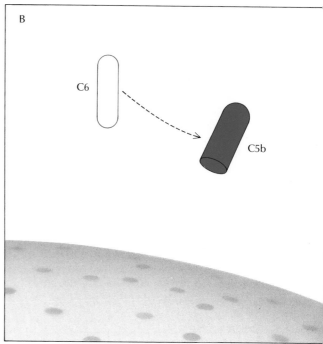

Just as C4-C2 serves as a C3 convertase, so the trimolecular C4-C2-C3b functions as a C5 convertase, cleaving C5 and liberating a second anaphylatoxin, C5a (A). C5b serves as the focal point for the membrane attack complex. Activation of C5b opens up sites that permit fusion with C6, C7, and C8, and the tetramolecular complex attaches to the cell membrane (B and C). C9 then joins this complex (D) and is polymerized by C5b-C8. Poly C9 then opens a transmembrane channel to the cell interior (E). This channel provides sufficient permeability for water and ions. Potassium leaves the cell, and water and sodium enter. The cell swells, and a much more gross disruption of the cell membrane occurs (F). Macromolecules can now escape and cell lysis is completed. However, cell membrane integrity is reestablished, with the membrane forming an empty sac (G), which subsequently is removed by phagocytosis.

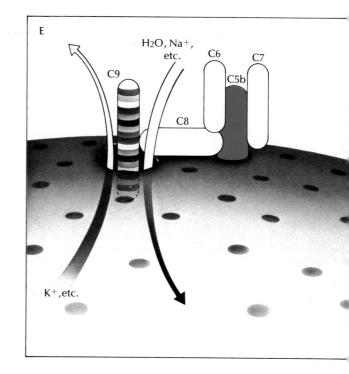

The Membrane Attack Unit— C5b, C6, C7, C8, C9

As soon as C5b dissociates in the reaction catalyzed by the convertase, it is inactivated in a manner that enables it to fuse with the next three complement components, C6, C7, and C8. Once this happens, the tetramolecular com-plex attaches to the target cell membrane; it then catalyzes the polymerization of C9 to a tubule 160 A in length by 100 A in width. One end of the tubule has a hydrophilic torus with an outer diameter of 200 A, while the other end is hydrophobic and binds to membrane lipids (see Figure 5, above). The ultrastructural image of polymer-ized C9 (poly C9) closely resembles that of the membrane lesion produced by complement. The poly C9 tubule consists of approximately 16 C9 molecules. The fully assembled membrane attack complex (MAC) is thus composed of poly C9 with C5b–C8 firmly attached.

Because of the intimate relation-ship among the five protein mole-

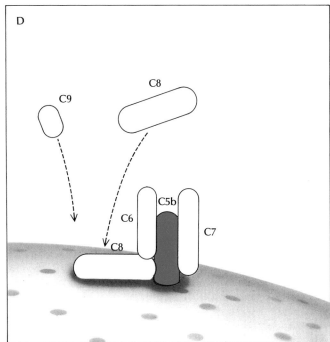

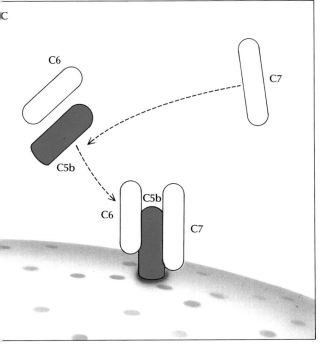

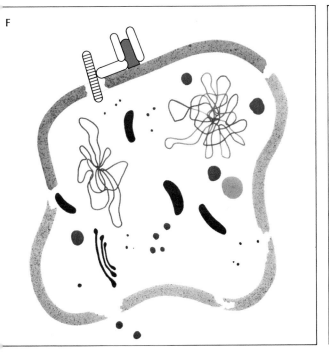

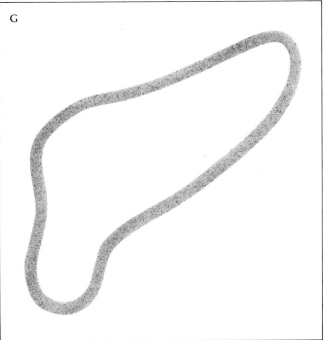

cules of the attack unit, it is difficult to dissect their relative contributions to the final lytic process. However, the evidence for each component's role is sufficiently firm to permit at least hypothetical descriptions of the same.

The initiating role of C5b has already been mentioned. Once the tetramolecular C5b–C8 complex is formed, it attaches itself, in a biochemically extremely intimate fashion, to the lipid moiety of the cell membrane. This very firm bond is established by the generation of hydrophobic forces in the course of the collision among the three molecules. On a physical basis, the most satisfactory explanation for the firmness of attachment relates to these forces and the hydrophobic nature of the interior of the cell membrane. Just such a phenomenon can be observed in systems employing synthetic membranes.

It had been previously assumed that all five MAC precursor proteins contribute to the structure of the MAC as visualized in the electron microscope. When it was realized that the ultrastructural image of the membrane-bound MAC was evoked by poly C9, the question arose as to the ultrastructural identity of the C5b–C8 complex. Careful electron microscopic studies could identify C5b–C8 as an elongated, clublike structure extending by more than 100 A beyond the upper rim of the poly C9 tubule. This structure had escaped detection in earlier investigations. The manner in which the tetramolecular C5b–C8 complex catalyzes poly C9 formation is unknown. Poly C9 within the MAC is assumed to constitute the major transmembrane protein channel (previously postulated by Manfred Mayer). This channel permits bidirectional ion and water flow. It is the beginning of the end for the target cell.

It is important to realize that the poly C9 channel is not the only type of membrane lesion produced by the MAC. In the absence of C9, C5b–C8 tends to aggregate within membranes. The effect is a weakening of the membranes so that they become leaky. Aggregation of C5b–C8 appears to be enhanced by a low dose of C9, one that is insufficient for poly C9 tubule formation. In other words, membrane damage can be inflicted upon a cell by a physical form of the MAC that lacks the poly C9 channel. That C5b–C8 aggregates are of biologic significance is evidenced by the fact that individuals with homozygous C5, C6, C7, or C8 deficiency are usually susceptible to Neisseria infections. In contrast, individuals with homozygous C9 deficiency, who by definition cannot make poly C9, are reported to enjoy a normal life. Therefore, the full biomedical significance of poly C9 remains to be determined.

Regardless of its biologic role, poly C9 is of considerable theoretical interest. It represents a model for the transition of a water-soluble glycoprotein to an integral membrane protein. Even in the absence of C5b–C8, C9 will polymerize and form tubules. Tubule formation appears to involve constrained unfolding of the molecule, because the long axis of the pro-

tomer measures 80 A and that of the tubule, 160 A. These observations may be relevant to mechanisms of membrane biosynthesis.

The actual mechanism of cell lysis has not yet been fully settled. However, the preponderance of evidence militates against the release or activation of lytic enzymes. Rather, the process appears to be dependent on physicochemical gradients. The cellular interior is of course far denser in its protein content than the extracellular fluid, so that the colloid osmotic pressure from the interior to the extracellular space is considerable. This will in turn lead to the attraction of water. Similarly, the potassium and sodium gradients result in an egress of potassium and an influx of sodium, which carries water with it. The summation of these influx forces results in gross swelling of the cell; with this swelling, the membrane becomes permeable to macromolecular substances, including intracellular proteins and nucleotides. Once the intracellular contents have diffused out, the membrane seals again and effectively becomes an empty sac. The cellular remnant is removed from the circulation by phagocytosis.

Having reviewed the molecular and cellular events that are involved in the immune lysis of a cell via the classic complement pathway, I would like to return to a formulation employed just before launching into that review: "the complexity and inherent beauty of the complement system." Anyone who has read this far probably needs little convincing with respect to the "complexity" moiety of that formulation. Is the "inherent beauty" simply in the eye of the enthusiast-beholder?

Perhaps the most convenient way of addressing this question is through an effort to answer a related inquiry. Is the complement sequence efficient or inefficient? In one sense, it is certainly efficient; a single lesion apparently suffices to lyse a cell. This 1:1 relationship is in accordance with the so-called one-hit theory of immune cytolysis first set forth by Mayer. However, if

one looks at the "molecular ecology" of the pathway, one can easily come to the conclusion that nature is being profligate indeed. For example, about 400 molecules of C4 are required to get one molecule into a position on the cell surface from which it can be instrumental in the formation of a cytolytic lesion. With C2, the number is even greater. The classic complement system is quantitatively efficient only at three points, all of which approach a 1:1 molecular-to-function ratio, C1, C5, and C8. To be sure, these are critical points, assuring as they do the optimal probability for recognition by the effector system, for launching of the operative or membrane attack portion of the sequence, and for achieving the final, irreversible lytic lesion.

Why then the complexity?

Obviously there is no way to answer this question definitively, but it is one we have thought about and discussed a great deal in our laboratory and with colleagues. Our starting point has often been the proposition: If one were to set about designing a cytolytic mediator system, what would its prerequisites be with respect to functional competence and safety? First of all, there are two obvious needs: the detection of antibody bound to a cellular surface at one end of a reaction and the capacity to attack target cell membranes at the other. Certainly the complement system meets these needs. But it must be kept in mind that we are conjuring up a lytic system—destructive by definition—so that it cannot be allowed to exist in the circulation with its molecular components in their active forms. Thus the precursors must be inactive. This need immediately creates another: for molecules that function as activators when the system is functionally evoked.

There is a third requirement as well: a means of localizing the attack to the target cell, to prevent it from being directed against, say, capillary walls 1,000 A downstream from the antigenic bacteria or viruses. The manner in which this localization function is subserved in the complement system is an extremely cogent example of the biologic elegance. Localization is basically realized through the great lability of the binding sites generated for four of the complement components: C2, C3, C4, and C5. These proteins are recruited by enzymatic activation not of enzyme sites but of binding sites. The binding sites are hydrophobic in nature so that they originally are located inside the molecule. Enzymatic attack on the molecule brings the binding sites momentarily to the surface, where their functional activity is temporally sharply limited by exposure to an aqueous medium. In this way, function is lost almost instantaneously after activation unless the molecule comes in contact with a binding site on the surface of the cell. It does not have time to get to an "innocent" host cell from the target cell on whose surface activation has been generated.

It is observation of this kind of phenomenon that has caused those of us working with the complement system to conclude that it is as efficient as it can be and no more complex than it needs to be to fulfill its biologic functions safely.

The Alternate (Properdin) Pathway

In this context the alternate, or properdin, pathway of complement activation may seem to add to the complexity of the complement system. Actually, however, it reflects the evolutionary development of the most simple humoral cytolytic analogue operating in the absence of complement-fixing antibody. For example, the alternate pathway converges with the classic pathway at a point that makes possible utilization of all the components of the latter's membrane attack unit.

Because so much of our understanding of the alternate pathway is the product of very recent and continuing research—and is therefore in a state of flux—I will content myself with a relatively brief exposition of the initiation, target deposition, recognition, and ampli-

Figure 6

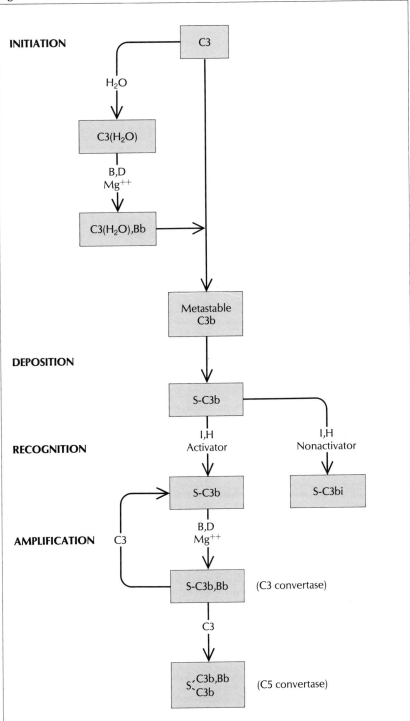

Diagram schematizes the functional stages of the alternate pathway starting with initiation by nonenzymatic hydrolysis, producing C3b-like molecule from native C3, and by the binding of Factor B, which is activated by Factor D to form a C3 convertase $C3(H_2O),Bb$. This enzyme catalyzes synthesis of metastable C3b and its deposition on the surface of target cells. On such surfaces, C3b fulfills a recognition function involving interaction with Factors H and I. Such interaction, if it occurs on, for example, bacterial cells, will lead to formation of a second C3 convertase (C3b,Bb), which enzymatically provides remarkable amplification, specifically mediated by a multiplicity of C3b molecules. These molecules facilitate both phagocytic digestion and mobilization of the complement membrane attack complex.

fication functions of the alternate pathway.

Initiation of the alternate pathway occurs in the fluid phase as the result of spontaneous hydrolysis of the internal thioester of native C3. This is a nonenzymatic reaction that yields a C3 molecule that is functionally C3b-like. When C3 is modified at the thioester site [C3(H$_2$O)], it acquires the capacity to bind another molecule, Factor B, which in turn is activated by Factor D. The reaction product is a C3 convertase, also a fluid-phase enzyme incapable of binding to a cell surface. As shown in Figure 6 on page 137, the convertase—C3(H$_2$O), Bb—catalyzes the deposition of C3b on biologic targets of complement. It does so by acting on native C3 to cleave a peptide bond in its α chain. What is cleaved off is the activation peptide C3a, and the functional product is a metastable C3b with a half-life in microseconds. Its carbonyl group becomes highly reactive and is capable of forming either an ester bond or an amide bond with hydroxyl and amino groups, respectively. These bonds provide the C3b with covalent linkage to the surface of biologic particles.

Once C3b is deposited on target cells, it apparently fulfills a recognition function. Two other alternate-pathway components are then mobilized—Factors H and I—to rapidly degrade C3b on the surfaces of host cells. Factor H binds to C3b and in doing so blocks the binding of Factor B and renders the molecule susceptible to enzymatic degradation by Factor I. If this occurs on the surface of foreign cells, such as gram-negative bacteria, there is a conformational change in the C3b molecule that greatly reduces its affinity for Factor H. Now C3b can bind Factor B again. As a result, a second C3 convertase (C3b,Bb) is synthesized. It is this enzyme that accounts for the remarkable amplification of the alternate pathway.

Because C3b is an essential subunit of the enzyme that cleaves native C3 to produce C3b, the convertase generates a positive feedback effect provided that control is restricted. Consequently, a particle that is an activator of the alternate pathway becomes covered with a multiplicity of C3b molecules. There are several consequences importantly relevant to host defense. First of all, since phagocytic cells have C3b receptors on their surfaces, particles bearing C3b molecules are susceptible to ingestion and intracellular digestion. Additionally, since C5 is cleaved and activated by the C3/C5 convertase only when it is in association with C3b, the plethora of C3b molecules facilitates formation of the membrane attack complex; thus, extracellular killing is also facilitated.

Finally, it should be noted that the role of properdin protein is stabilization of the alternate pathway C3/C5 convertase. Properdin physically binds to the enzyme complex, thereby increasing the association of its subunits. Similar stabilization of C3b,Bb can be achieved in vitro by employing nickel instead of magnesium in the formation of the enzyme.

This essentially completes the review of our current (and ever-changing) understanding of the chemistry and the function of the complement system. The primary importance of this system lies, of course, in its ability to function as an effector mechanism in the destruction of pathogens. Conversely, abnormalities in this system are being increasingly appreciated as major etiologic contributors to a wide range of immunopathologies. This is the subject of Chapter 15 in this volume.

The Biology of C-Reactive Protein

HENRY GEWURZ   *Rush Medical College*

Such stimuli as cellular injury, inflammation, and even pregnancy evoke production of a heterogeneous group of proteins, the so-called acute phase reactants. Examination of the properties and functions of these proteins has focused first and foremost on the C-reactive protein (CRP), which increases particularly dramatically (up to a thousandfold) and has been found in certain inflammatory deposits.

As will be discussed later, CRP is functionally integrated with the effectors of the immunologic and inflammatory responses, even as other acute phase proteins act in the coagulation processes (fibrinogen), as circulatory proteinase inhibitors (α-1 antitrypsin), in metal transport (ceruloplasmin), as hemoglobin scavengers following erythrocyte lysis (haptoglobin), as the fulcrum of the complement pathways (C3), in the modification of inflammation (α-1 acid glycoprotein), or in ways not yet defined (serum amyloid A protein). These acute phase reactants are just a sampling of a much larger group. Some, but by no means all, of the others are listed in Table 1 on page 140. However, even this very abbreviated list suggests that the heterogeneity of the acute phase proteins is teleologically very efficiently related to the spectrum of biologic activities required in response to insult and injury.

CRP was the first appreciated acute phase reactant and has been studied most intensively as prototypically representative of this class of proteins. Biomedical research attention to CRP has waxed, waned, and recently waxed again. During the past half century, substantial attention was paid to CRP because it helped diagnose the presence and extent of inflammation or tissue necrosis. CRP was first described in 1930. Levels were soon being measured in a variety of illnesses. The acute phase changes, however, seemed to be nonspecific, in the sense that they occurred to about the same extent in a number of diverse diseases. This contrasted with the extreme specificity of the immune response, and as interest in immunity accelerated during the 1950s, interest in the acute phase reactants waned. Recently, a number of laboratories have turned back to studies of the acute phase, with intriguing basic and often clinically relevant findings.

Experimental evidence suggests that CRP is a fundamental, multifunctional host component that has recognition capacity and can initiate and, perhaps, modulate a broad range of interactions. Moreover, since CRP levels in the body intimately follow the course of the acute phase, monitoring CRP seems to provide a valuable clinical barometer of illness. In this respect, CRP measurement can be considered in many ways a refined quantitative alternative or supplement to the erythrocyte sedimentation rate (ESR). Indeed, it is now appreciated that an elevated ESR is in large part a phenomenon secondary to enhanced activity of certain acute phase proteins.

Specifically, an increased ESR (originally, elegantly investigated and reviewed by R. Fahraeus in relation to the history of the acute phase response) is caused by enhanced erythrocyte aggregation, and this, in turn, results from increased levels of fibrinogen and other, still unidentified, globular proteins in the blood. One factor that influences erythrocyte aggregation is the charge-dissipation capacity of the plasma (its dielectric constant). This is influenced by the concentration and degree of asymmetry of the molecules dissolved in the plasma—the more asymmetric a molecule is, the more likely it is to become polarized by the surface electric charges of the red cells. When many asymmetric molecules are present, the plasma's charge-dissipation capacity is high. This dampens the repulsive effects of the like charges on the surface of the red cells and makes the cells more likely to aggregate. The cells form stacks, or rouleaux. The most asymmetric of the acute phase proteins that are present in significant concentrations in the plasma is fibrinogen, which thus has the greatest effect on the ESR.

Formation of rouleaux elevates the ESR because the stacked cells have a higher ratio of mass to surface area than single cells and, therefore, will fall out (sediment) from the plasma more rapidly. Abnormalities in the size and shape of the red cells, as in acanthocytosis and poikilocytosis, physically interfere with the formation of rouleaux. Such conditions can result in an ESR that appears normal while high concentrations of acute phase reactants are present. Conversely, certain other conditions, such as anemia, may be associated with ESR levels that are dispropor-

tionately elevated in relation to concurrent inflammatory reactions. More typically, however, the events that elevate ESR are chronologically paralleled by a primary manyfold elevation of CRP, and CRP levels more closely approximate the degree of ongoing tissue damage.

For these reasons, monitoring serum CRP provides a sensitive and quantitative index of acute changes in the body. We regard CRP as an alternative that is, in some cases, superior to the ESR for the detection of such changes, although it is equally nonspecific. As shown in Figure 1 (opposite page, top), CRP levels rise precipitously within hours of surgery, for example, and subside after a few days in the absence of further inflammation or necrosis. Measurement of both a patient's ESR and CRP level may be redundant, and recognizing that not every physician now has access to a laboratory that can perform CRP measurements rapidly, we currently recommend the use of either one of these values in the prophylactic screening of healthy patients or in charting the recuperative progress of those who are ill. Perhaps future investigations will define profiles of acute phase changes

that are characteristic for given inflammatory processes or diseases.

CRP or ESR measurement is useful in certain microbial infections, rheumatoid arthritis, systemic lupus erythematosus, neoplastic diseases, and other conditions (see Table 2, opposite page, bottom). It must be kept in mind that a high ESR or CRP level will not necessarily be due to the disease that is being investigated. Discovery of the acute phase in a patient who lacks a clear-cut clinical picture would make diagnosis of, say, an isolated psychogenic malady less likely and an underlying process associated with inflammation and/or tissue necrosis more likely. Therefore, a CRP rise in such circumstances should trigger an intensive clinical search for cause and, when a cause is not immediately discernible, careful observation of the patient. The acute phase measurements also can be used to monitor a therapy's effectiveness.

At the time CRP was first identified in 1930 in the Avery laboratory of the Rockefeller Institute, polysaccharides had recently been discovered to act as antigens, a property previously assigned exclusively to proteins. It was therefore feasible to prepare polysaccharide–antibody precipitates. Because such precipitates were protein–polysaccharide complexes, it was relatively straightforward to separate the two moieties and thus obtain a good preparation of a specific antibody. Medical researchers conceived of isolating polysaccharides from the surface of bacteria (particularly pneumococci), defining their relationship to serologic specificity and biologic activity, and using them to "fish" in a serum bank for material that could be used in antibacterial serum therapy.

It was within this context that W. S. Tillett and T. Francis found that serum from acutely ill individuals contained a substance that precipitated with the C fraction (termed C-polysaccharide, or CPS) of pneumococci. This factor was subsequently named C-precipitin or C-reactive substance. It was ultimately determined that it was a

Table 1. Acute Phase Proteins in Humans

	Electrophoretic Mobility on Paper	Molecular Weight	Normal Plasma Concentration (mg/dl)	Selected Biologic Functions
Concentration may increase by about 50%:				
Ceruloplasmin	α_2	151,000	15–60	CW transport, free radical scavenger
C3 (complement component)	β	180,000	80–170	Modification of inflammation, host defense
Concentration may increase twofold to threefold:				
α_1-Acid glycoprotein	α_1	40,000	55–140	Modification of inflammation
α_1-Antitrypsin	α_1	54,000	200–400	Protease inhibition
Haptoglobin	α_2	100,000	40–180	Hemoglobin transport
Fibrinogen	β	340,000	200–450	Coagulation
Concentration may increase a hundredfold to a thousandfold:				
C-reactive protein	γ	~105,000	< 0.5	Inflammation, host defense
Protein SAA	α_1	12,000	< 10	Unknown

protein—hence, its permanent (to date) designation as C-reactive protein.

CRP has an isoelectric point of 6.2, has a molecular weight of approximately 110,000, and was shown by A. P. Osmand et al in our laboratory to be composed of five noncovalently bound identical subunits, each with a weight of 21,500 (see Figures 2 and 3, pages 142 and 143). The complete amino acid sequence of the human CRP subunit was reported by T.-Y. Liu and colleagues (see Figure 4, page 143). It contains 187 residues, with one disulfide bond and no detectable lipid or carbohydrate. In serum, CRP has been found associated with lipoproteins of the very low-density (VLDL) and low-density (LDL) fractions, which affect the protein's precipitability and electrophoretic mobility.

Electron micrographs indicate that each CRP subunit is spherical and that the five units are arranged with cyclic symmetry. Of the more than 200 proteins whose structure has been determined by electron microscopy, only a handful have shown this form. One is CRP, and another is the serum amyloid P component (SAP), a molecule that we found shares remarkable amino acid sequence homology and a number of other properties with CRP, as will be discussed later in this review. A third is the hamster female protein (FP). We have called these proteins "pentraxin," based on the Greek for a cluster of five berries, and have proposed that they comprise a new, distinct, structurally and functionally related family of serum proteins. Two other pentameric proteins are enzymes that are otherwise unrelated to CRP and SAP. (Investigators have questioned whether CRP might have an enzymatic function, but no evidence for enzymatic activity by either CRP or SAP has been presented.)

Measurement of CRP levels in the blood was originally based on precipitation of CPS or the ability of CRP to swell the capsules of certain pneumococci (the quellung reaction). In 1950, widely utilized immunoassays involving capillary

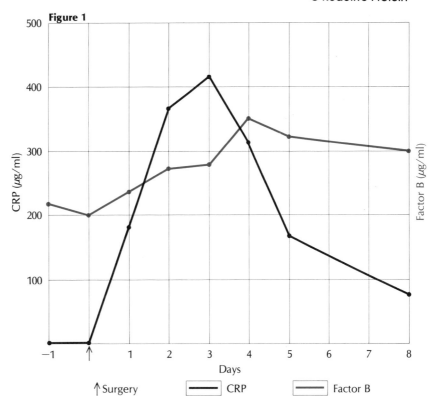

Figure 1

Postcholecystectomy rise in CRP was more than two hundredfold by postoperative days 2 and 3. Complement component (factor B) rose by less than 75%, although increase was more prolonged. Clinical uses of CRP measurement are tabulated below.

Table 2. Measurement of Serum C-Reactive Protein in Clinical Practice

Screening for organic disease
General screening aid for inflammatory diseases, infections, and neoplastic diseases or tissue injury

Detection and evaluation of inflammatory disorders (> CRP)
Rheumatoid arthritis
Seronegative arthritides (e.g., Reiter's syndrome)
Rheumatic fever
Vasculitic syndromes (e.g., hypersensitivity vasculitis)
Inflammatory bowel disease

Detection and management of infections (> CRP)
Neonatal infections
Postoperative infections
Intercurrent infections in leukemia
Bacterial infections in systemic lupus erythematosus
Pyelonephritis

Detection and evaluation of tissue injury and neoplasia (> CRP)
Myocardial infarction
Embolism
Transplant rejection
Certain tumors (e.g., Burkitt's lymphoma)

Aid in differential diagnosis
Systemic lupus erythematosus versus rheumatoid arthritis and other arthritides (< SLE)
Crohn's disease versus ulcerative colitis (< Crohn's)
Pyelonephritis versus cystitis (> pyelonephritis)
Bacterial versus viral infections (> bacterial)
Acute bronchitis versus asthma (< asthma)

Adapted from M. B. Pepys: *Lancet* 1:653, 1981, and I. Kushner: *Textbook of Rheumatology*, 1981

Figure 2

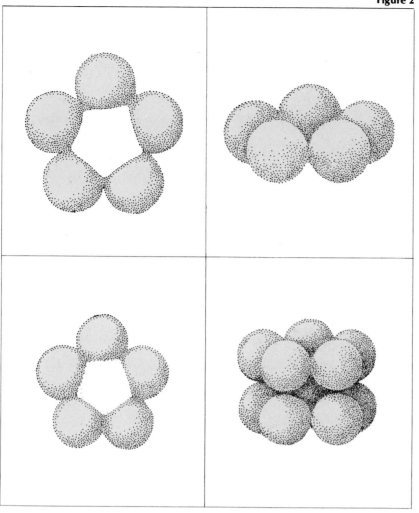

When viewed "from above," both human CRP (top left) and human SAP (bottom left) molecules show virtually identical pentameric structure characteristic of pentraxin protein class. However, in the side view, the SAP is revealed to be a decamer.

There is good evidence that at least one multifunctional factor released by macrophages has this capacity, and this substance has been independently recognized and given a variety of names reflecting these various functions: interleukin-1, lymphocyte-activating factor, leukocyte endogenous mediator (LEM), and endogenous pyrogen. For example, D. L. Bornstein and coworkers isolated an endogenous pyrogen preparation from rabbits and found that when it was infused back into these animals, it elicited a CRP response; R. F. Kampschmidt et al performed parallel experiments, and K. P. W. J. McAdams and colleagues used a similar approach to induce the synthesis of serum amyloid A. The work of these investigators and of P. A. Murphy, J. D. Sipe, M. B. Sztein, and their colleagues indicates that this molecule, now commonly termed interleukin-1, induces the production of amyloid A component (to be discussed) and other acute phase proteins in the liver.

There also is evidence that prostaglandins can mediate the synthesis of CRP and other acute phase proteins. J. T. Whicher and coworkers induced CRP production in humans by using PGE_1, whereas B.-S. Shim raised haptoglobin levels in rabbits by using PGE_1, PGE_2, $PGF_{2\alpha}$, and PGA_2. It is possible, however, that prostaglandins are only stimulating macrophages to release interleukin-1 or another mediator of the acute phase.

In short, it is currently unclear how many mediators trigger the production of CRP or any other acute phase protein. Nor is it known whether a mediator becomes consumed during the course of induction. Not unexpectedly, anti-inflammatory drugs diminish CRP production, but it is not yet known whether any of these agents influence CRP biosynthesis directly.

CRP, as well as the other acute phase proteins, is made predominantly in the liver by hepatocytes, as shown by Kushner and his colleagues. The first hepatocytes to produce CRP are in the periphery of the portal lobules; during a sus-

precipitation with monospecific antisera were introduced by H. C. Anderson and M. McCarty. Today four more sensitive immunologic methods are employed: Radial immunodiffusion in gel, which allows detection of 3 µg/ml CRP in overnight assays, is most widely used. Radioimmune assays are the most sensitive and precise—able to detect as little as 3 ng of CRP in a milliliter of fluid—but they are relatively slow and expensive. A more rapid method is nephelometry, one form of which involves detection of aggregates of CRP and antibody by their scattering of light (for example, from a laser source). Enzyme-linked immunosorbent assays (ELISA) are just now being developed for CRP and promise to combine sensitivity with speed and low cost.

The application of these assays has revealed that everyone has a low basal blood level of CRP (a median of about 600 ng/ml). No one yet has been found to lack the capacity to produce CRP. During the acute phase, CRP levels can rise by up to a thousandfold within two days, reaching concentrations as high as 500 µg/ml. The mean doubling time of CRP in humans is about eight hours, and a similar rate has been found in rabbits, as well as in isolated perfused livers in the definitive studies of I. Kushner and his colleagues.

The triggers of elevated CRP synthesis remain mostly unidentified.

tained response, cells that are closer to the center of the lobule also make CRP. It also is possible that small amounts of CRP are produced by cells outside the liver. Indeed, as will be detailed later in this review, there is recent evidence for the presence of CRP on the surface of certain lymphoid and phagocytic cells, although it is not clear whether this CRP is ever released.

Relatively little research has been done on the molecular biology of CRP or on the mechanisms of its enhanced release. However, recent work on the molecular biology of two other acute phase proteins is of interest. John Morrow isolated the messenger RNA and cloned the genes that code for mouse serum amyloid A from liver cells in the acute phase. He found that the level of serum amyloid A–specific mRNA rose in these cells during the acute phase. In a similar study, John Taylor isolated the mRNA and cloned the genes for the acute phase reactant α-1 acid glycoprotein (AAG) in the rat. He found that as AAG-specific mRNA increased (by as much as ninetyfold), there was a concurrent drop in the amount of albumin-specific mRNA in acute phase hepatocytes. Apparently, during the acute phase, there is not a marked change in the total amount of protein produced by the liver; rather, there are specific shifts within the protein profile. To our knowledge, similar studies have not yet been undertaken in a species known to produce a vigorous, rec-

Figure 3

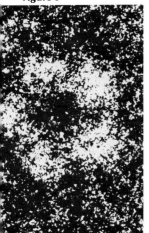 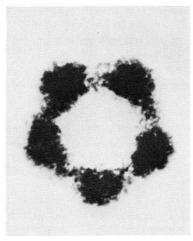 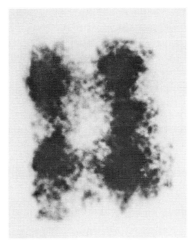 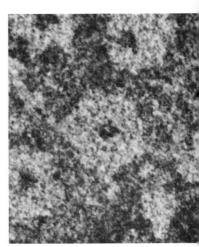

From left to right (above) are electron micrographs of human CRP, human SAP (top and side views), and hamster female protein. (CRP courtesy A. P. Osmand et al: Proc Natl Acad Sci USA 74:739, 1977; SAP, L. Pinteric, R. H. Painter: Can J Biochem 57:727, 1979; FP, J. E. Coe et al: J Exp Med 153:9777, 1981) Diagramed below are amino acid sequences of amino terminal

portions of human CRP, rabbit CRP, human SAP, and hamster FP. Note extensive homologies reflecting common evolutionary ancestry and high degree of conservation. Color is used to highlight specific homologies between human CRP and other protein sequences. (Diagram based on data from E. B. Oliveira et al: Proc Natl Acad Sci USA 74:3148, 1977, and papers cited above)

Figure 4

1	2	3	4	5	6	7	8	9	10	11	12	13	14	15	16	17	18	19	20	21	22	23	24	25	26 →
PCA	Thr	Asp	Met	Ser	Arg	Lys	Ala	Phe	Val	Phe	Pro	Lys	Glu	Ser	Asp	Thr	Ser	Tyr	Val	Ser	Leu	Lys	Ala	Pro	Leu

Human CRP H$_2$

1	2	3	4	5	6	7	8	9	10	11	12	13	14	15	16	17	18	19	20	21	22	23	24	25	26
X	Ala	Val (Gly)	Met	His	Lys	Lys	Ala	Phe	Val	Phe	Pro	Lys	Glu	Ser	Asp	Asx	Ser	Tyr	Val	Ser	Leu	Asx	X	Gly	Leu

Rabbit CRP

1	2	3	4	5	6	7	8	9	10	11	12	13	14	15	16	17	18	19	20	21	22	23	24	25	26
His	Thr	Asp	Leu	Ser	Gly	Lys	Val	Phe	Val	Phe	Pro	Arg	Glu	Ser	Val	Thr	Asp	His (Tyr)	Val	Asn	Leu	Ile	Thr	Pro	Leu

SAP

1	2	3	4	5	6	7	8	9	10	11	12	13	14	15	16	17	18	19	20	21	22	23	24	25	26
PCA	X	Asp	Leu	Ser	Gly	Lys	Val	Phe	Val	Phe	Pro	Arg	Gln	Ser	Glu	Thr	Asp	Tyr	Val	Asn	Leu	Ile	X	X	Leu

FP

X = Either lack of identification or deletion of residue; PCA = pyrrolidinecarboxylic acid ognizable CRP response.

In turning to a description of the functional activities of CRP—the major area of interest in our laboratory—it can be noted that a fairly broad picture of potential biologic activities, albeit one that still has many gaps, is evolving.

CRP has a considerable number of binding specificities, which fall into three categories: 1) It attaches to phosphate esters and, as defined by J. E. Volanakis and M. H. Kaplan, particularly to phosphocholine, which constitutes the CRP-binding site on the pneumococcal CPS; 2) it also recognizes galactosyl polymers involving two sugars, galactose and galactosamine; and 3) it reacts preferentially with various polycations (see Figure 5, opposite). CRP also reacts with certain lipids and lipoproteins, either by one of the aforementioned mechanisms or, conceivably, through still another binding site. CRP–lipid–lipoprotein relationships are being studied in our laboratory by V. Cabana and J. Siegel.

Before CRP will bind to phosphocholine, calcium must attach to the protein. Each CRP subunit has at least one calcium-binding site. For CRP to precipitate CPS, at least 0.9 mM of calcium is needed. This compares with a normal physiologic level of 1.0 to 1.2 mM of ionized calcium in serum. It appears that when the calcium cation binds to CRP, it significantly changes the protein's phosphate ester–binding site; the molecule undergoes a significant conformational alteration, as shown by circular dichroism studies by N. M. Young and R. E. Williams. And Volanakis and his colleagues have shown antigenic alteration in this ligand-binding site. The evidence is that CRP binds to phosphate esters at their phosphate group. Thus, free choline and analogues of phosphocholine that have a substituted phosphate group are not CRP ligands.

Phosphocholines are widely distributed in microbial products. CPS is in the cell wall of pneumococci, and the capsule of *Streptococcus pneumoniae* type 27 contains available phosphocholine as well. Type 27, therefore, is a particularly powerful binding target of CRP. Phosphocholine also has been found on the surface of fungi, lactobacilli, parasites, and dermatophytes by use of antiphosphocholine myeloma proteins as well as with CRP. Interestingly, Volanakis and his colleagues recently have shown that the idiotype for one of these proteins and the CRP-binding site for phosphocholine show antigenic cross-reactivity—i.e., they are structurally similar.

Two phospholipids that are widely distributed in human cell membranes, phosphatidylcholine and sphingomyelin, also contain phosphocholine. The phosphocholine in these molecules is not exposed in unaltered membranes, so CRP does not bind to these surfaces. However, during trauma, when the bilayer is disrupted, it has been hypothesized by Volanakis and Kaplan that the phosphocholine groups can become exposed and provide CRP with an attachment site. The regions where cellular injury has occurred, therefore, might acquire CRP deposits.

The binding of CRP to galactose and galactosamine is equally calcium-dependent. If the type 4 pneumococcal polysaccharide, which does not contain phosphocholine but does contain galactose and galactosamine, is depyruvated, it becomes a target for CRP binding. Galactosamine also may contribute, along with the phosphocholine, to the binding of CRP to CPS. In addition, CRP was shown to exhibit weak binding to agarose, which was attributable to its galactosamine-binding activity.

CRP reacts with many synthetic and natural polycations, such as L-lysine and L-arginine polymers, protamine, myelin basic protein, leukocyte cationic proteins, and histone proteins. It is interesting that the reactivity of CRP with lecithin liposomes, previously shown by us with C. R. Alving et al to require the presence of the cationic lipid stearylamine, involved binding to this latter positively charged component rather than to the unavailable phosphocholine. Calcium is not needed for this activity and, in fact, inhibits the binding. This inhibitory role may be due to competition for a common site on the CRP molecule or to a significant alteration in the polycation-binding site as a result of calcium attachment. The polycation-binding site on CRP appears to be distinct from the phosphate ester site because the two ligands do not cross-interfere in certain experimental systems but seem to be proximal, since L. A. Potempa has shown that haptenic phosphocholine can markedly influence the CRP–polycation reaction in the presence of calcium.

In deriving a synthesis for some of these observations, we have postulated that during cell injury, cationic proteins are released, e.g., from whole-cell granules (leukocyte cationic proteins) or cell nuclei (histones). Cell surfaces contain many anionic sites to which free polycations can bind and provide electrostatic loci for CRP fixation in a region of cellular injury. Indeed, we recently have observed that incubation of certain particles or unmodified cells with CRP and given polycations results in substantial CRP deposition on the polycation-reactive surface.

It appears that once CRP binds to a ligand, it initiates and modulates the inflammatory response in a manner analogous to, but distinct from, the activity of antibody (see Figure 6, pages 146, 147). The most significant currently appreciated aspect of this activity by CRP is its recruitment of complement, as shown by Kaplan and Volanakis (and extended in our laboratory). We have observed that CRP is as efficient as IgG in initiating classic-pathway complement activity.

For a CRP-ligand complex involving CPS to lead to the fixation of complement, two CRP molecules are required. These, presumably, allosterically modify the C1 component into a form that will attach and result in activation. Interaction of CRP with C1 requires the participation of C1q, even as antibody-induced activation does. Deposition of the C4, C2, and C3 components follows. This interaction is

Figure 5

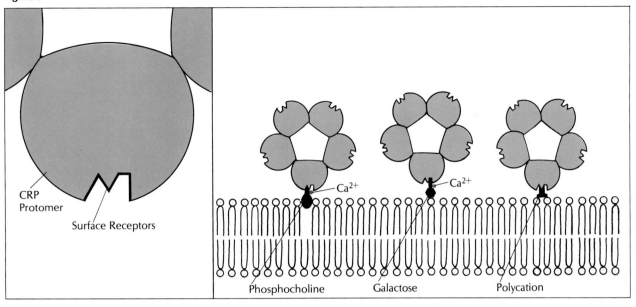

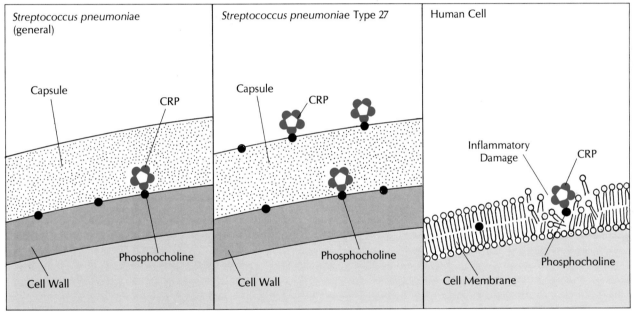

Schematized above are some of the binding characteristics of CRP. The first drawing (top left) shows a CRP protomer with its intimately related surface receptors for phosphocholine (PC), galactose, and polycations. Adjacent is a representation of CRP binding to appropriate ligands on an idealized cell membrane. Note calcium ion requirement for binding PC and galactose but not for polycations. At bottom left is generalized scheme of

CRP binding to S. pneumoniae. With S. pneumoniae type 27, however, phosphocholine is found in both the cell wall and capsule (center), perhaps accounting for enhanced reactivity with CRP. Finally, in human cell membrane, phosphocholine is not exposed. Therefore, CRP binding may first require exposure of phosphocholine by inflammatory damage. CRP may also bind to membrane-acquired or passively acquired polycations.

sufficient to permit complement-dependent cell adherence, in which macrophages are particularly active. In addition, of course, once C3 is activated, the lytic C5–C9 sequence is capable of initiation, and we have shown CRP-initiated lysis of both CPS-coated erythrocytes and appropriate liposomes. CRP recruit-

ment of complement also produces the split fragments that are active chemotactic agents in the plasma. Thus, CRP can initiate all the major known complement-dependent reactivities.

If, after complement deposition at a certain CRP-ligand complex, the CRP is removed and the resul-

tant complex (complement and ligand alone) is incubated with macrophages, the leukocytes adhere to but do not ingest the target. Only when CRP is restored does phagocytosis proceed. CRP, therefore, may have a dual role in phagocytosis: It leads to complement deposition, which is required for leukocyte attachment, and it also is required for ingestion. Also implied is that macrophages have a specific receptor for complexed CRP.

The ability of CRP to bind to a ligand, to cause deposition of complement, and to facilitate attachment and function of phagocytes is again reminiscent of antibody activity. It will be interesting to determine whether CRP can move from ligand to ligand, fixing complement as it goes.

We have performed a variety of experiments to explore the consequences of CRP's binding to a ligand and the resultant deposition of complement as just outlined. One line of investigation pursued by R. F. Mortensen, then in our laboratory, used sheep erythrocytes coated with CPS (E–CPS) as targets for phagocytosis by human monocytes (Figure 7, page 148). E–CPS by itself or in the presence of CRP (E–CPS–CRP) was not phagocytosed by the monocytes. The addition of both CRP and complement (E–CPS–CRP–C), however, triggered a high level of ingestion. In contrast, IgG

directed against CPS (E–CPS–IgG) could by itself induce a high level of phagocytosis, not further enhanced by the addition of complement when sufficient amounts of antibody were used.

When CRP was removed from an E–CPS–CRP–C complex (with EDTA), the amount of phagocytosis was reduced to nearly background levels. Readdition of CRP restored full phagocytic activity.

Mortensen later showed that uptake of E–CPS–CRP–C was inhibited by E–CPS–IgG or by 2-deoxyglucose (which blocks phagocytosis of E–CPS–IgG by monocytes). Conversely, CRP–CPS inhibits E–CPS–IgG uptake. These observations suggest that the macrophage Fc receptors for IgG, or closely related receptors, are also involved in CRP-mediated phagocytosis.

In vivo experiments by S. Nakayama et al in our laboratory revealed that the site of uptake of E–CPS is markedly affected by CRP and complement (see Figure 8, page 149). Mice with normal levels of complement clear about twice as

much E or E–CPS to the liver as to the spleen. Treatment of the complex with CRP, IgM, or IgG lowered hepatic clearance slightly while significantly raising splenic clearance, so that the amount absorbed by each organ became about equal. When mice were depleted of endogenous complement (using cobra venom factor), this change in clearance was not observed when either CRP or IgM was added but was still observed upon addition of IgG. If complement was restored to these animals, clearance of E–CPS–CRP and E–CPS–IgM again was divided in half between the liver and spleen. Removal of CRP from the erythrocyte complex also eliminated the enhanced splenic clearance.

These results indicate that phagocytic cells in the spleen require both complement and either CRP or IgM to ingest a target, whereas IgG alone is sufficient. The findings are remarkably consistent with our in vitro observations. However, it should be noted that the biologic significance of CRP's directing such complexes to the spleen

Figure 6

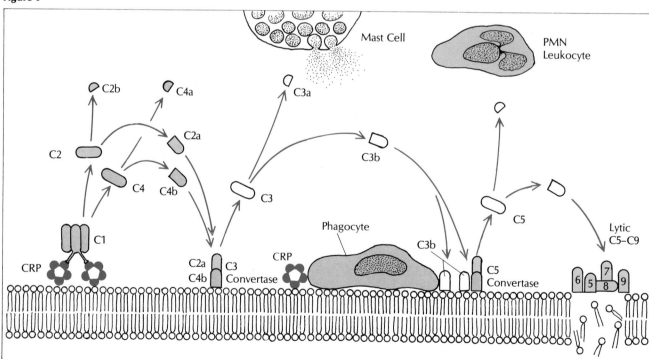

Among the depicted biologic functions of CRP complexes are complement activation (above), platelet aggregation (near right), and binding to large granular lymphocytes (LGLs, far right). With complement, CRP is effectively a surrogate for immunoglobulin in activating the classic pathway (but it inhibits the alternative pathway). CRP triggers the full C sequence, in-

rather than to the liver is not yet understood; it will be interesting to determine whether this is associated with a significant effect on antibody formation.

In the effort to examine circumstances that more closely reflect an actual physiologic response, C. Mold also led a group of studies on the ability of CRP to promote phagocytosis of bacteria. It will be recalled that although CRP binds to many types of pneumococcus, presumably to the phosphocholine in their cell walls, the amount of CRP that binds to *S. pneumoniae* type 27 is fivefold to tenfold higher than for any other pneumococcal type studied. This avidity is attributable to the phosphocholine in the capsule of type 27.

Experiments were designed by K. Edwards to compare various pneumococcal types with regard to the effects of CRP on complement consumption and binding, complement-dependent adherence, and phagocytosis (in this case, to neutrophils). With all types studied, CRP enhanced the amount of complement consumed.

In exploring quantitative aspects of pneumococcal phagocytosis by human neutrophils in vitro, we compared activity in the presence of either normal human serum or hypogammaglobulinemic serum. CRP greatly enhanced phagocytosis of type 27 when added in the presence of either serum type. In contrast, CRP had no effect on the ingestion of type 6 and inhibited the ingestion of *S. pneumoniae* type 3 when tested using normal serum. If the IgG-deficient serum was used, the background level of ingestion of each of these two pneumococcal types was lower, and a twofold enhancement resulted from the addition of CRP. These experiments obviously suggested that CRP can bring about the phagocytosis of certain bacteria in the absence of an IgG-immune response. As for the powerful CRP effect on phagocytosis of type 27, this could be due to the large amount of CRP adhering to the bacterium, or it could derive from the unique binding of CRP to the bacterial capsule. Ob-

viously, the quantitative and qualitative factors are not mutually exclusive.

Further experiments designed by Mold examined the effects of CRP on protection from pneumococcal infection in mice in vivo. To eliminate the effects of natural antibody, we developed BALB/c mice tolerant to CPS. These mice are particularly susceptible to infection by pneumococci. Injection of these mice with 200 μg of CRP 30 minutes prior to intravenous infection with pneumococcus type 3 significantly enhanced survival of the mice. Further studies showed that CRP was protective against pneumococcal infection even in the presence of natural antibody to phosphocholine, increasing the LD_{50} from 4×10^4 CFU to 2×10^5 CFU *S. pneumoniae* type 3, with comparable results when type 4 pneumococci were used (see Figure 9, page 150).

These studies thus demonstrate a second biologic property of CRP in vivo: In addition to initiating complement-dependent opsonization with preferential clearance to

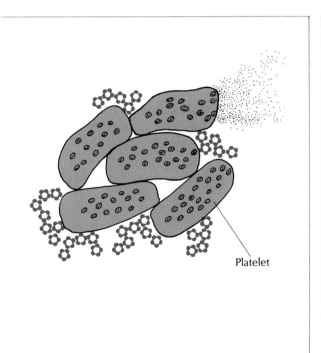

Platelet

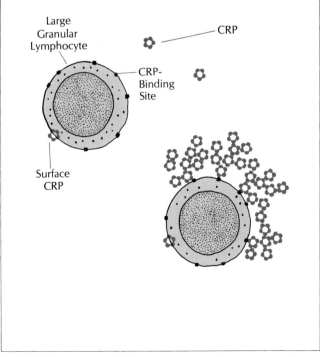

Large Granular Lymphocyte

CRP

CRP-Binding Site

Surface CRP

cluding opsonization for phagocytes, generation of anaphylatoxins and chemotactins, and assembly of the terminal lytic complex. CRP complexes also will cause platelet degranulation as well as aggregation. With respect to LGLs, it is noteworthy that they have been found to bear CRP and that CRP complexes bind to the cells, although not at the surface CRP sites.

Figure 7

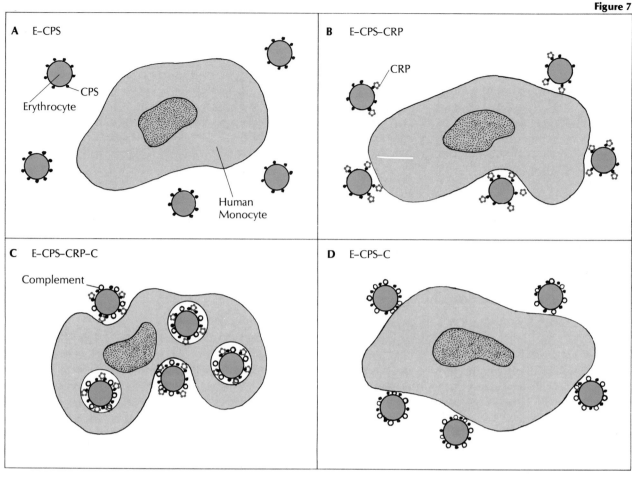

Experimentally, when erythrocytes were coated with pneumococcal C-polysaccharide and incubated with human monocytes, there was no attachment or ingestion (A). If CRP was added, there was attachment to monocyte surface (B), but ingestion did not take place until complement was activated and bound to the erythrocyte surface (C). When CRP was removed after C binding, red cell coated with CPS and complement attached to, but was no longer ingested by, the monocyte (D).

the spleen, CRP is protective against pneumococcal infection in normal as well as antibody-suppressed mice. The ability of CRP to react with and protect against infection with other organisms is under investigation by Mold and her colleagues. It is clear that CRP reacts preferentially with the pneumococcus, as compared with other organisms tested to date, and fails to react with some bacteria at all. Whatever the final correlation, it is apparent that CRP is selective rather than universal in its contribution to protection against infection by bacteria.

We have already noted that the activation of complement by CRP is similar to its activation by antibody. However, Mold has found that CRP is distinguished by being specific for the classic complement pathway and actually being an inhibitor of the alternative (properdin) pathway. Specifically, CRP inhibits activation of the alternative pathway by liposomes and pneumococci. When it binds to either of these ligands, it can convert a surface that is activating the alternative pathway into a surface that activates only the classic pathway. Other materials also activate the alternative pathway—erythrocytes, zymosan, lipopolysaccharide, and *Escherichia coli*—but none of these is interfered with by CRP. We know of no other molecule that shares CRP's ability to inhibit the alternative pathway in a particle-specific manner.

Although antibody is involved in alternative-pathway activation by pneumococci, it has nothing to do with activation by liposomes utilized in the study just cited. The inhibitory effect of CRP, therefore, most likely does not involve interference with an antibody. Instead, we suggest that CRP and the alternative-pathway proteins compete by binding to some other type of ligand and/or to each other in a way that impedes alternative-pathway activation.

The biologic ramifications of substituting classic-pathway for alternative-pathway activation are not known. From an investigative point of view, the CRP system provides a means by which the differences between the two complement pathways can be more fully explored. What is clear is that when CRP is appropriately bound, it can, in turn, activate the classic complement pathway, thereby inducing complement-dependent phagocytosis and cytolysis and generating complement-derived, biologically active peptides.

Aside from complement activation, CRP shares certain other properties with antibody: the ability to bind to lymphocytes and the ability to activate platelets.

Purified CRP will not bind to lymphocytes, but in the presence of calcium and small quantities of a multivalent phosphocholine-containing molecule (i.e., CPS), binding will occur, as shown by Karen James of our laboratory. Immunofluorescent labeling studies have revealed that CRP complexes attach to a small percentage of peripheral blood lymphocytes (3.0% ± 1.7%) and a substantially greater percentage of monocytes.

Characterization of the lymphocytes that bind CRP showed that 70% of these cells from normal donors and 90% of these cells from cancer patients possess IgG Fc receptors. Of all those cells with the Fc receptor, however, only 12% bind CRP, suggesting that CRP attaches only to a subset of these cells. This is in agreement with the earlier studies of Ralph Williams and his colleagues in New Mexico, who observed EDTA-elutable (and therefore, presumably, complexed) CRP preferentially on the surface of a subpopulation of lymphocytes bearing IgG Fc receptors from patients with acute rheumatic fever or even following streptococcal infections with the nonsuppurative sequelae.

The lymphocytes that bind CRP in our hands have the large granular lymphocyte (LGL) morphology (see Figure 10, page 151). This observation and the fact that the CRP-binding lymphocytes also have Fc receptors suggested that the lymphocytes that bind CRP are natural killer cells. Recent observations in other laboratories show that LGLs are responsible both for natural killer activity (a spontaneous, cytolytic response to tumor and microbially infected cells) and for killer activity (also known as antibody-dependent, cell-mediated cyto-

Figure 8

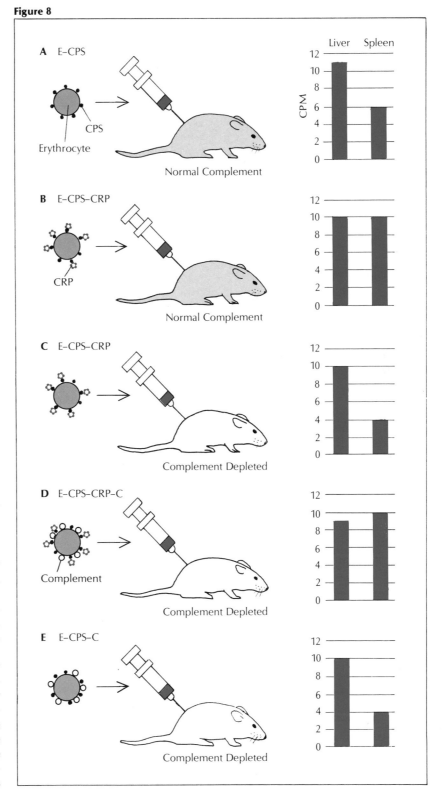

Enhanced clearance to the spleen is seen upon the binding of both CRP and complement. In mouse with normal complement levels, ^{51}Cr-labeled erythrocytes coated with pneumococcal C-polysaccharide were dominantly cleared by the liver (A). But when CRP was added, an increased splenic clearance was seen (B). In C-depleted animals, hepatic clearance was again dominant (C), unless C as well as CRP was added to the red cells (D). Enhanced splenic clearance was no longer observed when CRP was removed after C binding in the C-depleted animals (E). (Data from S. Nakayama)

Figure 9

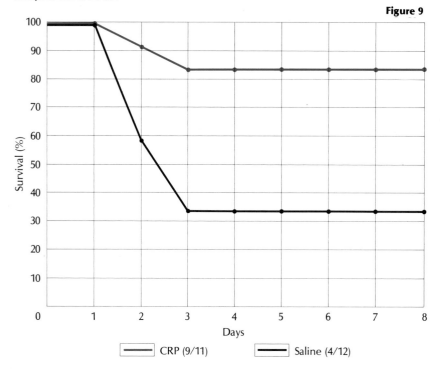

Experiments by C. Mold and colleagues showed that treatment with CRP dramatically increased the survival of mice injected with S. pneumoniae type 4.

toxicity) that acts via the IgG Fc receptor (see R. B. Herberman, "Natural Killer Cells"). For the sake of clarity, we shall refer to this lymphatic population as LGLs.

The relationship between CRP and LGLs is turning out to be quite intimate. Linda Baum of our laboratory examined the natural killer activity of LGLs after they were incubated with antibody directed against CRP. It should be emphasized that these LGLs were isolated from healthy human donors and had not been previously exposed to CRP in vitro. Treatment with anti-CRP serum, particularly in the presence of complement, markedly reduced the natural killer activity (see Figure 11, page 152).

This observation was extended by James, utilizing fluorescent labeling of the antibody used to generate the LGL-anti-CRP complexes. We discovered that 46% of LGLs have CRP on their surface that was not elutable with EDTA. These CRP molecules can be "capped," or clustered together, by anti-CRP, as can the absorbed CRP-CPS complexes, but they cap at different rates and may be capped independently.

We are left with the inference that at least certain LGLs contain endogenous CRP molecules on their surface membrane, and these are proving not to be identical with sites that bind exogenous CRP complexes. In this respect, CRP is, again, strikingly similar to immunoglobulin. Certain cells have surface immunoglobulin, whereas other cells have Fc receptors that bind soluble immunoglobulin. The relationship between the binding site for CRP complexes and the IgG Fc receptor has yet to be established.

What is the relationship between the LGL surface CRP and the CRP receptor? What is the biologic role of CRP in LGL function? As of now, we do not know the answer to either question, although we are wondering whether CRP might have a recognition function in keeping with its apparent role in natural immunity. It also might play a modulatory or regulatory role, as had previously been postulated. Marsha Vetter, working with Linda Baum, has observed that complexed CRP enhances the cell-mediated cytotoxicity potential of cytolytic T lymphocytes by twofold to thirty-

fivefold. Complexed CRP also slightly enhances the blastogenesis of resting lymphocytes and the responsiveness of allogeneic cells in a mixed lymphocyte culture. We are not sure why the LGLs from subjects in the acute phase (in our work, people with cancer) are more effective binders of CRP. One explanation is that LGLs become more active during the acute phase. Alternatively, the acute phase may stimulate the growth of a more active subpopulation of lymphocytes.

The interactions of CRP with the platelet have been extensively investigated by Barry A. Fiedel of our laboratory. As with its other antibodylike properties, CRP needs to be modified or associated with an appropriate ligand to activate platelets. When heated, CRP aggregates, and in this form it induces platelet aggregation and secretions, the way IgG does when it is aggregated by heat, antigen, chemical treatment, or coating to inert particles. A maximum response of platelets occurs in the presence of $> 50 \mu g/ml$ of heat-treated CRP. Indeed, on a weight basis, CRP is a tenfold to twentyfold more potent platelet activator than IgG.

Heated CRP behaves synergistically with other platelet stimulators, such as ADP, arachidonate, and acid-soluble collagen. This observation is important since it has been hypothesized that in vivo platelet activation reflects the interactive involvement of many activators.

Complexes of CRP and certain of its polycationic ligands (i.e., poly-L-lysine and protamine) are also effective platelet activators, but for reasons not yet clear, CRP-CPS complexes do not share this property. CRP activation requires ATP and calcium and is inhibited by cAMP, which indicates that the stimulation is an active process.

Among the substances released by CRP-activated platelets is thromboxane A_2, a powerful platelet-activating substance that also causes vasoconstriction. This may be a means by which complexed CRP activates and supports the inflammatory and hemostatic processes.

It can be noted parenthetically that several years ago, CRP preparations were found to inhibit, rather than stimulate, platelet activation. This has been attributed recently to a low-molecular-mass factor (8300 to 12,500 daltons) that binds to and frequently copurifies with CRP. When this factor is separated out, the inhibitory effects—and the paradox—are removed. Surely, biologic as well as chemical definition of the various molecules associated with CRP, CRP complexes, molecular forms of the protein, and cellular binding sites for these various expressions of CRP is of the greatest importance for interpreting the reactivities of CRP with the platelets as well as with leukocytes, complement, and altered cells.

CRP does not leave behind as many traces of its presence as one might expect. Kushner and Kaplan used indirect immunofluorescence to detect CRP deposits in the necrotic skeletal and cardiac muscles, apparently on the sarcolemma, of rabbits. Terry DuClos of our laboratory has found CRP deposited in the spinal cord lesions of rabbits with experimentally induced allergic encephalomyelitis. The pattern of CRP deposition in this instance suggested that the protein was inside the cells, perhaps reflecting phagocytic ingestion of CRP bound to necrotic tissue. W. E. Parish detected CRP and complement deposits in the cutaneous lesions of patients with vasculitis. CRP also has been found in the synovial mesothelium of rheumatoid arthritis patients. What is striking, however, is how often CRP is not seen at all or only in meager quantities, as compared with the amount of antibody and complement that can be seen in inflamed or necrotic tissues in certain diseases. It is not yet known whether this is due to quick catabolism of CRP, to combination with lipid and consequent sequestration of the protein, to lack of binding, or to some other cause.

The studies of CRP that we have described have focused predominantly on human CRP. Pentraxin molecules, however, are widely distributed through phylogeny. Phosphocholine-binding proteins that are structurally homologous with human CRP occur in many vertebrates, including mammals, birds, and fish (as defined by B. A. Baldo, T. C. Fletcher, and M. B. Pepys), and even in an invertebrate, the horseshoe crab, in the recent, most provocative definition by Liu et al. Rabbit CRP has been the most extensively examined animal form of the protein, beginning with the classic studies of McCarty and his colleagues. The N-terminal amino acid sequences of rabbit and human CRP were shown by Osmand et al to be very similar, and the molecules show antigenic cross-reactivity, although there are subtle differences between the two in terms of binding reactivities. Among the other pentraxins, SAP is of particular interest because of its relationship to human amyloid. Intriguingly, a hormone-related "female protein" has been discovered and investigated in certain species of hamster by John Coe. This protein has structural and immunologic similarity to SAP while expressing clear affinity for phosphocholine. Perhaps like the structural similarity between the phosphocholine-binding sites of certain myeloma proteins and CRP, CRP exhibits limited structural or functional relationships with the other phosphocholine-binding proteins.

There is no evidence for the existence of antibodies in invertebrates. Since CRP shares many properties with antibody (see Table 3, page 153), while reacting with a much more limited, if nonetheless widely distributed, group of targets, and since it appears earlier in phylogeny, it is tempting to speculate that CRP is a primitive forerunner of immunoglobulin. But because CRP, or a like molecule, is found in so many higher species and apparently performs a wide range of potentially useful functions, we like to think of it as being more than an appendix that evolution neglected to eliminate when antibodies arrived on the scene. Nevertheless, it is true that certain higher species do not produce CRP or any currently recognized related protein other than SAP. It also is intriguing that certain species—mice, for example—produce a protein that behaves quite similarly to CRP but is different. A description of this protein brings us to the final class of acute phase reactants to be discussed here: amyloid proteins. The CRP-like protein that mice produce is the serum amyloid P component, or SAP.

Amyloid is a proteinaceous substance that is deposited between cells and tissues during certain disease states. The function (if any) of amyloid is not clear, and although one may wonder whether it may be used to "wall off" certain regions when they are infected, no evidence for survival value of this material has been brought forward to date. As amyloid accumulates, it can encroach on and produce pressure atrophy of cells. There are two major types of amyloid, as well as many minor types: One major type is found in association with plasma cell dyscrasias and consists predominantly (about 90%) of immunoglobulin light chains; the other major type is found in association with chronic inflammation and consists predominantly (about 90%) of the acute phase protein serum amyloid A component (SAA).

Figure 10

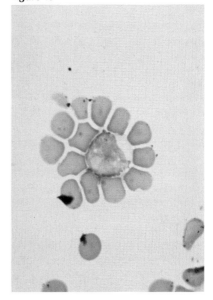

In rosetting experiments, cells binding CRP complexes showed large granular lymphocyte morphology.

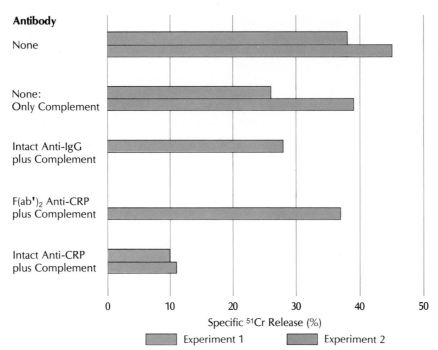

Antibody

(Bar chart)

Categories (top to bottom): None; None: Only Complement; Intact Anti-IgG plus Complement; F(ab')₂ Anti-CRP plus Complement; Intact Anti-CRP plus Complement

X-axis: Specific ⁵¹Cr Release (%) — 0, 10, 20, 30, 40, 50

Legend: Experiment 1, Experiment 2

The effector activity of natural killer (NK) cells was markedly diminished by treatment with intact antibody to CRP in the presence of complement. In a series of experiments by L. Baum et al, similar reduction of NK cell activity was not observed with anti-IgG antibody, with the F(ab')₂ fragment of anti-CRP antibody, or in the absence of antibody with or without complement.

SAP makes up about 10% of both these types of amyloid. Amyloids also have been found in the heart, endocrine glands, and elsewhere. Each contains a unique predominant protein as well as about 10% SAP.

As was mentioned previously, Osmand had observed in our laboratory that the first 30 N-terminal amino acids of SAP are about 60% homologous to the same region of CRP, but the two proteins have not been immunologically cross-reactive with the antisera reported to date. SAP has not been considered an important human acute phase reactant since its level in the blood, at most, only doubles and generally increases only 10% to 40%. However, in mice, as reported by Pepys, the biosynthetic patterns of CRP and SAP seem reversed: SAP levels rise a hundredfold to a thousandfold during the acute phase, whereas CRP levels rise only marginally.

SAP is composed of 10 noncovalently associated subunits, each with a molecular weight of about 23,500. As stated earlier, the sub-units arrange into pentameric discs that have the appearance of CRP—except SAP, which is a decamer composed of two rings back to back. The protein that appears in amyloid deposits seems identical to the SAP that is found in serum. In addition to similarity in ultrastructural appearance and amino acid sequence homology, both molecules show significant calcium dependence; are synthesized by hepatocytes; and, as mentioned previously, even seem to share certain binding reactivities and biosynthetic patterns across the species.

The function of SAP is unknown, although there is some evidence that it has a role in amyloid formation. Pepys and coworkers have demonstrated SAP in human vascular basement membrane and in association with elastic fibers, and they have shown that in the presence of calcium, SAP binds to isolated amyloid fibers and to certain insoluble polysaccharides, including zymosan and agarose. Strong reactivity with heparin and certain other polyanions has been demon-

strated. In collaboration with Pepys, we have shown that purified human SAP agglutinates sheep erythrocytes coated with C3. Further investigation indicated that SAP particularly binds to C3bi (a cell-bound breakdown product of C3), and aggregation of SAP seems to be required for this reaction to occur. While the significance of this binding is unknown, it suggests a possible physiologic role for SAP. Although SAP has this binding activity, it has not been shown to activate complement. Aggregated SAP also has been shown by Pepys to bind to fibronectin (which can react with the complement component C1q) and C4-binding proteins. It seems likely that SAP and CRP function in some coordinated or overlapping way.

Unlike SAP, SAA does not resemble CRP, but it does closely follow CRP's appearance and disappearance. SAA is the other, well-studied acute phase reactant that rises to quantities a hundredfold to a thousandfold over basal levels. Also in contrast to SAP, SAA exists in either of two forms, depending on whether it is in serum or deposited in amyloid. SAA purified from serum has a molecular weight of 12,000. The amyloid form, properly called the amyloid A component, is about two thirds this size. SAA is found in the lipoprotein fraction of serum and is believed to associate with HDL. Experimental induction of SAA in mice has shown that the amount of amyloid deposited does not directly reflect the amount of amyloid in the serum. The only biologic function reported for SAA to date is that it appeared to suppress the in vitro antibody response to T cell–dependent antigens. Studies by M. D. Benson and coworkers suggest that this effect is due to alteration of T cell–macrophage interactions by SAA.

This review should make it apparent that investigation of the biology of the acute phase is only beginning. We can be sure that we do not yet recognize everything that occurs during the acute phase, and our understanding of the changes that we are aware of is incomplete.

What we have learned is that the acute phase is an important physiologic state that warrants further examination and exploitation.

Our understanding of the acute phase has ramifications for the experimental immunologist. Usually, in vivo research of immunity takes no notice of the inflammatory state of a test animal. In vitro experiments usually use highly purified reagents that would not contain, for example, acute phase reactants. Obviously, these conditions do not represent or account for what actually goes on in the animal. Although simplicity has been required to establish an initial understanding of immunity, we should be striving to elucidate the phenomenon as it exists in a natural setting, which would suggest reevaluating many fundamental precepts under conditions that are operative during the acute phase.

Of all the acute phase proteins, we know the most about CRP, but we also have many unanswered questions about what this protein does and how it does it. Experimental evidence suggests that CRP recognizes foreign or altered substances. After combining with such a ligand, CRP reacts with complement, mononuclear leukocytes, neutrophils, and platelets to initiate immune-related as well as "non-immune" activities at an early stage of the inflammatory response, before specific antibody is produced. CRP not only appears to respond earlier than antibody but also seems to have developed first. In short, CRP and related acute phase pro-

Table 3. Activities and Reactions of CRP and CRP Complexes

With complement system
    Activation of classic complement pathway
    Inhibition of alternate complement pathway
    Initiation of C-dependent lysis

With macrophages
    Binding to membranes
    Initiation and mediation of C-dependent ingestion

With PMN leukocytes
    Binding
    Enhancement of migration
    Initiation of C-dependent opsonization

With peripheral blood lymphocytes
    Binding to subset of IgG Fc-receptor cells (LGLs)

With platelets
    Initiation of aggregation
    Initiation of degranulation

Other observed phenomena
    Protection against pneumococcal infection in mice
    Induction of cutaneous reactions in humans
    Deposition at inflammatory sites

Color code:
    In vivo reactions in color
    In vitro reactions in black

teins may subserve functions of a second language—one that may provide recognition and/or modulation designed to mobilize host defenses through inflammatory effectors.

Our experiments, which demonstrate the protection by CRP against certain fatal bacterial infections, underscore its physiologic value. It is now reasonable to consider CRP as a potential tool for therapy or prophylaxis. There is, however, a way to promote CRP activity that is more generalized and natural than injecting the protein. All one need do is induce an inflammatory response by, for example, adjuvant therapy. Since we know of no one who lacks the capacity to make CRP, inducing an acute phase should automatically boost CRP. Perhaps we should begin to devise additional ways in which a good inflammatory response can be promoted.

14

Leukocytes as Secretory Organs of Inflammation

GERALD WEISSMANN *New York University*

The physiologic term "secretion" almost automatically calls to mind the endocrine and exocrine glands – organs as diverse as the thyroid, pancreas, and pituitary. All these tissues, in response to stimuli of various kinds, manufacture chemicals that subserve important functions elsewhere in the body, and liberate them into the bloodstream or into other body regions such as the alimentary canal. All of them, moreover, can damage the body or derange its functioning if their secretions get out of control.

Like the tissues just mentioned, leukocytes (specifically, the granulocytes or polymorphonuclear leukocytes that play a central role in the body's defenses against foreign substances and organisms) can also be viewed as secretory "organs." They too manufacture and liberate substances that subserve an important physiologic function – the mobilization of the body's defenses against invasion, sometimes launching the process we call inflammation. Equally, their malfunction, like that of other tissues conventionally considered secretory, can produce serious pathologic consequences, as in immune complex diseases. Under these circumstances enzymes inadvertently secreted from lysosomes attack the tissues of the host instead of degrading antibody-coated bacteria or viruses. Since granulocytes recognize "foreign" particles mainly when such particles have been tarred with a brush of antibody, granulocytes possess surface receptors (Fc receptors) which function like hormone receptors in other secretory cells.

Therefore it was not surprising that recent work in our laboratory and elsewhere has revealed that the mechanisms of leukocyte secretion, as we are coming to understand them, bear a remarkable resemblance to those previously described in the endocrine and exocrine glands. For all the innumerable innovations it has generated over the past several billion years, evolution appears in certain respects very conservative. Having devised an efficient, or reasonably efficient, way of carrying out a particular type of process, it tends to stick to that pattern, though naturally modifications occur as appropriate for specific physiologic functions.

The relationship between leukocytes and inflammation has been known since 1882, when Elie Metchnikoff stuck a rose thorn into a starfish larva. Under his microscope, he observed leukocytes gathering at the point of invasion, while, at the same time, the larva underwent an inflammatory reaction very like that which occurs in human beings at the site of (say) a splinter in a finger. In further experiments, using soluble or finely divided substances, he was able to observe the process of phagocytosis, in which the "intruders" are found by the leukocytes, seized "after the manner of the amoeba," and digested within intracellular vacuoles by "cytases" – what we would now call lysosomal enzymes. Metchnikoff recognized eight different cytases; we now know there are more than 40.

The basic characters of the cytases were defined when Metchnikoff "fed" phagocytes the red cells of a goose, which, unlike mammalian erythrocytes, possess nuclei. The digestion of the goose cells established that phagocytes must produce at least three basic types of cytases: a lipase, which breaks down the lipid cell membrane; an acid protease, which breaks down hemoglobin; and nucleases, which break down the nucleic acids RNA and DNA.

The mechanism by which the cell digests these substances "outside the alimentary canal," said Metchnikoff, "is not as yet sufficiently known . . . but we know very definitely that each injection of serum, whether white of

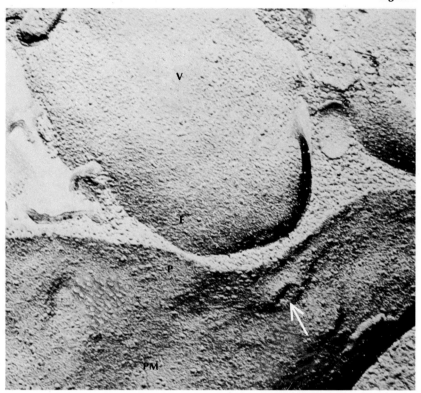

Incipient fusion between plasma membrane (PM) of polymorphonuclear leukocytes and a lysosomal vacuole (V) is shown in freeze-fracture electron micrograph by Sylvia Hoffstein. Fracture plane exposes protoplasmic (P) layer of plasma membrane and ectoplasmic (E) layer of vacuole membrane, which face interiors of cell and vacuole, respectively. Arrow shows channel opening formed where membranes fuse.

egg, milk or fatty matter [we would say foreign proteins or antigens], is followed by a rather considerable aseptic inflammation at the point at which these substances are introduced. We might conclude from this that the organism digests the food substances . . . by means of the inflammatory reaction." He summed up his findings in the statement: "There is no phagocytosis without inflammation."

Metchnikoff's conclusions were both true and untrue. As a rule there is indeed "no phagocytosis without inflammation," but inflammation is not the means by which the organism digests foreign bodies. Rather, it is a concomitant of such digestion, serving to attract leukocytes from elsewhere in the body to deal with the invasion and to wall off the invasion site. However, the inflammatory reaction does liberate cytases, which digest the body's own cells as efficiently as they do foreign cells and can also damage adjacent tissues.

Metchnikoff, along with several generations of physiologists after him, was misled by the observation that the cytases were liberated by killed or injured phagocytes – from which he concluded that they were liberated *only* in this manner. Only as recently as the late 1960s was it determined that phagocytes can and do liberate their cytolytic enzymes in the normal course of business, thereby triggering the inflammatory reaction.

To see how this occurs, let us take a closer look at the process of phagocytosis. As we know, this begins when the phagocyte, a polymorphonuclear leukocyte (PMN), "recognizes" a foreign particle in its vicinity, by virtue of the coating of the material by immunologic ligands or opsonins. Most of the ligands are either antibodies (IgG) that are keyed to surface components of the particle or derivatives of the complement system, specifically the substance C3b. The opsonins engage a receptor on the surface of the

PMN, causing it to invaginate and form a phagocytic vacuole that engulfs the particle. The mouth of the vacuole is then pulled shut, through formation of microfilaments in the adjacent cytoplasm that act as a sort of purse-string suture. Once pulled into approximation, the membranes around the mouth fuse, and the vacuole itself floats off into the cytoplasm. Meanwhile, membranous secretory granules containing digestive enzymes fuse with the vacuole membrane (see Figure 1 on this page) in order to release their enzymes into the vacuole where these can hydrolyze the foreign particle or antigen.

Now if these processes operated in a strict sequence (*first* the closure of the vacuole, *then* degranulation into the vacuole), there would be no release of the enzymes into the extracellular space and no inflammation. In fact, however, the timing is not always so precise, so that degranulation begins before closure, with an inevitable release of some degradative enzymes into the ambient area (see Figure 2 on page 157).

Such release will obviously occur if the foreign particle is too big to be phagocytosed, as in the case of a large ameba or a small worm. Here the PMN, unable to swallow the intruder, will nonetheless release its enzymes and other inflammatory products as long as it is in contact with the foreign organism, bombarding it with these substances rather as old-time warships used to fire broadsides at their enemies. Peter Henson has called this "frustrated phagocytosis."

Even with much smaller particles, enzyme release can occur, especially if the ratio of particles to phagocytes is high, calling for ingestion of a number of particles by a single phagocyte more or less simultaneously. Since the formation of each vacuole involves internal loss of a portion of the phagocyte's plasma membrane and a simultaneous increase in its internal contents, the result is a drop in the ratio of surface to volume. The most obvious sign of this is a loss of the phagocyte's normal ameboid shape and a rounding up into a roughly spherical form (a sphere, of course, has the lowest surface-to-volume ratio of any geometric form). At the same time, increased tension

Figure 2

on the plasma membrane requires the microfilaments to engage in more "pulling and hauling" to close the mouths of the vacuoles. This means that before closure is complete, degranulation is already well under way, and some cytolytic enzymes inevitably escape.

From a functional standpoint, this makes a good deal of sense, since some of these enzymes serve to mobilize the body's defenses against the invasion, both locally and at more distant sites. Clearly, if the invaders are so numerous as to overtax the capacities of the front-line phagocytes already on the scene, the chances are high that additional defenders will need to be mobilized if the attack is to be contained. Unfortunately, the mobilizing enzymes, along with others released with them, can also attack the body cells in the immediate vicinity. This is part of the price the body pays for defending itself against invasion. As we know from innumerable historical examples, even a necessary, defensive military action is likely to do some damage to innocent bystanders.

Evidently, then, secretion of cytolytic, inflammatory enzymes is a normal and indeed necessary part of the phagocyte's activities, at least under certain circumstances. Let us now take a closer look at these secretory processes in an attempt to elucidate their physical and chemical nature.

A more or less standard way of studying PMN secretion is to treat the cells with the reagent cytochalasin B, which (by mechanisms to be discussed later) prevents closure of the phagocytic vacuole, thereby producing copious and consistent secretion into the ambient medium. The extent of such secretion can be measured by assays of various cytolytic enzymes, notably, beta-glucuronidase.

Secretion under these circumstances can be triggered by a surprising variety of stimuli. Most obvious among these are antigen-antibody complexes (e.g., bovine serum albumin and its antibody), since it is such complexes that normally engender phagocytosis in vivo: i.e., complexes formed on the surfaces of foreign organisms or by reaction with foreign proteins engage the so-called Fc receptors on the PMN surface and

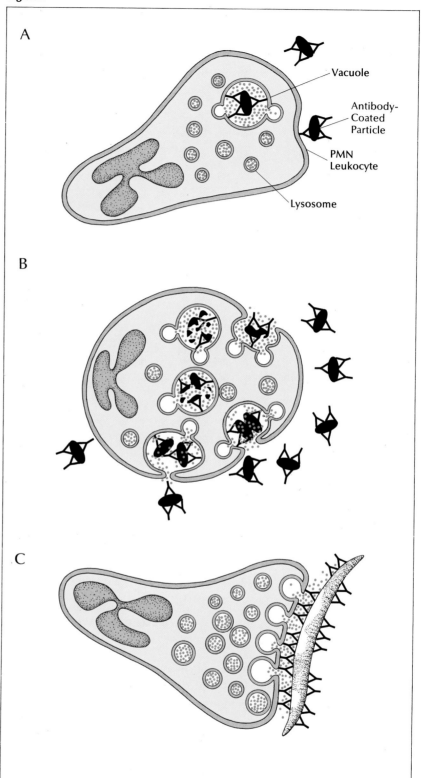

Phagocytosis of foreign substances by polymorphonuclear leukocytes (PMNs) can occur in three ways. Under "normal" conditions (i.e., a low particle-to-cell ratio) lysosomal enzymes (color) are released into closed phagocytic vacuole (A). With high particle-to-cell ratio, release occurs before closure, with escape of enzymes into ambient area where they can damage tissues (B). Release also occurs when foreign body is too large for ingestion: PMN attaches and "bombards" it with enzymes (C).

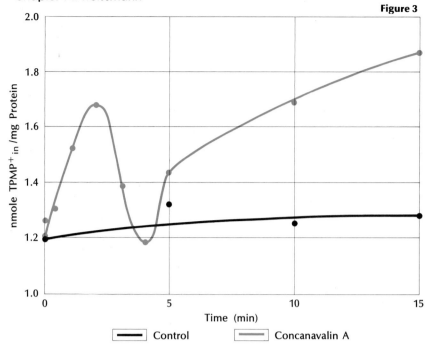

Figure 3

Hyperpolarization of PMN plasma membrane is first identifiable event in the phago-cytic process. Cell stimulated by concanavalin A shows hyperpolarization, reflected by sharp increase in the intracellular concentration of the reagent TPMP⁺ within min-utes. Equally sharp depolarization is followed by slow repolarization.

thereby set off the phagocytic process. Equally expectable is the triggering of secretion by heat-aggregated IgG, which forms a sort of pseudocomplex that engages these same receptors.

Rather more surprising is our dis-covery that the complement compo-nent C5a can also trigger secretion. This minor moiety of the C5 mole-cule, cleaved from it in the course of various immune reactions, has been known to subserve a number of func-tions, but these did not include affect-ing the internal processes of cells, or even binding to them. We have still not proved that the substance actually binds to PMNs, but there is every rea-son to think that it does. Early in this century, Paul Ehrlich enunciated the dogma *corpora non agunt nisi fixata* (substances do not act unless at-tached), and no exceptions have turned up in the meantime. I should note that the PMN response to C5a has thus far been observed only in cytochalasin B-treated cells in suspen-sion; however, when the cells are on a surface, C5a induces degranulation.

Other secretion-producing stimuli include the lectin concanavalin A,

which is known to bind to surface sug-ars (as opposed to the Fc receptors), and the cocarcinogen and potent inflammatory agent phorbol myristate acetate. Both of these, however, are classed as incomplete stimuli, in that they trigger certain PMN secretions (those of the so-called specific gran-ules) but not others (those of the azu-rophil granules). These two types of granules contain different enzyme complements subserving different functions. The fact that some reagents can stimulate release of one type but not the other suggests that the releas-ing processes involved may be some-what different for the two types. The physiologic significance of this obser-vation is unclear, since under normal conditions both types are released al-most simultaneously.

A rather different type of trigger is an ionophore, any one of several lipid-soluble substances that can promote the passage of calcium ion (Ca⁺⁺) into cells from the medium and also from intracellular calcium depots into the cytoplasm. This finding was not very startling, since the role of Ca⁺⁺ in secretion has been known for some

time, but it confirmed our feeling that we were dealing with a true secretory process.

Ionophore, we found, could trigger secretion even in the absence of ex-tracellular Ca⁺⁺ (i.e., when the ion was segregated by a chelating agent in the medium), meaning that it must be producing ionic redistribution within the cell. In this case, the mitochondria did not seem a likely source of the ion (as they are in other secretory cells studied), since PMNs seldom contain more than a few of these organelles. By using specific cytochemical tech-niques for the calcium ion, we were able to show that at least one source is the plasma membrane, which evident-ly contains Ca⁺⁺ within its structure or adsorbed to its inner surface.

Further experiments showed that the same translocation of calcium oc-curs in response to other secretory stimuli and that calcium is lost *only* from the invaginating area of the membrane, i.e., only at the point where the stimulus is acting. What happens to the "lost" calcium is not yet known.

All these activities going on in or around the membrane naturally fo-cused our attention on precisely what was happening there. Studies of other cells (e.g., lymphocytes and thyroid secretory cells) had already shown that one very early event was hyperpolar-ization of the cell. All cells under most conditions maintain a negative charge on the intracellular side of the plasma membrane with respect to their sur-roundings. They do so mainly by pumping cations such as sodium out of the cell. It has long been known that neurons are activated by depolar-ization – the sudden rise in plasma membrane permeability that allows an influx of cations, which momentarily abolishes the difference in charge across the membrane.

Lymphocytes and thyroid cells, however, are known to undergo the inverse of this process: a sudden *jump* in membrane potential, followed by a drop in potential (depolarization) and a slow rise in potential as the cell re-covers. It seemed likely that a similar hyperpolarization process was going on in polymorphonuclear leukocytes but this remained to be demonstrated.

Figure 4

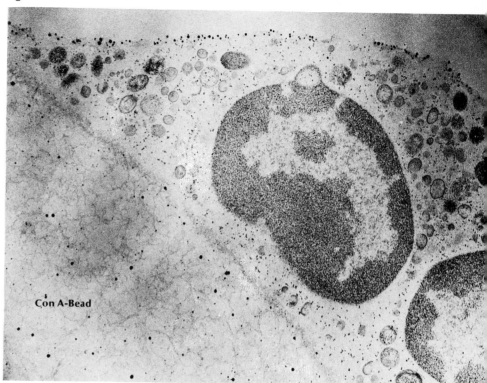

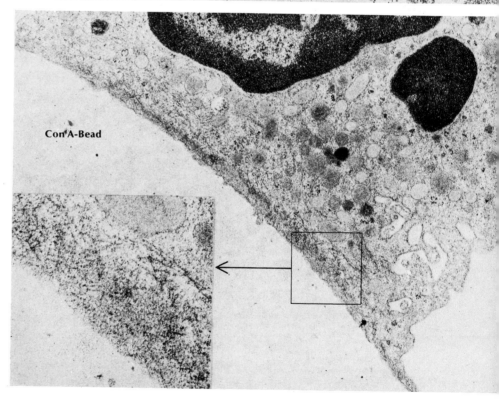

In relatively large cells, potential across the membrane can be measured directly by inserting a micro-electrode into the cell and another into the immediately adjacent medium. PMNs, however, are too small to receive even the smallest microelectrodes, so we were forced to measure membrane potential indirectly. This can be done by adding tritiated triphenylmethyl phosphonium (TPMP$^+$) to the medium; this cation is taken up by the cell to a degree that closely reflects the membrane potential, and the ^{3}H label makes it easy to measure its concentration. Through this technique we demonstrated that PMNs do indeed undergo hyperpolarization in the same manner as lymphocytes and thyroid cells (see Figure 3 on page 158).

Precisely how this occurs is not yet known. What is significant is that it represents the earliest known response of a nonmuscle cell to an external stimulus, since it occurs within five seconds after binding of a ligand, such as an immune complex, to the plasma membrane.

Following membrane hyperpolarization, and possibly (we do not yet know) as a result of it, another key event in phagocytosis occurs: the generation of toxic oxygen products, such as superoxide anion (O$_2^-$). This happens between 30 and 42 seconds after the triggering stimulus is received, in other words, well after the hyperpolarization and more or less simultaneously with the release of calcium ion into the cytoplasm (see Figure 4 on this page). Though we do not know what sets off either process, it seems likely that neither causes the other for at least two reasons. First, superoxide can be generated by stimuli (C3b, C5a), which do *not* trigger the release of secretory granules, a process in which calcium ion is believed to be deeply involved. More important, superoxide is generated at the exterior surface of the plasma membrane, whereas calcium ion, as noted, is released either from within the membrane or from its interior surface.

Superoxide is formed by a surface oxidase, which induces molecular oxygen (dissolved in the serum) to pick up an electron from the electron-carrier NAD(P)H, the latter being con-

Electron micrographs by Sylvia Hoffstein illustrate events in phagocytic process that follow hyperpolarization. Upper photo shows PMN stimulated by concanavalin A attached to sepharose beads and specifically stained to localize calcium; calcium ions within or on plasma membrane (black dots) are "lost" from stimulated portion of membrane in contact with bead (below). Later, microfilaments assemble in stimulated area (below). Under physiologic conditions, microfilaments help pull membranes inward to form phagocytic vacuole. Inset shows higher magnification of microfilaments.

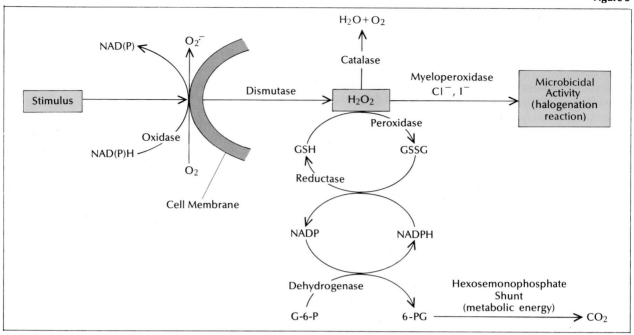

Formation of superoxide ion (O_2^-) in response to a phagocytic stimulus sets off two important processes. Superoxide reacts with water to form hydrogen peroxide (H_2O_2), which reacts with halogen ions to form microbicidal substances within the phagocytic vacuole. The peroxide also triggers a complex metabolic chain, activating the hexosemonophosphate shunt, which supplies energy for phagocytic activities. H_2O_2 is detoxified by catalase within the cytoplasm.

verted into NAD(P) plus one hydrogen ion. Most of the superoxide is further converted, by means of another enzyme, into hydrogen peroxide (H_2O_2), which is intensely active, as is superoxide itself. Since these two processes begin before invagination gets under way, simply in response to contact with a triggering stimulus, it follows that some superoxide and peroxide will be left outside the PMN (the consequences will be discussed later). The remainder will be carried into the cell as invagination occurs, with more being produced by the inside surface of the vacuole membrane, which, of course, originated as the outside of the plasma membrane. To further complicate matters, both peroxide and superoxide can migrate into the cytoplasm through the plasma membrane or the vacuole membrane.

Depending on where the peroxide is located, various things now happen. Within the phagocytic vacuole, hydrogen peroxide, in the presence of the granule enzyme myeloperoxidase, reacts with chloride ion (Cl^-) to form hypochlorite ($Cl_2O_2^{--}$). As we all know, this is a potent bactericide, the active agent used in chlorinating

drinking water and swimming pools. (The peroxide can also react with any other halide ion such as iodide that happens to be present, with the same bactericidal results.)

To the extent that the hydrogen peroxide migrates into the cytoplasm, or is formed there by superoxide that has so migrated, it is rapidly broken down by an intracellular enzyme (catalase) into water and molecular oxygen, both of which are harmless to the cell interior, as peroxide definitely is not. In the breaking-down process, however, a complicated series of events is set in train, the ultimate result of which is a stepping up of the cell's oxidative metabolism (see Figure 5 on this page).

The significance of superoxide in the body's defenses can be seen in chronic granulomatous disease (CGD) of childhood, in which the PMNs lack the surface oxidase that generates superoxide. Thus the phagocytes cannot kill catalase-positive bacteria such as *Staphylococcus aureus* very efficiently, because they cannot generate hypochlorite. Catalase-negative bacteria (pneumococci) produce enough H_2O_2 to commit suicide.

In vitro, the deficiencies of such cells can be corrected by adding particles coated with H_2O_2-generating enzymes to the CGD cells.

Let us return now from the scene of these purely chemical events to the better understood mechanical aspects of PMN secretory function. As previously related, the mechanical events proceed in three stages: invagination, in which an area of plasma membrane is pulled inward toward the center of the cell; closure, in which the mouth of the invagination is pulled shut; and degranulation, in which the azurophil and specific lysosomal granules fuse with the invagination, either before or after it has become a vacuole.

The first two steps are, and must be, sequential, since closure cannot take place until invagination has occurred. Steps two and three (closure and degranulation) are usually sequential, but may overlap. Degranulation may begin before closure is completed or (in the cytochalasin B-treated cell) without closure occurring at all.

All three processes involve the assembly of microfilaments. These are tiny bodies about 6 nm in diameter, which are polymers of the contractile

Figure 6

protein actin. In conjunction with the other contractile protein, myosin, these microfilaments can exert the forces necessary to produce invagination, closure, and degranulation (see Figure 6 on this page). In invagination and degranulation, they are assisted by microtubules, much larger bodies (about 30 nm diameter) formed by polymerization of another, noncontractile protein, tubulin. The microtubules, as it were, provide the microfilaments with an internal skeleton to pull against. In closure, microtubules are not needed; the filaments are pulling in the plane of the plasma membrane and attached to it (See Figure 7 on page 162).

It should be noted that although microtubules are helpful in both invagination and degranulation, they do not appear to be absolutely necessary. In experimental systems where microtubule assembly is blocked (e.g., by colchicine), these two processes continue, albeit at greatly reduced efficiency. This inefficiency can be observed clinically in Chediak-Higashi disease, in which the patient's PMNs for some reason are unable to assemble microtubules and thereby cannot complete the normal fusion processes of phagocytosis.

The assembly of both microfilaments and microtubules is believed to be in some sense related to the release of calcium ion from the PMN plasma membrane. More definitely, we can say that microtubule assembly, at least, is stimulated by (and probably controlled by) the "second messenger" cyclic GMP (cGMP). Conversely, it can be inhibited by the other second messenger, cyclic AMP (cAMP), which in this as in so many physiologic processes acts in an opposite sense to cGMP. This has been demonstrated in vitro by adding agents that raise intracellular levels of one or the other messenger molecule, and also clinically by a group at the University of Connecticut. Giving children with Chediak-Higashi disease substances such as carbamylcholine or ascorbic acid, which are known to increase cellular levels of cGMP, normalizes the bactericidal potency of their PMNs.

Microfilament assembly may or may not be controlled by cGMP, but in any case it seems to be a somewhat more

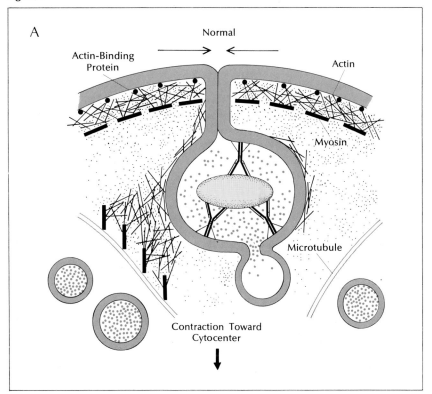

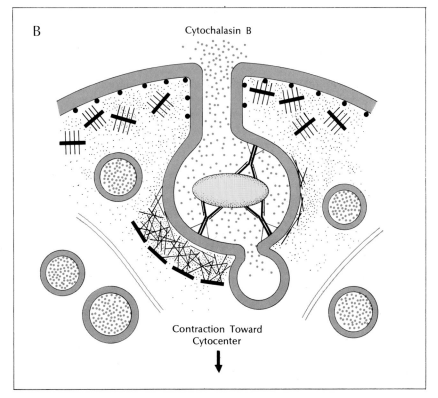

Membrane deformation during phagocytosis is induced mainly by microfilaments of actin and myosin. Vacuole is formed by inward pull of filaments attached to plasma membrane and perhaps to microtubules; closure occurs when filaments attach to actin-binding protein (ABP) anchored in membrane and pull parallel to membrane plane (top). Cytochalasin B interferes with proper interaction of actin and ABP and thereby prevents closure while leaving vacuole formation unaffected (bottom).

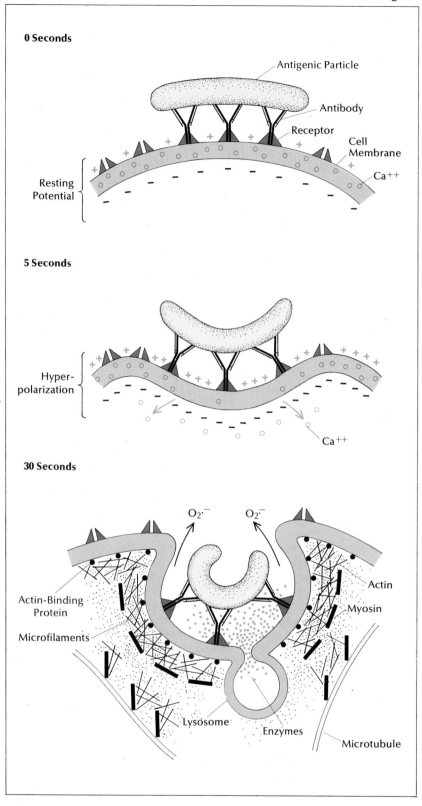

0 Seconds

Antigenic Particle

Antibody

Receptor

Cell Membrane

Ca^{++}

Resting Potential

5 Seconds

Hyper-polarization

Ca^{++}

30 Seconds

O_2^- O_2^-

Actin-Binding Protein

Microfilaments

Actin

Myosin

Lysosome

Enzymes

Microtubule

Sequence of events in phagocytosis begins with attachment of antibody-labeled antigen to receptors on plasma membrane of phagocytic cell (top). At 5 sec (center) membrane is hyperpolarized and calcium ions within are released into cytoplasm. At 30 sec (bottom) superoxide ion (O_2.-) has formed and microfilaments and microtubules are assembled. Contracted microfilaments help membrane invaginate.

complex process than microtubule assembly. Whereas microtubule assembly involves polymerization of only one (noncontractile) protein, tubulin, microfilament assembly involves actin, myosin, and a third, noncontractile, protein called actin-binding protein (ABP). ABP is attached to (or projects from) the interior surface of the plasma membrane and anchors the filaments to the membrane, thereby enabling them to exert force against it and deform it as phagocytosis requires. Finally, for contraction to be completed, a cofactor (whose exact nature has yet to be determined) must be present in the cytoplasm.

The function of ABP has been definitely demonstrated in the process of vacuole closure; in fact, the inhibition of closure by cytochalasin B results from its interference with the association between actin and ABP. One would expect that some ABP-like "anchor" would also be required for invagination and perhaps also for degranulation, but this has not yet been demonstrated. Assuming that one or more such substances exists, it (or they) must evidently be of a somewhat different nature from ABP, since, as already noted, neither invagination nor degranulation are inhibited by cytochalasin B.

Having elucidated the events of the phagocytic-secretory process as well as we can, let us now consider the products of secretion. The first of these are superoxide and its successor, hydrogen peroxide, which, in turn, forms hydroxyl radical (OH•) and singlet oxygen. As we have seen, some superoxide is routinely released into the immediate neighborhood of the PMN, where it (or one of its successor products) can react with the membrane lipids of nearby cells, damaging or even destroying them.

However, there is reason to suspect that superoxide also participates in other, more "constructive" activities (though some of the latter may have destructive consequences as well), for example, the formation of several types of chemoattractants through the direct oxygenation of membrane arachidonic acid. One of the metabolic pathways involving superoxide or one of its successor compounds leads to formation of a chemotactic sub-

Figure 8

Leukocytes and Inflammation

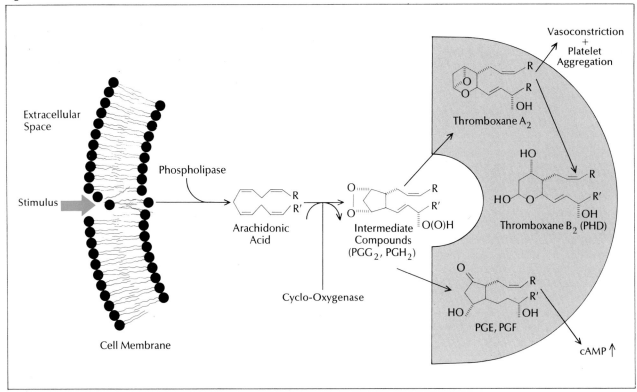

Secretion, in response to surface stimulation of the PMN, is accompanied by formation of prostaglandins and thromboxanes through oxidation of membrane arachidonic acid. A metabolic pathway, mediated by cyclo-oxygenase, leads first to short-lived intermediate prostaglandins (PGG$_2$ and PGH$_2$). These endoperoxides are metabolized to thromboxanes A$_2$ and B$_2$. Both (particularly A$_2$) are vasoconstrictors and platelet-aggregating substances. Other endoperoxide prostaglandins proceed via a different pathway to form stable prostaglandins (PGE and PGF) that moderate the inflammatory response of neighboring PMNs by enhancing intracellular cAMP. The 5 and 15 lipoxygenase pathways are not illustrated.

stance that attracts additional PMNs to the invasion site, in effect, bringing in more troops to deal with the enemy.

A more important metabolic pathway is mediated by the enzyme cyclo-oxygenase and leads to formation of the endoperoxide prostaglandins PGG$_2$ and PGH$_2$, which are in part further metabolized into yet other prostaglandins, the thromboxanes B$_2$ and A$_2$. All these substances, and especially thromboxane A$_2$, are vasoconstrictors and platelet-aggregating agents, and they thus serve to wall off and localize the invasion and its inflammatory consequences. Meanwhile, however, some of the endoperoxides are metabolized via a different pathway into the stable prostaglandins PGE and PGF. These are not notably inflammatory; they serve rather to moderate the inflammatory response of neighboring PMNs by raising intracellular levels of cAMP (see Figure 8 on this page).

In a quite different category from superoxide, part of which is routinely released from the cell surface where it is formed, are the contents of the secretory granules. As we have seen, under certain circumstances these can escape from an imperfectly closed vacuole, whereby they produce both destructive and constructive effects.

In this context, we must distinguish sharply between the specific and the azurophil granules. The former contain a variety of substances, not all of them having known functions, but none of them, so far as we know, exerting destructive effects on surrounding tissues when and if released. The azurophils, by contrast, contain several strongly proteolytic enzymes. Normally, i.e., within the closed vacuole, these serve to degrade foreign proteins, including the protein components of ingested organisms, but when released outside the cell, they can attack tissues. They include collagenase

and elastase (which can break down collagen and elastin) and cathepsin G, a chymotrypsin-like enzyme that attacks cartilage.

Cathepsin G and elastase, however, also can subserve useful functions. They can, for example, generate kinins from kininogen; by increasing vascular permeability, these permit PMNs to escape from the circulation and deal with invading organisms that have similarly escaped. Cathepsin G can also cleave the complement component C5 into C5a and C5b, substances whose role in PMN secretion has already been described. Finally, cathepsin G and elastase can activate resting lymphocytes, in effect (to continue with our military analogy) not calling in additional troops, as do the chemotactic substances formed from arachidonate, but mobilizing fresh reserves that presumably will be called up in their turn.

These potent roles of neutral proteases in immune reactions, such as the Arthus, which depends on granulocytes, may explain why the normal circulation contains inhibitors of these enzymes, the best known inhibitors being alpha-1-antitrypsin and alpha-2-macroglobulins, which can moderate if not wholly prevent their attacks on adjacent tissues. In this context, it will be recalled that patients with alpha-1-antitrypsin deficiency tend to get lung disease; unopposed by inhibitor, the enzymes spewed out by the PMNs in an ordinary respiratory infection act to degrade the matrix of the lung itself.

As our knowledge of the complexities of phagocytosis and inflammation has expanded, it has become clear that compounds exerting anti-inflammatory effects operate in many different ways. Broadly speaking, they can be divided into two classes: those that modulate the release of lysosomal enzymes by influencing degranulation and/or microtubule assembly, and those that inhibit formation of thromboxanes and prostaglandins.

The first class of compounds can be subdivided into two subclasses. One of these operates by raising intracellular levels of cAMP, which, as already noted, inhibits, as cyclic GMP promotes, degranulation and microtubule assembly. These agents include exogenous cAMP (plus theophylline), prostaglandin E_1, and isoproterenol. Colchicine and vinblastine, by contrast, promote the *dis*assembly of microtubules directly, although their other mechanisms of action are not completely known.

Anti-inflammatory agents, such as aspirin and indomethacin, on the other hand, have only modest effects on degranulation and enzyme release. They inhibit the cellular enzyme cyclo-oxygenase, which mediates the first step in converting arachidonic acid into endoperoxides and thromboxanes.

The corticosteroids do not fall neatly into either category, since they seem to affect the overall functions of PMNs, rather than individual aspects of PMN metabolism. At least some of their anti-inflammatory effects in immune reactions seem due to inhibition of all PMN activities: the production of toxic oxygen products, release of thromboxanes and prostaglandins, phagocytosis, and degranulation. The exact mechanism by which they accomplish this inhibition is not known, but it appears to involve membrane stabilization; more particularly, they may inhibit the fusion between membranes that is necessary for the enzymatic granules to empty into the phagocytic vacuole and release their contents.

As noted at the beginning of this article, the similarity between the mechanisms of PMN secretion and those of more "conventional" secretory cells testifies to the parsimony of evolution once it has got hold of a reasonably good thing. One might even note a certain similarity between PMNs and neurons, since in both cell types the initial response to stimulus involves a change in membrane potential, albeit in an opposite sense.

One might perhaps wonder why, since PMNs have probably been evolving for several hundred million years at least, they do not operate more "efficiently." Granted that they are very necessary parts of the body's defenses, but why, in defending the body, must they at times damage the very tissues they are defending? In fact, however, to assume that the products of evolution, whether individual cells or organisms, are bound to operate at 100% efficiency is to substitute teleology for science. Evolutionary survival has never required that successful species or metabolic mechanisms be wholly efficient – merely that they be efficient enough for population gain to balance population loss. So long as the evolutionary books balance, it does not matter how much red ink shows up in the ledger: what counts is the bottom line.

A moment's reflection will show that the human animal, like all other animals, is equipped with all sorts of evolutionary inefficiencies. The vermiform appendix is surely one, and the hyperuricemia consequent on renal tubular reabsorption of uric acid, unique to our species, is almost certainly another. Yet humanity has survived both appendicitis and gout – and seems likely to do so indefinitely. We may grumble at these and other ills with which an imperfect evolution has saddled us, but like Napoleon's grenadiers, though we keep grumbling, we keep marching.

Section III
DISEASE-SPECIFIC IMMUNOPATHOLOGIC PROCESSES

Complement Abnormalities In Human Disease

HANS J. MÜLLER-EBERHARD   *Research Institute of the Scripps Clinic*

We have previously presented a review of the chemistry and function of the complement system (Chapter 12). It is, however, necessary to fill in some gaps before launching into the major theme of this article: the ways in which complement or selective deficiencies in complement components may lead to pathologic states or events. In addition, although the biologic role of complement in the defense against pathogens, the major thrust of the earlier chapter, will not be rediscussed, some space will be devoted to several biologic oddities that may have important implications with respect to the protective functioning of complement in certain special situations, notably parasitic infestations and viral oncogenesis.

Two pathways of complement activation have been defined, the classic and alternate, or properdin, pathways. Both eventuate in a common terminal pathway of membrane attack. The classic pathway (see Figure 1 on page 168) of complement activation is initiated by C1, a trimolecular complex in which the collagen-like C1q fulfills the recognition function, becoming fixed by attachment to the complement receptors on the Fc fragments of immunoglobulin molecules. The other two C1 proteins, C1r and C1s, are zymogens or proenzymes, as is the next component, C2. All three are serine esterases.

Among the recently identified complement reaction products is a C2-derived kinin-like peptide, released from C1s-cleaved C2 by action of plasmin. C2 kinin is trypsin-labile, a property that distinguishes it from classic kinin.

C1s cleaves C4 and C2, after itself being cleaved through a complex sequence by C1r. The major fragments of the cleaved components—C2a and C4b—form a bimolecular complex that functions enzymatically as C3 convertase to activate C3, the most important protein of the entire complement system. In addition, C4b has been shown to promote immune adherence (see Figure 2 on page 169).

Designation of C3 as the major protein of the whole system rests both on quantitative considerations and on the multiplicity of functions it subserves. Not unexpectedly, C3 is the precursor of a number of physiologically active fragments. First there is the activation peptide, C3a, which is one of the anaphylatoxins of the C system. C3a can be assayed in vitro on the basis of its ability to trigger histamine release from basophils and mast cells and to induce smooth muscle contraction. In vivo, the anaphylatoxin will elicit an immediate erythema and edema when injected into human skin.

The next fragment, C3b, is *the* opsonin of the complement system. In its bound form it can react with specific cellular receptors on lymphocytes and phagocytic cells, including monocytes and neutrophils, and thereby function as a ligand to facilitate involvement of these cells in immunologic and inflammatory responses. This fragment also participates in the activation of the alternate pathway in the form of a subunit of that pathway's C3 convertase. In addition, C3b is the source of several other physiologically active fragments—C3c, which in turn is the precursor of C3e, and C3d, which, like its parent fragment, can react with specific cellular receptors on lymphocytes and other cells and thereby serve as a ligand. C3e systemically liberates or mobilizes polymorphonuclear leuko-

Figure 1

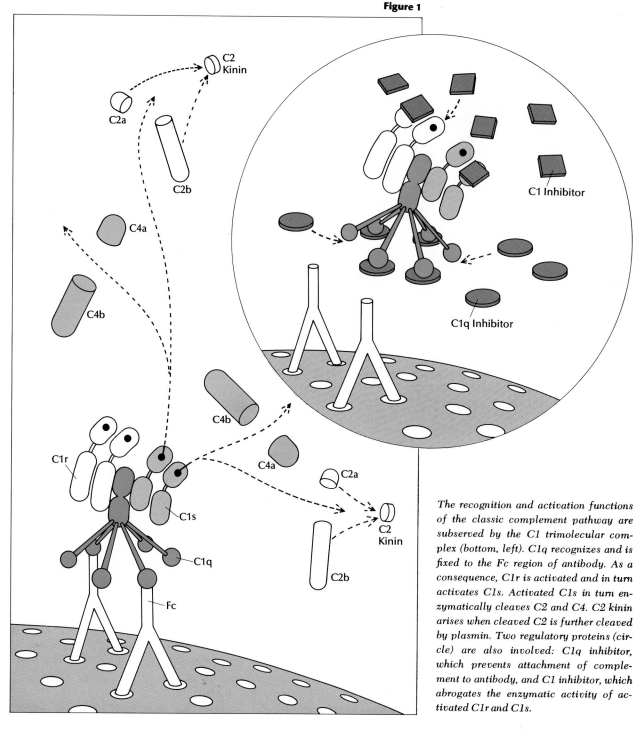

The recognition and activation functions of the classic complement pathway are subserved by the C1 trimolecular complex (bottom, left). C1q recognizes and is fixed to the Fc region of antibody. As a consequence, C1r is activated and in turn activates C1s. Activated C1s in turn enzymatically cleaves C2 and C4. C2 kinin arises when cleaved C2 is further cleaved by plasmin. Two regulatory proteins (circle) are also involved: C1q inhibitor, which prevents attachment of complement to antibody, and C1 inhibitor, which abrogates the enzymatic activity of activated C1r and C1s.

cytes from bone marrow. An example of the relationship between the complement system and clinical disease is worth citing at this point. It has been found that individuals homozygously deficient in C3 will not mount a leukocytosis response to even the most severe bacterial infections. While the genetic defect relates to the entire C3 molecule,

one can deduce that the lack of white cell elevation is directly related to the deficiency in C3e activity. Figure 3 on page 170 schematically summarizes the functional roles of C3 and its various fragments.

C3b is noteworthy in two additional respects. One is its ability to associate with the C3 convertase (C4b-C2a) to form a trimolecular

complex that is the C5 convertase, and thus trigger the terminal, lytic sequence common to both complement pathways. The other is its role in the initiation of the alternate pathway. Here we have to supersede the concept, proposed in my earlier article on the complement system, that a separate protein designated as Factor I sub-

Figure 2

Complement Abnormalities

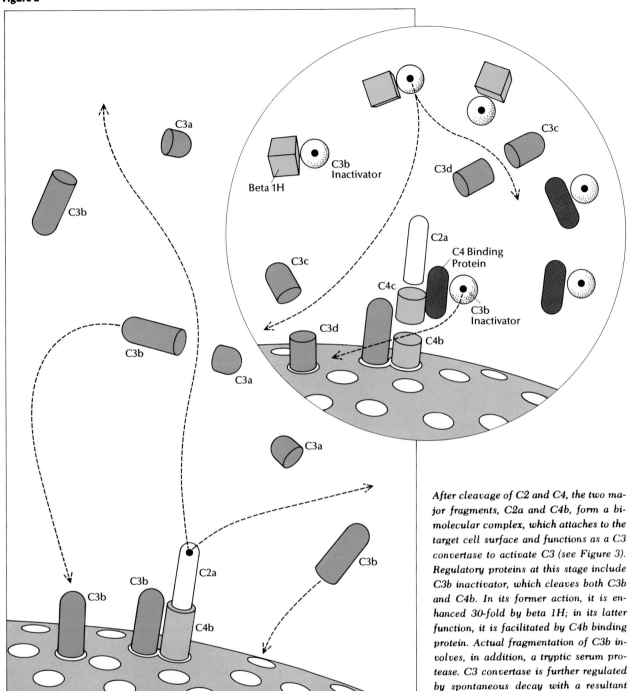

After cleavage of C2 and C4, the two major fragments, C2a and C4b, form a bimolecular complex, which attaches to the target cell surface and functions as a C3 convertase to activate C3 (see Figure 3). Regulatory proteins at this stage include C3b inactivator, which cleaves both C3b and C4b. In its former action, it is enhanced 30-fold by beta 1H; in its latter function, it is facilitated by C4b binding protein. Actual fragmentation of C3b involves, in addition, a tryptic serum protease. C3 convertase is further regulated by spontaneous decay with a resultant dissociation of C2a in inactive form.

served the recognition function of the alternate pathway in a manner analogous to C1q and antibody in the classic pathway. The evidence now is that recognition is achieved by C3b's attachment to a target surface. If that surface contains structures capable of activating the alternate pathway, the molecular sequence to be described is set in motion. If not, then two important regulatory proteins are brought into the picture. It can be noted that the regulatory proteins play an extraordinarily significant role in the alternate pathway.

The alternate pathway is initiated by nonenzymatic hydrolysis of native C3 in solution. A detailed description of this and subsequent events is presented in Chapter 12 and need not be reiterated here.

Having discussed the initiation and assembly phenomena of the two pathways, we can turn now to a brief review of the terminal proteins. The first of these is C5, a molecule strikingly similar to C3. The homology in primary structure between the two suggests that they may have arisen in evolution by gene duplication. C5 is activated by the C5 convertase of either pathway. During activation, a peptide fragment, C5a, is cleaved off. It is the second anaphylatoxin of the complement system and is even more potent than C3a. Both have the ability to induce release of hydrolytic enzymes from leukocytes and histamine from mast cells and basophils. C5a has the additional property of being chemotactic for PMN leukocytes and monocytes. Together, the two anaphylatoxins are extremely powerful phlogogenic substances.

In its nascent state C5b has a transient ability to serve as a focus for the formation of the tetramolecular complex that consists of C6, C7, and C8, in addition to C5b. This complex, in turn, polymerizes C9, the complement component now believed to be directly involved

in creating the lytic membrane lesion that is the raison d'être of the membrane attack complex.

The regulatory or controlling proteins of the classic and terminal pathways are perhaps less dramatic than the analogous molecules of the alternate pathway, but they are biomedically important. Two such proteins have been identified for C1. One is a C1 inhibitor that binds to activated C1r and to activated C1s and, in doing so, completely abrogates their enzymatic activities. C1 inhibitor also binds and inactivates other serum enzymes in the Hageman factor system. The second C1 regulator is the C1q inhibitor; it binds physically to C1q and abrogates its biologic activity. Similarly, the C3b inactivator acts on the classic pathway by cleaving and inactivating C3b and C4b. Its activity on C3b is enhanced about 30-fold by beta 1H,

and its cleavage of C4b is facilitated by C4b binding protein.

Another controlling factor is the anaphylatoxin inactivator, or serum carboxypeptidase B. Its enzymatic activity results in the removal of basic amino acid residues from the carboxyl terminal of peptides. Since both complement anaphylatoxins, C3a and C5a, have C terminal arginine residues, they will be attacked by the inactivator, with a resultant abrogation of their anaphylatoxic activity. Interestingly, even after the removal of its C-terminal arginine, C4a continues to function in chemotaxis of PMNs.

We know of three regulatory proteins that function at the level of the membrane attack complex, in each case by insertion into the complex as it is forming, competitively occupying a combining site and preventing the attachment of the complex to a target membrane

Figure 3

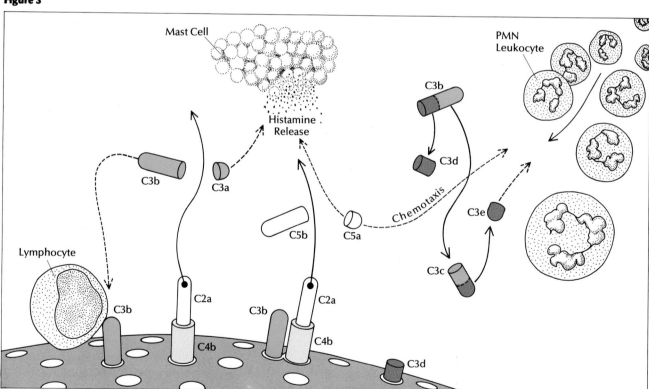

After native C3 has been cleaved by C3 convertase, one fragment, C3a, acts as an anaphylatoxin and triggers the release of histamine from mast cells and basophils. C3b, when bound to a cell surface, interacts with lymphocytes and polymorphs to facilitate their involvement in immune and inflammatory responses. C3b also associates with C3 convertase (C2a-C4b) to form a C5

convertase. In addition, C3b acts to help in the initiation of the alternate pathway. Finally C3b gives rise to at least three other active fragments. These are C3c, which is a precursor of C3e, and C3d, which like C3b reacts with specific cellular receptors and functions as a ligand. C3e liberates or mobilizes PMN leukocytes from bone marrow. C5a, in addition to being ana-

surface. The membrane attack complex (MAC) inhibitor (or S-protein), antithrombin III (ATIII), and lipoprotein are proteins that must bear structural resemblance to the surfaces of biologic membranes.

Clearly, then, the complement system involves a formidable array of 21 serum proteins. At this time, defects, i.e., deficiencies, have been identified clinically for many of these proteins, including some of the regulatory proteins. The proteins for which clinical deficiencies have *not* been found to date are Factors B and D, properdin, C9, C1q inhibitor, anaphylatoxin inactivator, beta 1H, and the MAC inhibitor. Most of these anomalies are genetically based and are expressed only in homozygous individuals, although there are exceptions, as will be noted further on.

Genetic deficiencies have been described for C1r, C2, C3, C4, C5,

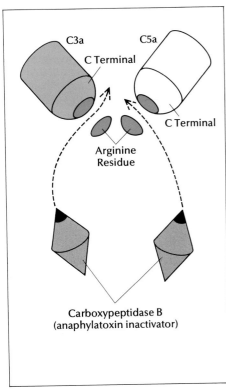

phylatoxic, causes chemotactic migration of leukocytes. The regulator, carboxypeptidase B (right), cleaves arginine residues from the carboxy terminals of C3a and C5a, abolishing their anaphylatoxicity but not altering C5a chemotaxis.

C6, C7, C8, C1 inhibitor, and C3b inactivator. The clinical pictures for patients with homozygous deficiencies in C1r, C2, C4, and C5 of the classic pathway are strikingly similar. The salient feature in these patients is a marked increase in the incidence of autoimmune disease, notably of the systemic lupus erythematosus type. The expression includes all of the classic manifestations of lupus—skin lesions, renal disease, and serologic manifestations, such as anti-DNA and antinuclear protein autoantibodies. In addition, these patients manifest other clinical disorders—chronic glomerulonephritis, arthritis, recurrent systemic and skin infections, various dermatitides, and vasculitis.

While the frequency of autoimmune disease in individuals with these early-component deficiencies is immensely enhanced over that in a normal population, it should be stressed that such clinical manifestations do not appear in all persons with these deficiencies. For example, about half of the affected individuals with C2 deficiencies have autoimmune disease, but the other half are normal except possibly for some increased susceptibility to bacterial infection. This may be surprising when the defect is homozygous. However, careful evaluation of these people reveals that they do have trace amounts of the deficient complement protein in their serum. These traces, when calculated out for the total plasma volume, may well cumulate to a quantity that has considerable biologic activity. This observation, taken together with in vitro evidence that cells from these deficient individuals will make some of the missing components, suggests that the genetic defects involved relate to regulatory rather than structural genes.

Clinically, C3 deficiency is the most severe of all complement defects. The first patient to be identified with the defect was in South Africa and presented with the signs and symptoms of a Bruton-type agammaglobulinemia, including frequent severe bacterial infections.

However, it was found that he had normal immunoglobulin levels and was able to respond normally to antigenic challenge. While this patient was under observation and the specific nature of his defect remained unidentified, Alper and Rosen at Harvard published a paper in which they described a patient with a very similar clinical picture who had been found to suffer from a C3b inactivator deficiency. The South African physicians suspected that their patient's problem might be the same and sent a serum sample to Boston. It was there that the diagnosis of C3, rather than C3b inactivator, deficiency was made.

The apparent paradox—similar manifestations for deficiencies in C3 and C3b inactivator—is explicable in the light of our current understanding of the molecular mechanisms of the alternate pathway. As we now know, C3b inactivator deficiency will result in hypercatabolism of C3. When C3b arises in the serum, it is normally limited by the inactivator. This effectively curbs the amount of alternate-pathway C3 convertase generated as the result of the sequence previously described (in which C3b collides with Factor B, facilitating the cleavage of Factor B by Factor D) as necessary for the formation of active C3 convertase. This enzyme turns over additional C3 and thereby produces more C3b, which in turn cycles again to yield further C3 convertase. If this process is not arrested by C3b inactivator, eventually all of the available Factor B will be consumed. And when this happens, further formation of the convertase is precluded. Therefore, what one finds in patients with C3b inactivator deficiency is depletion of intact C3, much C3b, and absence of Factor B.

The clinical severity of C3 deficiency (one of the four patients so far studied has died of overwhelming infection) clearly relates to the protective functions of this component. Obviously, in the absence of C3, both pathways leading to complement-dependent phagocytosis or lysis of bacterial cells will be impaired. Additionally, as mentioned, C3e is needed for mobilization of leukocytes from the bone marrow, and patients with C3 deficiency are unable to mount a leukocytosis response to infections.

In an in vitro system, phagocytosis will take place without complement if immunoglobulin, say IgG, is complexed with a bacterial cell in the presence of macrophages or other phagocytes. The antibody will attach to the macrophage via that cell's Fc receptor, and this will serve to activate the macrophage and initiate ingestion of the antigen-antibody complex. However, in an in vivo situation one has the added complication of free or uncommitted immunoglobulin that can preempt the Fc receptor of the phagocyte and prevent attachment of the opsonized bacterium. In these circumstances, C3b on the bacterial surface provides an additional site for attachment, since macrophages and other phagocytes have C3b, as well as Fc, receptors. Normally antibody is then required for activation of the macrophage. However, if the phagocyte is activated by some other stimulus or is a neutrophil, phagocytosis can take place through C3b opsonization without the participation of antibody.

Although individuals deficient in C3 are effectively deprived of their complement defense along both pathways, some modulation of this defect may be derived from the immune adherence activity of C4b. It has been shown that persons with a C3 deficiency will respond to antigen challenge by activation of C1 and the placement of C4b on target cells. A few families have been identified with individuals lacking C4 activity due to a homozygous defect. Clinically, the deficiency is expressed by the increased incidence of SLE typical of early component abnormalities. We have not yet found a combined C3-C4 deficiency, but in theory such a combined defect would abolish all known complement defense.

The next group of deficiency disorders involves C5. Here again, autoimmune diseases such as SLE are seen, but equally prominent is increased susceptibility to bacterial infections. As with the early component defects, no explanation has yet been found for the lupus or for the bacterial susceptibility, which is manifest despite the presence of adequate C3 concentrations. However, one can postulate that the absence of the chemotactic activity of C5a and the resultant failure to mobilize PMN leukocytes at the site of a bacterial infection could provide the explanation.

Let us turn now to the effects of absence of C5b, which serves as the nucleus for formation of the membrane attack complex (C5b through C9). Because the first individuals found to have C6 and C7 deficiencies were clinically healthy, an impression began to develop that perhaps the membrane attack complex was not really all that important in the defenses against bacteria. Indeed, the major emphasis so far as complement's role in the defense against infections was concerned was placed on the opsonic action of C3 and to some extent of C4. It was then established that patients with C5, C6, C7, and C8 deficiencies are highly susceptible to infections, particularly to diseases caused by *Neisseria gonorrhoeae* and *Neisseria meningitidis*. Retrospectively, it was realized that the first patient seen with a C6 deficiency had a disseminated gonococcal infection, which had been discounted with respect to a possible role of the complement defect. Subsequently, a number of patients with MAC deficiencies have required treatment for overwhelming gonococcal infections and/or for recurrent meningitides. It is now widely accepted that there are certain bacteria that can only be combated in vivo with the aid of complement-mediated lysis. The particular need for complement lysis for Neisseria destruction has been explained by the fact that these species are not effectively killed by intracellular enzymes. This may be true for some other bacteria, but to date these have not been studied systematically.

We have already discussed the effects of deficiency in one of the regulatory proteins—C3b inactivator—in the context of C3 deficiency. Another genetically determined regulatory-protein deficiency is C1 inhibitor deficiency, and it occurs more frequently than any other inherited complement defect. Estimates are that C1 inhibitor deficiency is found in about one individual per thousand. Clinically, C1 inhibitor deficiency is expressed as angioedema, with localized swelling of tissues sequential to trauma or without apparent cause. The edema may be in one of the extremities, in the intestine where it can readily mimic appendicitis, or in the oropharyngeal structures where it can present as or evolve into a life-threatening compromise of airway patency. At the molecular level, two forms of the deficiency have been identified. In one, no C1 inhibitor is made; in the other, inhibitor is made but it is faulty and ineffective.

I would note parenthetically that the ability of this deficiency to cause pharyngeal edema has led to suspicion that it might be involved in sudden infant death syndrome. However, in the 12 or so SIDS cases that we have investigated here at Scripps, no complement abnormalities have been identified.

The working hypothesis to explain the connection between C1 inhibitor deficiency and angioedema is that the effects are caused by excessive release of C2-derived kinin (see Figure 4 on page 173). Studies of individuals with C1 inhibitor deficiency and clinically manifest angioedema have shown that their sera have enhanced activation of C1r and C1s and are almost totally lacking in C2 and C4, although they synthesize both of these components normally. Starting with continuous activation of C1 in the absence of inhibitor and consequent excessive activation of C2 and C4, what appears to be happening is cleavage of C2 by the excessive C1s. This is followed by interaction of plasmin with C2a or C2b, further cleavage that releases the C2 fragment having kinin activity, and eventually the expectable, kinin-induced release of his-

Figure 4   Complement Abnormalities

tamine and other vasoactive substances that provoke edema.

Of clinical interest is the fact that testosterone analogues provide effective treatment and prophylaxis for angioedema caused by C1 inhibitor deficiency. It was observed some time ago that testosterone markedly enhances C1s inhibitor levels in the serum. When administered to persons with the type of deficiency that involves the synthesis of a faulty inhibitor, testosterone causes production of normal inhibitor along with the faulty product. For those who do not make any inhibitor, the treatment induces normal protein production. By using an analogue of testosterone that has no virilizing effects, one can employ the approach on a prophylactic as well as on a therapeutic basis.

Another complement abnormality for which effective therapy appears available is in Leiner's disease, which is associated with C5 dysfunction; whether this association is primary in the etiology of the disease or secondary to the disease is not known. Patients with this relatively rare condition are highly susceptible to infections, particularly bowel and skin infections. Quantitatively, they have normal serum levels of C5, but there seems to be a failure of the component to promote phagocytosis. Correction can be achieved by the administration of fresh plasma. The use of fresh plasma infusions has also proved useful in the management of acute infectious episodes in patients with C3b inactivator deficiency. In these situations, the plasma provides C3b inactivator and in this way temporarily normalizes both C3 and Factor B levels.

In addition to the genetic complement deficiencies, there are also some acquired or idiopathic deficiencies, notably with respect to the C1 components. Thus, some individuals with chronic urticaria have been found to lack C1q even though they have normal amounts of C1r and C1s and have no discernible synthetic defect. Why this anomaly should be associated with

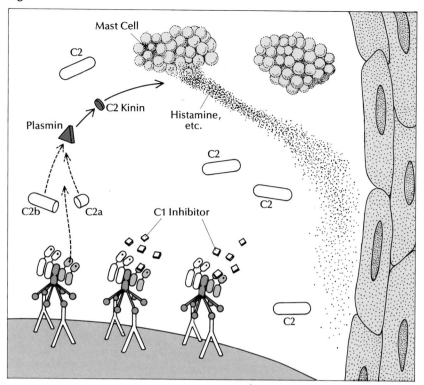

The hypothesized role of C1 inhibitor deficiency in the pathogenesis of angioedema is schematized. In the normal individual (above), the amount of C2 kinin liberated is effectively controlled by turning off the enzymatic activity of C1s and thereby limiting the cleavage of C2 (and C4). When C1 inhibitor is not available to exert this regulatory effect (below), C2 will be cleaved until all molecules are consumed. As a result, the concentration of C2 kinin will be enhanced. In turn, kinin-mediated release of mediators from mast cells will escalate and angioedema will eventuate.

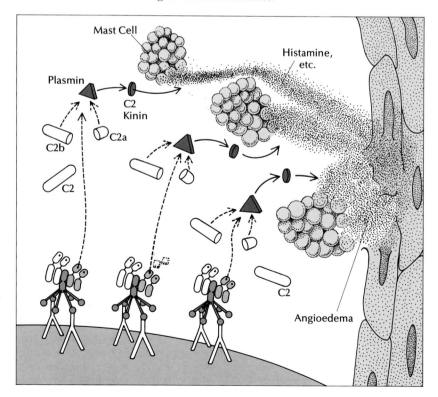

a collagen vascular disease is unknown. C1q can also be exceedingly reduced in agammaglobulinemia patients. This was originally thought to relate to synchronous production of the immunoglobulins and the C1q, which as noted is the Ig-recognition molecule. However, it is now known that this is not the explanation. Rather, it turns out, gamma globulin levels in the serum are a determinant of C1q's biologic half-life. C1q and gamma globulin are in continuous reversible interaction. This interaction occurs even with monomeric gamma globulin, which does not lead to complement activation. As a result of the interaction, C1 is held in the circulation far longer than it would be otherwise. Effectively, its biologic half-life is prolonged. Conversely, any reduction of circulating immunoglobulin proportionally decreases interaction with C1 and accelerates the in vivo turnover of this complement component.

Turning now from complement deficiency diseases to the role of complement in immunopathology—i.e., as an aberrant or inappropriate phenomenon that leads to tissue injury rather than defense against bacterial or other foreign antigens—we now recognize a number of situations where complement plays a very significant role. Included are many of the so-called autoimmune diseases, those marked by immune complex deposition. Many of the collagen vascular diseases, such as SLE, rheumatoid arthritis, and many of the nephritides, are encompassed, as are myasthenia gravis and a host of dermatoses.

A great deal of our understanding of the ways in which complement causes injury in these diseases comes from studies with two classic animal models, nephrotoxic nephritis and the Arthus phenomenon (see Figure 5 on page 175). In nephrotoxic nephritis, an antibody is produced in one animal against the kidney tissue of another (e.g., rabbit antibody to rat kidney antigens). The antibody is then injected into the animal against whose kidney antigens it has been raised. The antibody will localize in the kidney, and within minutes, complement deposition will be seen at the site of antibody localization. Within a few hours, PMN leukocytes will invade the rat glomeruli and a full-blown glomerulitis will ensue. The role of complement is sharply delineated if the animal is treated with cobra venom factor. Cobra venom contains a factor that associates with Factors B and D to form a stable C3 convertase. This will result in rapid consumption and total depletion of C3. If the anti-kidney antibody is injected in this period of C3 depletion, no deposition of C3 in the glomeruli takes place and PMN leukocytes are not mobilized. In these circumstances, there is no subsequent glomerulitis—a clear demonstration of the need for and participation of complement in this experimental disease.

In the Arthus phenomenon model, antibody is injected into the animal's circulation and its antigen is injected locally into tissue. As the two diffuse toward each other, a meeting takes place in the blood vessel wall, with precipitation of antigen and antibody and activation of complement. Vasculitis and then necrosis result. Once more, injection of cobra venom factor will abort the inflammatory response, although the immune complex precipitates can be seen under the microscope.

These two models provide strong evidence that similar mechanisms are operating in many of the clinical immune complex diseases. Recently, a third model has been developed (in rats) that is specifically pertinent to myasthenia gravis. In this model the receptor at the neuromuscular junction is used as the antigen. The protein is prepared in a way to stimulate the formation of autoantibody when it is injected into the animal. It has been shown that this autoantibody will interact with antigenic structures on the motor end plates at the neuromuscular junctions. The resulting antigen-antibody complexes activate complement, and the activation leads in turn to membrane lysis. When these events occur, the animal's signs and symptoms are indistinguishable from those of naturally occurring clinical myasthenia. Again, the process can be aborted by cobra venom factor.

These models certainly support the plausibility of assigning to the complement system a major role in the immunopathogenesis of autoimmune and complex diseases. However, plausibility is not enough, and it is necessary to be extremely cautious in attributing pathologic phenomena to complement in human disease. Three criteria must be met.

• Complement deposition should be present at the site of the tissue lesion.

• Both enhanced complement activation and increased turnover of complement proteins in the circulation should be demonstrated.

• Increased levels of the reaction products of complement should be present in the circulation or in the tissues.

To satisfy the first of these criteria, either biopsy or autopsy material must be examined. Such studies have been done for almost all forms of glomerulonephritis, and a virtually universal finding is deposits of complement in the glomerular capillary walls.

To determine the circulatory turnover of complement proteins, one must inject radiolabeled isolated human complement components into the circulation and measure their half-life or plasma disappearance time. With such measurements, one can calculate the rates of both synthesis and catabolism. This has now been done for a variety of diseases, including lupus and rheumatoid arthritis, and for dengue hemorrhagic shock, which is, of course, an acute immunologic disease. Among the proteins that were labeled and studied were C1q, C3, C4, C5, C7, and Factor B. In each of these situations, an increased catabolic rate was found, often accompanied by an increased synthetic rate as well. This evidence is entirely consistent with greater than normal activation of the complement system. To some extent, this increased activation has

Figure 5

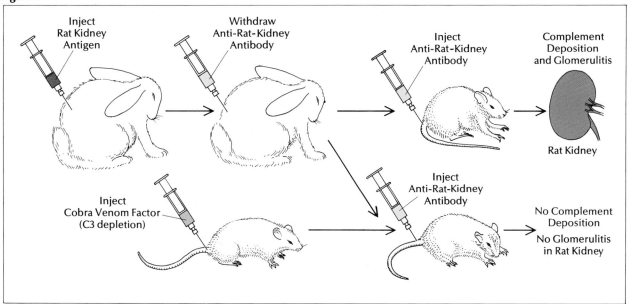

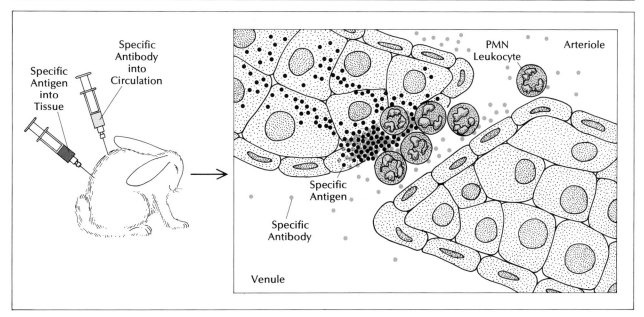

Two animal models can be used to demonstrate the immunopathologic role of complement. In the nephrotoxic nephritis model (top), glomerulitis can be produced in rats by raising an antiserum to rat kidney tissue in a rabbit, then injecting it into the rat. In the Arthus phenomenon model (bottom), antigen is inject-ed into tissue, and antibody is introduced into the circulation. The two diffuse toward each other and combine within a vessel wall, causing vasculitis. In both of these models, injection of cobra venom factor will abort the pathologic response, since the factor inactivates complement.

been specifically correlated with pathologic phenomena. For example, in rheumatoid arthritis patients, a disproportionately large fraction of the labeled C3 will be recovered from the synovial fluid. A positive correlation is also found between the abnormal distribution of labeled proteins and disease activity, certainly an important consideration in an episodic disease like RA.

Finally, increased levels of products of complement activation have been demonstrated in several diseases. In patients with certain types of nephritis, it has been possible to show enhanced circulating C3d, for example. C3d is a useful monitor because it persists in the serum longer than the other C3 fragments. Studies of synovial fluid in RA patients have provided evidence of increased C5a, still in its active, chemotactic form, as well as of increased levels of various C3 and C4 catabolic products.

There is, of course, a fourth criterion one would like to meet in order to establish unequivocally the role of complement in pathogenesis—demonstration that *decomplementation* obviates or inhibits inflammatory responses. At present, we simply do not have a means to achieve this in humans. Cobra venom factor cannot be employed in people because it is immunogenic and can produce serum sickness. Eventually, a means will be devised for testing this criterion, but meanwhile it can be stated that there is a spectrum of diseases, including almost all autoimmune processes, in which the weight of evidence justifies the conclusion that complement is a major contributor to pathogenesis. In these diseases, the common pathway starts with the formation of immune complexes between an endogenous antigen and its autoantibody, continues with the activation of complement, and eventuates in inflammatory processes mediated by complement activity.

In the introduction to this discussion of the relationships between the complement system and human disease, it was noted that some observations related to "biologic oddities" would be appended. Before doing so, I would emphasize that the word oddities should not be equated with trivialities. Indeed, the areas to be discussed are of potentially great significance. The first may provide an explanation for why RNA tumor viruses, so frequently associated with neoplasia in animals, have never been detectable in human cancers.

The relevant development here is the finding in our laboratories that RNA tumor viruses are attacked directly by human C1. This attack occurs without the presence of IgG or IgM antibodies usually needed to activate the classic complement pathway and involves recognition by C1q of a viral coat protein characteristic of RNA tumor viruses, P-15E. The result of this recognition is activation of the classic complement pathway, with formation of the membrane attack complex and the destruction of the virus. Particularly intriguing is the fact that while human or primate complement does this, complement from all other mammalian species studied to date does not. Here we have not only a difference between human complement and that of other species but also a system that seems to be designed to destroy RNA tumor viruses without any need for antibody and before any oncogenic events can occur.

This delineation of a role for the complement system that logically, at least, would seem to constitute a defense against cancer leads to an area that must remain speculative for another decade or so, but which is worthy of surveillance in the intervening years. In observing individuals with deficiencies of the components making up the membrane attack complex, C5b through C9, one wonders whether in the long run these people will manifest an increased frequency of malignant disease. Certainly, it could be expected that complement would be required to mediate any humoral component in the host's antitumor defenses. And the existence of humoral antibody as an adjunct to cell-mediated defenses has been demonstrated for malignant melanoma and very possibly for other cancers as well. How important are these humoral defenses? Will persons deprived of or deficient in these defenses be more susceptible to neoplasia? These are questions that time and continued observation will answer.

Another important group of studies involves the role of complement in defense against parasitic infections. A paper published by investigators at the British National Institute for Medical Research (Ramalho-Pinto, McLaren, and Smithers) in the *Journal of Experimental Medicine* 147:147, 1978 describes the activation of complement via the alternate pathway by *Schistosoma mansoni*. In the course of this activation, which does not involve immunoglobulin, the parasites become coated with the host's C3b, and the eosinophil chemotactic factor is released. The attracted eosinophils appear capable of killing the parasites. Incidentally, as the schistosomula age, they seem to adapt and no longer activate the alternate complement pathway. However, biologically and teleologically it is interesting that the alternate pathway provides an initial defense against parasites that does not require antibody.

In concluding, one last set of biologic phenomena is worth touching upon. Until relatively recently, little work had been done on the biosynthesis of complement. However, studies done in the past few years make it clear that cellular capability for complement production is quite ubiquitous. We now know that macrophages can make at least 10 of the C proteins, that fibroblasts make some complement, and so do established tumor (melanoma) cell lines. It appears that the complement structural genes can be turned on in many different cell types.

For a number of years there has been an interest in our laboratory in the question of how cells kill other cells. This interest has been focused on various types of cytotoxic lymphocytes. It now can be stated on the basis of firm evidence that lymphocytes, most probably including the K cells of antibody-dependent cellular cytotoxicity, can synthesize complement. In actual fact, K cells bear on their surfaces the hallmark of C membrane attack complex, a specifically associated neoantigen. What is more, when the K cells are in the process of killing target cells, one can by immunofluorescent antibody techniques actually see antibody to this neoantigen at the site of the cytotoxic event. This evidence bolsters experiments showing that lymphocytes incorporate radiolabeled amino acids in synthesizing complement.

In other words, there seems here to be a demonstration of the elegant efficiency of a biologic system. In response to the need to destroy foreign invaders, as well as to eliminate internal threats to homeostasis, two apparently separate immunologic defense systems evolved. It may turn out that they can both use the same set of protein molecules to accomplish the ultimate destruction of their targets.

16

HLA Relationships to Disease

JANE G. SCHALLER *and* JOHN A. HANSEN   *University of Washington*

A basic question in medicine is why some people get certain diseases and others do not. Geneticists have tried for years to associate measurable genetic traits with disease susceptibility. For instance, attempts were made to relate red cell antigens with specific diseases, and associations, albeit weak ones, were found between ABO types and risks of gastric carcinoma and duodenal ulcers. In 1963, F. Lilly, L. J. Old, and E. A. Boyse reported that susceptibility to spontaneous leukemia in the mouse was associated with certain antigens of a multigene system known as the H-2 histocompatibility complex. Since the discovery of the human leukocyte antigen (HLA) system in the 1950s, for which Jean Dausset was awarded a share of the 1980 Nobel Prize for Physiology or Medicine (along with George Snell and Baruj Benacerraf), a great deal of attention has been focused on the HLA system as the human equivalent of the mouse H-2. Thus, there was great excitement when J. L. Amiel in 1967 described a significant association between certain HLA antigens and susceptibility to Hodgkin's disease. Since then, a number of other diseases have been related to HLA genetic factors. The best known of these is the association between ankylosing spondylitis and HLA-B27. First reported simultaneously in 1973 from Los Angeles and London, this remains the strongest known association between a genetic trait and a human disease.

Many other diseases now have been related to the HLA system. Associations are particularly strong for certain rheumatic diseases and for a group of diseases that are characterized by chronic inflammation and aberrant immunologic reactions. However, before getting down to the specifics of HLA-disease associations, a word should be said about the antigens themselves and the genes that control them.

Genetic differences between donors and recipients of foreign tissues can cause immunologic reactions leading to graft rejection, or in bone marrow transplant recipients, to graft-versus-host disease as well. The HLA system plays the major role in effecting such transplant reactions, and for this reason the HLA system also is known as the human major histocompatibility complex (MHC). When an individual is exposed to foreign cells, the predominant host immune response is directed to the donor's MHC antigens. The concept of an MHC, developed by Snell and Peter A. Gorer, derives from experimental studies in mice (later confirmed in several other species), showing that although many different genes can influence a transplantation reaction, one system of genes, the MHC, always has the strongest effect.

The genes of the HLA system are located in close proximity to each other on human chromosome 6 (see Figure 1, page 178). To date, four gene loci (HLA-A, B, C, and D) controlling histocompatibility determinants have been defined. Alternative genes that may occur at each gene locus are known as alleles. Each of these HLA gene loci has multiple alleles and thus controls a highly polymorphic series of gene products, the HLA antigens. Only the gene products of the HLA-A, B, and C loci are well defined. The HLA-A, B, and C genes control the biosynthesis of two glycoproteins, one heavy chain and one light chain, that together form a heterodimer on the surface of the cell.

HLA-A, B, and C antigens are detected by a standard microcytotoxicity typing assay (see Figure 2, page 179). Lymphocytes to be typed are incubated with human sera containing HLA antibodies of known specificity, exposed to complement, and then exposed

Figure 1

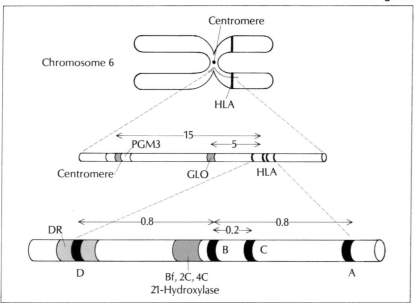

Genes controlling the human leukocyte antigen (HLA) system are located on chromosome 6 (top). Genes linked to the HLA system (center) include those for the enzymes phosphoglucomutase-3 (PGM3) and glyoxalase-1 (GLO). PGM3 locus at centromere is about 15 recombination units from HLA region. Map of HLA region (bottom) shows HLA-A, B, C, and D with relative distances (recombination units) between each locus. The HLA-DR (D-related) region is closely associated with the D locus; genes for complement components Bf, 2C, and 4C, and a gene for 21-hydroxylase, with the B locus.

to a vital dye; cells bearing antigens recognized by the HLA test antibodies will suffer membrane damage, which is noted by uptake of the dye. The HLA-A, B, and C antigens have been called serologically defined, since they react with test sera containing specific antibodies.

The fourth HLA locus, HLA-D, marks a region that probably contains more than one histocompatibility gene. HLA-D is detected by the mixed lymphocyte culture (MLC) assay. When cells from identical twins or HLA-identical siblings are tested in mixed lymphocyte culture, there is no reaction. However, when cells from unrelated individuals are tested, the MLC reaction is generally positive, and the resulting increased rate of responder lymphocyte proliferation can be measured (as DNA synthesis, reflected by incorporation of tritiated thymidine [3H-Tdr]). The degree of cellular proliferation correlates with the degree of HLA-D disparity between responder and stimulator. HLA-D antigen specificities are determined by an adaptation of this standard MLC assay (see Figure 3, page 180). Lymphocytes from the individual being typed comprise the responder-cell panel; HLA-D typing cells (cells obtained from selected individuals known to be homozygous for specific HLA-D types), the stimulator-cell panel. Responders react vigorously to test cells expressing foreign HLA-D antigens but react weakly or not at all to test cells that express D antigens similar to their own. Since both the procurement of HLA-D typing cells and the HLA-D typing procedures are difficult, HLA-D typing is not available widely.

Closely related to the HLA-D region is a series of serologically defined antigens that are distinct from HLA-A, B, and C antigens. These antigens, present on the surface of B lymphocytes and commonly known as B-cell antigens, are formally designated as "D-related," or DR, antigens. HLA-DR antigens are found not only on B cells but also on monocytes, macrophages, and some bone marrow cells; they are not, however, detectable on most T cells. DR types are determined by the microcytotoxicity typing assay, using the patient's B lymphocytes (separated from peripheral blood) and test sera of known DR specificity. Exact relationships between HLA-D and HLA-DR remain to be determined. HLA-DR rather than HLA-D typing has been used in many recent studies of disease associations because it requires less cumbersome laboratory procedures.

The HLA system is highly polymorphic with many alleles existing for each locus. Twenty alleles have been identified for the A locus, 42 for the B locus, 8 for the C locus, 12 for the D locus, and 10 for DR. Each individual expresses one allele for each of these loci. The group of HLA alleles on a single chromosome is called a haplotype; an HLA haplotype is inherited from each parent. Most individuals are heterozygous for HLA, that is, they have five different alleles in the HLA region of each chromosome.

The closer two loci are on a chromosome, the more closely linked they are said to be, and the less likely that crossing over or exchange of homologous genes between paternal and maternal chromosomes will occur when the cells divide in meiosis. The result of the crossing-over phenomenon is called recombination. Because the genes in the HLA complex are closely linked, recombinations between alleles at the A and B loci or B and D loci occur at a frequency of <1%. HLA haplotypes are, therefore, almost always transmitted from one generation to another without change.

It has been estimated that 80 additional genes are located between the HLA-A and HLA-B loci; 100, between HLA-B and HLA-D; and as many as 1,500 between HLA-B and the locus for the enzyme phosphoglucomutase-3 (PGM3), which is also on chromosome 6. It is likely that traits determined by these intervening genes, most of which have not been identified, are inherited along with HLA haplotypes. Among the genes on chromosome 6 that have been identified are several known to be closely linked to the

HLA gene complex. These include the gene determining properdin factor B (Bf), also called C3 proactivator; genes controlling the second and fourth components of complement; and a gene for the enzyme 21-hydroxylase.

The prevalence of individual HLA antigens varies considerably from one population to another. For example, HLA-A30 is found in 28% of blacks, only 5% of whites, and has not been found in Japanese; HLA-Aw24 occurs in 58.5% of Japanese, 18% of whites, and only 6% of blacks; HLA-B8 occurs in 16% of whites but rarely (<0.5%) in Japanese; HLA-A1 occurs in 28% of whites and 1% of Japanese.

The frequency of HLA haplotypes also varies in different populations. Haplotypes that are very common in whites include A1, B8, Dw3, DR3; A3, B7, Dw2, DR2; and A2, Cw3, B15, Dw4, DR4. In other population groups, these same haplotypes might not be found, and completely distinct sets of alleles might appear together as common haplotypes. Sometimes the alleles of two or more loci, for example, A1, B8 and A1, B8, DR3, occur together on the same haplotype with a frequency that is greater than would be expected if their association was only random. This is known as linkage disequilibrium. If one calculates the expected frequency of the A1,B8 haplotype on the basis of the known gene frequencies, A1 and B8 should appear together in the North American white population at a frequency of 1.7%. The observed frequency of the A1,B8 haplotype in the North American white population, however, is about 68/1,000 (6.8%). Another common haplotype in whites that shows strong linkage disequilibrium is A3,Bw35,Cw4. (No C-locus antigen has been identified for the A1,B8 haplotype.) Certain D and DR alleles also appear to occur preferentially with certain HLA-A and B alleles. For example, Dw2,DR2 occur with B7 and Dw3,DR3 with B8 more frequently than would be expected.

Several explanations for linkage disequilibrium have been offered. The most popular is the concept that at some time in the course of evolution, a certain combination of alleles (e.g., A1, B8, DR3) may have conferred a selective advantage. Although the concept cannot be proved, it is supported by the observation that the frequency of certain alleles and haplotypes differs for population or ethnic groups from different environments. Thus, for example, the haplotypes that commonly show linkage disequilibrium in West African blacks are completely different from those that occur in European whites.

Another explanation is that some

Figure 2

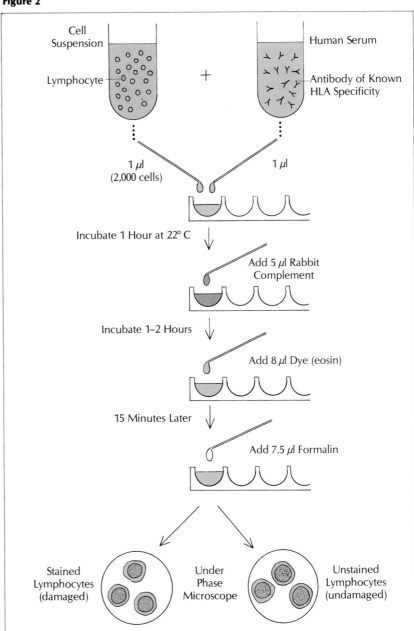

To identify the HLA-A, B, and C antigens on human lymphocytes, the lymphocytes are added to human serum containing HLA antibodies of known specificity and incubated in the presence of complement. Cells bearing antigens recognized by the HLA antibodies are damaged in the presence of complement and will be stained by vital dyes. Formalin is added to stop the reaction, and the cells are examined by phase-contrast microscopy. Stained cells are the end point of a cytotoxic reaction and indicate that the cells express the same HLA specificity as the typing serum used.

Figure 3

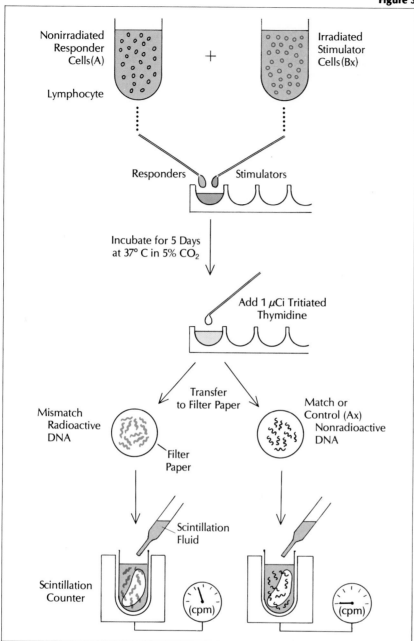

Compatibility for HLA-D is assessed by the one-way mixed lymphocyte culture (MLC) assay. Lymphocytes from the designated responder (individual A) are incubated with an equal number of irradiated lymphocytes from the designated stimulator (individual Bx). Reactivity of the responders is reflected in cellular proliferation, which can be estimated radioisotopically by the counts per minute (cpm) of tritiated thymidine incorporated into the DNA of experimental (A+Bx) versus control (A+Ax) cultures.

disequilibrium is the so-called founder effect, which postulates that, as a result of migration, a foreign gene or haplotype is introduced into a population, resulting in linkage disequilibrium in the genetic pool of that population. Many generations of random breeding and recombination may be required to neutralize the effect of the mutant haplotypes.

Recognition of foreign histocompatibility antigens on transplanted tissue is a function of an individual's genetically determined immune responsiveness. An unanswered question, which may be significant in relation to disease susceptibility, is whether the immune response (Ir) genes are controlled by, linked to, or actually part of the human MHC. Ir genes are, of course, known to determine or limit host response to bacteria, viruses, and other pathogens and foreign antigens. From analogies with data obtained from animal experiments and from preliminary human studies, it seems likely that the two systems are in fact linked, as they are, for example, in the H-2 system of the mouse.

For one thing, the HLA-A, B, and C antigens in the human and the murine MHC (the H-2K, D, and L antigens) show profound structural and biochemical homology (see Figure 4, page 183). In both species, these antigens appear on the surfaces of cells as two polypeptide chains; a heavy chain that is a glycoprotein of 44,000 MW is actually inserted into the cell membrane; and a light chain of 12,000 MW that is known to be β_2-microglobulin is found noncovalently bound to the heavy chain (see Figure 5, page 184). The amino acid sequence of the heavy chain contains constant domains that show strict conservation between species, but the heavy chain also contains hypervariable regions in which the amino acid sequence varies among individuals and species. The heavy chain, therefore, has preserved the overall integrity of its structure through evolution but, at the same time, contains a high degree of polymorphism. In fact, the polymorphism

haplotypes have arisen relatively recently and have not yet reached a random distribution. It is possible that the C2-deficiency gene, for example, occurred relatively recently in human history, as a result of mutation in a gene present on a chromosome expressing the A10, B18,DR2 haplotype. Because there has been an insufficient amount of time for equilibration by random recombination, the C2-deficiency gene still appears to be in linkage disequilibrium with the antigens of the mutant haplotype.

A third explanation for linkage

within the hypervariable regions of the heavy chain is so great that it has been conservatively estimated that more than 35 million HLA phenotypes are possible. The light chain, which appears not to be polymorphic, is controlled by a gene found on human chromosome 15.

Similarities are also found between human DR antigens and mouse immune-associated (Ia) antigens. In the human and the mouse, these antigens consist of two polypeptide chains, one heavy (34,000 MW) and one light (29,000 MW), each having carbohydrates on them. The genetic control of these antigens in both the human and the mouse is complex.

In the mouse, the Ir genes are located in the I subregion of H-2. For his discovery of Ir genes, Benacerraf shared in the Nobel Prize for Physiology or Medicine in 1980. Ia (I subregion-associated) antigens may be related to Ir genes. Ia antigens are expressed selectively on mouse B cells and not on T cells. Functionally, Ia antigens appear to regulate cell-to-cell interactions. The I subregion of H-2 also controls the determinants that cause strong reactions in mixed lymphocyte culture, and I-region incompatibilities cause strong graft-versus-host reactions.

In the human, the DR region of the HLA complex controls the B-cell alloantigens, and the D region itself controls the reaction in mixed lymphocyte culture. Direct evidence that the D region controls Ir genes is lacking, but by analogy with the I region in the mouse, it seems probable.

In any discussion of genetics and disease risk, the terms linkage and association are often confused. *Linkage* refers to the proximity of gene loci on a particular chromosome. Linkage can be identified only by family studies of more than one generation to determine if certain traits are transmitted together. Few human diseases have been clearly linked to the HLA complex. These include 21-hydroxylase deficiency with resulting congenital adrenal hyperplasia, deficiencies of the second and fourth components of complement, hemochromatosis, and, possibly, the predisposition to ragweed hayfever. In contrast, many human diseases have been found to have associations with various HLA antigens. *Association* refers to a relationship between two separate traits or findings. Associations can be found by examining sufficiently large study and control groups. An example of association is the occurrence of B27 antigen more often in patients with ankylosing spondylitis than in a randomly selected control population.

Two major disease groups that have shown associations with the HLA system are the rheumatic diseases and a group of diseases characterized by chronic inflammation and aberrant immunologic reactions. The rheumatic diseases can be subdivided into those that show associations with B27 and those that show D and DR associations. The group of diseases characterized by chronic inflammation and aberrant immunologic reactions are associated with B8, Dw3, and DR3. A number of other diseases have been associated with yet other HLA antigens.

Of all the disease associations, the most striking is that of the spondylarthropathies with HLA-B27. No D-locus associations have been found. The spondylarthropathies are several disease states characterized by arthritis of the spine and sacroiliac and axial joints, often with rheumatoid factor–negative peripheral arthritis as well. Ankylosing spondylitis is the prototype; other related conditions include Reiter's disease, the spondylitis of inflammatory bowel disease, psoriatic spondylitis, reactive arthritis, one subgroup of juvenile rheumatoid arthritis, acute iridocyclitis, and some instances of backache.

The B27 antigen is found in more than 90% of white patients with classic ankylosing spondylitis, but in fewer than 10% of white control populations. An individual with the HLA-B27 antigen has an 80 to 90 times greater relative risk of having ankylosing spondylitis than one who does not have the B27 antigen. However, a person with the B27 antigen probably has no more than a 5% to 20% chance of ever developing spondylarthropathy. Ankylosing spondylitis is known to be familial. Among first-degree relatives of B27 patients with ankylosing spondylitis, 50% have HLA-B27 antigen, and as many as 30% of these have either ankylosing spondylitis or some other manifestation suggestive of spondylarthropathy.

The prevalence of B27 correlates with that of ankylosing spondylitis in certain population groups. For example, the Japanese have virtually no B27, and ankylosing spondylitis is very rare in that population; it is of some interest to note that for the few Japanese who do carry B27, the relative risk for the disease is extremely high (306). On the other hand, the Haida Indians of British Columbia have more than a 50% prevalence of B27, and also a very high prevalence of ankylosing spondylitis.

Ankylosing spondylitis is found 5 to 10 times more often in males than in females, although B27 is distributed equally between the sexes. The reasons for this sex difference are not known, but it seems that maleness either increases susceptibility to or enhances severity of disease or that, contrariwise, femaleness confers resistance to either susceptibility or to severity; or alternatively, the sex difference may result from differential exposure to an environmental agent.

Other spondylarthropathies are also associated with HLA-B27. These diseases may coexist with ankylosing spondylitis in the same families. Some cases of seronegative peripheral arthritis, generally affecting only a few joints, also occur in this context; the term "partial Reiter's syndrome" has been used to designate such patients. The relative risks for the other spondylarthropathies in patients with HLA-B27 are somewhat lower (15 to 40) than for ankylosing spondylitis. Patients with Reiter's disease appear to have an increased prevalence of B27 whether or not there is associated spondylitis. Individuals who develop reactive arthritis as a sequela to gastrointestinal infection caused by Yersinia, Salmonella, or Shigella also have a high prevalence of HLA-B27, whereas those who do not, have no more B27 than would be found in the general population. Patients with the peripheral arthritis of psoriasis or inflammatory bowel disease do not have an increased prevalence of HLA-B27.

Classic adult-onset rheumatoid arthritis has been associated with Dw4 and DR4. These types have been found in 47% of patients with disease as compared with 25% of controls. No A, B, or C associations have yet been found. The DR4 association is strongest for severe erosive rheumatoid factor–positive adult rheumatoid arthritis in whites.

Juvenile rheumatoid arthritis (JRA), or juvenile arthritis, denotes the condition of chronic synovitis in childhood and has been known on clinical grounds to include several subgroups that differ in clinical and laboratory findings and, indeed, are now being shown to differ in HLA associations as well. HLA-B27 is strongly associated with pauciarticular arthritis in older children, primarily boys; many of these children have early spondylarthropathy that becomes apparent with years of follow-up. DR4 is associated with a subgroup of children who have positive tests for rheumatoid factors and generally severe polyarthritis; this subgroup is probably the childhood equivalent of classic adult rheumatoid arthritis. Another subgroup, young children with pauciarthritis who frequently have chronic iridocyclitis and positive tests for antinuclear antibodies, has strong associations with both DR6 and DR8 and an additional association with DR5 in those children who acquire associated iridocyclitis. There have been suggestions of yet other associations, for example, of BW35 and DR8 with systemic-onset JRA; these remain to be firmly established.

The HLA studies in rheumatic disease provide evidence that there are indeed genetic differences between patients who express different kinds of arthritis, whether the expression be classic adult rheu-

matoid arthritis, ankylosing spondylitis, childhood pauciarthritis with chronic iridocyclitis, or childhood pauciarthritis with sacroilitis. These studies support the concept (based on clinical observations) that what we call rheumatoid arthritis is, in fact, a heterogeneous disease.

An interesting group of diseases, characterized by chronic inflammation and aberrant immunologic reactions, is associated with HLA-B8, Dw3, and DR3. These diseases are at times familial. In general, the relative risks are lower (3 to 10) than for HLA-B27 and the spondylarthropathies. These diseases include gluten-sensitive enteropathy (celiac sprue), dermatitis herpetiformis, chronic active hepatitis, myasthenia gravis, insulin-dependent diabetes mellitus, Graves' disease, Addison's disease, thyroiditis, Sjögren's syndrome, childhood dermatomyositis, and perhaps lupus erythematosus. For example, several studies have reported that 62% to 81% of adults with celiac sprue are HLA-B8 positive, whereas only 16% to 22% of normal controls in the same populations have B8. Thus the relative risk for B8 is 9. At least two DR antigens are also associated with susceptibility to celiac disease. A strong association is seen with DR3, which is found in 79% of patients (relative risk, 18), and a lesser association is seen with DR7, which is found in 45% of patients (relative risk, 4). Thus the association with B8 is probably due to the high linkage disequilibrium with DR3. The enteropathy of celiac sprue is due to the effect of gliadin, a component of gluten, on intestinal mucosa. Of patients with dermatitis herpetiformis, 70% have a gastrointestinal lesion that appears to be identical to that of celiac sprue, and 85% of this subgroup (but only 30% of those without the gastrointestinal lesion) are positive for B8,Dw3. The HLA associations appear, therefore, to be with the gastrointestinal lesion rather than the skin lesion.

Chronic active hepatitis is a form of chronic liver disease characterized by hyperimmunoglobulinemia; formation of aberrant antibodies,

such as antinuclear antibodies; and occasional rheumatic symptoms. Thirty-seven percent of patients, but only 16% of controls, are positive for B8 antigen (relative risk, 3), whereas 37% of patients, but only 21% of controls, are positive for DR3 (relative risk, 2.2). Graves' disease, Addison's disease, thyroiditis, and juvenile diabetes mellitus are characterized by formation of antibodies reactive with tissues of the target endocrine organ. Patients with these conditions also have an increased prevalence of B8 and DR3/Dw3 antigens.

HLA typing has suggested that there are genetically distinct forms of several diseases. For example, myasthenia gravis with onset at an early age, thymic hyperplasia, and formation of autoantibodies is associated with B8,DR3 antigens, whereas adult-onset myasthenia gravis characterized by thymoma is not. Sjögren's syndrome occurring as an isolated condition is associated with B8,DR3, whereas Sjögren's syndrome associated with rheumatoid arthritis is not. Insulin-dependent diabetes mellitus (often of childhood onset and thus called juvenile diabetes mellitus) is HLA associated, whereas adult-onset, insulin-independent diabetes is not. The HLA associations in juvenile diabetes are even more complex. This condition is associated with two haplotypes: B8, DR3 and B15, DR4. The relative risks appear to be stronger for the DR antigens than for the B antigens. The relative risks for DR3 and DR4 are 3.3 and 6.4. The association with DR4 is strongest for young children. If an individual is homozygous for DR3 or DR4, the relative risks increase to 10 and 16, respectively. The highest relative risk is found for individuals who carry both DR3 and DR4 (relative risk, 33), suggesting that these two genetic determinants represent independent risk factors. Whether DR3 and DR4 are directly related to disease susceptibility or are distinct markers associated by linkage disequilibrium with separate susceptibility genes is not known. There is, for example, a report that a very strong association of juvenile dia-

Figure 4

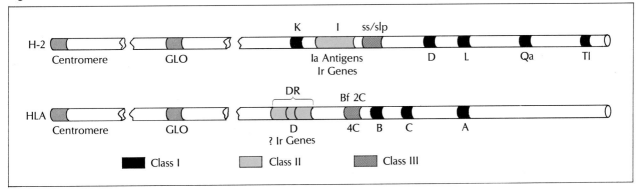

Comparison of the major histocompatibility complex (MHC) in the mouse (H-2) and in the human (HLA) reveals many similarities. Class I loci control the human HLA-A, B, C antigens and the mouse H-2-K, D, L antigens. Class II loci code for immune *response genes in the mouse, and by analogy, in the human, and they control Ia antigens in the mouse and DR (B-cell) antigens in the human. Class III loci code for complement components in both species.*

betes also exists with an allele of Bf(Bf-F1), suggesting that a susceptibility gene is closely linked to the Bf locus, which is known to be linked to HLA.

An intriguing study has shown an association of HLA-B8,DR3 antigens with toxic reactions (expressed as proteinuria) to gold and D-penicillamine therapy in patients with rheumatoid arthritis. The relative risk for renal toxicity, generally thought to take the form of immune complex nephritis, is 32 for rheumatoid arthritis patients with this haplotype who receive gold or D-penicillamine.

Other diseases with HLA associations include pemphigus, multiple sclerosis and optic neuritis, pernicious anemia, and psoriasis. DR4 has been found in increased frequency in patients with pemphigus (relative risk, 32). B7 (relative risk, 1.7) and Dw2 (relative risk, 4.3) have been associated with multiple sclerosis and optic neuritis. Patients with psoriasis have an increased frequency of B13, B17, B37, and Bw39, as well as DR7. The relative risk for psoriasis in individuals who are positive for any one of these antigens is 3 to 4. However, recent findings suggest that the common HLA factor may be a C-locus antigen, specifically Cw6 (relative risk, 4.8). The apparent increase in other HLA antigens in patients with psoriasis is probably due to linkage disequilibrium with Cw6.

Few firm associations have been made with A-locus antigens. Perhaps the best example is hemochromatosis. HLA-A3 is increased in this disease as well as B7 and B14. Family studies indicate that the susceptibility gene for idiopathic hemochromatosis is, in fact, HLA-linked, probably closely to the A locus.

From the above discussion, it is apparent that there are many associations of human diseases with antigens determined by the HLA gene loci. If the loci for Ir genes are in close proximity to the HLA system in the human, as they have been shown to be in the mouse, it seems likely that genes controlling immune function may be involved in the pathogenesis of at least some of these associated diseases. Indeed, since most of these diseases appear to be characterized by either chronic inflammation or by immune aberrations, a role for Ir genes in their causations would seem appropriate. It is also likely that some of these associations of diseases with HLA haplotypes are explained because a gene (or genes) determining disease occurrence or susceptibility is, in fact, linked to the HLA gene complex.

Nevertheless, genetic factors do not completely account for disease susceptibility. Even the close association between B27 and ankylosing spondylitis is far from absolute. There are substantial data indicating that environmental factors can trigger the occurrence of disease in susceptible hosts. The en-

vironmental agent theory postulates that individuals with genetic susceptibility to the disease may develop it only when exposed to an environmental agent (or agents), whereas those without genetic susceptibility may not develop the disease with similar exposure, or perhaps only when environmental exposures are great. For example, individuals with HLA-B27 may develop sterile arthritis when infected with the environmental agents Yersinia, Shigella, or Salmonella (reactive arthritis), and individuals with HLA-B27 may develop Reiter's syndrome when infected with the environmental agent Shigella. These are excellent examples of disease occurring when a genetically susceptible host (marked by HLA-B27-positivity) encounters an environmental agent or trigger (in these cases, bacteria that infect the bowel). Recent work done in Australia suggests that Klebsiella infections in individuals who are B27-positive may be implicated in ankylosing spondylitis.

The presence of additional genes also may influence associations between HLA antigens and disease susceptibility. For instance, the DR3 and DR4 genes associated with diabetes mellitus may determine susceptibility, or perhaps these genes may be linked to some as yet unidentified gene that is, in fact, the true susceptibility gene. It is probable that many diseases result from interactions between multiple ge-

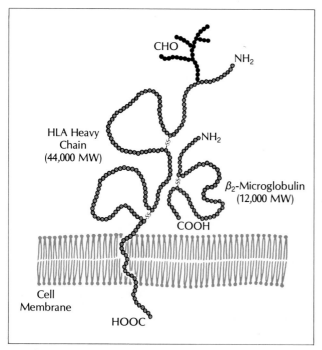

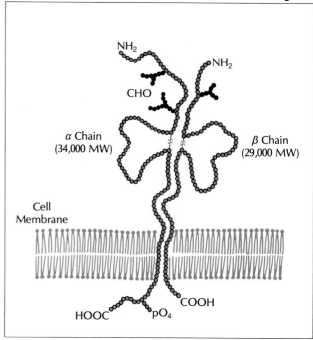

The molecular structure of the class I major histocompatibility antigens, HLA-A, B, and C in the human and H-2-K, D, and L in the mouse, is the same. These antigens consist of a heavy chain inserted through the cell membrane and β₂-microglobulin (left). The class II histocompatibility antigens, HLA-DR in the human and Ia in the mouse, are also similar (right).

netic and environmental factors, most of which are still unrecognized.

Possible heterogeneity of disease must also be considered in making disease associations. Failure to delineate diseases accurately according to their clinical and laboratory manifestations may result in obscuring potential associations. For example, the strong association between B27 and spondylitis might never have been recognized if spondylitis had remained lumped diagnostically with rheumatoid arthritis, as it was until recent years in the United States. In this regard, HLA typing has proved valid in distinguishing subgroups of patients within heterogeneous diagnostic categories, such as insulin-dependent from insulin-independent diabetes, and dermatitis herpetiformis with gluten enteropathy from dermatitis herpetiformis without the gastrointestinal component.

It is also possible that Ir- or D-locus genes are more directly involved in the pathogenesis of some diseases than are other HLA genes, but because of linkage disequilibrium, significant associations with HLA-A, B, or C antigens also may be found. If this is true, one would expect HLA-D typing to reveal stronger associations; this has indeed proved to be the case with many diseases, including multiple sclerosis, diabetes, and Addison's disease. Adult rheumatoid arthritis appears to have only a D association, with no known A, B, or C associations.

Various hypotheses have been developed to explain the mechanism of the association between HLA type and disease susceptibility. One is the molecular mimicry hypothesis, according to which histocompatibility antigens and such etiologic agents as bacteria and viruses might be molecularly similar, or might cross-react. Another hypothesis is that cell-surface antigens may be modified as a result of such events as viral infection, exposure to toxins, or neoplastic change. Such modification of HLA antigen structures might allow host immune cells to attack the altered cells, no longer recognized as "self."

Another theory proposes that Ir genes are involved in disease susceptibility. The most direct evidence comes from studies of ragweed hay-fever. Family studies suggest that the immunologic findings (high titers of anti-IgE antibodies) and clinical phenomena (ragweed hay-fever symptoms) are linked to HLA. The immunologic hyperreactivity of the several diseases associated with the HLA-B8, DR3 haplotype also suggests that Ir genes may be involved in pathogenesis. For example, in celiac sprue, Ir genes may determine aberrant reaction of the gastrointestinal mucosa to gliadin; and in Addison's disease, thyroidosis, Graves' disease, and juvenile diabetes mellitus, Ir genes may be responsible for the antiorgan antibodies and the chronic end-organ damage that have been observed.

Studies of the HLA system have clearly been of great research interest. What are the present uses of the HLA system for physicians in the practice of medicine? To date, the most fruitful clinical use of HLA typing has been in selecting donors for transplantation. An HLA identical donor, that is an identical twin, shares the entire HLA complex of the recipient. For most transplants, serologic typing is carried out for HLA-A, B, and DR antigens. In kidney transplants from identical donors, 90% to 95% of grafts survive for two years or more. If the donor is a haploidentical family member (either a parent or a sibling who shares only one of the recipient's two HLA-A, B haplotypes), two-year graft survival drops to 75%. With a graft from an unrelated donor, the probability of two-year graft survival drops to 50%.

Until recently, bone marrow transplants required an HLA-identical sibling donor. There is now evidence that some degree of HLA incompatibility will be tolerated by the bone marrow recipient, but the limits for incompatibility are not known. A major HLA incompatibility probably would lead to graft rejection or serious graft-versus-host disease.

HLA typing for A, B, and C antigens is done in some cases to select donors for blood platelet transfusions. Individuals who have had multiple transfusions of blood and blood products can become sensitized to further platelet transfusions. This problem can be eliminated by selecting HLA-A- and B-compatible platelet donors.

Another clear application of HLA typing is in establishing paternity. The use of HLA typing in paternity cases in the last several years has increased significantly as a result of legislation that affects the responsibility of the biologic father. Law enforcement and social service agencies are finding it economically worthwhile, in terms of savings in the cost of care for dependent children, to establish paternity in cases where child support is contested.

The place of HLA typing in clinical medicine, other than the uses cited, is somewhat controversial at present. Theoretically, HLA typing could be helpful in establishing a diagnosis, in identifying individuals at risk for developing a particular disease, in genetic counseling, and in prenatal diagnosis.

So far as diagnosis is concerned, only the association between B27 and ankylosing spondylitis is strong enough to be considered for this purpose, and many rheumatologists are of the opinion that even this association is not close enough to

be useful in the individual case. HLA typing for B27 antigen is a nonspecific test and cannot take the place of a thorough physical examination. Furthermore, reliance on HLA typing as a diagnostic test can lead to misdiagnoses, such as occurred in the case of a boy with hip pain seen at our clinic. The child had both HLA-B27 and an uncle who had ankylosing spondylitis. He was referred to this clinic with a presumed diagnosis of ankylosing spondylitis, but when he was properly evaluated, it was discovered that his hip pain was due to a large congenital bone cyst that had fractured, and that he had no evidence whatsoever of rheumatic disease. Similarly, it is not safe to assume that a 40-year-old man with back pain and HLA-B27 has ankylosing spondylitis; despite the B27, accurate clinical assessment is still needed to be sure he does not have another condition, such as disc disease. On the other hand, HLA typing of a large series of patients has already proved valuable in identifying subgroups of patients within diagnostic categories; and as a research tool, HLA typing may lead us to a better understanding of etiology and pathogenesis of many important human diseases, such as diabetes and rheumatoid arthritis.

At the present time, the use of HLA typing to identify patients at risk for particular diseases is not practical, since no means of disease prevention are yet at hand. For example, although it is possible to predict from available knowledge that persons with certain HLA types are at risk for juvenile diabetes, probably no purpose is served by such information. If the environmental agent or agents against which the susceptible host could be protected were known, then identification of persons at risk through HLA typing might be worthwhile. Such possibilities of disease prevention, however, currently await identification of environmental agents precipitating disease in susceptible hosts or perhaps of mechanisms of obliterating the specific host immune responses

(such as production of anti-islet cell antibodies).

Probably none of the diseases associated with HLA to date are either strongly enough associated or severe enough to warrant using HLA typing in genetic counseling. For example, one would not advise people to avoid having children simply because they have either HLA-B27 or ankylosing spondylitis.

HLA typing can, however, be of great potential use in the prenatal diagnosis of conditions linked to the HLA system, among them the complement component deficiencies (C2 and C4) and 21-hydroxylase deficiency. Although rare, these conditions may have severe consequences for affected individuals, and they can be identified prenatally by HLA typing of fetal cells in the amniotic fluid.

In summary, studies in recent years of the HLA system in humans have provided exciting insights into basic mechanisms of immunology and genetics. The associations and linkages that have been established between a number of human diseases and the HLA system may ultimately help us to answer the age-old question: Why do certain individuals get diseases while others do not? Research studies indicate that occurrence of HLA-related human diseases may be determined by genes closely linked to HLA, determining disease susceptibility or host immune responsiveness; it is also likely that environmental agents are important in triggering many of these diseases. Hopefully, future studies along these lines will provide some important answers concerning etiology and pathogenesis of such important human diseases as rheumatoid arthritis and diabetes. At the present time the chief roles of HLA typing in clinical medicine are to match donors and recipients of tissue grafts and to establish paternity. Several rare human diseases are amenable to prenatal diagnosis by HLA typing of fetal cells. The role of HLA typing in diagnosis of disease and genetic counseling at this time, however, is minimal.

Immunologic Aspects of Cancer

HERBERT F. OETTGEN   *Memorial Sloan-Kettering Cancer Center*

As is well known, immunology originated in the study of infectious diseases, and the control of these diseases with specific vaccines remains immunology's greatest clinical triumph. The field of cancer immunology is relatively young, and the prospects for immunotherapy of cancer—through any of a variety of possible approaches—remain distant and ill defined. In order to reach such an ambitious goal, we must be able to answer three fundamental questions: Do tumor-specific antigens exist? If so, does the host respond to them immunologically? And how might that response be manipulated to the host's benefit? This discussion will review some of what we have learned so far about these points; by necessity, however, the first question will consume most of our attention. As might be expected, some of the discussion will concern the results of animal studies—particularly those in the inbred mouse, in which identification and characterization of tumor-specific antigens are relatively easy.

The field of tumor immunology began in the 1950s, when it was shown by Foley, Prehn, Main, and others that sarcomas induced by carcinogenic polycyclic hydrocarbons, such as methylcholanthrene, expressed strong transplantation antigens that caused rejection of tumor grafts in mice of the same inbred strain. In subsequent studies with tumors induced by oncogenic viruses, such as polyoma virus, Sjögren, Hellström, Klein, and Habel showed that these tumors were also marked by antigens that elicited transplantation resistance in syngeneic mice. In this early stage in the development of the field, tumor immunologists noted a striking difference between sarcomas induced by chemical carcinogens and tumors induced by viruses. Each chemically induced sarcoma had individually distinct antigens, that is, the antigens generally elicited transplantation resistance to that tumor but to no other tumor, not even to different tumors induced with the same carcinogen in the same mouse. In contrast, immunization with a tumor induced by an oncogenic virus led to the development of resistance to grafts of any other tumor induced by that virus. While it appeared at first that these phenomena delineated a sharp distinction between chemically induced and virally induced tumors, it has since been found that this distinction is not absolute. Some virally induced tumors have been shown to have antigens that do not cross-react; some chemically induced tumors appear to share cross-reacting antigens.

In the effort to understand their chemical nature and genetic origin, much work has been devoted to defining tumor-specific transplantation antigens by in vitro techniques. It has been demonstrated that for tumors and leukemias induced by oncornaviruses, such as the murine leukemia virus, viral structural components incorporated into the cell surface appear to be the transplantation antigens. Tumors induced by DNA viruses, such as polyoma virus, do not express viral structural components, but there is growing evidence that a virus-specified nonstructural component, the T antigen, may be expressed on the cell surface and be responsible for their immunogenicity.

The origin of the highly restricted antigens of chemically induced tumors is unknown. However, in vitro methods for detecting these antigens have been developed only recently, so that the relative lack of progress in this direction is explicable. The major difficulty has been that these antigens generally do not elicit a humoral immune (antibody) response, even though they induce marked resistance to tumor grafts. Again, however, recent work indicates that this lack of a humoral response is not absolute. DeLeo and Old have defined two antigens with an exceedingly restricted distribution on methylcholanthrene-induced sarcomas that will evoke detectable antibody in hyperimmunized mice. They thus have provided the first serologic probes for investigation of the nature of these antigens. The introduction of the hybridoma technique for producing monoclonal antibodies is a highly promising approach to the definition of the surface antigens of chemically induced sarcomas. Given the evolving technology, investigators can hope to obtain answers to a number of basic immunologic questions: Do the serologically detectable antigens correspond to the transplantation antigens? What is their genetic specification? Are they causally related to the malignant phenotype, or do they represent an extremely polymorphic class of normal cell surface markers that distinguish one cell from another but fail to induce tolerance because of their restricted nature? If the hypothesis inherent in the last question proves valid, the antigens might only be recognized as foreign when malignant transformation causes clonal expansion of cells bearing them.

Tumors induced by chemical carcinogens or oncogenic viruses vary greatly in their capacity to render mice immune to subsequent challenge with the same tumor. Naturally occurring tumors of mice have, in transplantation experiments, generally been found to be only weakly antigenic, and in certain studies they do not appear to be antigenic at all. These findings and the observation that athymic nude mice do not have a high incidence of chemically induced or spontaneous tumors have led some to argue that the immunosurveillance theory of cancer is incorrect and that transplantation experiments demonstrating immunogenicity of certain tumors are artifactual. Even if one accepts the initial premise, the conclusion need not follow. The basic tenet of the field is that cancer cells are antigenically distinguishable from their normal progenitors—whether this leads to immune recognition or not. There-

Figure 1

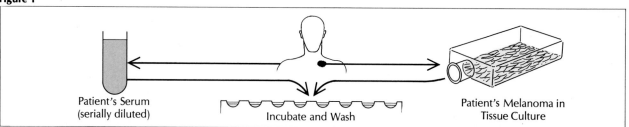

Autologous typing system developed by Old et al detects antibodies against tumor cell surface antigens. Patient's tumor cells (e.g., melanoma) are cultured and then mixed with autologous serum (above). In each of four assays (below), attachment of *autologous antibody to the melanoma cells is indicated by adherence of red blood cells to the tumor cell surface. In combination, the assays detect antibodies belonging to different immunoglobulin classes and subclasses.*

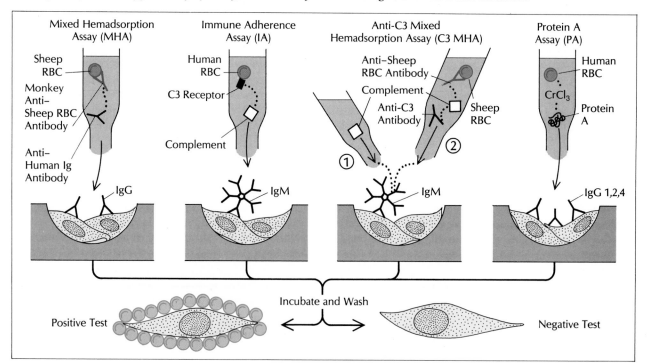

fore, the value of immunologic approaches to cancer does not depend on the validity of the immunosurveillance theory. Indeed, there is no reason to believe that all cancer antigens are recognizable as transplantation antigens capable of eliciting rejection. Considering the many known routes by which cancer cells can escape immunologic destruction, it is almost surprising that they are ever demonstrable by transplantation experiments.

While transplantation experiments have been enormously important in the initial detection of tumor-specific antigens, they are cumbersome, time consuming, and obviously not ultimately applicable to human cancer. The in vitro techniques for the demonstration of immune reactions to tumor antigens can be classified as those that use antibody as the analytic probe and those that measure cellular reactivity. The former are currently more advanced, better understood, and easier to use. While development of methods to demonstrate cellular immune reactions in vitro can be expected to greatly enhance their utility, serologic techniques for analysis of cell surface antigens of tumors have yielded most of our present knowledge of these antigens. What serologic analysis can accomplish is best exemplified by our knowledge of the surface antigens on murine leukemia cells.

Of the various types of mouse tumors, our knowledge of the surface antigens of mouse leukemia is most advanced. Leukemia cells have been the object of intense interest for two reasons. First, leukemia cells can be easily obtained in cell suspension, thus greatly facilitating serologic analysis. Second, most mouse leukemias arise in the thymus, providing the serologist with an easily accessible normal counterpart, thymocytes, to study comparatively with the leukemic cell population. As a consequence of these advantages, more is known about the surface antigens of normal and malignant T cells than almost any other cell population. Several categories of cell surface antigens on mouse leukemia cells have

been defined and shown to reside on normal thymocytes as well as on leukemia cells. They include antigens coded for by the major histocompatibility (H-2) complex and differentiation antigens, such as Thy-1 and Lyt, which are indicative of thymic derivation. In addition, a system of antigens has been discovered by Old, Boyse, and Stockert that shows the characteristics of leukemia-specific antigens in some mouse strains and normal differentiation antigens in other strains.

These antigens have been called TL (thymus leukemia) because the only types of cells on which they are found are mouse thymocytes and leukemia cells. Mouse strains can be classified as TL-positive or TL-negative, depending on whether their thymocytes express the antigen. The locus controlling expression of the TL trait is on chromosome 17, closely linked to the H-2 complex. The surprising feature of TL is that leukemias may express TL even when they arise in mice that lack TL on their thymocytes. This has been interpreted as indicating that all mice have the structural genes for TL but that expression of these genes is normally repressed in TL-negative strains. Leukemogenesis disturbs this genetic repression. The appearance of TL antigens on the leukemia cells of TL-negative mice is the clearest example of a qualitative change in gene expression associated with malignancy. The occurrence of fetal antigens or inappropriate histocompatibility antigens in experimental tumors has also been ascribed to genetic derepression. Further work is needed to establish this possibility.

A similar mechanism appears to be involved in the frequent appearance of another category of mouse leukemia cell surface antigens in leukemias of strains that normally do not express these antigens. These antigens are specified by the murine leukemia virus (MuLV). Much of what is known about the biology of the virus and the leukemias it induces was learned through the application of serologic techniques. The range of antigens that has been identified includes structural

components of the virus particle and viral antigens that are incorporated into the cell surface, as well as soluble antigens shed by MuLV-infected cells. We know from the work of Rowe that the genetic information for MuLV is carried by all mice as an integral part of their genome. Old and Stockert have shown that viral gene expression relates to the probability of developing leukemia and is profoundly influenced by genetic factors and by the state of cellular differentiation. Low-leukemia strains express only few MuLV-related antigenic systems on their thymocytes (or none at all). High-leukemia strains, on the other hand, express the full range of antigens. Because the leukemia arises exclusively in the thymus (even though MuLV genes are probably incorporated into the genome of every cell of the mouse), only cells that differentiate in the thymus appear to be susceptible to the leukemogenic effect of the virus. How does differentiation control expression and function of MuLV genes? This is a central question, and its answer(s) remains speculative. The appearance of MuLV antigens in leukemias of mice that do not normally express these antigens suggests that tumor-specific antigens may appear as a consequence of activation of normally silent genes.

It is important to note that, to date, antigens have not been found that are, in the strictest sense, leukemia-specific, that is, found only on leukemia cells. What has been encountered instead are antigens that behave as normal differentiation antigens in some mouse strains and as tumor-specific antigens in strains that do not normally express these antigens. Coding genes for TL and MuLV antigens are universal but in some strains never activated. As malignant transformation leads to expression of these normally silent genes, the gene products (restricted to tumor cells in these strains) have the appearance of transformation-specific products. While a good start has been made, our understanding of the great variety of surface antigens on normal and malignant cells

Figure 2

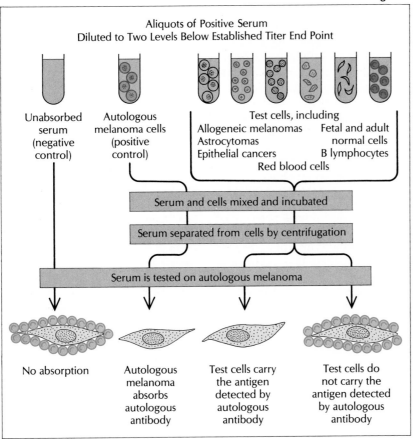

Aliquots of Positive Serum
Diluted to Two Levels Below Established Titer End Point

Unabsorbed serum (negative control)

Autologous melanoma cells (positive control)

Test cells, including
Allogeneic melanomas   Fetal and adult
Astrocytomas   normal cells
Epithelial cancers   B lymphocytes
Red blood cells

Serum and cells mixed and incubated

Serum separated from cells by centrifugation

Serum is tested on autologous melanoma

No absorption

Autologous melanoma absorbs autologous antibody

Test cells carry the antigen detected by autologous antibody

Test cells do not carry the antigen detected by autologous antibody

To determine the specificity of the antigen recognized by the patient's antimelanoma antibody, the serum is appropriately diluted and then incubated with various types of cells and centrifuged. The supernatant serum is tested for antibody against the patient's melanoma (as shown on page 188). If the antibody assay is negative, the cells used for absorption carry the same antigen as the autologous melanoma (positive absorption test). If the antibody assay is positive, the cells used for absorption do not carry the antigen (negative absorption test).

of the mouse is still fragmentary. Other antigens that have been identified require more precise characterization before they can be categorized. The goal of this research is not the development of a catalogue of cell surface antigens. Rather, it is to understand how the surface is constructed, how neoplastic transformation affects that structure, and how the immune system responds to these changes.

Let us now turn to human cancer antigens. Although the literature on the subject is voluminous, the existence of specific human cancer antigens must still be considered uncertain. The general view that tumor-specific antigens have been demonstrated in many types of human cancer is simply not justified.

The critical issue is specificity, and defining the specificity of a serologic or cell-mediated immune reaction is much easier in mouse than in man. The difference derives from the availability of inbred murine strains that have permitted the transplantation studies that first established the existence of tumor-specific antigens and made possible the production of the reagents required for the serologic definition of these antigens. In the absence of this advantage, human cancer immunologists are still attempting to develop approaches that can cope with the issue of specificity.

Much of what is known at present about human cancer cell surface antigens is derived from testing heterologous antisera raised in animals against human cancer cells and from testing allogeneic sera and lymphoid cells from cancer patients and other human donors on fresh cancer cells or a few established cancer cell lines. So far, candidate tumor-specific antigens defined by heterologous sera have turned out, on careful analysis, to be differentiation antigens, that is, antigens characteristic of some normal cells at some stage of development, rather than antigens restricted to cancer cells. Tumor antigens detected by reaction with human sera have been found to fall into several categories. The best studied examples have been alloantigens (particularly products of the HLA complex and ABO locus), antigens related to the Epstein-Barr virus, and antigens related to the sera used in culturing human cancer cells. The unknown participation of normal alloantigens in studies involving sera or lymphoid cells from one individual and tumor cells from another poses a critical problem, so most surveys for humoral or cell-mediated immunity to cell surface antigens of human cancer cells could not distinguish tumor-specific reactions from reactions against other categories of antigens.

To develop as unambiguous a serologic typing system as possible, our group (Old, Carey, Shiku, Takahashi, Pfreundschuh, Ueda, and Oettgen) turned several years ago to analyzing autologous serum reactivity to cell surface antigens of human cancer. The decision to stress the serologic approach in no way indicates that we regarded humoral immune reactions against cancer antigens as more important than cellular immune reactions. It was made simply because defining the specificity for serologic reactions is far easier than it is for reactions involving lymphoid cells. The autologous typing procedure has several essential features (see Figure 1, page 188):

First, the reagents involved are limited to serum and tumor cells from the same individual; this eliminates the contribution of alloantibodies and facilitates detection of antigens belonging to the individually distinct, or unique, category. Second, only tumor cells established in continuous culture are used as target cells; this permits repeated serologic tests and ensures reproducibility. As it is difficult to establish the most common cancers—lung, breast, colon—in culture, initial emphasis was placed on malignant melanoma, astrocytoma, and renal cancer. Third, several serologic techniques (mixed hemadsorption, immune adherence, anti-C3-mixed hemadsorption, protein A assay) are used in order to reduce the possibility that antibody of a particular immunoglobulin class might be missed; together, the four assays detect IgM and IgG antibodies, both complement-fixing and non-complement-fixing. Finally, absorption analysis is used to define specificity, as it has been used in the analysis of tumor antigens of the mouse. Since normal cells from individuals with genetic identity to the tumor donor are not available, as many normal cell types as possible are cultured from the tumor donor, including skin fibroblasts, B cells, T cells, and skin epithelium. These autologous normal cells (including noncultured peripheral blood cells), as well as a wide range of allogeneic and xenogeneic normal and malignant cells, make up the panel of absorbing cells used in our analysis.

Over the past seven years we have investigated more than 200 patients by autologous typing (see Figure 2, page 190). These studies have revealed three classes of cell surface antigens: Antigens of the first class are restricted to the autologous tumor and cannot be detected on autologous normal cells or on any other normal or malignant cell type; these antigens are reminiscent of the highly restricted antigens of chemically induced sarcomas. Antigens of the second class are shared tumor antigens, expressed by autologous as well as some allogeneic tumors of similar and in some cases dissimilar origin but not by a wide range of other tumor types or by normal B cells, kidney cells, or fibroblasts. Antigens of the third class are widely distributed on autologous, allogeneic,

and xenogeneic normal and malignant cells. The largest number of reactions detected by autologous typing is due to antibodies against the third class. Together with alloantibodies, these antibodies probably account for most of the positive reactions recorded in past serologic studies of human cancer. Absorption analysis is essential, particularly for defining antigens of the third class, which may seem tumor-specific in direct tests because tumor cells may express higher levels of these antigens than normal cells.

To illustrate some of the observations made on the basis of autologous typing, let me briefly review our findings with malignant melanoma. We have established melanoma cell lines from 160 patients; with few exceptions, the lines derive from recurrent or metastatic melanomas. In many cases, companion cell lines of normal skin fibroblasts and Epstein-Barr-virus-transformed lymphocytes have also been established from the same patients (melanocytes have been difficult to culture). Autologous typing of 75 melanoma patients has shown IgG or

IgM antibodies in 56; thus far, the antibodies in 30 of these patients have been characterized: They were directed against individually distinct antigens in four, against shared tumor antigens in five, and against widely distributed antigens in 21 (see Figure 3 on this page).

The individually distinct antigen that has been studied most is the antigen detected on the melanoma of patient AU, a 51-year-old man whose tumor showed unexpectedly slow progression. The patient had IgG antibody that reacted with his own melanoma; titers rose when the tumor recurred and fell when the recurrent tumor was removed. The antibody was absorbed only by the patient's own melanoma and not by any other malignant or normal cell in the large panel tested. It was possible to solubilize the AU antigen by limited papain digestion, and it was shown by Lloyd to be a glycoprotein with a molecular weight in the range of 25,000 to 40,000. The solubilized antigen was not related serologically to normal cell surface components, such as HLA, Ia, or β_2-microglobulin. A first

Figure 3

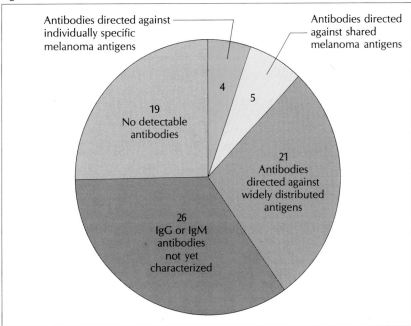

Autologous typing of 75 melanoma patients at Memorial Sloan-Kettering detected antibodies in 56. Of 30 patients sufficiently analyzed, four had antibodies recognizing individually specific melanoma antigens, five had antibodies recognizing shared melanoma antigens, and 21 had antibodies against widely distributed antigens.

indication of the locus that specifies the AU antigen was obtained in experiments using the technique of somatic cell hybridization. Fusion of AU melanoma cells with Chinese hamster cells resulted in hybrids expressing the AU antigen; results obtained by Resnick and Pravtcheva in an extensive analysis of one hybrid series indicate that the antigen is coded for by a locus on chromosome 19. Further studies should tell us whether these individually distinct melanoma antigens represent a family of polymorphic but structurally related molecules coded for at a single locus or totally unrelated molecules coded for at many loci.

An example of a shared melanoma antigen was found in patient AH, a man with recurrent melanoma, who has been free of recurrence in recent years. IgM antibody in the patient's serum recognized an antigen on his melanoma that was also found on other melanomas and on astrocytomas but not on epithelial cancers, B-cell lines, or fibroblasts. Physically, this antigen appears to be a glycolipid, but its structural characterization is still incomplete. One important question about this antigen (and the class it represents) is whether antibody directed against it occurs as a consequence of cancer. A provisional answer comes from the results of Houghton's survey of over 100 nontransfused, apparently normal males; five had IgM antibody to an antigen related to the AH system, suggesting that overt melanoma is not necessary for the development of AH antibody.

A new dimension has been added to serologic analysis of human cancer cells by the development of the hybridoma methodology (see Figure 4, page 193). So far, hybridomas secreting monoclonal antibodies to human cancer cell surface antigens have been produced by immunizing mice with human cancer cells and fusing their spleen cells with mouse myeloma cell lines. Several groups, including our own, have used monoclonal antibodies to define various systems of antigens on the cell surface of malig-

nant melanomas and some other human cancers, each with a characteristic cellular distribution. A glycolipid antigen defined by Dippold and Lloyd in our group shows the most restricted distribution; it is found on melanomas, astrocytomas, and melanocytes but not on epithelial cells, fibroblasts, or cells of hematopoietic origin. None of the antibodies developed so far, however, recognize components that are specific for cancer cells. Murine monoclonal antibodies can only tell us, of course, what the mouse recognizes on human cancer cells. As human myelomas are now becoming available for fusion with human lymphocytes, we will be able to produce human monoclonal antibodies and more precisely define the cancer cell surface antigens that can be detected by the human immune system. Once correlations of certain clinical features with the presence or absence of cell surface components detected by these antibodies have been established, this work may eventually lead to new classifications of tumors. Apart from their use as analytic probes, monoclonal antibodies may also find applications in diagnosis, in prophylaxis, and in therapy.

Given the human cancer cell surface molecules that can be defined by serologic analysis, one of the current challenges is to determine which of them are, or can be made, immunogenic in man. Since some of the antigens are known to elicit an immune response in the autologous host, and serologic methods to monitor that response and define its specificity are available, it is justifiable to determine whether cancer patients can be immunized with these antigens. The idea of a human cancer vaccine is, of course, not new; many patients have been injected with autologous or allogeneic tumor cell preparations over the past 60 years. The complexity of these studies, however, makes any assessment of the value of this approach to cancer therapy exceedingly difficult.

A fundamental problem has been the lack of rapid and precise methods of monitoring the persistence of

relevant antigens during vaccine construction and of assessing the immunogenicity of these antigens in patients receiving the vaccines. In the development of vaccines against infectious diseases, serologic responses to bacterial or viral antigens have provided this essential guidance. The lack of comparable serologic tests to monitor the effectiveness of cancer vaccines has been a major impediment to investigating this approach to cancer therapy. Now, with the development of serologic typing systems for defining cell surface antigens of melanoma and other cancers, we do have tests that can be used to gauge the immunogenicity of cancer vaccines. With these methods, we have begun the process of assaying a number of different melanoma vaccines.

The first vaccines were prepared from irradiated but otherwise unmodified autologous or allogeneic melanoma cells. Autologous melanoma cells were used because the unique antigens are restricted to autologous melanoma. The definition of shared antigens provided the rationale for using allogeneic melanoma vaccines. When the patients' serologic response to these vaccines was analyzed, however, Livingston found that a response to unique or shared melanoma antigens was induced only in exceptional cases. While it was encouraging that the desired serologic response was induced at least occasionally, the rarity with which this occurred points to the need for increasing the immunogenicity of the "weak" tumor antigens in the vaccines. There are a number of ways to attempt this that have adequate experimental precedent. They include the introduction of "helper" determinants by infecting the vaccine cells with certain nonpathogenic viruses, fusing them with cells carrying foreign determinants by the technique of somatic cell hybridization, or modifying them chemically. As progress is made in isolating and characterizing unique and shared human cancer antigens, it will be possible to use vaccines containing purified antigens. The development of powerful new adjuvants has opened yet another area for exploration in this context.

The way cancer antigens are presented is not the only factor, however, that determines the immunogenicity of cancer vaccines. Basic immunology has revealed several ways in which the response to immunization is determined by the recipient's immune system rather than the immunizing agent. One is based on an individual's genetic constitution. Immune response genes determine whether or not an individual's immune system can recognize a given antigen at all; nothing is yet known about immune response genes that govern the immune response to human cancer antigens. Other regulatory factors (helper cells, suppressor cells, soluble factors, idiotype-anti-idiotype networks) have been shown to control the magnitude and duration of the immune response.

Eliciting a maximal response to cancer vaccines may depend on developing strategies by which genetic restriction of the immune response can be overcome, or the balance of regulatory circuits can be shifted in the direction of induction as opposed to suppression. The latter has been attempted experimentally in various ways: administration of antibodies thought to be specific for suppressor cell surface antigens, chemical modification of antigens to favor inducer over suppressor cells, and chemotherapy or irradiation to reduce suppressor cells. While the effectiveness of any of these approaches is not yet certain, there is no doubt that attempts at immunization with cancer antigens will have to take into account host factors that regulate the response to these antigens.

One way to overcome limitations posed by the host's immune system would be to transfer immunity to cancer antigens with antisera or sensitized lymphocytes. While this approach has been used successfully in the mouse, it has not been applied to human cancer because specific antisera and sensitized lymphocytes have not been available. This may change if monoclonal antibodies of requisite specificity

Figure 4

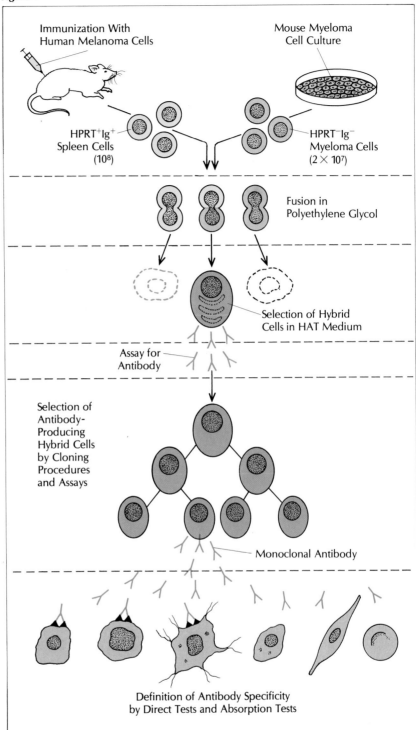

Production of hybridomas secreting monoclonal antibodies to human melanoma cell surface antigens is initiated by immunizing mice with human melanoma cells. The immunized spleen cells—positive for both immunoglobulin and the enzyme hypoxanthine phosphoribosyl transferase (HPRT)—are fused with cultured mouse myeloma cells (Ig- and HPRT-negative). Hybrid anti-human-cancer-antibody-secreting cells are selected out in the HAT medium, which permits survival only of cells that are HPRT-positive. By successive cloning, a population of hybrid cells that secrete monoclonal antibodies to the melanoma originally used for immunization is selected. A large panel of cells is then used to delineate the cellular distribution of the antigens detected by the monoclonal antibodies in direct tests and absorption tests.

can be developed and if stable clones of sensitized cytotoxic T cells can be cultured in T-cell growth factor.

Because serologic methods offer the most precise and versatile tools to test the immunogenicity of vaccines in cancer patients, we consider an optimal antibody response to unique or shared cancer antigens a valid criterion by which vaccines can be selected for therapeutic trials. There is, of course, a general impression that increased cellular rather than humoral immunity is the desired end point of immunologic manipulation in cancer patients. We know too little about this, however, to form a judgment in the matter. There has also been concern that immunization may result in augmented rather than restricted tumor growth, particularly if the procedures used induce increased humoral immunity. Once again, we do not know if this possibility exists in man; there is no evidence that enhancement of tumor growth has been observed in any patients receiving cancer cell vaccines (or, for that matter, in any animal experiment with strictly syngeneic tumors). Nevertheless, we will have to remain alert to this possibility.

In clinical practice, the field of immunotherapy has been dominated by nonspecific approaches. BCG and *Corynebacterium parvum* are two agents that have been used widely on the premise that they potentiate immunologic reactivity on a global basis, which results in a more effective immune reaction against cancer. While the concept is appealing, its general validity remains to be proved. The overall results of clinical trials with these agents have led to a disenchantment with this approach to cancer therapy. Nevertheless, a body of solid observations remains that requires continued exploration, beginning with Coley's observation, around the turn of the century, that cancers may regress during bacterial infections or after injection of bacterial vaccines. To be sure, some of the early reports may not satisfy modern criteria for convincing documentation. However,

Kempin and colleagues have developed additional evidence for a therapeutic effect of Coley's toxin in a recent trial at our hospital. Patients with nodular non-Hodgkin's lymphoma were randomized into two groups. Both received the same chemotherapy, and one was also treated with a mixed bacterial vaccine. The frequency of complete remission, as well as remission duration, was greater in the vaccine-treated group.

Other convincing examples of successful application of this approach include the destruction of skin tumors induced by Klein by topical application of agents causing delayed hypersensitivity reactions and the regression of melanoma metastases after intratumoral injection of BCG, first described by Morton. More recently, several groups have reported success in the treatment of superficial bladder cancer with BCG administered by intravesical instillation and simultaneous percutaneous vaccination. A pilot study by Morales suggested that the approach was successful, and this suggestion has been confirmed by Pinsky and Lamm in two prospectively randomized trials comparing the results of surgical treatment alone with the results of surgery followed by BCG. A significant delay of recurrence was seen in the BCG-treated group, and the number of recurrent tumors was smaller in patients who developed recurrence. Only patients who received BCG showed conversion to negative cytology.

It has turned out far more difficult than initially expected to learn how these agents work and what role specific immune reactions play in the process. There is evidence that some of the antitumor effects are caused by mediator molecules released by host cells. The best known of these endogenous mediators are the interferons. Another mediator of much interest is a factor found in the serum of mice treated with endotoxin. Intravenous injection of tumor-bearing mice with endotoxin has long been known to cause, within hours, acute hemorrhagic necrosis of tumor

grafts, often followed by complete regression. Although extensively investigated over the past 40 years, the way endotoxin causes acute tumor destruction remains unknown. Direct action is unlikely because endotoxin is not toxic for tumor cells in vitro. The suggestion that a mediator molecule was involved was derived from Old's finding that acute hemorrhagic tumor necrosis could be induced not only by injection of endotoxin but also by injection of serum from mice that had been treated with endotoxin after priming with BCG. The tumor-necrotizing factor (TNF) in the serum has been shown to be a glycoprotein with a molecular weight of 40,000; it causes tumor necrosis in vivo and is cytotoxic or cytostatic for a range of mouse and human cancer cells in vitro. It originates from the macrophage.

When TNF-containing serum from endotoxin-treated mice was examined in immunologic systems by Hoffmann, it was found to have striking effects on the maturation and function of lymphocytes. With further purification, the immune response–enhancing activity was found not to reside in TNF but in a different molecule now known to be interleukin-1 (IL-1), a protein with a molecular weight of 13,000. IL-1, also a macrophage product, plays a central role in the regulation of the immune response. It induces maturation of T- and B-cell precursors and stimulates T cells to produce interleukin-2, also known as T-cell growth factor. One can speculate that TNF and IL-1 are involved in two distinct phases of tumor rejection. TNF causes the primary event of acute necrosis, which is known to be independent of an immune response; it can be induced even in severely immunosuppressed hosts. IL-1, on the other hand, may play a role in the secondary phase, the rejection of residual tumor cells, which is known to depend on an immune response.

Many points remain to be explored, such as the basis of TNF's tumor-cell selectivity, its possible involvement in the cytotoxic effect of activated macrophages and other killer cells, and the relation of TNF to other endotoxin-induced serum factors, particularly a factor that enforces differentiation of leukemia cells, recently described by Metcalf and Burgess. Yet another potent antitumor factor has been discovered by Kassel and Old in normal plasma. It was first recognized in experiments concerned with antitumor effects of interferon in leukemic mice. The surprising finding was that normal plasma was as effective as the interferon preparation. Subsequently, striking regression of lymphomas was also induced in cats and dogs by treatment with normal plasma. Purification of the factor from plasma has

shown that it shares several characteristics with cold insoluble globulin, also called fibronectin. For this reason, Mosessohn suggested that the cryoprecipitated fraction of plasma might be active because it is rich in cold insoluble globulin. Taking up this suggestion, MacEwen found that cat cryoprecipitates were in fact as effective as whole plasma in inducing regression of cat lymphomas. Clinical tests are now under way with human cryoprecipitate.

Over the next few years, we can expect a better understanding of the nature of human cancer antigens and the immune response they elicit. With the recognition that immunologic reactions are con-

trolled by genes, the genetic control of immune response to cancer now needs definition. To prevent tumors from escaping immunologic destruction, we have to learn how to overcome genetic restrictions on immune responses and how to force the regulatory inducer-suppressor network into a balance favorable to tumor destruction. We will require, among other things, more detailed knowledge of the action of immunomodulators and their endogenous mediators. Neither uncritical optimism nor paralyzing pessimism is justified. We can expect that immunology will continue to make important contributions to our understanding of cancer.

Cellular Differentiation Markers In Lymphoproliferative Diseases

FREDERICK P. SIEGAL   *Mount Sinai School of Medicine*

As is true in cancer generally, attempts to classify the malignant lymphoproliferative diseases are motivated by the hope that such classification will afford the clinician more reliable means to evaluate prognosis and to arrive at an optimally rational form of therapy. The ultimate goal, of course, is to match specificity of diagnostic capabilities with specificity of therapeutic modalities.

Until not much more than 15 years ago, classification of both the lymphomas and the leukemias was dependent almost entirely on morphologic observation. From the point of view of the pathologist, purely morphologic criteria proved difficult to apply consistently. Furthermore, nomenclature was confusing because assignment of cell type on the basis of morphology was sometimes inappropriate. For example, we have learned that most lymphomas categorized as histiocytic (implying derivation from malignant expansions of cells of the monocyte-macrophage line) are not histiocytic at all, but lymphocytic. There were several reasons for this confusion, one being the fact that lymphocytes tend to be extremely polymorphic; they circulate as small, round cells but change drastically in both size and nuclear characteristics when stimulated by antigen or mitogen. A somewhat parallel polymorphism exists for monocytes and macrophages.

In 1966, Henry Rappaport published the AFIP fascicle that introduced a revised classification of lymphomas. This system is still the standard by which all other schemes are evaluated and continues in revised form to be a useful system for classifying these disorders. The first differential criterion of the Rappaport classification depends on whether the histologic architecture of the tumor is nodular or diffuse. Further classification is dependent on cytologic characteristics of the malignant cells: e.g., size, nuclear morphology, presence or absence of nucleoli.

Since Rappaport's classification, a number of newer classification schemes have been proposed, most based on a combination of morphologic and clinical features of each type of lymphoma. An international expert committee recently developed a "working formulation" of non-Hodgkin's lymphomas that may improve comparability of studies in these diseases (see table on page 205). The scheme includes concepts based on recent information on cell lineage, when the cell type can be deduced from morphology. Unfortunately, certain lymphomas in the scheme are heterogenous with respect to lineage, despite morphologic similarities.

As understanding of the lymphoproliferative diseases has developed, a number of deficiencies in these classification systems have surfaced. For one thing, the use of cell size as a criterion of cellular differentiation led to a number of categorizations that no longer seem valid. Although the Rappaport classification includes both lymphomas and leukemias, it tends to treat the two classifications as discrete. On the other hand, one of the major contributions made by studies of lymphoproliferation using cellular markers is the documentation of the continuum between various leukemias and the non-Hodgkin's lymphomas. Certainly, this concept is consistent with the known behavior of lymphocytes. They are not sessile cells attached to lymphoid organs, but rather they constantly circulate through blood and lymph, percolating through lymph nodes, splenic stroma, and other lymphoid organs. Normally, the lymphocyte will remain at a particular site only if it encounters something that specifically retains it, presumably through cell-surface interactions. For example, T-lymphocyte precursors in the blood apparently remain in contact with thymic epithelium because of cell-cell contact phenomena mediated by receptors. Similarly, specific antigen-reactive cells remain at a site where antigen has been localized (e.g., in a lymph node). The normal lymphocyte is thus in constant traffic between and through lymphoid organs. In a pathologic setting, it may well be that every lymphoma has its corresponding leukemic manifestation, and vice versa.

This concept is best exemplified by chronic lymphocytic leukemia (CLL) and the so-called well-differentiated lymphocytic lymphomas. Clinically, when biopsies have been done on the lymph nodes of CLL patients, lymphomas have been found with considerable frequency. In the past, this was often regarded as an association between two different diseases—a reasonable assumption, especially since in most cases when a diagnosis of CLL is made, the physician sees no need to biopsy. It is only when the patient presents with "bulky disease" that biopsy is standard. The critical point is that when one studies the marker characteristics of the malignant cells in well-differentiated lymphocytic lymphoma, these cells are indistinguishable from the leukemic cells of CLL. Both are B lymphocytes with the same panoply of markers.

If lymphoma and leukemia are two expressions of the same type of neoplastic cell, why is the clinical expression in some individuals dominated by solid tumors and in others by leukemic manifestations? No answer is yet available, although very probably the differences relate to factors on the cell membrane that mediate the cell's trafficking through the body. As already noted, lymphocytes are circulating cells,

with the lymphoid organs as way stations on their rounds. Moreover, with appropriate stimuli, such as infection and chronic inflammation, it is not uncommon to see aggregations of lymphoid tissue in a wide array of "nonlymphoid" structures, such as the lungs and lamina propria of the gut.

K. J. Gajl-Peczalska and her colleagues at the University of Minnesota performed a number of studies on patients with solid non-Hodgkin's lymphomas using cell markers. They demonstrated with these methods that one could find a substantial proportion of patients with such tumors whose peripheral blood contained an abnormally enlarged cohort of monoclonal lymphoid cells that were probably related to the solid malignancies.

More recently, K. Ault has used computer-assisted analysis of fluorescence intensity patterns (cytofluorography) to define lymphoid clones in the blood of patients with various lymphomas. All in all, the evidence seems to be mounting that, from a clinical point of view, it is necessary to consider lymphomas as diseases to be treated as disseminated from their onset.

To those used to thinking in immunobiologic or immunopathologic terms, the lymphomas and leukemias are widely considered to be diseases involving monoclonal expansions of the various B and T lymphocyte classes and subclasses in several states of differentiation and activation. The lymphoproliferative diseases can be regarded, as can the immunodeficiency diseases, as disorders localized to one or another compartment of the lymphoid system. Therefore, just as we can characterize Bruton's agammaglobulinemia as a B-cell defect or the Di George syndrome as primarily affecting T cells, so should we be able to classify the lymphoid malignancies by the cell types involved. Marker analysis facilitates such classification.

The insights underlying our current ability to classify lymphoid malignancies by the involved lymphocyte type actually long antedated our recently acquired capacity

to identify lymphocyte populations and subpopulations by various differentiation markers. As early as 1944, McEndy, Boon, and Furth at Columbia were able to demonstrate that leukemias in an inbred (AKR) mouse strain were of thymic origin. In the 1960s, Peterson, Cooper, and Burmester, working with Good at the University of Minnesota, demonstrated the association between avian leukosis in chickens and the bursa of Fabricius. More recently, R. L. Lukes and his colleagues at the University of Southern California and K. Lennert and his group in Germany observed that certain lymphomas shared the cytologic features of cells normally found in the germinal centers of lymph nodes (particularly cleaved or dented nuclei). From the fact that these germinal centers are foci for B-cell localization, they reasoned that these tumors should be B-cell proliferations. They also noted that tumors with nodular (the term "follicular" is now used) architecture ought to be of B-cell origin, since architectural organization into nodules is characteristic of B, but not of T, cells. This was the first recognition that most, if not all, nodular lymphomas involve B lymphocytes. By correlating these observations with the localization patterns of various lymphomas, Lukes and Lennert independently developed classification systems that incorporate lymphocyte characterization. Figure 1, page 199, provides a cutaway map of the lymph node with various anatomic areas correlated with lymphocyte localization patterns.

The term "differentiation marker" provides a clue to the approach taken in current efforts to define and classify malignant lymphoproliferative diseases. The strategy is to identify molecules or phenomena that discriminate between lymphocytes and histiocytes, between B cells and T cells, and among maturational phases of lymphocytes within the various classes.

Many of these differentiation markers have been discussed in other contexts in previous chapters in this volume. An example is the

Thy-1 marker universally present on T lymphocytes in mice and absent on B cells. Cytoplasmic and surface immunoglobulins serve as the most useful markers of the B-cell lineage. In addition to observing such specific and serologically detectable markers, we are also able to take advantage of certain discriminatory in vitro phenomena. An important example of this is the ability of human T cells to form rosettes with sheep erythrocytes. Some B lymphocytes, on the other hand, rosette with mouse erythrocytes but not with sheep red blood cells (see Figure 2 on page 200). Finally, enzymatic markers have been found that are relatively specific for the various cellular cohorts involved. Thus far, perhaps the most useful enzymatic marker has been terminal deoxynucleotidyltransferase (TdT), which appears restricted to cells associated with the early phases of the differentiation pathways of the lymphocyte. This, as will be discussed, seems to have particular significance in defining

a number of the leukemias.

Which are the markers of these different lymphocyte subsets that have been used in identifying, classifying, and defining the lymphoproliferative diseases? Figures 3 and 4 on pages 201 and 202 depict currently reasonable schemes for the differentiation of T and B lymphocytes, respectively. Both start with an essentially hypothetical entity, the lymphoid stem cell, and propose the Ia-like B-cell alloantigens as markers common both to cells destined to function as B cells and to those that will differentiate into T cells. These markers are surface molecules analogous to the factors identified as Ia antigens in mice (see D. H. Katz, "Genetic Controls and Cellular Interactions in Antibody Formation"). They have been shown by B. Benacerraf, H. McDevitt, Katz, and others to be products of genes in the I region of the murine major histocompatibility region. Functionally, the Ia antigens have been found to be involved in such lymphocyte interac-

tions as B-cell–T-cell cooperation.

About 80% of human blood lymphocytes are cells that have differentiated in the thymus and under thymic influence. The T cells can be subdivided on the basis of differential stages into lymphoid stem cells, pre-T lymphocytes, thymic T cells (thymocytes), and peripheral T cells. The last can again be subdivided into helper, suppressor, and cytolytic T cells.

The lymphoid stem cell is itself derived from a precursor cell, a stem cell from which not only lymphocytes are derived but also most (if not all) of the other hematologic cell types including erythrocytes, platelets, histiocytes, and granulocytes. In the T lineage, the next stage after the lymphoid stem cell is that of the pre-T lymphocyte, a term applied to cells committed to the thymic differentiation pathway before their arrival in the thymus. Once in the thymus, marker characteristics begin to develop. The thymocyte acquires TdT activity. Its surface becomes recognizable as

Figure 1

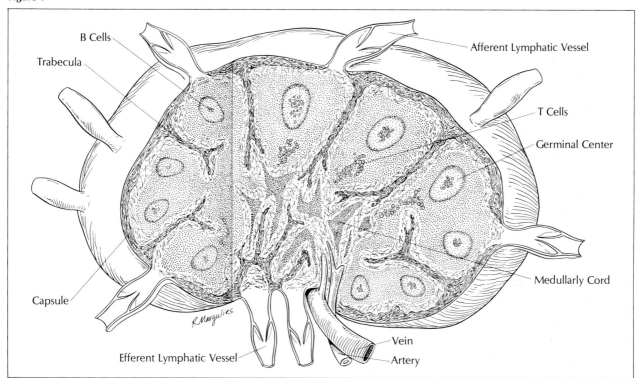

Cutaway drawing of a normal immunized human lymph node emphasizes B and T lymphocyte localization patterns. The B cells are seen to be concentrated in the germinal, or follicular, centers located on the periphery of the node. In contrast, the so-called thymus-dependent, or T-cell, areas are found to predominate in the deep cortical areas of the node.

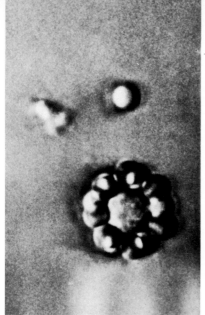
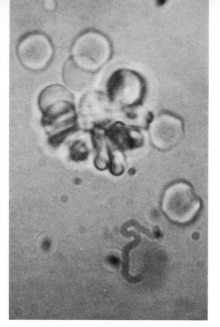

Figure 2

A sheep erythrocyte rosette, a characteristic marker for T lymphocytes, is seen at left. The adjoining micrograph shows a mouse erythrocyte rosette, a B-cell marker. It was formed by lymphocytes from a patient with chronic lymphocytic leukemia.

that of a human T cell. Thymic lymphocytes acquire the ability to form rosettes with sheep erythrocytes at both 37° C and 4° C. They also develop characteristic surface antigens, somewhat analogous to the differentiation antigens so well defined for murine thymocytes. These antigens can be defined by both conventional and monoclonal antibodies. This latter type of reagent has revolutionized analysis of cellular differentiation markers in the past few years.

Differentiation through the thymus can be followed by observing the gradual loss of TdT activity and the sequential gain or loss of several antigenic structures. Monoclonal antibodies have permitted subdivision of thymocytes into several sequential compartments. Ultimately, more mature thymocytes diverge into two major subsets characterized by specific differentiation antigens, as in the mouse. These cells then lose thymus-specific antigens as they become peripheral T cells.

When thymocytes are exported from the thymus and become functioning peripheral T lymphocytes, they lose their ability to form sheep erythrocyte rosettes at 37°, but still make rosettes at 4°. Their surface complement of differentiation antigens is altered; differentiation

among the functionally distinct suppressor/cytotoxic and helper/inducer T-cell subpopulations can now be made on this basis. Although TdT activity is lost to some extent, other enzymatic markers can be recognized, specifically acid phosphatase, adenosine deaminase, and alpha-naphthylesterase (assayed under acid conditions). The acid alpha-naphthylesterase provides a neat differentiation marker among monocytes, T cells, and B cells. Monocytes will stain for this enzyme diffusely and uniformly; T cells will show only a discrete "spot"; B cells will not stain at all.

B lymphocytes constitute about 10% of the blood lymphocyte pool. In the differentiation of B cells from lymphoid stem cells, Cooper, Raff, and Owen showed that the first development is the acquisition of cytoplasmic IgM (mu) heavy chains. Cooper's group and Janossy and colleagues pointed out that TdT is present early in the B-cell, as well as in the T-cell, lineage. Thus, pre-B cells in normal bone marrow having Ia antigens on their surface and cytoplasmic mu chains express nuclear TdT. Cells that have cytoplasmic IgM and Ia-like antigens have been classified as pre-B lymphocytes. The mature, circulating B lymphocyte has a much wider array of markers. These include

surface immunoglobulin, most commonly both IgM and IgD, sometimes alternatively IgA or IgG. Some mature B cells also form rosettes with mouse erythrocytes. This marker appears early in the differentiation of B cells and may be lost in subsequent stages, since the germinal center cells do not seem to make mouse rosettes well. B lymphocytes retain Ia-like antigens on their surfaces and also express a number of specific receptors in the membranes. They efficiently bind aggregated or complexed IgG as well as structures in the third component of complement (C3b and C3d). Epstein-Barr virus is selectively bound by B cells but not by T or other hematopoietic cells. Monoclonal antibodies are described that define other antigens restricted to certain B-cell subsets.

The next differential stage of the B-cell lineage is the plasmacytoid B cell. This concept of a transitional cell between the B lymphocyte and the antibody-secreting plasma cell is interesting because it exemplifies the value of studies of lymphoproliferative diseases in adding to our understanding of normal lymphocyte physiology; its existence was first appreciated through observations in patients with Waldenström's macroglobulinemia. Plasmacytoid B cells, as the name implies, begin to take on some of the characteristics of plasma cells. They have increased rough endoplasmic reticulum and a significant portion will stain for cytoplasmic Ig, a phenomenon that is quite rare in normal peripheral blood B cells. They also continue to have some surface immunoglobulin.

The fully developed plasma cell has lost these receptor molecules. It is rich in cytoplasmic immunoglobulin and probably has some unique surface antigens. An important and characteristic plasma-cell marker is immunoglobulin J chain, apparently occurring in association with all Ig classes. This is noteworthy because in circulating immunoglobulins, J chain is usually identified only in IgA and IgM.

The "third population" of lymphocytic cells, recognized by Froland and Natvig in Oslo, is less well defined with respect to origins, functions, and stages of differentiation. The marker characteristics of these cells have not yet been well correlated with the several functionally distinct cell types. These cells include "K" cells that participate in antibody-dependent cytotoxicity (see J.-C. Cerottini, "Lymphoid Cells as Effectors of Immunologic Cytolysis") and natural killer (NK) cells involved in resistance to tumor or organ grafting and certain infections. Third population cells tend to be morphologically distinct from other lymphoid cells and have come to be referred to as "large, granular lymphocytes" because of their relatively abundant cytoplasm with visible organelles. These cells do have defined surface molecules, such as receptors for immunoglobulin Fc and for complement components, but these are not sufficiently unique to serve as markers in this context.

The third population cells bear superficial morphologic and structural resemblances to monocytes

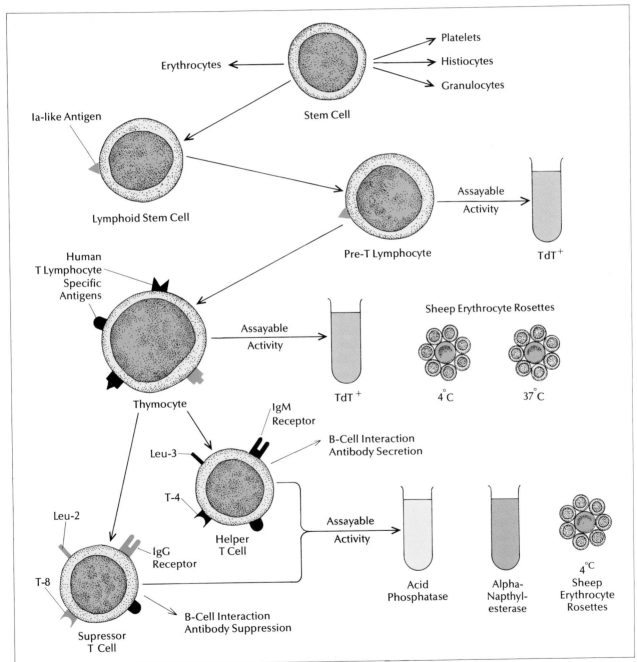

In this diagram of T-lymphocyte differentiation, the starting point is a stem cell from which various blood cells are derived. This, in turn, gives rise to a lymphoid stem cell which, when it differentiates along the T-cell pathway, evolves sequentially to pre-T cell, thymocyte, and functionally specific peripheral T cells. Marker characteristics of each are indicated.

but probably represent distinct lineages. In their possession of receptors for immunoglobulin and complement components, the third population lymphocytes are like monocytes. However, there are significant differences that can be used to segregate the two. The lymphocytes are not phagocytic as, of course, monocytes are; they usually lack the lysosomal and other enzymes generally associated with monocytes. For marker purposes, alpha-naphthyl-acetate-esterase staining patterns can be used to distinguish the monocyte component.

Although we have already alluded to the significance of certain aspects of lymphocyte trafficking through the body and localization in various lymphoid structures in the development of our current approaches to the classification of lymphoid malignancies, some additional comment here might prove helpful as a prelude to a systematic discussion of the application of markers to lymphoma/leukemia differentiation.

Figure 4

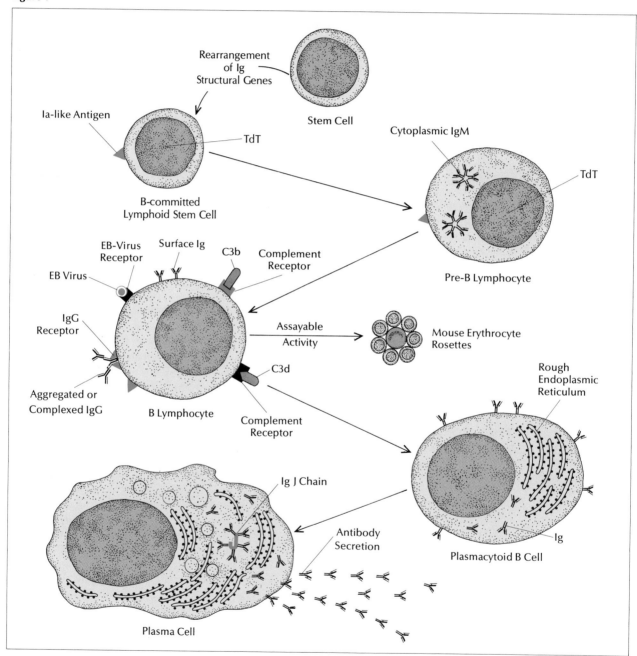

In the B-lymphocyte pathway, the appearance of cytoplasmic IgM in the pre-B lymphocyte is the first distinctive marker. Subsequent stages are shown with their marker characteristics.

With respect to both the T and B pathways, malignant proliferations have been identified that appear to correspond to each of the stages of lymphocyte differentiation.

Lymphocyte traffic is not random. T cells migrate to various areas of the spleen, lymph nodes, and other lymphoid tissues. These have come to be designated as thymus-dependent areas, since in neonatally thymectomized or congenitally athymic (nude) mice, these deep cortical areas are relatively depleted of lymphocytes. A parallel phenomenon occurs in patients with the Di George syndrome.

There are also segments of lymphoid tissues, termed thymus-independent, in which B cells "home." Most characteristically, they are the germinal centers (or primary follicles) of the lymph nodes. In the cross-sectional map of the lymph node (Figure 1), these areas can be seen around the periphery of the node.

As previously pointed out, Lukes and Lennert applied this knowledge of lymphocyte localization to the development of morphologic criteria for classification of lymphomas, and their postulates have held up extremely well as we have learned to use markers for the same purposes. Thus, a follicular architecture in a lymphoma is in effect the pathologic analogue of the normal germinal center. Lukes observed that in the group of lymphomas that had been designated by Rappaport as nodular, poorly differentiated lymphocytic lymphomas, the nodules often include large numbers of cleaved small cells, previously recognized as characteristic of normal germinal centers. These tumors also were likely to contain larger cells with round nuclei, previously identified as histiocytes. It seemed reasonable that both cell populations in nodular lymphomas should be B cells. Subsequent research appears to have confirmed this hypothesis; virtually all nodular lymphomas studied to date with marker techniques have the characteristics of B-cell tumors, at least in adults. In children, the picture is less clear-cut.

Another important B-cell trait is the tendency to aggregate. Maria de Sousa at the Sloan-Kettering Institute showed that if B lymphocytes were purified in vitro, they would spontaneously agglutinate. Such aggregation occurs at different rates with T lymphocytes, and when T and B cells are mixed, aggregation is inhibited. This observation may be applicable in the identification of chronic lymphocytic leukemia as a B-cell disorder, since CLL cells tend to aggregate in vitro. From a biologic point of view, de Sousa has suggested that B-cell aggregation helps to create the germinal center, with B lymphocytes migrating to loci where there are other B cells.

Having summarized the cellular markers, we can now turn to the different lymphoproliferative diseases and describe the ways in which the markers can help identify them. For historical reasons, it is appropriate to start with Burkitt's lymphoma. In 1968, Eva Klein and her colleagues in Stockholm first reported the finding of IgM on the surface of Burkitt's lymphoma cells. At the time, it was not clear that surface Ig was a discriminant for B cells. However, when subsequent work by Martin Raff in London showed that most mouse lymphocytes could be separated into two populations on the basis of immunoglobulin or theta (Thy-1) antigen on their surfaces, the work in Klein's laboratory took on seminal significance in understanding the biologic specificity of lymphocyte classes.

The next of the lymphoproliferative diseases to be well characterized by markers was chronic lymphocytic leukemia. It is now generally accepted that in all but 2% or 3% of the cases, this is a B-cell disease. Interestingly, until we had the ability to identify lymphocytes by their marker characteristics, the cellular nature of CLL was controversial. Many workers maintained that it was T-cell proliferation because of certain kinetic observations. However, experiments by a number of groups, including those of Nossal in Australia, J.-L. Preud'homme and M. Seligmann in Paris, B. Pernis and his colleagues in Milan, Henry Kunkel's group at Rockefeller University, and Howard Grey and his collaborators in Denver, showed that most CLL proliferations involved cells with an IgM heavy chain and a light immunoglobulin chain on their surfaces. Later, IgD was found to be characteristic of B lymphocytes, and CLL patients with IgD heavy-chain determinants on their involved cells were also identified. At any rate, the association of CLL with monoclonal B-lymphocyte proliferation is now firmly established. Recent analysis with hybridoma-derived antisera shows the CLL B cell to share some cell surface antigens with normal T cells. There are some CLL cases in which the T cell is the dominant pathologic component, and, interestingly, such cases seem to cluster geographically (e.g., on islands in Japan), but they nevertheless represent a small minority.

As this work has progressed, we have also come to realize that CLL, Waldenström's macroglobulinemia, and multiple myeloma are part of a spectrum of B-lymphocyte proliferations. An interesting and still unresolved question with respect to these diseases is: At what level of differentiation does the malignant transformation arise? There is evidence that in some cases it can occur as early as the stem cell. The fact that the leukemic cells of CLL are usually monoclonal and express unique Ig heavy-chain and light-chain components—in other words, have a specific variable region—suggests that the malignancy arises in cells that have already been committed not only to the B-differentiation pathway but also to reactivity with a particular antigen. The tendency of the CLL cells to form mouse erythrocyte rosettes and their relative paucity of surface immunoglobulin contrast with the surface characteristics of follicular center-cell neoplasms. The B cell of diffuse, well-differentiated lymphocytic lymphomas appears by marker criteria to be identical to the CLL cell.

Analogous to these B-cell disorders is a spectrum of T-cell diseases that includes Sézary's syndrome and mycosis fungoides. In these disorders, there is localization of neoplastic lymphocytes to

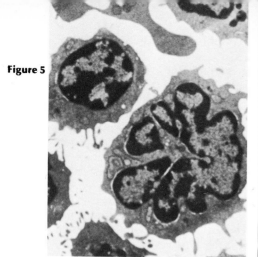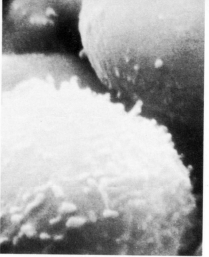

Figure 5

Transmission and scanning EMs (by Etienne de Harven of Sloan-Kettering Institute) show characteristic morphology of T lymphocytes in Sézary's syndrome, one of several T-cell malignancies that appear to have a tendency to involve cutaneous tissue.

skin. Parenthetically, it might be noted that the predilection of the malignant lymphocytes of these T-cell tumors for the skin remains an unexplained phenomenon. Functionally, the dominant cell type in Sézary's syndrome has been identified in some cases as exemplary of the helper T cell; at least a portion of the pathologic cells found in this disease make sheep erythrocyte rosettes in the cold (4° C), express OKT4 or Leu3a determinants, and respond to the mitogenic stimulation of phytohemagglutinin. Mycosis fungoides is characterized by a very similar T cell (see Figure 5, this page). Many investigators feel that this lymphomatous disease and Sézary's are really variants of the same disorder.

An RNA virus containing a reverse transcriptase and presumed to be oncogenic has recently been detected in leukemic T cells of patients with T-CLL in Japan and in the cutaneous T-cell lymphomas in the United States (MF-Sézary). Such an agent has not yet been observed in B-cell lymphomas in humans.

Another extensively studied lymphoproliferative disease is so-called hairy-cell leukemia, which characteristically in its early stages affects B-cell (thymus-independent) areas of the spleen, and which often expresses a unique enzymatic activity, that of a tartrate-resistant acid phosphatase. The highly "ruffled" surfaces of the cells seen under the scanning electron microscope are similar to those of normal monocytes, rather than of lymphocytes, and there is good evidence that these pathologic cells can be phagocytic. Nevertheless, most studies have shown that typical hairy cells synthesize and display monoclonal immunoglobulin (IgM or IgD), a characteristic that would seem to define them as B cells of some sort. The issue is further complicated by the fact that no one has yet identified a normal counterpart of the leukemic hairy cell.

Recognition of the virtual identity by marker criteria of the CLL cell and the B lymphocyte of diffuse, well-differentiated lymphocytic lymphoma, on one hand, and the difference between this cell type and the B lymphocyte of most nodular lymphomas, on the other, was one of the factors that led Daniel Filippa, Benjamin Koziner, and the author, working with several other colleagues at the Memorial Sloan-Kettering Cancer Center, to group the non-Hodgkin's lymphomas into several categories based on nodal architecture, cytology, and cell markers (see table on page 205 and Figure 6, page 206). Essentially what we were seeking was to approach lymphoproliferative disorders by relying on multiple immunologic and cytochemical markers. We would ascertain how well the cell characterization by these relatively objective criteria relates to conventional morphology. At the same time, we could begin to as-

sess a therapeutic approach based chiefly on differentiation markers and could relate the marker-based cellular identification to various classification systems currently in use. In addition, we were taking into account the growing body of knowledge with respect to the continuum between the lymphomas and the leukemias.

Our approach required first of all a discrimination between the two different pathologic expressions of B lymphocytes. We designated as type I the B cell that is exemplified in the majority of cases of CLL. In addition to the marker characteristics mentioned above—the tendency to form mouse erythrocyte rosettes and the relatively faint immunofluorescent staining for surface Ig—one should note that on this cell the surface immunoglobulin is monoclonal, possessing either kappa or lambda light chains and a heavy chain constituent usually of IgM, with or without IgD. Morphologically, the cells are small, round, and uncleaved. Their cytoplasm is scanty, their nuclear chromatin clumped, and their nucleoli inconspicuous. The type I B cell is the marker-defined counterpart of the non- or prefollicular center cell defined by Lukes and Collins.

Type II B cells include two morphologic subtypes with identical surface markers. Both subtypes stain brightly for surface immunoglobulin, and in further contrast with the type I cells, they form mouse rosettes only infrequently. The two subtypes are differentiated basically by size, one consisting of small cells, often with cleaved nuclei, the other being larger and generally having the morphologic appearance of "activated" lymphocytes or lymphoblasts. In short, lymphomas consisting of type II B cells seem best to fit into the concepts of Lukes and Lennert of follicular or germinal center-cell neoplasms. Although the type II cells are not associated with any of the more prevalent varieties of leukemia, they are very likely the same cells as those long ago recognized by Rosenthal and Isaacs as leukemic-phase lymphoma cells and more recently defined by A. C. Aisenberg and his colleagues at Harvard as those of chronic lymphosarcoma cell leukemia that stain especially brightly for surface immunoglobulin.

With respect to solid tumors, type II B cells can be associated with either "histiocytic" or poorly differentiated lymphocytic lymphomas. The larger "activated" cells correspond to the cells of some tumors designated as histiocytic in the Rappaport scheme, while the smaller B cells fit into the poorly differentiated lymphocytic group. In a lymphoma categorized as "mixed histiocytic-lymphocytic," both large and small cells have the same markers. As a general rule, those lymphomas that have nodular architecture consist of type II B cells, whether they are "histiocytic" or poorly differentiated lymphocytic. On the other hand, the diffuse lymphomas of both "histiocytic" and poorly differentiated lymphocytic types are less predictable, although they too are most often made up of type II B cells, especially in adults. When cells of the diffuse poorly differentiated lymphocytic type have cleaved nuclei, they appear likely to be B-cell proliferations and probably have the same marker characteristics as the prototype type II B cell. Among other diffuse lymphomas, it is much more difficult to identify with any degree of certainty the cell type on the basis of morphology.

In a marker-based approach to classification, one can readily realize that only some of those lymphomas previously classified as "histiocytic" are truly histiocytic. Among the true histiocytic proliferations, the characteristic markers are those previously listed for the monocyte. Of these, phagocytic ability and the presence of nonspecific esterases, peroxidase, and lysozyme have proved helpful in identifying malignant proliferations. In addition, these cells share with B cells receptors for complement and for IgG. One can easily appreciate how the confusion between monocyte and B lymphocyte came about, especially since monocytes and macrophages can morphologically resemble the larger type II B lymphocytes. In addition to the infrequently occurring true histiocytic solid tumors, histiocytic malignancy may, of course, present as monocytic leukemia with lymphadenopathy or as histiocytic medullary reticulosis.

Marker-Based Differentiation of Lymphomas and Leukemias

Cell Type	Cell Characteristics	Lymphomas	Leukemias
B lymphocytes (I)	Sparse surface monoclonal Ig; tendency to form mouse erythrocyte rosettes; small, round uncleaved nuclei; scanty cytoplasm	Well-differentiated lymphocytic (diffuse)	Chronic lymphocytic
B lymphocytes (plasmacytoid and plasma cells)	Increased rough endoplasmic reticulum; frequent cytoplasmic Ig; Ig J chain; may be Ig secretors (plasma cells)	Multiple myelomas and tumors associated with Waldenström's macroglobulinemia and heavy-chain disease	Leukemic expression of myelomas; Waldenström's macroglobulinemia
B lymphocytes (II)	Plentiful surface Ig; mouse erythrocyte rosettes infrequent; small with cleaved nuclei (IIa) or large "activated" (IIb)	Most nodular tumors included but also may be diffuse; poorly differentiated lymphocytic (IIa) or "histiocytic" (IIb) or mixed	Rare variants including chronic lymphosarcoma-cell leukemia
B lymphocytes (unspecified)		Burkitt's leukemic reticuloendotheliosis	B acute lymphocytic; hairy-cell
Thymocytes	Medium-sized round cells; dispersed chromatin; round or convoluted nuclei; nuclear TdT; form sheep erythrocyte rosettes at 37°C and 4°C; a few have C receptors; acid phosphatase positive	Poorly differentiated lymphocytic (diffuse); malignant lymphoblastic (often with mediastinal "bulky" disease)	Acute lymphocytic
T lymphocytes	Small cells; sheep erythrocyte rosettes at 4°C only; acid phosphatase positive		T chronic lymphocytic
T lymphocytes	Large cells; cerebriform or round nuclei; aneuploid; sheep erythrocyte rosettes only at 4°C	Sézary's syndrome; mycosis fungoides	Sézary's syndrome
"Null" or "non-T, non-B" lymphocytes	Characterized by markers not clearly definitive of cellular commitment to a particular differentiative pathway	Poorly differentiated (diffuse)	Acute lymphocytic and blast crises of chronic myelogenous
Monocytes	Phagocytes with nonspecific esterases, peroxidase, lysozyme; receptors for complement and Ig	True histiocytic; histiocytic medullary reticulosis	Monocytic with lymphadenopathy

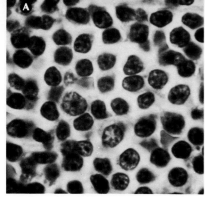

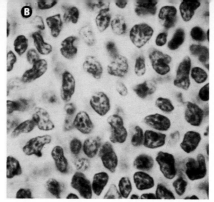

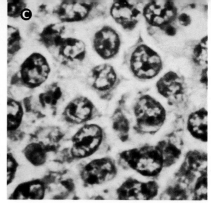

A number of different cell types represented in the marker-based classification on the preceding page are exemplified in photomicrographs provided by Dr. D. Filippa of Memorial Sloan-Kettering Cancer Center: A, type I B cells typical of well-differentiated diffuse lymphomas and chronic lymphocytic leukemia; B, type IIa small B lymphocytes with cleaved nuclei, found in poorly differentiated lymphocytic lymphomas; C, large type IIb B cells seen in so-called "histiocytic" lymphomas; D, undifferentiated B lymphocytes typical of Burkitt's; E, monocytes involved in true histiocytic lymphomas; F, T lymphocytes characteristic of a variety of tumors, including lymphoblastic malignant lymphoma, and of acute lymphocytic leukemia.

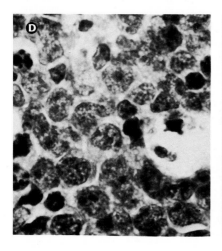

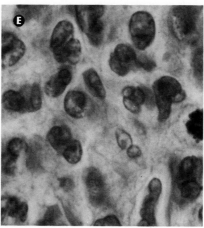

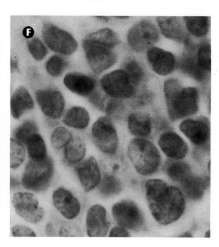

In this scheme, certain other tumors formerly defined morphologically as diffuse, poorly differentiated lymphocytic lymphomas consist of T cells. Microscopically, these cells are most commonly medium-sized round cells, with dispersed chromatin and round or convoluted nuclear morphology. They, of course, carry T-cell markers, including nuclear TdT, and have the ability to form sheep erythrocyte rosettes, both at 37° and at 4°, suggesting their derivation as proliferations of thymic T cells (thymocytes). In some cases, the involved cells also have complement receptors; this may be significant in that C receptors have been found to be present on normal fetal thymocytes.

Lukes and R. D. Collins considered a group of lymphomas seen most commonly in childhood and adolescence and frequently associated with convoluted nuclear morphology to be distinct from most other diffuse poorly differentiated lymphocytic lymphomas. Rappaport, B. N. Nathwani, and their colleagues widened this category by inclusion of patients whose malignant cells had nonconvoluted nuclei, recognizable through T-cell surface markers and acid phosphatase staining. These patients frequently present with mediastinal "bulky" disease. With the increasing use of additional T-cell markers, especially TdT, it now seems clear that this group (malignant lymphoma, lymphoblastic) is part of a continuum with T-cell acute lymphocytic leukemia (ALL), and clinically it has the same tendency as childhood T-ALL to affect the CNS. In childhood, these ALL cells, which bear the marker characteristics of thymocytes (and may be the human counterpart of Furth's mouse thymus-derived leukemia) account for about 20% of ALL cases, and these may have a somewhat poorer prognosis than those ALLs in which the cells do not form sheep erythrocyte rosettes. Stuart Schlossman in his laboratory at Harvard has applied hybridoma reagents to the lymphoblastic lymphomas of thymocytes. They showed that different stages of the thymocyte differentiation pathway can be represented by different cases of these disorders. Tendency to become leukemic, or to remain as bulky disease, may be determined to some extent by the stage of intrathymic differentiation represented.

Still another group of diffuse lymphoproliferations includes cells that appear to be at a very early stage of differentiation from the stem cell. Because these cells lack the markers of either mature T cells or mature B cells, they had been designated as "null" cells, or "non-T, non-B cells." However, they do contain nuclear TdT and bear Ia-like antigens as well as characteristic surface antigens and a hexoseaminidase isoenzyme defined by Melvin Greaves and his colleagues in London. Greaves developed conventional (and, later, monoclonal) antisera that detected a leukemia-associated antigen on these cells. Because the null ALL were the most common type seen in about 80% of children at the time, he called the antigen cALLA (common-ALL antigen). Greaves soon discovered that cALLA is not, however, a leukemia-specific antigen. It is expressed on the surface of a sizable proportion of lymphoid cells in normal bone marrow, including those having cytoplasmic mu chains and clearly committed to the B-cell lineage. Most non-T ALL cells express cALLA, as well as Ia and TdT, as do their normal counterparts.

Korsmeyer, T. A. Waldmann, and P. Leder, working at the NIH, recently analyzed common ALL cells for evidence of early commitment to differentiation along the B-cell lineage. They found rearrangements of the immunoglobulin structural genes in cells that had previously been seen in B cells and plasma cells but not in T cells or any other somatic or germ-cell line. These excisions of genetic material, which prepare lymphoid cells to eventually secrete immunoglobulin, are probably the earliest detectable events in commitment to become B cells and indicate that most null ALL are very early B cells. In their solid-tumor expression, cells of this type most commonly form diffuse, poorly differentiated lymphomas.

It was also recognized that about 20% of acute leukemias of childhood could be segregated out from the non-T, non-B category through the use of special anti-IgM reagents developed by Alexander Lawton at the University of Alabama. Working with M. D. Cooper, Lawton, and other investigators, L. B. Vogler has shown that these ALL lymphocytes contain cytoplasmic mu and therefore might be the neoplastic counterparts of pre-B cells. These leukemic cells also carry Ia-like antigens and TdT.

Although the application to the lymphoproliferative disorders of the newer marker systems has tended to rationalize, and to some extent to modify, our present classifications of these disorders, a critical question remains for physicians: Have the results significantly enhanced ability to diagnose, manage, and evaluate prognosis?

In dealing with this question, one must first take into account what was known before there was any appreciation of marker characteristics. Thus, it was long ago observed by Brill et al and Symmers that patients with nodular disease had a better prognosis than those with diffuse lymphoma. The issue may be whether diffuse lymphomas can be separated prognostically on the basis of B- or T-cell origins. This has, so far, been hard to settle, in part because T-cell lymphomas are relatively rare, at least in adults. Most non-Hodgkin's lymphomas in adults consist of B cells, whether the tumors are nodular or diffuse. What we may be en route to finding out is that localization in nodules is still the most important clinical marker for a relatively favorable prognosis in lymphoma. And if this should be established, it may follow that a tendency to tissue localization, as in nodular tumors, is simply a characteristic of relative normality for B cells of the follicular-center type. In other words, a cell that tends to behave in a physiologic way with respect to its neighbors may also be "less malignant."

Perhaps of more immediate clinical applicability is the recognition of the continuum between lymphoma and leukemia. Some attention has already been paid in this review to the cellular identity of diffuse, well-differentiated lymphocytic lymphomas and chronic lymphocytic leukemia. Another noteworthy association is that between acute lymphoblastic leukemia and some of the poorly differentiated lymphocytic lymphomas. Different cell types may be involved. Often these lymphomas are separable on clinical grounds by the presence of bulky mediastinal tumors, by the age of the patient, and by nuclear convolutions. At least in the group of young adult patients in whom the thymic T cell is often the dominant lymphocytic type, the tumor is cytologically indistinguishable from ALL, and indeed the disease often evolves clinically into ALL. With this in mind, the lymphoma group at Memorial Sloan-Kettering (Koziner, Clarkson, and Lee) has adopted a policy of treating such patients aggressively from the start, using an ALL protocol even before leukemic manifestations are present.

Marker approaches can be used to elucidate equivocal clinical situations. For example, one can discriminate between benign lymphocytosis and early CLL (as Rudders in Boston has done). A recent case comes to mind in which a child was seen with a round-cell bone tumor. The differential question was one of Ewing's sarcoma vs lymphoma, two entities for which treatment approaches are quite different. Studies directed at detection of lymphocyte markers permitted the diagnosis to be made.

Another example relates to the long-observed phenomenon of blast crisis in chronic myelogenous leukemia. In such crises, the malignant cells take on the morphologic and behavioral characteristics of blast lymphocytes. Marker analysis in several cases has shown that the cells contain terminal transferase and cytoplasmic mu chains expressing a pre-B-cell stereotypic pattern. Biologically, this raises investigative questions with respect to the differential level at which malignant transformation takes place while it sheds light on the differentiation potentials of stem cells. Clinically, the marker studies have facilitated treatment by providing guidelines for an appropriate shift from chemotherapeutic regimens directed at myeloid leukemia to regimens appropriate to lymphocytic leukemia.

Perhaps even more important is that by studying the lymphoproliferative diseases in this sharpened focus, we are likely to enhance greatly our understanding of normal lymphoid cells. One must keep in mind the tremendous advances in knowledge about normal immunoglobulins and antibodies that came from the discovery and study of the monoclonal expansions of immunoglobulin molecules that we call myeloma proteins. Equal benefits can be expected from the studies of monoclonal expansions of lymphoid cells. A good example of this is the analysis of suppressor cells and their interactions, already carried out by S. Broder and T. A. Waldmann at the National Cancer Institute. This analysis was based on studies of a child with ALL and hypogammaglobulinemia. They were able to show that the ALL cells were functionally suppressor cells and had characteristics similar to normal suppressor T cells. Their exploitation of these cells in in vitro analyses enabled them to demonstrate that suppression was a product of cooperation between two distinct types of T cells, one of which was represented by the ALL cells (as a T-cell analogue representative of normal T cells, even as myeloma proteins are representative of normal antibody structure.) Thus, it is not unrealistic to predict that just as expanding knowledge of the lymphomas has resulted from advances in immunobiology, we will be able to complete the circle and use the expanding knowledge of lymphoid malignancies to deepen our comprehension of normal lymphocyte physiology.

19

Immunologic Mechanisms In Nephritogenesis

CURTIS B. WILSON *and* FRANK J. DIXON   *Research Institute of the Scripps Clinic*

Two major mechanisms in which antibody plays a role have been identified in the etiology of renal disease or injury in humans. These pathways involve either antibodies specific for structural components of the kidney or antibodies that form immune complexes (IC) with nonglomerular antigens in the circulation, which then lodge in the kidneys in continuing equilibrium with antigen, antibody, and additional IC from the circulation. The latter—the IC disease mechanism—is the more common (possibly 70% vs 5%) of the two immunologic causes of kidney disease.

In humans, anti-kidney antibody disease has been limited to reactions against antigenic components of the renal basement membranes (in animals, reactions have been observed to non-basement membrane glomerular capillary wall antigens and to foreign materials that become trapped or "planted" within the glomerulus). Immune responses to basement membrane can lead to a variety of nephritic syndromes, including anti-glomerular basement membrane (GBM) glomerulonephritis, anti-GBM antibody-induced Goodpasture's syndrome, in which the glomerulonephritis is combined with pulmonary hemorrhagic disease that results from involvement of alveolar basement membranes, and anti-tubular basement membrane (TBM) antibody-induced tubulointerstitial nephritis. Not infrequently, anti-GBM and anti-TBM disease occur concurrently. IC disease is less specific in terms of target and can be precipitated at any kidney site at which the complexes lodge and trigger various phlogogenic and histiolytic processes. Most commonly circulating IC are localized in glomerular capillaries or glomerular mesangial cells with resulting glomerulonephritis (GN). Or, occasionally, the complexes can accumulate in tubular interstitial tissue and/or along the

TBM to bring about a tubulointerstitial nephritis.

The initiation or perpetuation of renal disease whether through anti-kidney antibodies or IC may involve a number of mediator systems. These include, of course, humoral factors such as complement and polymorphonuclear and mononuclear leukocytes with their phlogogenic lysosomal contents. A possibility that has aroused considerable interest is that the nephritides can be initiated and perpetuated by several mediator systems without the participation of antibody. Various studies have implicated complement and the coagulation proteins. The former may have a part in the production and/or perpetuation of hypocomplementemic membranoproliferative glomerulonephritis in children, and the latter are believed to play some role in the glomerular injury observed in the so-called hemolytic uremic syndrome in kidney disease associated with systemic coagulopathies and possibly in eclampsia.

On the other hand, so far as cellular mechanisms of immunity are concerned, there is little evidence to implicate any immunologically specific role for direct involvement of T lymphocytes, at least with respect to GN. Experimentally, GN can be transferred with antibody alone. In tubulointerstitial nephritis, mononuclear infiltration tends to be a more prominent sign, however, and there is some evidence to suggest a role for cellular immunity in anti-TBM antibody disease.

Anti-basement membrane antibody and IC diseases can be differentiated by the patterns produced by the immunoglobulin and complement deposits, and both immunofluorescent and enzymatic techniques have been employed to demonstrate this variation. These differences are depicted schematically in Figure 1 on page 210 and shown micrographically in Figures 2 and 3 on page 211. Anti-GBM or anti-TBM antibodies distribute uniformly all along the affected basement membrane and form a characteristically linear pattern. IC antibodies, on the other hand, will deposit irregularly from the circulation and tend to form granular lumps distributed in and about the glomerular capillary wall or mesangium. The direct binding of antibodies to irregularly localized structural or planted glomerular antigens as seen experimentally can also result in granular immunoglobulin deposits. The exact definition of the mechanism then requires identification of the antigen-antibody system involved.

In arriving at our current understanding of both major forms of immunologically mediated nephritis, a great deal of information has been derived from animal models. Much of this knowledge can be summarized through a more or less chronologic review of these model systems. As far back as the early years of this century it was first observed that if heterologous anti-kidney antibodies were injected into an appropriate host, kidney injury would result. By the mid-1930s, Masugi had refined this model into what is still sometimes referred to as Masugi nephritis. Subsequently, it was shown that the GBM was in fact the site of the antigens against which the heterologous antibodies were directed, and that the nephritic process induced by the foreign immuno-globulin-GBM interaction was amplified by a homologous antibody raised against the heterologous antibody or gamma globulin fixed in the glomerulus. This observation was the first example of a foreign or planted antigen in a nephritogenic immune response.

Since this model of anti-kidney antibody nephritis required initiation by heterologous antibody, it was obviously an artificial one. However, Steblay and his coworkers, working with sheep, showed that animals could, upon relevant immunization, make antibodies reactive with their own basement membrane structures, and that this actually caused an autoimmune form of anti-GBM nephritis. A variety of autoimmune models of anti-basement membrane antibody-induced nephritis have now been developed using immunization with GBM or TBM. The severity and clinical manifestations vary with the animal species used for immunization. A few years after Steblay's animal experiments were reported, the same mechanism of autoimmune anti-basement membrane nephritis was described in spontaneous clinical disease.

Certainly, experimental anti-GBM antibody-induced nephritis and its variants have provided a most fruitful environment for the study of the mechanisms of renal disease caused by the interaction between fixed antigens and circulating antibodies. We will return shortly to discussion of anti-basement membrane antibody disease, but first let us interpose a parallel discussion of the equally fruitful line of animal-model research related to immune complex diseases. This is a line that again can be traced back to the turn of the century and to the clinical observation that a common complication of serum therapy in patients was a generalized illness involving the kidneys, the heart, and a number of other organs and tissues. It was early

Figure 1

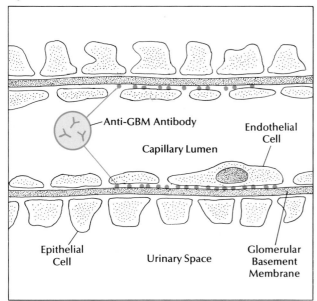

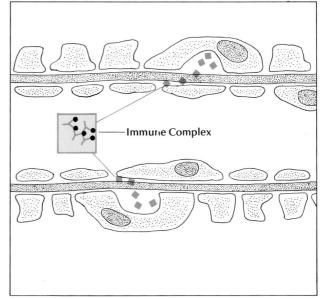

Schematically shown are the patterns of deposition of immuno-reactants in anti-kidney antibody nephritis (left) and in immune complex (IC) nephritis (right). In anti-kidney antibody disease, specific antibodies are directed against antigenic determinants (e.g., on the glomerular basement membrane) and deposited in a linear pattern along the endothelial surface of the membrane. In IC nephritis, complexes are formed in the cir-
culation as a result of immunologic responses to a wide variety of antigens. The complexes circulate to the glomerular capillaries, pass to the glomerular basement membrane, and accumulate in subendothelial, epithelial, and intramembrane areas. In either situation an array of cellular and soluble phlogogenic mediators is mobilized or activated, causing nephritogenic disruption of the glomerular basement membrane.

appreciated that so-called serum sickness results from the host's immune responses to foreign serum proteins. The advent of appropriate methodology applied to animals made it possible to demonstrate that the equilibrium reaction of the host's antibodies with foreign proteins occurred in the circulation, and the antigen-antibody complexes thus formed did accumulate in target organs, particularly in the kidneys where deposition led to glomerulonephritis.

This mechanism was first demonstrated in acute experiments involving single injections of large amounts of foreign serum protein (one-shot serum sickness). It was later shown that daily injections of small quantities of antigen produced a chronic serum sickness that more closely paralleled human disease. Still later, the system was adapted to the use of the host's own tissue as the antigen to produce IC kidney disease. Variants were developed in which animals were immunized with antigens such as thyroglobulin to produce an IC-type nephritis. Analogously in man, the immune response against thyroglobulin, a frequent occurrence in autoimmune thyroiditis, can infrequently lead to glomerulonephritis through deposition of the thyroglobulin-antibody complexes in the glomeruli.

In several other experimental situations kidney disease results from in situ complexes that are formed in response to either normal renal antigens or foreign antigens trapped or planted in the glomerulus. Foreign immunoglobulin, as already noted, would be an example of this latter type reaction. Materials taken up by the mesangium or products with an inherent ability to lodge in the glomerulus through direct binding, such as DNA or lectins, perhaps of bacterial or viral origin, have also been implicated. Does this happen in human disease, and if so, is it an important pathologic phenomenon? At the moment, these questions remain unanswered.

Turning back now to the nephritides caused by anti-basement membrane antibodies, it should be kept in mind that antibodies of at least two different basement membrane specificities can induce disease. One is

specific for antigens on the GBM and therefore produces glomerulonephritis; the other reacts with TBM antigens to cause tubulointerstitial nephritis. When the antibody is directed against GBM, complement is usually activated (see Figure 4, pages 212 and 213), and the complement chemotactic component, C5a, attracts polymorphonuclear leukocytes to the reaction site. There the PMNs release their lysosomes, and the lysosomal contents disrupt the permeability properties of the GBM. The rapidity and the intensity of the injury is directly related to the amount of antibody involved, with cumulative effects also dependent on how long the antibody is present at the reaction site. A proliferative response within the glomerulus may also be produced, along with extracapillary proliferation and accumulation of macrophages observable as crescent formation. In the most severe cases, the pathologic consequences include rapidly progressive nephritis that may lead to fulminant renal failure.

Studies of the specific events in this sequence have shown an impairment of salt and water transport that occurs immediately after antibody fixation. At the same time, or very closely thereafter, changes can be identified in the filtration properties of the glomerular capillary wall in part related to changes in its net electrical charge. This is important since the capillary wall is normally anionic. This serves to help retain albumin, a relatively small molecule that on the basis of size alone is near the limit of size discrimination provided for filtration of macromolecules and could diffuse across the wall. Albumin is normally retained because it is also an anion and therefore is repelled by the fixed negative charge. Accordingly, when the charge of the wall is altered, the effect is a rapid leakage of albumin into the urine.

The macromolecular leakage that results from the changed electrostatic properties of the capillary wall is accentuated as the process continues, and additional structural damage is done, altering the ability of the glomerular capillary wall to discriminate molecules on the basis of size as well as charge. Eventually the point is reached when effectively all of the se-

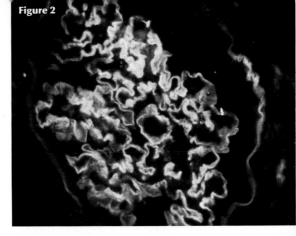

Immunofluorescence micrograph is representative of pattern in anti-basement membrane antibody disease. Linear IgG can be seen along the GBM, and to a lesser extent in Bowman's capsule. Patient had proliferative glomerulonephritis.

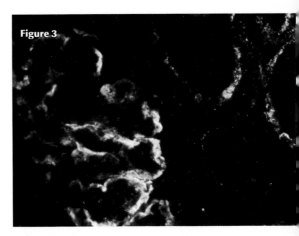

Immunofluorescence in immune complex disease specimen from patient with lupus shows heavy IgG granular deposits along the glomerular basement membrane (left) and diffuse, granular IgG along the tubular basement membrane.

rum proteins may pass from capillary to urine. Incidentally, although this process is being described in the context of anti-kidney antibody disease, it also occurs as a result of IC disease.

Although tubulointerstitial disease may be mediated by antibodies of different specificities from those attacking GBM structures, the pathogenic processes seem closely parallel, with deposition of antibody along the TBM, fixation and activation of complement, and chemotactic attraction of inflammatory cells, such as the PMN leukocytes, followed by a persisting mononuclear cell infiltration. The disease picture is somewhat dif-

The nephritogenic events initiated by immune complexes (ICs) or anti-kidney basement membrane antibodies are depicted sequentially. Either ICs or antibodies against membrane antigens are deposited on the GBM and/or the TBM (1), and complement may be activated either through the classic or alternate pathway (2A and 2B). As the complement sequence proceeds, its anaphylatoxic components (C3a and C5a) will produce increased membrane permeability and inflammation (3). Noncomplement mediators (e.g., vasoactive amines, coagulation proteins, kinins) may also contribute to the inflammatory process. In addition, the complement chemotaxins will atttract PMN leukocytes to the reaction site (4). At the same time, there is a marked enhancement of monocyte infiltration around the basement membrane and particularly in the mesangial stalk. C3b in proximity to the membrane surface provides an immune adherence site for the PMNs (5). These cells release lysosomal enzymes, causing disruption of the membrane.

Figure 4

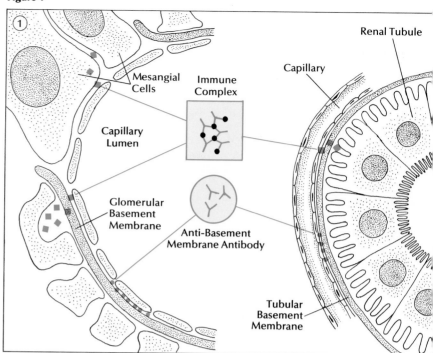

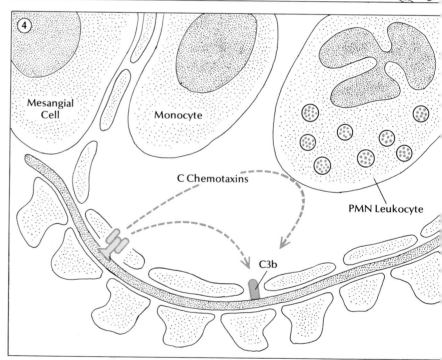

ferent since the tubules are surrounded by interstitial tissue, and it is in this tissue and its capillary network that the immunologic and inflammatory responses take place. Obviously, with tubular disease there is a predominance of defects associated with tubular function, such as aminoaciduria and glycosuria. These can occur without detectable disruption of glomerular filtration. However, it should be noted that there is very little "pure" anti-TBM antibody disease. About 70% of the patients with anti-GBM disease whom we have studied have anti-TBM antibodies and some tubular involvement.

Both anti-GBM and anti-TBM diseases raise an obvious question: What causes these normal structures to behave immunogenically?

We have no hard evidence that exogenous antigens are specifically involved in the breaking of self-tolerance. However, a number of years ago this laboratory showed that in normal individuals one could find antigens that cross-react with kidney basement membranes in both blood and urine. There have also been loose clinical associations between anti-basement membrane disease and influenza infection, exposure to hydrocarbon solvents, neoplasia, and prior renal trauma or ischemia. A stronger association exists with kidney transplantation, particularly with anti-TBM antibodies, but of course in this situation the possibilities of immunogenic introduction of basement membrane antigens is not mysterious.

Actually, specific association of anti-basement membrane disease and documented influenza is unusual. It is interesting, however, that about 40% of the patients we have studied with anti-GBM disease had given some history of a flu-like illness preceding the development of nephritis by two to six weeks. But it is not possible to say whether the illness was viral or bac-

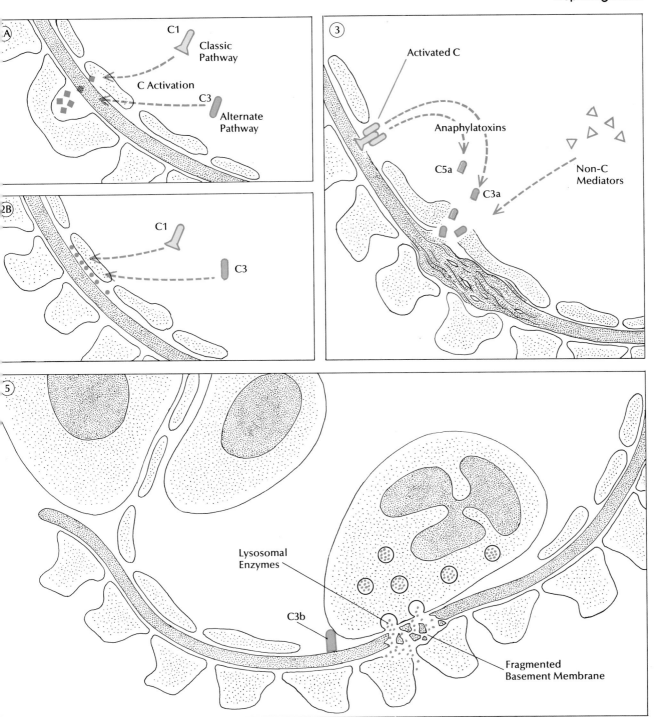

terial or whether it was simply a pro-dromal manifestation of the developing kidney disease. The generally transient nature of the anti-GBM antibody response suggests that an identifiable stimulus of relatively short duration is present and should be uncovered by painstaking clinical and epidemiologic studies.

Moving on now from disease caused by specific anti-basement membrane antibodies to that resulting from deposition of IC formed in the circulation, one can start by stating that two ingredients must come together intravascularly – antigen and antibody. Experimentally, this requirement can be met in a number of ways, such as the injection into an animal of foreign serum protein. In "real life," the evidence suggests that, for endogenous antigens, formation of IC is most likely to result if a previously sequestered cellular antigen is exposed or released into the circulation. This appears to happen, for example, in patients with systemic lupus erythematosus (SLE) when normal cell death and disruption spills nuclear antigens into the bloodstream and these antigens complex with antinuclear antibodies characteristic of SLE. A situation involving exogenous antigens that might favor the formation of circulating ICs is chronic administration of drugs that possess antigenicity. Another source of IC antigen is viral products, or virions themselves, that are shed into the circulation for long periods in the course of chronic viral infection.

Once the complexes are formed, size is probably the parameter most important in determining whether or not they will reach the kidney basement membranes and what will happen to them in the membranes. And size, in turn, is largely dependent on the quantitative relationships between antigen and antibody in the serum (see Figure 5, page 215). At one extreme is the situation of a very large excess of antibody over antigen, in which several antibody molecules combine with one antigen molecule. In turn, these antibody molecules may attach to other antigens, so that a lattice consisting of multiple antigen-antibody combinations evolves. Such an aggregate can become so large that it will be rapidly phagocytized. These aggregates do fix complement and therefore have phlogogenicity, but they are catabolized very quickly and lose their phlogogenic potential.

At the other extreme are the very small complexes formed in large antigen excess. These typically contain a single antibody molecule divalently attached to two antigen molecules. Such complexes usually will not fix complement and by and large cannot initiate inflammatory processes.

The real pathologic potential seems to lie between these two extremes of complex size, i.e., in complexes formed when antigen excess is modest. These complexes are of intermediate size, and they are soluble. Although they are not rapidly phagocytized, they are large enough to fix complement and are phlogogenic. It is this type of complex that we now see as responsible for nephritis, arteritis, and other manifestations of IC disease. However, there is probably one significant exception to the generalizations relating complex size to pathogenicity. This pertains to situations in which the antigen itself is very large, as might occur with intact viruses or

macromolecules like DNA. Here a single antigen unit may be complexed with a large number of antibodies, the result being a large complex. Whether because such complexes are not readily phagocytized or whether other unknown factors are operating, there is substantial evidence that these do produce IC disease. In the case of viruses, peptides rather than intact virions may be involved in true nephritogenic IC.

Let us now examine in some detail the way in which size functions as a determinant of pathology, and particularly of the site of injury, focusing on the intermediate range of mobile, phlogogenic IC. The largest of these intermediate aggregates, if they escape the circulating phagocytes and the reticuloendothelial system, tend to lodge in the mesangium that lies in the glomerular stalk between the capillaries, outside the capillary endothelium. Cells in this area can be phagocytic, and when they ingest complexes, hypertrophy and proliferation can follow. Monocytes may also accumulate in this area.

Smaller intermediate complexes tend to lodge beneath the endothelium. From the subendothelial sites, they are capable of migrating through the capillary wall. The dynamics of the antigen-antibody reaction with continually changing IC composition may contribute to this movement. After the smaller complexes pass through the basement membrane to its epithelial aspect, they accumulate to form large aggregates or lumps in the subepithelial space.

These IC deposits cause injury to the glomerular capillary wall, and one usually finds some alteration of renal function, manifested as proteinuria, shortly after deposition is detectable. More profound damage probably results from complement-mediated attraction of PMN leukocytes, with enzymatic damage, glomerular cell proliferation, infiltration of macrophages, and other events similar to those causing tissue injury in anti-basement membrane antibody disease. In other words, the result is severe glomerulonephritis.

Although for clarity we have described the mesangial and endothelial attack by IC in sequence, it should be stressed that actually the two are likely

to occur simultaneously. When phlogogenic IC are formed in the circulation, they are likely to arrive at the glomerulus in assorted sizes. At the same time that the larger particulate complexes produce mesangial hypertrophy, smaller complexes are likely to be deposited beneath the capillary endothelium. A number of other factors also are involved in determining the site, extent, and character of nephritic lesions. Taken together, these variations have permitted the classification, largely on the basis of light microscopy, of different expressions of immunologically produced nephritic injury. (Such a classification is presented in Table 1, page 216, and a number of the entities are pictured in the micrographs that comprise Figure 6, page 219).

In the foregoing discussion, emphasis has been placed on two mediators of renal tissue injury: one, a soluble system – complement; the other, cellular – polymorphonuclear and mononuclear leukocytes and macrophages.

In this context, it should be noted that models have been developed in which anti-GBM antibodies do not fix complement but nevertheless lead to renal damage. Indeed, approximately one fourth of the cases of anti-GBM disease in humans appear to be unrelated to complement fixation.

There are probably other soluble and cellular mediators that contribute to a lesser degree to immune injury in IC disease. These could well include vasoactive substances that are known to increase vascular and membrane permeability, such as kinins, histamine, SRS-A, and serotonin, and which may enhance tissue damage and also the cells that secrete them, e.g., basophils, mast cells, and platelets.

In attempting to put the knowledge gained from animal-model systems of IC disease into a clinical context, an appropriate starting point is a review of the antigens that have been associated with IC nephritis. The listing of such antigens in Table 2 on page 217 is reasonably complete, although as studies continue, additions are frequent. Exogenous and endogenous antigens are listed in the table, with clinical disease correlations for both. The first subcategory under the exogenous antigen group is that of phar-

Figure 5

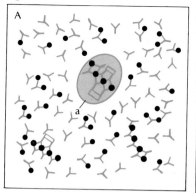

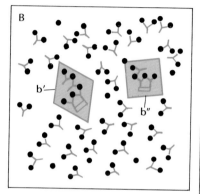

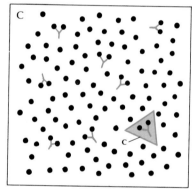

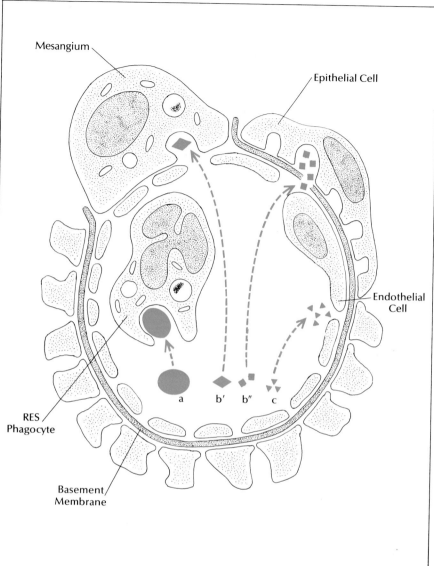

A key factor in determining whether immune complexes initiate kidney disease is the relative concentrations of antigen and antibody in the serum. The small panels depict the effects of this relationship. At one extreme (as shown in A), a large antibody excess results in an extensive lattice and large complexes that come out of solution and/or are phagocytized before reaching the kidney. At the opposite extreme (C), if there exists a large antigen excess, complex size is held below the requirement for fixing complement; such complexes are not phlogogenic. In between, when there is modest antigen excess (B), the complexes formed are large enough to fix complement but not so large that they are rapidly intercepted by RES phagocytes. Within this nephritogenic range, as schematized in the large panel, size is a determinant of where complexes will become localized; the larger complexes (b') are most likely to be taken up by phagocytic cells in the mesangium, the smaller ones (b'') are most likely to pass through glomerular or tubular basement membranes and to be trapped by epithelial foot processes.

maceuticals, and here we include foreign serum, in large part because serum sickness is the classic example. Actually, serum sickness is a rarity in this day and age, and when it does occur clinically, the kidney manifestations are not likely to be as severe as they are in rabbits.

Somewhat more significant is the IC disease that may follow the admin-

istration of drugs, where either the drug or its metabolites may combine as haptens with serum proteins and circulate. Thus, an antibody response to the drug can result in circulating complexes. Repeated immunization, for example, can result in IC glomerulonephritis.

Gold and other heavy metals used in therapy (e.g., mercury) are also associ-

ated with IC disease. Several key questions remain to be answered: Is the gold itself acting as the antigen or is the exogenous gold damaging tissues and causing the release into the circulation of previously sequestered endogenous antigens? And since gold is administered to rheumatoid arthritis patients who have underlying immunologic derangements, how much of the IC formation should be attributed to the gold, how much to the disease for which it is given? Irrespective of the answers, the fact is that kidney disease is a very common toxic response to gold therapy, and in this disease extremely dense glomerular deposits suggestive of IC are seen by electron microscopy.

From the clinical point of view, certainly the most interesting exogenous antigens are those derived from a variety of infectious agents. Most intriguing of all, perhaps, are the streptococcal antigens. The concept that post-streptococcal nephritis is an IC disease is supported by considerable evidence. One can see streptococcal antigens in complexes deposited in the glomeruli, particularly if the study is done shortly after the appearance of lesions. Later, the antigens become more difficult to identify, possibly because they become covered by excess circulating antibody.

This phenomenon is related to the equilibrium that exists between deposited complexes and circulating antibody, antigen, and complex. Deposited complexes can interact either with circulating antibody or, through unoccupied antibody-combining sites, with free antigen. This is clinically important because it may account for the perpetuation of disease even after the original antigenic source (infection) is no longer operative.

The therapeutic potential of this situation is intriguing. In experimental models, it has been possible to manipulate antigen and antibody to effectively dissolve the complexes. When this is done in a system in which a single antigen has precipitated disease, the pathologic process is aborted. Unfortunately, most IC diseases are not referable to single antigens but rather to multiple immunogens and their corresponding antibodies. It has not yet proved feasible clinically to "dissolve away" mixed agglomerations of antigen-antibody.

In studying the antigens associated with IC disease, it is obvious that representatives of virtually every type of pathogen known to infect and infest humans are included. There are bacteria (e.g., streptococci and *Treponema pallidum*), parasites (malarial and schistosomal), and viruses (hepatitis B, measles, Epstein-Barr). Renal IC disease can be secondary to many infections and infestations, and in many cases the "complication" is more serious and severe than the primary infection.

The endogenous antigens that have been associated with IC kidney disease are similarly varied. The nuclear antigens of SLE and the thyroglobulin of thyroiditis have been well studied. Conceptually, tumor antigens are particularly interesting, and it is noteworthy that in a small but significant minority of patients with bowel cancers, lymphomas, and some other cancers, there is enough tumor-associated antigen shed into the circulation to produce an antibody response and nephritic complications.

From such a heterogeneous roster of antigens – both exogenous and endogenous – it is difficult to pinpoint any characteristics that can be associated with development of IC disease in the kidneys. There does appear to be a requirement for the chronic presence of circulating antigen in a quantity appropriately related to the host's response. Obviously, appropriateness is a vague quality, but from what we know about the processing of antigen it would appear to relate

Table 1

A Summary of Glomerular Immunofluorescence Findings in Common Histologic Forms of Human IC GN	
Morphology	Immunofluorescence
PRIMARY GN	
Proliferative GN; variable proliferation of endothelial, epithelial, and mesangial cells	
Diffuse proliferative GN including poststreptococcal GN; electron-dense GBM deposits usually subepithelial	Diffuse granular IgG with variable IgA, IgM, and FRA*; C3 usually present, may predominate in poststreptococcal GN
Focal proliferative GN including mesangial hypertrophy; electron-dense mesangial deposits	Granular IgG and C3 often with prominent IgA or IgM in segmental GBM and mesangial deposits; FRA variable
Proliferative GN with crescent formation; electron-dense GBM deposits	Diffuse granular IgG and C3 with variable IgA and IgM; FRA striking in crescents
Membranous GN; thickening of the GBM with subepithelial spikes and diffuse electron-dense deposits	Diffuse heavy granular IgG and C3 with variable IgA, IgM, and FRA
MPGN; thickening of GBM with hypertrophy and interposition of the mesangium between GBM and endothelium – subendothelial and intramembranous-dense deposit subtypes	Prominent granular C3 along GBM usually accompanied with IgG, IgM, variable IgA, and FRA in subendothelial type; C3 alone in mesangium; GBM and TBM of intramembranous type
Focal sclerosing GN; segmental GBM thickening progressing to hyalinization, usually worst in juxtamedullary glomeruli	Granular IgG, IgM, and C3 may be present in sclerotic areas
Chronic GN; end-stage renal architecture	Granular C3 usually prominent with variable or absent IgG, IgA, IgM, FRA
IC GN of Systemic Disease	
SLE; membranous GN and focal, diffuse, and crescent-forming proliferative GN	Granular IgG, IgA, IgM, C3; FRA corresponding to histology; IgA often prominent
Henoch-Schonlein purpura; focal and diffuse proliferative GN	As described for focal proliferative GN; granular IgA, FRA often prominent
Glomerular Disease of Uncertain Immunologic Cause	
Lipoid nephrosis; no or minimal light microscopic abnormalities; foot process fusion	No immunofluorescence findings
Alport's syndrome; proliferative GN with electron microscopic evidence of GBM splitting	Usually no immunofluorescence findings
Wegener's granulomatosis; proliferative and crescent-forming GN; electron-dense GBM deposits	Variable granular IgG, IgM, C3, and FRA deposits
Fibrin/fibrinogen-related antigen	

to a quantity that would persist in the circulation without exhausting the host's complement of sensitized or sensitizable cells and in a relationship to antibody that would lead to the formation of complexes capable of being deposited in the kidneys. Regardless of the antigen involved, the steps in the pathogenesis of IC disease are relatively straightforward. An intravascular encounter between antigen and specific antibody leads to the formation of complexes that are deposited in the kidney as a concomitant of physiologically normal renal filtering functions.

From the discussion thus far, it is clear that immunologically mediated nephritis can be initiated by at least two major pathogenetic mechanisms, anti-basement membrane antibody formation and the deposition in renal structures of IC from the circulation. The clinical characteristics of either are likely to be determined by the logistics of the immune reaction, i.e., the amount of antigen-antibody participating and the duration of the reaction. With either of the two mechanisms, the pathology can present in varied ways, with a range that extends from the subtle and subclinical to the acute and catastrophic. In short, we are dealing with highly diverse and complicated diseases that will only be sorted out by meticulous immunologic studies.

Based on our observations of approximately 500 patients with anti-basement membrane antibody-induced disease, several interesting clinical features emerge. Approximately two thirds of the patients present with combined renal and pulmonary symptomatology consistent with a clinical diagnosis of Goodpasture's syndrome (see Figure 7, page 220). Roughly one third have glomerulonephritis alone and the remaining 1% to 2% have their disease confined to the lung, with a clinical presentation of idiopathic pulmonary hemosiderosis. The glomerulonephritis associated with anti-GBM antibodies is usually severe and rapidly progressive; however, as experience grows, milder and sometimes self-remitting forms of nephritis are being encountered with increasing frequency. Over 90% of the patients in this series are Caucasian,

Table 2

Antigens Involved in Human IC GN	
Endogenous	
Antigen	*Clinical Condition*
Nuclear antigens	SLE
? Renal tubular brush border antigens	Membranous GN in Japan, sickle cell anemia, renal neoplasia
Thyroglobulin	Thyroiditis
Tumor antigens	Neoplasms
Ig	Cryoglobulinemia
Exogenous	
Pharmaceuticals	
Foreign serum, toxoids, drugs	Serum sickness
Infectious Agents	
Bacterial	
Nephritogenic streptococci	Poststreptococcal GN
Staphylococcus albus, Corynebacterium bovis	Infected atrioventricular shunts
Enterococcus	Bacterial endocarditis
Salmonella typhosa	Typhoid fever
Treponema pallidum	Syphilis
Diplococcus pneumoniae	Pneumonia
Parasitic	
Plasmodium malariae, P. falciparum	Malaria
Schistosoma mansoni	Schistosomiasis
Toxoplasma gondii	Toxoplasmosis
Viral	
Hepatitis B	Hepatitis
Retroviral-related antigen	Leukemia
Measles	Subacute sclerosing panencephalitis, SLE
Epstein-Barr	Burkitt's lymphoma
Fungal	
Candida albicans	Candidiasis

and recent studies have suggested a segregation of the disease with DRw2 histocompatibility antigens. In patients with Goodpasture's syndrome nearly 70% are males. The sex distribution is more nearly equal in the patients with glomerulonephritis alone. The majority of the patients develop the disease during the second or third decades of life, although patients below 10 years of age and over 70 are identified. Of interest, a second grouping of patients in their 50s and 60s is becoming evident, particularly among females.

Renal failure used to develop in 70% of the patients with Goodpasture's syndrome and in 85% of the patients with glomerulonephritis alone. Recently, some improvement in outcome has accompanied the intensive therapies now being used. About 20% of each group has succumbed. A flu-like antecedent illness is observed in about 40% of each group and, interestingly, a few patients have presented with arthralgia or acute arthritis. An-

tecedent streptococcal infection is unusual, and a history of toxic exposure has been obtained in less than 20%.

Diagnosis of anti-basement membrane antibody disease is based on the immunofluorescent detection of classic linear deposits of IgG, and less frequently IgA or IgM, along the basement membrane. The diagnosis should be confirmed by elution study or detection of circulating anti-GBM antibodies, since nonimmunologic linear accumulations of IgG and other serum proteins are sometimes identified in kidneys from patients with diabetes mellitus, kidneys obtained at autopsy or following perfusion prior to transplantation, and relatively normal kidneys from persons in whom there has been no other reason to suspect anti-basement membrane antibody disease.

Circulating anti-basement membrane antibodies have classically been detected by indirect immunofluorescence using sections from normal human kidneys. The test has been helpful but is relatively insensitive and is hard to standardize, perhaps in part related to qualitative or quantitative differences in basement membrane antigens between individual kidney targets. The indirect immunofluorescent technique does detect anti-TBM antibodies, which accompany anti-GBM antibodies in about 70% of the instances. We have developed a radioimmunoassay for detecting circulating anti-GBM antibodies, using as an antigen the noncollagenous portion of the GBM remaining after collagenase digestion and extensive dialysis. Using this test on serum obtained from patients who have had extensive immunopathologic characterization of their renal disease, we have found that 76 of 78 patients with anti-GBM antibody-induced Goodpasture's syndrome and 43 of 52 patients with anti-GBM antibody-induced nephritis alone had detectable circulating antibody with this technique. Only two of 329 patients with IC glomerulonephritis had circulating antibody, and both developed the antibody during an accelerated phase of chronic membranous glomerulonephritis. Of interest, a few patients with SLE have had evidence of circulating anti-GBM antibody in addition to the numerous other autoantibodies these patients develop. Only one of over 200 patients with negative renal immunopathologic studies had detectable anti-GBM antibody. This patient subsequently developed anti-GBM antibody-induced nephritis in a transplant, suggesting that our original diagnosis had been inadequate to find the antibody.

The mean amounts of antibody measured by radioimmunoassay do not differ significantly between the patients with Goodpasture's syndrome and those with glomerulonephritis alone. The anti-GBM antibody response is usually transient, lasting only weeks to months, with only rare examples of recrudescence. There is little correlation between the episodes of pulmonary hemorrhage and the absolute amount of antibody present in the circulation, although pulmonary hemorrhages rarely occur in the absence of detectable circulating antibody. Anti-alveolar basement membrane antibody can be detected more frequently in patients with pulmonary involvement than in those with glomerulonephritis alone. Prior studies with antibodies eluted from the lungs of patients with Goodpasture's syndrome demonstrated cross-reactivity with the GBM. It often appears that some additional event, perhaps physiologic or infectious in nature, is necessary before the pulmonary damage, presumably mediated by the antibody bound along the alveolar basement membrane, becomes clinically overt. Nephrectomy has been suggested as beneficial to patients with severe pulmonary hemorrhage of the Goodpasture's type; however, favorable responses have not been achieved uniformly. Nephrectomy does not appear to have any immediate effect on the level of circulating anti-GBM antibody, although subsequent disappearance of the antibody may be more rapid. Since large doses of steroids are now considered therapeutic during acute bouts of pulmonary hemorrhage, nephrectomy is being considered only as a last resort.

The overall clinical outcome of patients with anti-GBM antibody-induced glomerulonephritis or Goodpasture's syndrome has improved. Improvements in diagnostic techniques, allowing identification of patients with milder and self-remitting forms of the disease, as well as more ready accessibility to dialysis therapy, and the now-common use of high-dose steroids in the management of severe pulmonary hemorrhage have contributed. Although techniques for manipulating the immunopathologic factors have been slow in coming, certainly much slower than our understanding of the phenomena, they are beginning to be available at the bedside. For example, there has been a good deal of interest and apparent success with the use of plasmapheresis coupled with intense immunosuppression to decrease levels of circulating anti-basement membrane antibodies. Since the production of anti-basement membrane antibodies is usually relatively short-lived, any maneuver to hasten disappearance or remove the antibody theoretically should have therapeutic benefit. The current impression is that the combined immunosuppressive and plasmapheresis therapy offers a further incremental benefit over that produced by immunosuppression alone. At least one controlled study is currently under way to assess this clinical impression, which is largely based on a compilation of small series and anecdotal reports of cases handled in a generally similar, but not identical, manner. It is apparent that the severity of the disease at the time of institution of therapy has a great bearing on the outcome, since patients not developing progressive renal failure initially may not do so and those with severe and irreversible failure at the time therapy is instituted would not be expected to recover. The best candidates for this new therapeutic approach, then, would be patients with mild-to-moderate renal failure that appears to be advancing. As the number of patients treated grows and follow-up becomes available, it is apparent that some patients may experience an eventual decline in renal function even after having had an initial improvement and apparent stabilization of their course with disappearance of detectable circulating anti-GBM antibody.

Anti-GBM antibody disease, as noted, is severe and is quite likely to progress to renal failure requiring either transplantation or dialysis. Renal transplantation during the active phase of anti-GBM antibody production generally results in a recurrence of severe anti-GBM antibody-induced nephritis in the transplant. Once detectable anti-GBM antibody has declined or disappeared, renal transplantation can generally be undertaken without great danger of recurrent nephritis in the immunosuppressed transplant recipient. Recently, we had the opportunity to study samples from a woman with Goodpasture's syndrome who, following nephrectomy, had been free of detectable circulating anti-basement membrane antibody for a period of two years prior to receipt of an identical twin kidney transplant. Within three months, this nonimmunosuppressed recipient again developed circulating anti-GBM antibody, with clinical, histologic, and immunofluorescent evidence of recurrent anti-GBM antibody-induced nephritis. Immunosuppressive therapy and plasmapheresis were instituted at that time, with a subsequent decline in antibody levels and retention of func-

Figure 6

Nephritogenesis

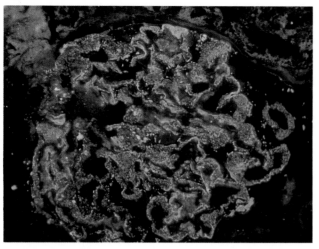

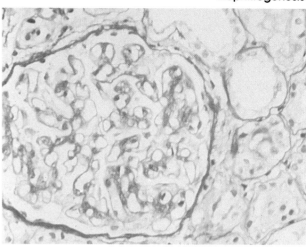

Micrographs on this page are representative of various types of IC kidney disease as visualized by immunofluorescent and by histologic techniques. Shown above is the immunofluorescent pattern of membranous glomerulonephritis with heavy, granular IgG deposits along the GBM. Accompanying histology reveals only some thickening of the glomerular capillary wall.

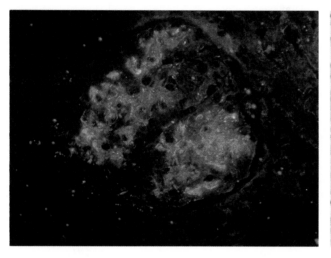

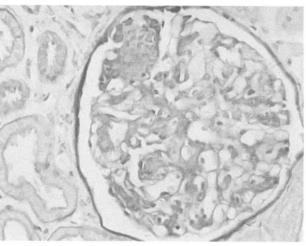

Immunofluorescently, the specimen above is consistent with IC nephritis with immunoglobulin dominantly concentrated in mesangial areas. Histology confirms diagnosis of proliferative glomerulonephritis largely confined to the mesangium. The paired slides below are from an even more focal mesangial IC nephritis. Granular deposits of IgG are highly concentrated in the mesangium. The histologic section shows that the pathologic changes are indeed confined to the mesangial stalk.

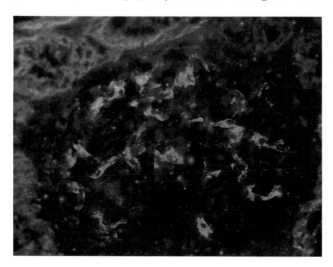

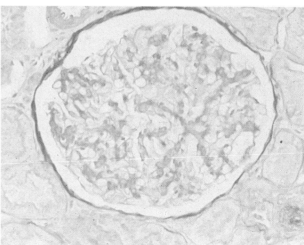

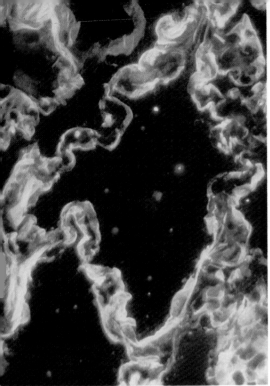

Figure 7

Immunofluorescence micrograph of a lung specimen from a patient with Goodpasture's syndrome shows very heavy linear IgG deposits along the alveolar basement membrane.

tion in the transplant. In this patient the antigenic stimulus appeared to reside in the kidney itself.

IC-induced glomerular injury, occasionally accompanied by IC-induced tubulointerstitial nephritis, is responsible for a wide variety of clinical and histologic types of glomerulonephritis in man. In many situations, the precipitating antigen or antigens cannot be identified, so that the IC etiology can only be presumed. The various forms of presumed IC nephritis can be classified on the basis of morphologic and immunofluorescent criteria. If one refers back to Table 1 and to the micrographs of Figure 7, it will become apparent that most of the glomerulonephritides are characterized by proliferation, meaning simply that there is an increase in the number of cells (intrinsic and/or inflammatory) in the glomerulus. Additional characteristics include accumulations of circulating polymorphonuclear and mononuclear leukocytes, various distortions of glomerular architecture, crescent formation, thickening of the GBM, and, eventually, sclerosis. The ICs are identified by im-

munofluorescence studies as scattered granular accumulations of immunoglobulin, complement, and antigen in deposits of various sizes and locations in and about the GBM. The IC deposits can also be identified through the electron microscope by their typical electron-dense appearance.

The pattern of IC deposition within the glomerulus (detected by immunofluorescence) generally correlates very well with the degree and type of histologic damage and the resultant clinical course of the patient. The dense accumulation of predominantly IgG accompanied by complement along the subepithelial aspect of the GBM seen in membranous glomerulonephritis is typical of this histologic and immunofluorescent correlation. In this disease, damage to the GBM results in striking urinary protein loss without early loss of renal function, leading to a clinical presentation of nephrotic syndrome. Diffuse deposits of IC within the mesangium and throughout the GBM typically lead to more proliferative forms of glomerular injury, which, because of their activity, generally cause a nephritic presentation with active urinary sediment and protein loss, with renal functional impairment relative to the degree of glomerular damage. IC deposits confined largely to the mesangium, sometimes of restricted immunoglobulin class, as in the instance of "IgG-IgA nephropathy," cause less histologic alteration and result clinically in only asymptomatic proteinuria or hematuria, with bouts of recurrent gross hematuria sometimes associated with respiratory infection. Another form of probable IC-associated nephritis is the so-called membranoproliferative hypocomplementemic nephritis seen in 10% to 15% of nephritic children. The disease can be subdivided into at least two types on the basis of localization of electron-dense deposits: in one, the deposits tend to be in a subendothelial position, while in the other, electron densities extend throughout the GBM and TBM. Immunoglobulin deposits are usually present in the former but are frequently overshadowed by C3 accompanied by other components of complement (C5-9), suggesting predominant activation of the alterna-

tive complement pathway in the latter. Of interest, a circulating factor has been observed in some of these patients that is capable of activating complement through the alternative complement pathway. Originally described as C3 nephritic factor, and subsequently as nephritic factor, or NF, the substance has been identified as an antibody reactive with conformational or neoantigenic changes in the bimolecular complex of C3 and activated factor B. It should be stressed that low serum complement is not an exclusive characteristic of membranoproliferative hypocomplementemic glomerulonephritis and can be associated with any disorder in which IC consumes large amounts of complement. However, in most situations other than membranoproliferative glomerulonephritis, the classic complement pathway is the major pathway involved, with early components C1, C2, and C4 also being consumed.

While in one sense one has to regard the classifications of IC glomerulonephritis as a continuum, it is also true that within each classification there is considerable stability. Patients who present with diffuse proliferative glomerulonephritis are likely to continue to have this picture until the disease is resolved. Although progression from mesangial IC localization and hypertrophy to more severe proliferative forms of glomerulonephritis does occur, there is a considerable probability that once the pattern is established it will persist. The most important determinant of severity and histologic damage is probably related to the quantity and tempo of IC deposition within the glomerulus.

As the detection of circulating antibodies has improved our understanding of anti-basement membrane disease, efforts have been intensified to develop techniques for the measurement and monitoring of circulating IC in patients with suspected IC-induced glomerulonephritis. A large number of assays have now been developed based on separation of IC immunoglobulin through physicochemical techniques or through its biologic functions, such as activation of complement or interaction with cells. In this regard, we have had the most experience with assays based on the interaction of IC with complement and Fc receptors present on cultured lymphoblastoid cell line Raji, and through the ability of IC to react in solid phase with C1q, the first component of the complement system. These radioimmunoassay techniques are capable of detecting 5 to 10 μg of aggregated human gamma globulin (AHG) per ml of serum, and the results are usually expressed in terms of AHG equivalents. Both assays are IgG-specific in that the amount of complexed IgG bound to the Raji cell or affixed to the solid phase C1q tube is quantitated. This property eliminates many nonspecific reactants, such as endotoxin, heparin, and DNA, which can cause false-positive results in certain IC assays.

Studies of serum from large numbers of patients with suspected IC nephritis have now been carried out and have proved of great interest. Those patients with IC disease associated with such systemic IC disorders as SLE are very often positive for circulating IC, with relatively large amounts of IC present. The amount of IC in the circulation correlates in a general way with the clinical activity of the disease process. In patients with primary IC glomerulonephritis, the frequency of detection as well as the quantity of circulating IC is generally less. Of even more interest, the frequency of detection is related to the type of IC glomerulonephritis under study; that is, patients with acute forms of IC glomerulonephritis, including acute poststreptococcal glomerulonephritis and certain forms of rapidly progressive nephritis, frequently have detectable circulating IC, while those patients with more indolent forms of IC glomerulonephritis, such as membranoproliferative, membranous, and chronic glomerulonephritis, are usually free of detectable circulating IC, in spite of often striking glomerular IC localization.

In explaining the apparent contradiction between circulating IC and glomerular localization in the more indolent forms of glomerulonephritis, questions arise about the sensitivity and specificity of the assays in detecting nephritogenic IC, as well as the timing of samples for study. As experience grows and similar results are found with more and more assays, one begins to wonder about other factors that may influence the nephritogenicity of low levels of IC. Certainly in diseases such as SLE, hepatitis, and other chronic infections, large amounts of antigen with excessive IC formation are expected, presenting the phagocytic system of the body with an unusually large load of material to process, probably resulting in a larger amount of material than normal escaping the clearance mechanism to lodge in vessels including those of the glomerulus.

In this context, it should be noted that the kinetics of IC diseases can be very puzzling. In some situations, e.g., SLE, the patient has extremely large quantities of circulating IC so that deposition in the kidneys is not surprising. However, in other forms of IC nephritis, the amount of circulating complex seems to be minimal and the presence of the complexes in the circulation episodic. In such situations, progression of disease is inclined to be slow, but it does occur. One wonders what the individual abnormalities are that cause a patient to develop IC disease in the absence of abnormal levels of circulating complexes. There is some evidence suggesting a cumulative effect resulting from chronic and episodic presence of complexes in the circulation in diseases such as SLE.

In those patients with low levels of circulating IC, however, one must question if other factors, perhaps genetic in origin, may result in inappropriate handling of more or less normal amounts of IC encountered or produced daily in our normal immunologic surveillance. Epidemiologic and family studies will be necessary to evaluate this possibility. One should also keep in mind that once the initial deposition has occurred, continued in situ modification of the IC could be taking place via interaction with antigen or antibody alone. In addition, the exact role of local or in situ IC formation is not yet well understood. When positive, the IC assays appear to be of use in monitoring the activity of a patient's disease process, particularly when therapeutic maneuvers such as intense immunosuppression and/or plasmapheresis are being applied.

The therapeutic modalities directed at IC-induced glomerulonephritis have relied heavily on nonspecific immunosuppressive regimens, generally including corticosteroids. Efforts should, of course, be made to identify the antigen(s) involved in the nephritogenic IC with a view toward its elimination. Such an approach has been shown to be fruitful in eliminating infections through specific antimicrobial therapy. Endogenous antigens, such as those related to the thyroid or neoplastic tissue, can be ablated. Removal of circulating IC through plasmapheresis as well as alteration in levels of serum mediators by this modality is being explored for its potential benefit. There are also reasons for optimism regarding both pharmacologic manipulation of mediators of the immunologic injury and improvements in physical techniques for design of extracorporeal systems that would permit blood to be treated by extraction of IC, antibodies, antigen, or activated mediators. Such alternatives would obviate full-scale plasmapheresis.

Tissue Mast Cells in Immediate Hypersensitivity

K. FRANK AUSTEN *Harvard University*

The functioning of tissue mast cells as effectors in the immediate hypersensitivity reactions to such insults as bee stings or penicillin injection or ingestion in the allergic individual has long been appreciated. However, in the light of our present knowledge, the concept that the mast cell functions essentially by releasing into the microenvironment granules containing histamine and perhaps other mediators can be characterized as highly simplistic.

The mast cells do degranulate when activated, and the granules do release histamine and other primary mediators in response to antigen bridging of surface immunoglobulin (IgE) molecules. However, in addition to this cytoplasmic response, there is a rapidly sequential alteration of the cell membrane that sets in train the oxidative metabolism of arachidonic acid. The resulting products include prostaglandin D_2 (PGD_2) and leukotrienes, which function as secondary, but highly potent, mediators of immediate hypersensitivity.

Recognition of the pluripotential nature of tissue mast cells has come only in the past few years. With this recognition has come not only a far more sharply focused understanding of immediate hypersensitivity phenomena but also a realization that the mast cell, rather than being simply a nuisance that can turn a mildly pathologic response (or no response at all) into a severe and even life-threatening reaction, has an important physiologic role.

Indeed, one can properly regard mast cells as "sentinels." This perception derives from two significant facts. Of all immunologically active cells, mast cells are the only ones that possess a recognition system that is already in the tissues. The system can recognize "nonself" the moment it enters the organism, without the need for recruitment from the blood circulation or from the lymphatics. Moreover, the distribution of mast cells is highly appropriate for sentinels. They are found on cutaneous and mucosal surfaces and around venules (see Figure 1, page 224). If any exogenous antigen is to penetrate the organism, it must enter either through the skin or through gastrointestinal or other mucosa. And if penetration to the circulation does occur, the mast cells stand guard at the interface between the arterial and venous vasculature. Finally, because they concentrate on their surfaces most of the body's IgE molecules (which, of course, are far fewer than those of the other immunoglobulin classes), tissue mast cells possess the specificities required for immune defense.

The distribution of mast cells also affords a clue to what in an evolutionary sense appears to be at least one of its homeostatic functions, protection against helminthic infestation. To a degree, this may be a somewhat obsolescent function in a modern industrialized society where parasitic worms have all but disappeared from the human environment. However, in the evolutionarily recent past, the human environment was certainly worm-infested, and to some extent it remains so in the undeveloped countries inhabited by most people.

Why have we been so late in arriving at an understanding of the behavior of mast cells?

In part, the answer is technologic. The methodology

for obtaining and working in vitro with dispersed mast cells has been available only in the past dozen years or so. And the ability to purify them to a degree that permits biochemical studies is even more recent than that. In addition, although taken together mast cells can be considered to have an organic function, they are not concentrated in any single "convenient" organ, a fact that no doubt has retarded study. Perhaps most importantly, interest in immediate hypersensitivity has historically been concentrated on its most dramatic expression—anaphylaxis. This has tended to divert attention away from effector mechanisms and toward the target organs and structures in which anaphylaxis is manifested. Anaphylaxis has traditionally been studied not on a cellular or molecular level but in the intact animal or through contractile effects on whole organs or parts of organs.

The phenomenon can be conveniently categorized as cutaneous or systemic. Cutaneous anaphylaxis has been traditionally demonstrated by the familiar Prausnitz-Küstner wheal and flare used in allergy testing. In laboratory animals, the analogue to the wheal and flare is the blue spot seen on the pelt when dye is added to the provoking antigen. Systemic anaphylaxis may present in one of three distinctive patterns, all of which are uniquely human phenomena. In some individuals, the elicited reaction is marked swelling of the upper respiratory tract with resultant airway obstruction and asphyxiation. As the reaction develops, the individual becomes aware that his or her tongue is swollen and protruding from the mouth and that the voice is hoarse or lost. The second pattern is also one of severe respiratory compromise leading to asphyxiation. However, the lesion is much lower in the respiratory tract,

Figure 1

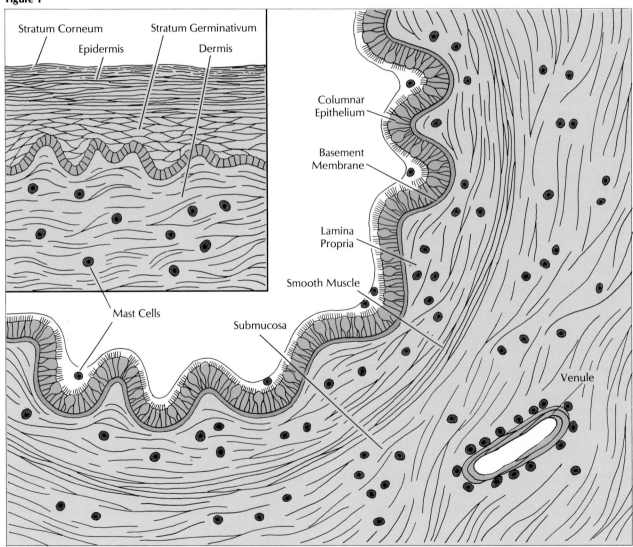

Mast cell distribution is appropriate for "sentinel" functions as schematized in bronchus and skin (inset). In the bronchial tissue, the mast cells are found near the mucosal surfaces and in the submucosa, as well as around venules. Skin mast cells are in the dermis. Thus they are near interfaces with external environment or between venous and arterial circulations.

involving spasm of the bronchioles. The patient can get air in but cannot move it out again. Clinically, the major sign is severe dyspnea. The third pattern in the human is one of primary vascular collapse without respiratory distress. It should be noted that only the first two patterns are easily related to the distribution of human tissue mast cells. In a clinical context, it should be pointed out also that the interventions for each of these three patterns are very different, although they all start with immediate administration of epinephrine.

Considerable research attention has been and is being paid to the question of why humans should have three different reaction patterns in contradistinction to experimental animal species, each of which manifests only one type of reaction. The differences could relate to the manner in which the individual encounters antigen, but it seems more probable that the answer will lie in the heterogeneity of our mast cell populations and of their products.

Before turning to the studies of the past decade that have elucidated this heterogeneity, let me just point out one more human/animal difference or possible difference. In most animal species, mast cells can be activated or fired by either IgE antibodies or by antibodies of a heat-stable IgG subclass. Thus far, only IgE antibodies have been implicated in human immediate hypersensitivity reactions. It remains to be determined whether there is a human counterpart to the heat-stable IgG-triggered animal reactions.

Once it was demonstrated that mast cells and histamine were involved in immediate hypersensitivity, it became feasible to develop in vitro systems using mast cell preparations to analyze the response on a cellular and subcellular basis. In order to investigate the biochemistry of the tissue mast cell or to identify the array of its products, it was necessary to have one or more cell systems that could be worked with in vitro. Two such systems

were developed for initial studies of this kind. Most were done with rat peritoneal mast cells. Rats, mice, and hamsters have mixtures of cells in their peritoneal cavities that include about 5% mast cells. Since these cells are free from tissues, they can be extracted by simple lavage. With density gradient centrifugation, a preparation that is about 98% mast cells can be obtained.

Other workers, anxious to study human cell populations, resorted to use of basophils, which, of course, are peripheral blood cells. Basophils resemble mast cells in that they have metachromatic granules and have both IgE receptors and IgE immunoglobulin on their surfaces.

Figure 2

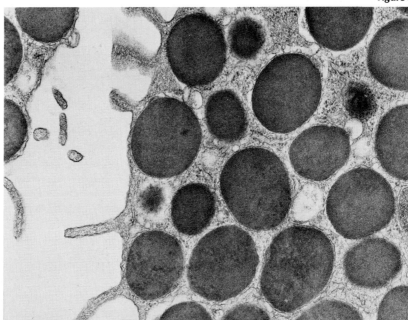

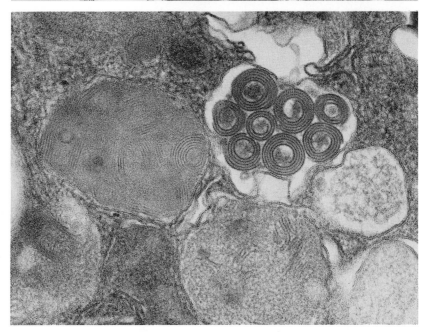

The amorphous internal structure of rat peritoneal mast cells (top, × 50,000) is in sharp contrast to the scroll-like crystalline structure of human mast cells (bottom, × 174,000). (All of the photomicrographs accompanying this article were provided through the courtesy of Drs. John P. Caulfield and Ann Hein.)

Figure 3

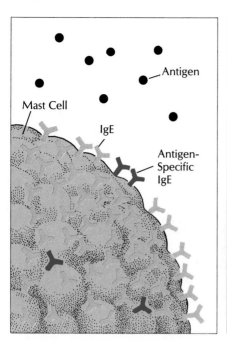
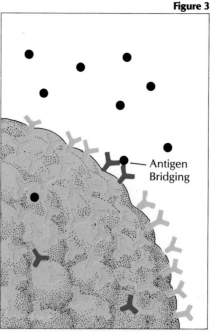

Because IgE constitutes a very small fraction of circulating immunoglobulin, it must be concentrated by receptors on the mast cell surface to subserve its function of cell activation. When two IgE molecules of the same specificity are in close proximity on the surface, the mast cell is effectively sensitized (left). Subsequent bridging by the appropriate antigen will entrain the activation-secretion response (right).

Thus, it was possible to gain a great deal of information about cells that are activated by IgE-antigen interaction and respond by degranulation and histamine release. Unfortunately, there was a tendency to forget that the basophils are not tissue cells; rather, they are polymorphonuclear leukocytes with functions appropriate to circulating cells and very different from those of mast cells, which mediate reactions that take place in solid tissues.

Whereas rat peritoneal mast cells are usable for investigating biochemical events, they are morphologically very different from human tissue mast cells. The rat cells have a granular infrastructure that is essentially amorphous, while the human mast cell granules have a remarkably perfect crystalline structure (Figure 2, page 225). The importance of this crystalline structure to the understanding of the events involved in immediate hypersensitivity will become clear later in this presentation. It was not until the mid-seventies that the means to obtain human tissue mast cells was developed. The source was lung tissue removed at surgery, usually for cancer—specifically, the apparently normal rim or margin of lung tissue that is customarily removed when a tumor is excised. With a four-step enzymatic procedure this lung tissue could be dispersed to lung cells, containing about 5% mast cells. Techniques for separating these cells on the basis of their size yielded human mast cell preparations of 60% to 80% purity. While this was not sufficient for biochemical studies, it did permit us to isolate the products of the human mast cell and to compare them with chemical substances elaborated by the purified rat mast cells. It should be noted that more recently, L. M. Lichtenstein and his colleagues at Johns Hopkins have developed techniques that produce human mast cell preparations with greater purity.

With this background and with the fact that the mast cell has an unusual pattern of localization in the body, we can begin to delineate the events that relate to its function. The first role that can be recognized is provision of a "stage" for IgE. It has been noted that IgE represents a very small fraction of the total immunoglobulin complement. For antigen to interact with antibody and produce a change in the mast cell, it must bridge two IgE molecules. The chances of this happening with IgE in the circulation would be vanishingly small. However, a mast cell has on its surface IgE antibodies of all specificities, thus greatly amplifying the probability of antigen bridging and of activating the effector functions of the cell (see Figure 3, at left). When a mast cell has enough IgE molecules on its surface to allow for the presence of two molecules of the same specificity side by side, the cell can be considered to be sensitized. In this context, sensitization does not imply any biochemical change in the cell; rather it merely describes the situation in which there is a mathematical probability that two IgE molecules of the same specificity are susceptible to antigen bridging.

Once antigen bridging actually takes place, the cell engages in a series of biochemical modifications that lead to what is termed the activation-secretion response. It is this response that leads to the firing of the cell and the release of the primary mediators, so called because they exist prepackaged in the cytoplasmic secretory granules and only require transport to the outside of the cell.

In parallel with this sequence is a complex series of biochemical events that lead to perturbation of the mast cell's phospholipid membrane. The result is the elaboration of a new set of soluble mediators, called secondary or lipid mediators. The lipid mediators are not derived from the secretory granules; rather, they are by-products of the oxidative metabolism of arachidonic acid occurring consequent to the perturbation of the cell membrane. The secondary mediators are the leukotrienes and PGD_2, metabolic products of arachidonic acid. The most intensively studied leukotriene mediator is SRS-A, the slow-reacting substance of anaphylaxis.

Figure 4

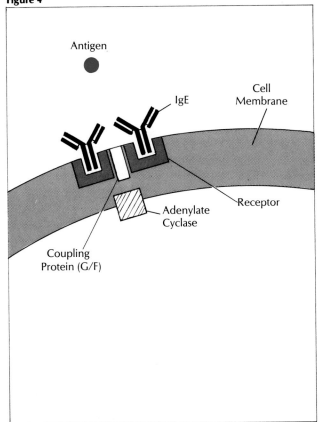

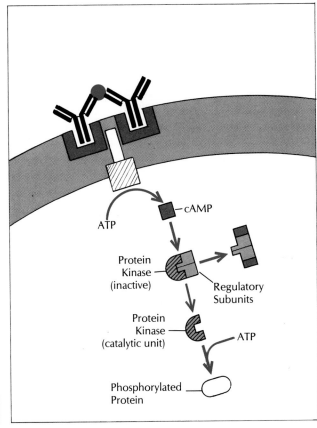

Mast cell membrane structures involved in the initial steps of the activation-secretion response include the IgE receptors linked to a transmembrane coupling protein (G/F) and the catalytic unit of adenylate cyclase (left). When two IgE molecules are bridged by a specific antigen, the G/F unit activates the adenylate cyclase (right) and cytoplasmic ATP is used to

produce cAMP, which then recruits a cytoplasmic, cAMP-dependent protein kinase. This it does by binding to the two regulatory units of the inactive kinase, liberating a catalytic unit that phosphorylates another, still-undefined protein, using additional ATP in the process. It is noteworthy that the biochemistry closely parallels that of endocrine hormonal release.

It is currently believed that perturbation of IgE-Fc receptors initiates parallel biochemical sequences, one leading to degranulation and release of primary mediators, such as histamine, and the other to the events in the lipid membrane that cause elaboration of the secondary mediators, such as SRS-A and PGD_2. The receptor also provides the transmembrane route for the biochemical message that causes release of the granules. Once the IgE molecules are bridged, the receptors are modulated so that the message is forwarded into the cell.

As shown in Figure 4 above, the IgE receptor is basically a binding protein. It is linked to a transmembrane coupling protein designated as G/F, because it is also activated by either guanine nucleotides, such as guanosine, or by fluoride.

When the IgE receptor is perturbed by antigen bridging, the coupling protein transmits a transmembrane activation of adenylate cyclase in the membrane; adenylate cyclase, in turn, acts upon cytoplasmic ATP to make cyclic AMP (cAMP). The cAMP now acts to recruit a cytoplasmic cAMP-dependent protein kinase. This it does by replacing the two regulatory units of the kinase, thus freeing the remaining catalytic unit(s). The catalytic unit, utilizing additional ATP, then phosphorylates another—still undefined—protein, which begins to move the granule toward the cell surface.

Although somewhat complicated in the recounting, this is really a rather simple biochemical chain reaction. Indeed, it is also a ubiquitous one in the sense that all known hormone-release mecha-

nisms work by a parallel receptor-adenylate cyclase-cAMP-protein kinase sequence. The recognition that this was the scenario for mast cell degranulation was slow in coming, largely because early studies with basophils and other impure or inappropriate systems suggested that immediate hypersensitivity reactions were only suppressed if cAMP levels were raised. We now know that it is not that simple. Rather, the cAMP appears to provide both a facilitative and then an inhibitive, or turnoff, regulatory signal.

A second major step forward in the understanding of the degranulation process was made possible by the availability of human mast cells for in vitro preparations. As already noted (and depicted in Figure 2), the rat mast cell has essentially amorphous granules, while those of the human cell have a clearly defined crystalline structure with a scroll shape and a regular periodicity of 75 A to 150 A. When a rat mast cell is fired, about all that is seen is swelling and fusion of the perigranular and cell membranes. However, due to its crystalline structure, with the human mast cell granule the entire sequence of events can be followed by electron microscopy (see Figure 5, at right.). Within 30 seconds after the human mast cell is fired in vitro, the crystalline structure has begun to disintegrate and amorphous debris appears within the granule. As the crystalline structure disintegrates completely, the granules double in size. As the granule swells and dissolves, it somehow signals organelles, known as intermediate filaments, which begin to surround the granule. Once the filaments have surrounded the granule, they begin to move with it toward the cell surface. When the swollen granule, now containing solubilized material, reaches the cell membrane, it fuses with the membrane, and its contents are released into the microenvironment. It is important to stress that what has just been described has been visualized morphologically (in collaboration with John Caulfield) but not characterized biochemically, except for the initial phase involving activation of adenylate cyclase and the cAMP-dependent protein kinase.

While all of this is happening within the cell, the cell membrane changes have also been proceeding apace. Indeed, there is reason to believe that the two processes are interdependent. Certainly, both are triggered by the aforementioned perturbation of the IgE receptor. Based on studies of T. Ishizaka and colleagues, the receptor activates not only cell membrane adenylate cyclase but also membrane phospholipase(s). There are actually two membrane phospholipases, designated as A_2 and C. It is not clear whether one or both are activated in the rat mast cell, and there is no information relevant to the human mast cell. The phospholipases act on phospholipid substrates to cleave arachidonic acid away, leaving behind a lysophospholipid. There are variations in the sequence depending on whether the A_2 or the C phospholipase is involved, but the end products are the arachidonic acid central to the synthesis of the lipid mediators and fusigenic moieties that facilitate the process of fusion between the granule and mast cell membranes.

In addition to this action of the phospholipases, there appears to be another enzymatic process that is important in the early stages of mast cell activation. Collaborative studies between J. Axelrod and F. Hirata and Ishizaka suggest that mast cell membrane phospholipids are also acted upon by methyl transferases and that the resulting methylation of the polar head groups alters the orientation of phospholipid molecules. These altered molecules are the substrate for the lipases in the reactions that lead to the generation of arachidonic acid and of the fusigenic molecules.

By way of summary of the various reactions that take place at the level of the cell membrane and in the cytoplasm, attention is called to Figure 6, page 230. This diagram also takes note of the current view that corticosteroids act on mast cells through the nucleus to generate a molecule called macrocortin (or lipomodulin). This has been proposed as a mechanism through which steroids might act chronically to down-regulate allergic disease.

Since the primary mediators are by definition contained in the secretory granules, and since the entire content of the granules reaches the extracellular environment during the course of an immediate hypersensitivity reaction, one can properly consider everything in the granules to have a mediator function in the reaction. To be sure, our understanding of the roles of histamine, the most dramatic of which are alteration of membrane permeability and contraction of smooth muscle, is extensive. However, as in vitro studies of mast cells have proceeded, it has become strikingly

Figure 5

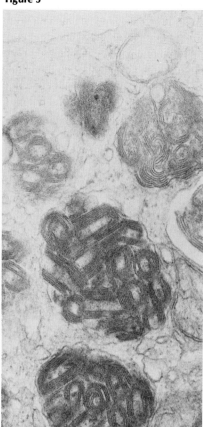

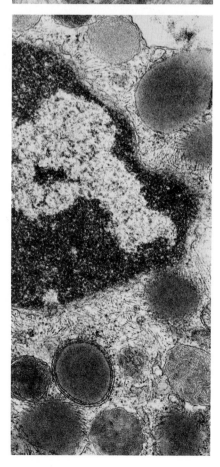

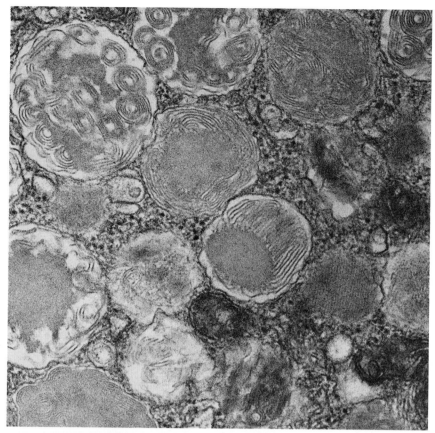

The crystalline structure of the human mast cell facilitates study of the events leading to degranulation of the cell and the release of primary mediators. In the unstimulated cell, crystalline structure of granule contents is seen (far left, × 60,000). Five minutes after stimulation of cell by anti-IgE, several granules can be seen to have solubilized amorphous material within the crystalline patterns (left, × 78,000). The next photo (below, far left) shows a mast cell with several granules having completely solubilized contents and with surrounding intermediate filaments (× 50,000). The adjacent EM shows granules being discharged from the mast cell surface. Those that remain in cytoplasm are completely amorphous, and intermediate filaments are very prominent (× 50,000). Finally, a largely degranulated mast cell with vacuoles communicating with the extracellular space is seen (× 12,000). All magnifications given are those of the original photomicrographs.

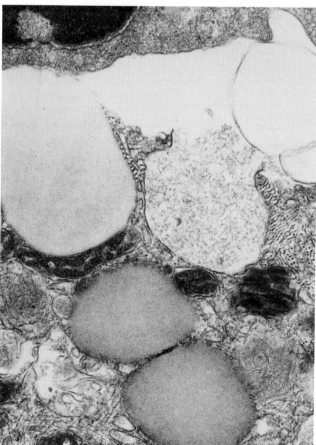

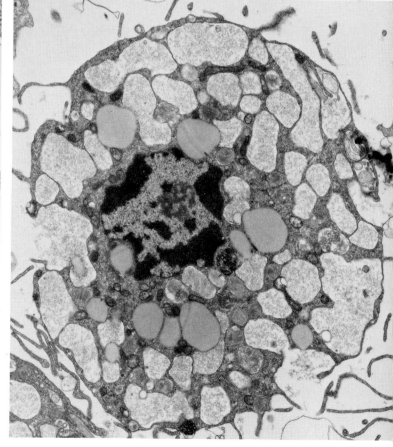

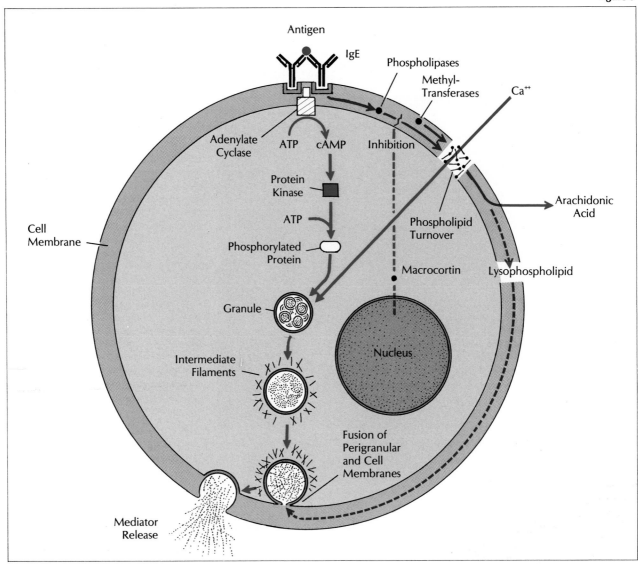

The protein phosphorylated by the early steps in the activation-secretion sequence (see Figure 4) initiates movement of the granules toward the cell surface. This movement is facilitated by the action of intermediate filaments. At the cell surface, there is fusion between the perigranular and cell membranes, and the granules secrete their contents into the extracellular space. In parallel with degranulation, there is perturbation of the phospholipids of the cell membrane, also initiated by antigen bridging of IgE pairs. Phospholipases and methyltransferases catalyze phospholipid breakdown and the release of arachidonic acid. Another product, a lysophospholipid, facilitates membrane fusion and therefore degranulation. Also shown is the suggestion that steroids act in allergic diseases by generating macrocortin, which in turn inhibits phospholipid turnover.

clear that the granules (both in rats and in humans) are extremely rich in protein and that the protein is dominated by enzymes of the neutral protease class. Indeed, it has been found that rat mast cells have about 30 μg of neutral protease per 10^6 cells and human cells, about 20 μg/10^6. Thus, mast cells appear to be not only the major source of histamine in the tissues, but also the major source of neutral proteases. For example, human mast cells contain about 10 times as much neutral protease as polymorphonuclear leukocytes, which have always been considered a very rich source of these enzymes. For example, all of the neutral protease that can be extracted from rat skin is derived from mast cells.

The nature of the proteases appears to be, to a considerable degree, species specific. In rats, the dominant protease has a chymotryptic activity with the same specificity for substrate digestion as pancreatic chymotrypsin. Rat mast cell secretory granules also contain carboxypeptidase A and a variety of acid hydrolases. In the human mast cell, the dominant neutral protease possesses tryptic activity similar to that of pancreatic trypsin, although structurally the two enzymes are very different.

The finding of such impressive reservoirs of neutral protease in mast cells permits some intriguing postulations about still-to-be-defined physiologic and pathophysiologic functions of this cell population. It seems plausible to speculate that normally these enzymes engage in tissue repair processes. For example, in the event of microbial damage to tissue, debridement has to take place before repair can start. Mast cell enzymes could be the agents for such debridement. On the other hand, inappropriate release of these proteases could well destroy normal connective tissue by digestion of the peptide core of the proteoglycans. The various proteoglycans (e.g., chondroitin sulphate proteoglycans) have long been recognized as among the most important molecules in relation to the integrity of connective tissue. One must consider the possibility that these proteases have the capacity to convert a reversible event into chronic tissue injury.

A critical group of primary mediators are the chemotactic factors. If the mast cells are to fulfill their sentinel functions, they must not only change mucosal and vascular permeability to facilitate the importation of plasma proteins, such as immunoglobulin and complement, but also bring phagocytes to the site of antigen incursion. To this end, potent chemotactic factors are released during mast cell degranulation. These factors attract eosinophils (of course, eosinophilia has long been recognized as one of the hallmarks of allergic reactions), neutrophils, and other phagocytic cells.

From a historic point of view, the first human chemotactic factor that was structurally characterized (as a tetrapeptide) was a molecule that selectively attracted eosinophils. Because of the association between eosinophilia and allergy, we assumed that mast cells should be able to elaborate this factor. This assumption proved correct, and two eosinotactic tetrapeptides were defined in the activity termed the eosinophil chemotactic factor of anaphylaxis; another component has now been recognized to be leukotriene B_4 (LTB$_4$).

The first of what are now known as the secondary or leukotriene mediators of immediate hypersensitivity was discovered in the early 1940s by two Australian scientists, C. H. Kellaway and E. R. Trethewie, while observing the allergic reaction in guinea pig lung preparations. They found that perfused lungs subjected to anaphylaxis contained in addition to histamine a second substance with spasmogenic or contractile activity. Because the second substance contracted smooth muscle more slowly than histamine, they called it slow-reacting substance of anaphylaxis. SRS-A was largely ignored for the next decade until W. E. Brocklehurst, in England, developed a bioassay for it by adding an antihistamine to the organ bath; the antihistamine blocked the action of histamine and therefore allowed measurement of the contractile activity of SRS-A in the mixture elaborated by the anaphylactic reaction in guinea pig lung tissue.

Brocklehurst also made another critical observation that in concert with the bioassay revived interest in SRS-A. He obtained a segment of lung tissue from an allergic patient undergoing surgery. This segment was large enough to contain a small bronchial tube, which he cannulated and attached to a manometer before subjecting it to a specific antigen-antibody reaction. The piece of human lung responded to antigen challenge by releasing not only histamine but large amounts of SRS-A. Moreover, the bronchiole in the presence of an antihistamine contracted, as recorded by pressure changes in the manometer. Thus, SRS-A could provoke bronchospasm and had to be reckoned with for its relevance to human asthma.

In 1974, Jeffrey Drazen and I administered partially purified SRS-A to guinea pigs and demonstrated a profound change in pulmonary function, with the major effect being on the peripheral rather than the central airways. The preparation used had been purified by techniques developed with Robert Orange and Robert Murphy, then at the Massachusetts Institute of Technology. Although we had developed a significantly purified preparation, it was not volatile when analyzed by mass spectroscopy with or without gas chromatography. Nonetheless, it was shown to be enriched for sulfur when analyzed by spark source mass spectroscopy and electron probe analysis. Subsequently, Charles Parker and his colleagues at Washington University, St. Louis, and M. K. Bach at The Upjohn Company, who had been in our laboratory, independently demonstrated that SRS-A molecules incorporated arachidonic acid in their biosynthesis. Murphy then went to work with Bengt Samuelsson at the Karolinska, who, of course, with Sune Bergstrom had been responsible for so much of our knowledge of the products of arachidonic acid metabolism (which we now know as the prostaglandins and the thromboxanes) and with P. Borgeat had described LTB$_4$. Together with E. J. Corey at Harvard, Samuelsson and Murphy identified the complete structure of SRS-A as an eicosatetraenoic acid linked to glutathione via a thioether bond. It was actually Corey's chemical insights that provided the final stereochemical structural information. Figure 7 on page **232** is a diagram of that structure and of its conversion products, LTD$_4$ and LTE$_4$. In all, it took more than three decades from the discovery of SRS-A to its full characterization. Possibly this lengthy time span can be explained, in part at least, by the fact that SRS-A is a most unusual chemical mediator. It is the first example of a mediator that is part sulfidopeptide and part fatty acid.

The metabolic pathways are also summarized in Figure 7. In brief, arachidonic acid is acted upon by 5-lipoxygenase to form an intermediate, 5-hydroperoxyeicosatetraenoic acid, which is converted to a molecule designated as leukotriene A$_4$. (If the fatty acid is instead metabolized by cyclooxygenase, the prostaglandin-thromboxane pathway is activated.) Leukotriene A$_4$ (LTA$_4$) then enters two different pathways, one yielding leukotriene B$_4$ (LTB$_4$), the other sequentially

Figure 7

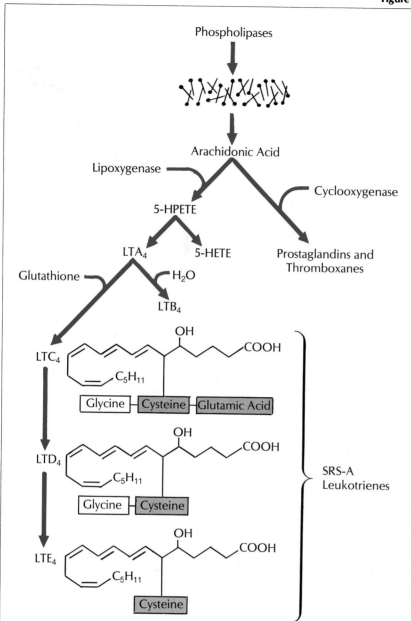

The oxidative metabolism of arachidonic acid can lead to the synthesis of prostaglandins, thromboxanes, and leukotrienes. LTC$_4$, LTD$_4$, and LTE$_4$ are believed to be mixed in the powerful secondary mediator of immediate hypersensitivity, SRS-A.

yielding leukotrienes C$_4$, D$_4$, and E$_4$ (LTC$_4$, LTD$_4$, LTE$_4$). Most SRS-A is a mixture of these last three.

Noteworthy is the fact that leukotriene B$_4$ is structurally very different from the molecules of the C$_4$ series. This difference is reflected functionally. Leukotriene B$_4$ is the most potent natural chemotactic factor identified to date, with chemotaxis for eosinophils, neutrophils, and monocytes. SRS-A is by

far the most potent vasoactive and spasmogenic mediator known. For example, with Drazen, Regis McFadden, and colleagues, we have shown that the leukotrienes C$_4$ and D$_4$ are on a molar basis 4,000 times as potent as histamine in compromising airway function in normal humans. In other words, one has to inhale a 10^{-2} molar solution of histamine to get the effect achieved with 10^{-6} moles of leukotriene. Clearly, the

secondary mediators generated by mast cells have an extremely important role in fulfilling the functions of those cells.

As early as 1960, Brocklehurst, J. H. Humphrey, and I found out that SRS-A could *not* be generated from rat peritoneal mast cells in measurable amounts (bioassay). One possibility was that this was a unique species peculiarity of the rat. However, it was subsequently shown that human mast cells yielded less SRS-A as they were dispersed and purified. This raised two possibilities. One was that human lung mast cells were releasing products that acted on other cell populations to elaborate SRS-A. The second was that there were really two different populations of mast cells, only some of which produced SRS-A. While this question has not yet been finally settled, the weight of evidence favors the multipopulation concept. In fact, our group has recently characterized a second species of mast cells from the bone marrow of mice.

Several laboratories had shown in 1981 that one could differentiate a population that was 98% mast cells if the marrow cells were treated in culture with T-cell growth and differentiation factors. Ehud Razin, Richard Stevens, and others in our group, in collaboration with Karl Schmid's laboratory, analyzed these cells and found that while they were morphologically characteristic of murine mast cells, they contained no heparin, and heparin has always been considered a sine qua non of the mast cell. These mouse bone-marrow-derived cells could be distinguished from basophils (which contain a conventionally sulfated chondroitin sulfate) and heparin-containing mast cells because they contained a proteoglycan called chondroitin sulfate E, which is highly sulfated and which previously had been identified only in squid cartilage.

This second population of mast cells elaborates extremely large quantities of LTC$_4$ when stimulated either immunologically or by the calcium inophore system. Whereas the conventional heparin-containing mast cell converts arachidonic acid to PGD_2, the atypical mast cell converts it to LTC_4.

It is important to note that although SRS-A has been generated from human mast cells, it is not known whether the cells producing the leukotriene are typical or atypical.

This mast cell heterogeneity may well have a clinical correlate. Patients with mastocytosis, which, of course, is a mast cell proliferative disease, do not have the manifestations of a possible leukotriene-mediated disease, such as bronchospasm, but rather those of a prostaglandin-mediated disease (D_2, as assessed in collaborative studies with John Oates and Jack Roberts). Treatment of mastocytosis by histamine blockade (H_1 and H_2 antihistamines) and PGD_2 blockade (aspirin) attenuates the disease and eliminates the elevated level of PGD_2 metabolites from the urine.

With the availability of synthetic leukotrienes, in collaboration with Corey, systematic studies were initiated to try to analyze the effects on the human lung. In the first phases of these studies, with N. A. Soter and R. A. Lewis, it was found that LTC_4, LTD_4, and LTE_4 were all extremely active in inciting the wheal-and-flare reaction—about 100 times more so than histamine, again on a molar basis. Perhaps more importantly, the leukotriene-induced reactions were much more prolonged than the usual histamine reactions. With the leukotrienes, the wheal lasted two to four hours and the flare, six to eight hours. At the same time, we looked at PGD_2 challenge. It also elicited a wheal-and-flare reaction,

which was not as persistent, resolving completely within two hours.

Cutaneous challenge with LTB_4 was also evaluated. It was found that for about four hours after administration nothing happened. Then, quite suddenly, a very sore spot developed at the site of injection. On biopsy, the area was found to be heavily infiltrated with neutrophils.

The leukotriene responses are particularly intriguing if one thinks about the various components of the inflammatory reaction. Both their strength and their duration suggest an important role in allergic inflammation. In addition, it was observed that the LTC_4 wheal has a white ischemic center, reflecting an arteriolar response. Apparently, SRS-A not only induces hyperpermeability but also constricts arterioles sufficiently to produce localized ischemia, while LTB_4 causes an influx of inflammatory cells.

After using cutaneous reactivity to establish tolerance of human subjects to the leukotriene preparations, we undertook inhalation studies to evaluate their effects on pulmonary function. Once again, the investigators served as volunteer subjects, first for trials with leukotriene C and more recently with leukotriene D. The pulmonary function response of the subjects was initially calibrated with histamine. The results, as noted, showed a 4,000 times greater respiratory compromise with the leukotrienes than with histamine.

On the basis of such findings as this, one can confidently propose the leukotrienes as major mediators of reversible airway disease. This is not to say that histamine

will not make a contribution, but certainly one must take into account, both pathogenetically and therapeutically, this set of remarkably potent molecules that are generated in the process of mast cell activation. Do the leukotrienes actually play a role in human asthma? There is not yet any direct evidence for this, but radioimmunoassays developed by Lewis may provide circumstantial evidence if these leukotrienes are produced in sufficient quantities to enter the blood plasma.

It is worth mentioning that the secondary mediators are highly likely to have roles other than those being postulated in immediate hypersensitivity and to involve cell lines other than mast cells. They will be elaborated by any cell type that possesses a membrane capable of metabolizing arachidonic acid upon perturbation. In that context, it has been shown that a number of different cell types each have their own preferred pathways of arachidonic acid metabolism. Mast cell products have been discussed in this review. Other cells make various prostaglandins and leukotrienes. Mouse macrophages, for example, elaborate large quantities of LTC_4 along with PGE_2, while human neutrophils elaborate mainly LTB_4. Basically, any time a cell membrane is perturbed, its environment will be enriched selectively by the various products of the oxidative metabolism of arachidonic acid. The program for selection largely resides in the enzymatic capabilities of the particular cell membrane. What seems clear is that qualitatively and quantitatively these products will profoundly influence the cell's role in biology.

Murine SLE Models And Autoimmune Disease

FRANK J. DIXON   *Research Institute of the Scripps Clinic*

The words "autoimmune" and "disease" are so inextricably linked for physicians that many might find paradoxical the statement that autoimmune responses are ubiquitous and only exceptionally disease producing in mammalian species. For the most part, autoimmune or immunologic self-recognition responses play a variety of roles that are either homeostatically essential or neutral rather than pathogenic. For example, the cooperative interaction between immunologically competent lymphocytes involved in the presentation of antigen required to initiate an immunologic response and the killing of virus-infected cells necessary to the completion of such reactions is dependent on the mutual recognition of cell surface markers present on both cell populations and coded for by genes in the major histocompatibility complex (MHC). Similarly, the response to idiotypic determinants on antibodies consists of the formation of anti-idiotypic antibodies that appear to play a critical role in regulation of the immunologic network.

If one starts from the premise that autoimmunity is usually physiologic, an obvious question arises: What factors determine and lead to the development of autoimmune diseases? In recent years, investigators have had available a sophisticated and highly rewarding system in their efforts to answer this question, i.e., mouse models for a disease that has long been accepted as the prototype of autoimmune pathology—systemic lupus erythematosus. Before describing these murine SLE models, let me briefly note some of the information and insights that have already been derived from them:

1. There is significant experimental support for the statement that the essential immunopathologic perturbation in SLE appears to be the hyperactivity of B lymphocytes with corresponding enhancement of serum antibodies, particularly IgG antibodies, and consequent antigen–antibody complex formation. As a corollary, the evidence argues against any consistent aberrations related to immunologic regulatory cells, such as the suppressor T cells. Although enhanced helper T-cell activity has been observed in one of the SLE models, this enhancement functions largely to implement a polyclonal B-cell proliferation.

2. There is loss of tolerance or of tolerizing responses. It has been demonstrated experimentally in all of the SLE murine models that when antigens are injected in forms that in normal animals cause specific tolerance, no such nonresponsiveness is induced.

3. No single gene or group of related genes that code for a generalized autoimmunity or a predisposition for autoimmunity can be identified. Rather, it appears that various individual genes or a cluster of genes determine specific autoantibodies, and the development of autoimmune disease depends on the additive effects of these genes' surpassing a "threshold" for disease. Interestingly, the genes that are involved in these autoimmune responses do not appear to be associated with the major histocompatibility complex.

4. A number of factors can accelerate the pathogenesis of SLE in the animal models. These factors vary from model to model, and none of them, including several viruses, induces significant pathogenic effects in normal (non-SLE) animals.

5. One of the murine SLE models also provides an animal model for rheumatoid arthritis that is strongly

correlated with the human disease.

6. A largely unexpected association has been shown between autoimmune phenomena and the formation of immune complexes and coronary artery disease with myocardial infarction.

The discussion that follows will deal in some detail with each of these salient points. First, however, it is appropriate to describe the various SLE murine models and their development, beginning with the now classic New Zealand black (NZB) × New Zealand white (NZW) hybrid that has represented the prototypical system for the study of lupus over the past 20 years. A great deal has been learned about immunopathology from this system, but in working with it, one has always been confronted with something of a dilemma, i.e., it has been difficult to differentiate between characteristics of disease and peculiarities that might be epiphenomena of these rather singular mice. The New Zealand mice are unusual animals with respect to both their virologic and immunologic traits. As long as we had only one mouse model to study, we could not unequivocally state that a particular phenomenon was attributable to autoimmunity rather than to other factors inherent in the model animal.

Now, largely as a result of the work of E. D. Murphy and J. B. Roths at the Jackson Memorial Laboratory in Bar Harbor, Me., we have two more murine models: the BXSB and the MRL/l. Both of these strains develop early in their lives a spontaneous acute lupus, and each has a counterpart that manifests a late chronic form of the disease. The MRL/l mouse genome includes a lymphoproliferative (lpr) gene that is recessive and that in homozygous animals codes for a tremendous lymphoid proliferation, notably, a T-cell expansion. Both male and female MRL/l mice get SLE early, beginning as early as the second or third month of life, and have 50% mortality points of five and six months for the female and male, respectively.

The MRL/l mouse has a congenic counterpart, designated the MRL/n, a strain that for all practical purposes is genetically identical to it except that it lacks the lpr gene. The MRL/n mouse also develops spontaneous lupus but does so late in its life, with 50% mortality reached at 18 to 20 months. Because the two MRL strains are congenic and identical for their major histocompatibility complex (H-2), one can transfer cells from

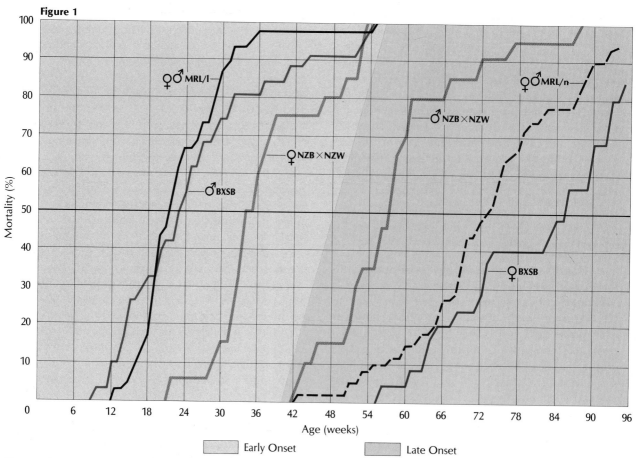

Figure 1

Mortality (%) vs Age (weeks)

Early Onset   Late Onset

Temporal patterns of murine SLE in various types of mice support the concept that accelerating factors operate on a background of lupus susceptibility. Thus, in MRL animals, the presence of lpr gene in "l" strain hastens onset of SLE, as compared with that seen in lpr-negative "n" strain. In both BXSB animals and NZ hybrids, sex determines the presence or absence of accelerating factors, although in opposite directions and for different physiologic reasons.

MRL/n to MRL/l mice freely, greatly facilitating study of the lupus and its associated phenomena. For unknown reasons, transfers in the opposite direction are not tolerated.

Like the MRL mice, the BXSB strain affords models of both early-onset and late-onset disease, but in this case the difference is dependent on the sex of the animal. Males spontaneously contract the early form, with the 50% mortality point at five to six months. Females develop late disease, with half dying by the latter half of the second year of life. Figure 1 on page 236 depicts the differing temporal patterns of disease in the various murine SLE models.

Also noteworthy is that the BXSB, MRL/l, and New Zealand mice all have very different breeding derivations. The BXSB strain is derived from a single cross between a C57 black female mouse and a satin beige (SB) male. The MRL/l animals have a much more complicated pedigree, having arisen, in the twelfth generation of MRL inbreeding, from a spontaneous mutation that gave rise to the lpr gene. The ancestry of the strain itself includes at least four different inbred strains, with estimated contributions to the MRL genome ranging from 0.3% to 75%. More important, as shown in Table 1 on this page, the three different murine models (MRL/l, BXSB, and NZ) have totally different genomal constitutions; each is of a different H-2 haplotype, and each has very different lymphocyte surface alloantigen repertoires and different IgG allotypes. The fact that SLE can arise spontaneously in animals of such varied and unrelated genetic constitutions may offer some insights into the failure to confirm speculations that human lupus susceptibility might be associated with a particular HLA serotype.

The finding that BXSB males develop SLE earlier than females of the same strain was somewhat surprising in view of the preponderance of human lupus prevalence in women. However, more recently R. G. Lahita and H. G. Kunkel have found that despite the

Table 1. Derivation of SLE Mice and Genetic Markers

Strain	Derivation	H-2	Lymphocyte Surface Alloantigens	IgG Allotype
NZB	Inbred for color from stock of undefined background	$H-2^d$	Thy-1,2, Ly-1,2, Ly-2,2, Ly-3,2, Qa-1[a], Mls[a]	e
NZW	Same as NZB	$H-2^Z$	Thy-1,2	e
BXSB	From (C57BL/6J × SB/Le) F_1	$H-2^b$	Thy-1,2, TL[−], Ly-1,2, Ly-2,2, Ly-3,2, Qa-1[b]	b
MRL/l	Genome = 75% LG, 13% AKR, 12% C3H, and 0.3% C57BL/6	$H-2^k$	Thy-1,2, TL[−], Ly-1,2, Ly-2,1, Ly-3,1, Qa-1[b]	a

truth of the generalization that SLE occurs more frequently in females than in males, the disease is not all that rare in males and there are families in which the disease occurs primarily in males and is transmitted through the fathers. It may well be that BXSB disease is a specific counterpart of one form of human lupus. This correlation is reinforced by the evidence that in the BXSB strain, lupus is specifically associated with the Y chromosome and is not hormonally mediated. Thus, castrated males do not differ from unmanipulated males in the temporal patterns of SLE onset or mortality. Even more convincing have been the results of cell transfer studies between males and females, as schematized in Figure 2 on page 238. If one transplants male bone marrow into lethally irradiated female recipients, the latter will develop "male disease," and vice versa.

The lack of direct hormonal influence on the pattern of disease development in the BXSB strain is in sharp contradistinction to the ability of female sex hormones to accelerate disease in the traditional New Zealand hybrid mouse. In these animals, females have a 50% mortality at around nine months of age, and the males reach this end

point at 14 to 15 months. These mortality rates can virtually be reversed by early castration plus appropriate sex hormone therapy. For example, a castrated and estrogen-treated male will have much earlier disease, and a castrated and androgen-treated female much later disease.

In the course of this review, we have thus far noted three distinct accelerating factors: the lpr gene in MRL animals; the Y chromosome, or gene(s) on the Y chromosome, in the BXSB strain; and female sex hormones in the New Zealand mice. Interestingly, each of these "normally" operate in very different autoimmune genetic backgrounds. However, crossbreeding studies show that these accelerating factors can operate in unfamiliar autoimmune backgrounds, as summarized in Figure 3 on page 238. Thus, when one crosses a BXSB female with a New Zealand male, the offspring will show the SLE patterns of the NZ animals. For example, the female offspring of the BXSB female × NZB male mating will get early disease, and the male offspring of the same cross will get late disease. Similarly, a BXSB male can convey, via transmission of his Y chromosome, the predilection for early disease to the male offspring

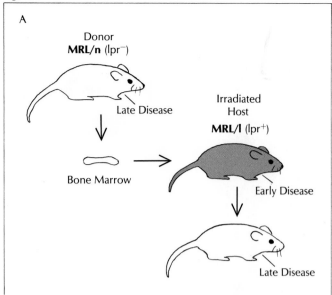

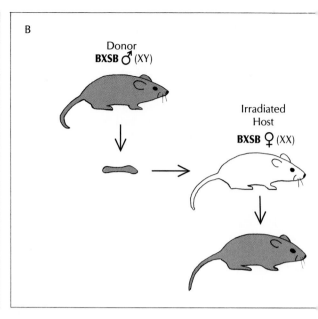

Bone marrow cell transfer experiments demonstrated that genomic constituents can be transplanted, with resultant alter- *ation of lupus-onset patterns. Marrow from MRL/n mice will delay SLE expression in MRL/l mice (A). In BXSB males and*

of his mating with an NZB or MRL female. Because the accelerating factor in the MRL/l animals is a recessive gene that is expressed only in homozygotes, one cannot test its expression by crossbreeding with other strains that do not carry the lpr. However, Murphy and Roths have engrafted the lpr gene into NZB mice and found that they get sick very early. Normally, NZB mice do not manifest SLE until the second year of life.

In summary, the accelerating factors can operate rather indiscriminately on any lupus background. However, it is important to stress that they have little effect on the normal mouse, i.e., one that will not spontaneously develop SLE. It would appear that a lupus genetic background is sufficient to assure the development of autoimmune disease late in the animal's life; early disease will develop only if an additional accelerating factor is present.

To this point, the discussion has been limited to endogenous accelerating factors. There is, in addition, one other kind of accelerating factor that is interesting in that it is completely exogenous: chronic lymphochoriomeningitis (LCM) virus infection initiated at birth. In normal, nonlupus animals, such

chronic infections predispose to a chronic, low-level antigenemia and to the formation of antigen–antibody complexes, and consequently to a mild, chronic glomerulonephritis. In any of the lupus mice, on the other hand, LCM virus infection at birth rapidly leads to a fulminant immune-complex lupuslike disease that is fatal within the first

few months of life. Once again, we have a situation in which an accelerating factor, this time an exogenous infectious agent, can dramatically alter the course of autoimmunity, changing a slow, rather indolent process into a rapidly lethal one.

Having discussed the genetic aspects of SLE in murine models,

Figure 3

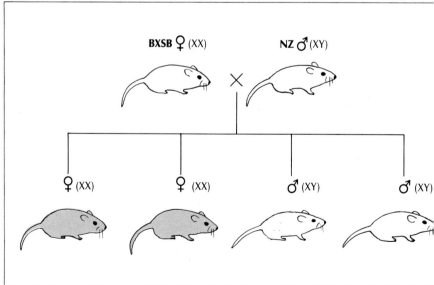

Offspring of BXSB females and NZ hybrid males will segregate, with respect to lupus patterns, on the basis of whether they carry the NZ X chromosome for early disease. Thus, females that get one X from each parent express disease in the second six months

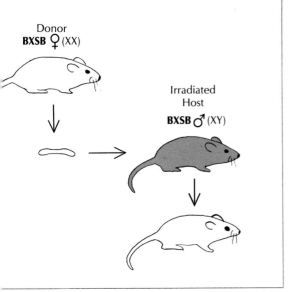

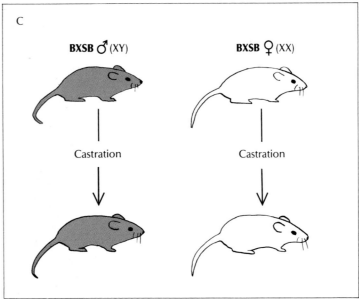

females, marrow transplants in either direction will result in either sex's having lupus typical of the other (B). Lupus expression in BXSB mice is not hormonally dependent, as shown by castration experiments (C).

and the apparent interrelationships between gene backgrounds and the factors that influence the age at which a genetic predisposition is likely to be expressed as autoimmune disease, we can turn now to some of the immunologic common denominators of the disease.

Constitutional differences notwithstanding, all SLE mice develop disease with striking immunopathologic similarities. Circulating immune complexes are found in the course of reactions between autoantigens and autoantibodies. In each strain, the circulating immune complexes are deposited in the kidneys and lead to a lupus nephritis; in all strains, there is also complex deposition in other vessels and, as will be discussed later, particularly in the coronaries. All have antinuclear antigen (ANA) antibodies that participate in immune complex formation. The animals also make antibodies to a glycoprotein identical to or closely resembling a molecule derived from retrovirus, the so-called gp70. However, it is worth stressing that gp70 is an invariable constituent of the sera of all mice, healthy and sick, and is never associated with virus production or viremia. The singular phenomenon in the lupus mice that distinguishes them from all other mice is the ability to react to gp70 immunologically, i.e., with specific antibody. This is not in itself surprising, particularly if one regards gp70 as a normal murine serum protein, since the lupus mice almost, by definition, make a wide variety of autoantibodies. Indeed, gp70 behaves in these mice very much like an acute-phase reactant and has the characteristics of a number of human acute-phase reactants, including C-reactive protein and serum amyloid protein. gp70 is stimulated by almost any inflammatory process.

The point worth emphasizing with respect to gp70 is that its presence, and the presence of its

of life (as in NZB×NZW), whereas males that, of necessity, get their X chromosome from the BXSB parent will develop late disease. If the sire is BXSB, offspring that receive his Y chromosome will develop the hyperacute form of lupus (as in male BXSB).

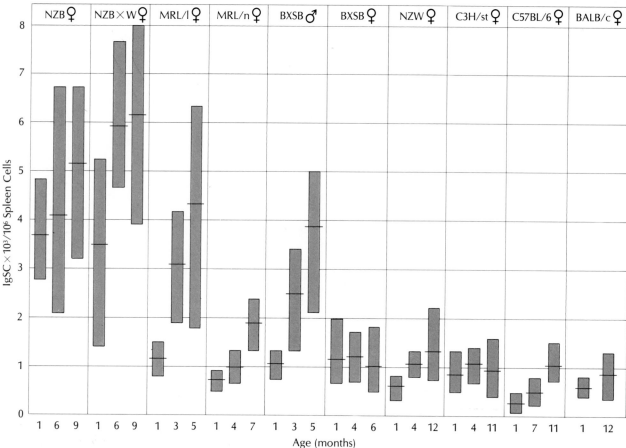

The importance of B-cell hyperactivity in susceptibility to murine lupus is supported by the fact that all of the autoimmune strains show higher frequency of immunoglobulin-secreting cells (IgSC) than do matched immunologically normal mice.

antibody, in lupus mice do not argue for direct viral participation in the pathogenesis of SLE. Its association with retrovirus could well be coincidental, or it might well be that the virus has acquired the glycoprotein from its mammalian hosts, rather than vice versa.

Clearly, murine SLE, like lupus and other autoimmune diseases in humans, is associated with more than one autoimmune response. In the light of this, it has been tempting to speculate that the whole immune system must be predisposed to hyperreactivity and autoimmune phenomena. This attitude has prevailed for many years, and more recently, with the growing knowledge of the modulation of the immunologic system by regulatory T cells—helper and suppressor—it was only natural to suspect that this autoimmune disease might well result from a breakdown in T-cell regulation, particularly from a lack of suppressor cells.

There have been numerous reports, related to both murine and human lupus, implicating defects in suppressor T cells. At least in our experience, this implication has not held up. We have now done extensive studies in the murine systems and have found few, if any, T-cell regulatory abnormalities, particularly early in life. In the young animal destined to develop SLE, B-cell abnormalities are clearly in evidence, whereas suppressor T cells react perfectly normally. A number of other investigators critically reexamining the suppressor T-cell situation in both humans and mice have reported similar results. We have found that employing either nonspecific mitogenic stimulation with concanavalin A or antigen-specific stimulation with urea-denatured ovalbumin, we could induce perfectly normal suppressor activity in all three strains of lupus mice.

As for helper T-cell activity, only one murine model, the MRL/l, shows abnormal helper T-cell function. It will be recalled that the factor in MRL/l mice that accelerates the disease is the lpr gene, which codes specifically for a helper T-cell lymphoproliferation. Therefore, in the MRL/l mice, one does see an enhancement of helper T-cell activity. This is not paralleled in the other models, which do not manifest the same kind of T-cell hyperplasia.

To make the T-cell story complete it should also be noted that R. M. Zinkernagel has shown that in lupus mice cytolytic T-cell activity is perfectly normal. We also have observed in the course of our studies on suppressor T-cell activity that the B cells of lupus animals are completely capable of receiving and responding to suppressor T-cell signals.

What has been consistently and repeatedly shown is that one of the most characteristic abnormalities of all lupus animals is a B-cell hyperactivity. Figure 4 on page 240 presents some of these findings. This hyperactivity can be detected soon after birth. It is reflected in a magnified response to lipopoly-saccharide, particularly in very young New Zealand animals; in increased IgM levels in unmanipulated animals; and in increased plaque formation to haptens to which the animals have not previously been exposed. The last is generally accepted as a response reflecting so-called polyclonal B-cell activation. It also has been shown that lupus animals are generally more resistant to the induction of tolerance (see Figure 5 on this page), and this would be an expected finding in the presence of B-cell hyperactivity since such hyperactivity implies the presence of more immunoglobulin-secreting and Ig-containing cells than normal. For example, if one presents a young lupus mouse with monomeric or deaggregated human gamma globulin in doses that could be expected to induce tolerance, the lupus animals will respond to the human gamma globulin.

In addition to these general indicators of B-cell hyperactivity in lupus mice, there are some rather more specific findings suggestive of an earlier-than-normal maturation of the B-cell system. For instance, it has been shown that the B lymphocytes switch from IgM to IgG secretion in lupus mice before they do so in immunologically normal animals. Furthermore, surface molecules, including receptors, mature at a younger age in the lupus models than they do in other mice. This is reflected in an increased IgD:IgM ratio and in the "premature" presence of complement (C3) receptors. All of these observations point to a polyclonal, nonspecific hyperactivity of B cells occurring in the first weeks or months of life in lupus animals. Finally, there is evidence that these phenomena are directly related to the age of onset of SLE; the premature maturation of the B-cell system will take place sooner in the mice destined to get earlier acute lupus than in the congenic or sex counterpart animals that do not develop SLE until late in life. When everything is taken together, the argument for the primacy of B cell-system abnormalities in the etiology of murine lupus is most compelling. One can start this argument at either end of the disease spectrum. The first immunologic abnormalities seen in the lupus animals consist of phenomena related to nonspecific B-cell hyperactivity. In full-blown disease, the immunologic pattern is one of hyperactive B-cell antibody secretion and consequent formation of immune complexes.

In contrast, the only T-cell regulatory function that differs in lupus mice from that seen in normal mice is the proliferation of helper T cells in the MRL/l strain. It should be emphasized that assigning a secondary role to T cells in the immunopathology of murine lupus does not preclude an important role for the thymus. Indeed, as summarized in Figure 6 on page 242, the thymus does appear to be a significant participant in the immunopathologic processes of autoimmunity, with the nature and direction of that participation showing interesting strain-to-strain variation. A number of studies have been done with early and late thymectomy in the New Zealand hybrid, and the weight of evidence suggests that neonatal or early thymectomy will accelerate development of the disease to some extent.

This is in direct contrast to observations in the MRL/l animals. Here early thymectomy will actually prevent development of lupus en-

Figure 5

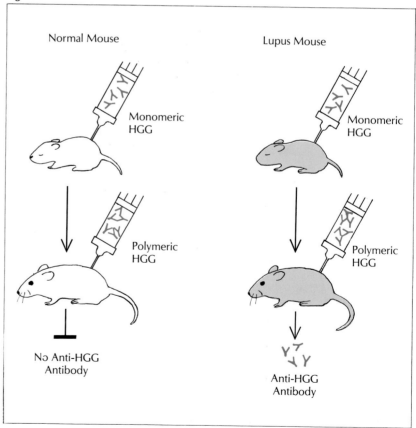

Normal Mouse

Lupus Mouse

Monomeric HGG

Monomeric HGG

Polymeric HGG

Polymeric HGG

No Anti-HGG Antibody

Anti-HGG Antibody

The resistance to specific tolerance in lupus mice can be shown by comparing their response to tolerogenic monomeric human gamma globulin with that of normal mice. The latter will show tolerance on subsequent challenge with immunogenic HGG; the autoimmune mice will respond to such challenge with detectable specific antibody.

Figure 6

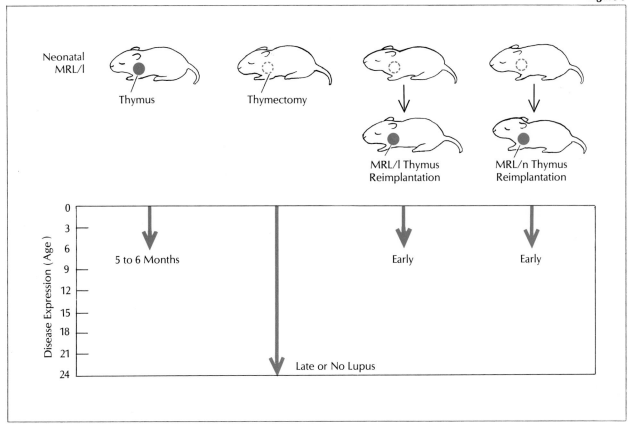

The thymus is necessary for early expression of lupus in MRL/l mice, but its role is apparently not strain-specific. Thus, neonatal thymectomy will delay or obviate the development of SLE in MRL/l mice. However, reconstitution with either an MRL/l or an MRL/n thymus will equally restore the capacity for early onset of SLE. Interestingly, neonatal thymectomy in (NZB×NZW) F₁ and in BXSB mice has no retarding effect on the lupus and in some instances may even slightly accelerate the disease.

tirely, or at least retard development until late in the animal's life. The thymus appears to be an essential element for pathogenesis. If one transplants a thymus back into the previously thymectomized MRL/l mouse, the animal will develop SLE in the same time frame and with the same severity as an unmanipulated animal. Interestingly, the thymus used for reconstitution need not be MRL/l in derivation. The thymectomized mouse can be given an organ from the congenic MRL/n mouse and still go on to a full-blown case of early, fulminant lupus. Thus, it can be concluded that there is nothing inherently abnormal in the MRL/l thymus, but a thymic environment is necessary for the autoimmune events that lead to SLE.

In addition to providing a set of models that permits study of the varied facets of lupus as an auto-immune disease, the mouse strains that we have been discussing may afford investigators models of two other important human diseases. The first of these involves the development of a vascular disease that had not previously been associated with immunologic events and phenomena. It is a noninflammatory, or at least nonexudative, degenerative vascular disease. Although it can occur anywhere in the vasculature, it is best seen in the coronary system and is associated with myocardial infarction.

The underlying lesion can be found in about 20% of the lupus mice if one looks for it when the animals are sacrificed late in their lives. It is associated with myocardial infarction at about the same frequency in all of the strains and seems to be no more frequent in mice with polyarteritis than in those without it. In some cross-breeding experiments, the frequency of infarcts in the myocardium have been extremely high. For example, in one cross involving an NZW female and a BXSB male, the coronary vascular disease with associated myocardial infarction was found at autopsy in 80% of the males and 30% of the females of the F₁ generation.

Typical lesions are illustrated in Figure 7 on page 243. Characteristically, one sees a deposition of immune complexes in which complement, gamma globulin, and gp70 antigen are localized in vessel walls. Incidentally, gp70 is the only antigen that has been systematically looked for in these lesions, so that one cannot exclude the possibility that other antigens are present. The immune complexes can be found in the coronary vessel walls but are not associated with cellular inflammation as a rule. The depos-

Figure 7

Murine SLE Models

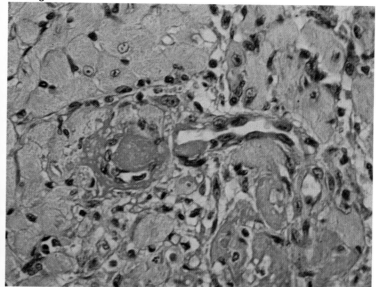

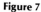

Coronary artery disease, often associated with myocardial infarction, occurs in about 20% of lupus mice. Micrograph at left shows degenerative disease of small coronary vessel (center) and myocardial infarction (lower right). Vessel wall contains PAS-positive immune deposits, and lumen is partially occluded by thrombus. Pair of photos directly below show immune deposits in a longitudinal section of a small coronary. Deposits are revealed by PAS staining and by immunofluorescent C3 stained with fluorescein-labeled antibody. This was early disease, and inflammatory response is lacking. At bottom left is a medium-sized coronary artery with substantial PAS-positive immune deposits in subendothelium and media. Alongside is corresponding fluorescein-labeled immunoglobulin-stained specimen.

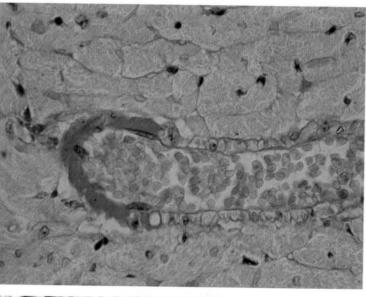

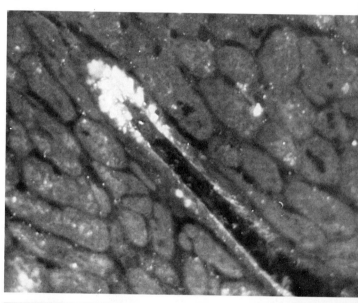

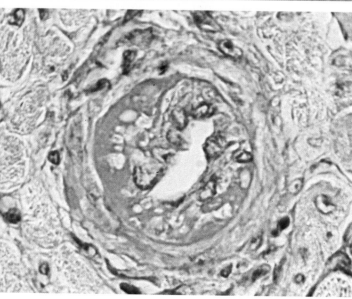

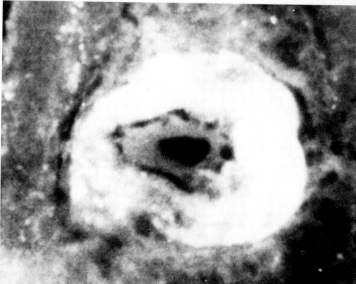

Figure 8

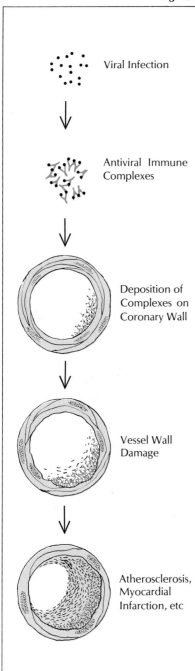

Viral Infection

↓

Antiviral Immune Complexes

↓

Deposition of Complexes on Coronary Wall

↓

Vessel Wall Damage

↓

Atherosclerosis, Myocardial Infarction, etc

A sequence for the development of early coronary disease in humans is suggested by the finding of immune complexes in coronary vessel walls in lupus animals that have a high frequency of myocardial infarction. The concept is that immune complexes formed in the wake of a viral infection or other antigenic exposure are deposited in vessel walls, with subsequent complement fixation and inflammatory damage to the intima and wall and, finally, superimposition of both atheromatous and thrombotic occlusive processes.

its are PAS-positive and identifiable by immunofluorescence. The coronary disease is virtually always associated with glomerulonephritis. The infarcts are frequently very large—sometimes extensive enough to cause ventricular rupture.

How does this experimental disease relate to human disease? As improved treatment has prolonged the lives of SLE patients, it has become quite clear that they are developing coronary disease with an increased incidence, as compared with persons without lupus. The disease in humans recently has been reported to be associated with the deposition of immune complexes in the vessel walls. However, the lesion in humans has largely been masked by atheroma, and it seems very likely that the atherosclerotic lesions are localizing at the sites of immune complex deposition. The mice are incapable of developing atherosclerosis because they lack lipid receptors on their vessel walls; therefore, one sees the pure immunologic disease in the mice, whereas in humans one sees the combined immunologic-atherosclerotic lesion.

These observations lead to the question: Could immune complex insult be responsible for some of the non-lupus-related coronary disease seen in humans?

We know that there are many situations in which immune complexes circulate temporarily following viral and other infections. There are also diseases characterized by chronic circulation of immune complexes. It seems entirely reasonable to hypothesize that deposits of these complexes in vessels generally, and in coronary vessels particularly, could lead to a chronic degenerative vascular process that in humans, in turn, might predispose to atherosclerosis. This hypothesis remains untested but could be particularly plausible in the instances of coronary disease in young people, who so frequently have viral infections—the common childhood diseases that may well be associated with elevated levels of circulating complexes. This concept is schematized in Figure 8 at the left.

There is still one more excursion away from SLE that is worth taking before returning to that disease. This one involves the rheumatoid arthritis model that has emerged almost serendipitously from these studies. In the MRL/1 mice only, it has been shown that more than 609 of the animals develop rheumatoid factor, and with it a rheumatoid arthritis that is clinically apparent in perhaps 20% of the older MRL/1 mice and microscopically detectable in 75% of them (see Figure 9 on page 245). It is, to my knowledge, the only spontaneous animal arthritis that is noninfectious in origin, has rheumatoid factor associated with it, and very closely resembles human rheumatoid arthritis in its manifestations: the vascular lesions, the synovial inflammation, the mononuclear infiltrates in the perisynovial and periarticular tissues, pannus formation, the destruction of cartilaginous joint surfaces, and, as a terminal event, the actual fusion of joints.

Returning now to lupus, brief mention of some of the observations bearing on treatment of the disease is merited. There are several manipulations that will delay the onset of lupus disease and/or slow its progression. Perhaps one of the more interesting is simple restriction of caloric intake. It has been found that animals that are on an approximately 50% reduced caloric intake will live about twice as long as those who feed ad libitum. It does not seem to matter what one does to curb calories, i.e., whether through fat restriction, carbohydrate restriction, or a combination of both. The restricted animals are smaller, but they are reasonably active and healthy looking. They do not get their SLE as early, and they do not contract kidney disease as quickly. Although the specifics of the effects of caloric restriction have not yet been closely studied, it has been shown that these regimens do delay the onset of autoimmune responses and, most specifically, delay the response to gp70.

It is possible that the caloric restriction may be essentially a form

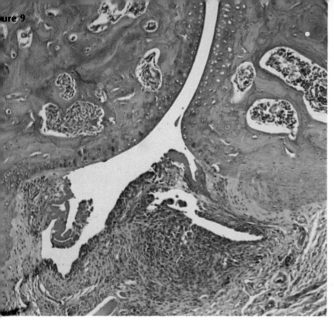
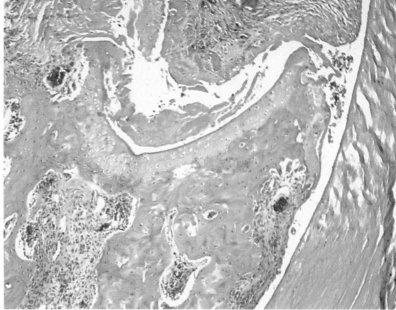

One lupus strain—the MRL/l mouse—has proved to be a rheumatoid arthritis model as well. Micrograph above shows section through knee joint of a five-month-old animal with inflammation of synovium and subsynovial tissue. Inflammatory process is beginning to extend along cartilaginous articular surfaces. The second photograph is of section through knee of 6½-month-old mouse. There is now almost complete destruction of joint surfaces, with partial fibrous ankylosis. Although a portion of the articular cartilage remains on the lower joint surface, the upper joint surface has been completely destroyed.

of immunosuppression, and indeed, almost any kind of nonspecific immunosuppression will delay or completely prevent SLE in the lupus mice. For example, cyclophosphamide will extend the lives of these mice for long periods of time. Perhaps the most effective and least injurious approach to treatment in mice has been the use of total lymphoid irradiation (see S. Strober, " Managing the Immune System with Total Lymphoid Irradiation"). Animals treated by TLI manifest little or no autoimmune responsivity and get little or no disease.

In conclusion, perhaps we could go back to the statement made at the outset of this review—i.e., auto-immunity is a generalized physiologic phenomenon that becomes pathologic only under specific circumstances. Are these circumstances defined by the quantity of reaction or by the target for the reaction? The answer probably is a little of each. If the target that the host recognizes and then responds to is not very critical to the whole organism, the process may well go unnoticed. If, on the other hand, inactivation or immobilization of the target would constitute a critical event for the host, then we are confronted with a clinical picture recognizable as autoimmune disease. Second, one can conceive of autoimmune responses to potentially pathogenic targets that are not quantitatively great enough to really produce disease, at least until a threshold level of response has been surpassed.

In murine lupus, and probably in human lupus, too, the quantitative pathogenic factor may well be the B-cell nonspecific hyperstimulation. Perhaps as an integral part of this hyperstimulation, and perhaps as a deviation within it, the B lymphocytes become particularly responsive to autoantigens. This possibility is certainly well within the framework of current immunologic thinking, since a hyperreactive B-cell system would have maximal opportunity to react to antigens that are ever-present.

22

The Immunopathology of SLE

HENRY G. KUNKEL   *The Rockefeller University*

Although not initially recognized as resulting from a reaction of autoantibody with tissue components, the lupus erythematosus (LE) cell phenomenon, first noted in the bone marrow of patients with systemic lupus erythematosus (SLE) by M. M. Hargraves et al in 1948, was the opening wedge for the current concept that at least some of the protean manifestations of the disease—most notably, lupus nephritis—are due to immunologically induced tissue injury. About 10 years later, when studies of sera from SLE patients identified gamma globulin (7S IgG) as the reactive serum fraction involved, and when specificity for deoxyribonucleoprotein was demonstrated, the immunologic nature of the LE cell phenomenon, observed in about 75% of patients with SLE, was established. But characterization of possible immunopathologic mechanisms in SLE had only begun. For example, immunofluorescence studies in the late 1950s also indicated the presence of gamma globulin and complement in vascular and glomerular lesions in the disease, but the relationship between these lesions and circulating antibody remained to be defined.

In the years since these early studies, perhaps the single most important fact to emerge from serologic investigations of SLE is that a *generalized* excessive autoantibody production characterizes the disease. The work of E. M. Tan, H. R. Holman, G. C. Sharp, M. Reichlin, and others has delineated a great number of different autoantibodies that may appear in the serum of these patients (see Table 1, page 250). Among the wide variety currently recognized in SLE are those directed against nuclear constituents (double- or single-stranded DNA, or both, deoxyribonucleoprotein, ribonucleoprotein, Sm antigen, and "carbohydrate-protein" antigens), cytoplasmic constituents (ribosomes, carbohydrate antigens, and lipid antigens), gamma globulin, soluble clotting factors, platelets, red cells, lymphocytes, and double- or single-stranded RNA.

Some of this antibody activity is also seen in other diseases, and some appears to be relatively specific for SLE. For example, the LE cell phenomenon, or anti-deoxyribonucleoprotein activity, occurs in about 15% of patients with other rheumatic diseases and predominates in drug-induced lupus-like syndromes; antibodies to single-stranded DNA (SDNA) can be found in rheumatoid arthritis, chronic active hepatitis, and primary biliary cirrhosis, and antibody to nuclear ribonucleoprotein in especially high titer is frequent in patients with so-called mixed connective tissue disease. On the other hand, although relatively low concentrations of antibodies to double-stranded, or native, DNA (NDNA) are present in other systemic rheumatic diseases, *high* titers of anti-NDNA are essentially seen only in SLE, and antibody to another nuclear constituent, Sm antigen, also seems to be highly selective for the disease. The exact cellular source(s) of the antigens against which these many antibodies are directed is unknown. Recent evidence by Schwartz and associates indicates that some monoclonal anti-DNA antibodies also react with phospholipids, such as cardiolipin, suggesting a relationship to the antibodies against clotting factors. Some of the antibodies—notably, those reactive with double-stranded RNA—cross-react with bacterial or viral polynucleotides, causing some to raise the possibility that exogenous agents may act as immunogens in the disease.

Reports of high titers of antibodies to certain herpesviruses or myxoviruses in patients with SLE and detection of viruslike structures in kidney, skin, and peripheral lymphocytes of affected patients support this view. However, some of the antibodies reactive with double-stranded RNA have also been shown to cross-react with single-stranded RNA and DNA, indicating that polynucleotides other than viral RNA may act as immunogens, and the virus-like structures, which also have been observed in other conditions, are widely in-

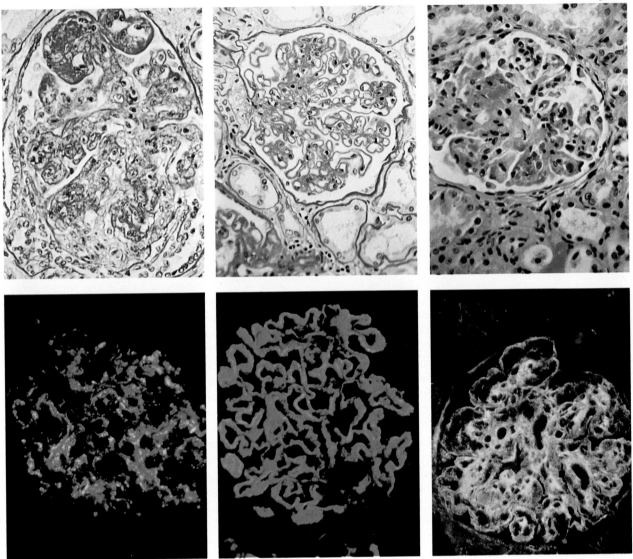

Three types of glomerular lesion commonly seen in lupus nephritis are represented in photomicrographs prepared by histologic (top) and fluorescent-antibody staining. In focal disease (left), one sees irregular thickening of the membrane and fusion of capillary tufts, with irregular deposits of immune complexes in the capillary walls. In membranous disease (center), the GBM thickening is more pronounced, and so-called wire-loop deposits are seen. In diffuse disease (right), structural damage is marked, and the immune deposits are massive so that normal glomerular architecture is obliterated. (Courtesy D. Koffler)

terpreted as representing intracellular degeneration. The great variety of antibodies found in SLE, moreover, would seem to argue against the viral infection hypothesis, especially since some of the antibodies present are directed against nuclear constituents seen only in mammalian cells. Nevertheless, the role of infection in the pathogenesis of SLE remains open to further study. Direct evidence linking other exogenous factors to a mild form of the disease, particularly such drugs as procainamide, provides support for the concept that environmental agents may serve as haptens and induce SLE or an SLE-like syndrome.

Circulating antibodies against NDNA were among the first to be described in patients with SLE. Aside from the usefulness of high titers in the diagnosis of the disease, measurements of anti-NDNA activity are also useful in monitoring patients, because markedly increased titers correlate closely with the onset of periods of clinical exacerbation. In terms of elucidating SLE immunopathology, however, one of the most important observations concerning NDNA antibodies is that increased titers are also closely correlated with depression of serum complement levels in patients with active (acute systemic, renal, or extensive skin) disease. Circulating immune complex formation has been implicated by the detection of NDNA itself in SLE sera, in the presence of anti-NDNA in some studies and alternating with anti-NDNA in others.

In the last few years, a large number of methods for the detection of immune complexes have been developed. All of these show marked elevations in SLE sera during acute episodes of the disease. This was first apparent in C1q agar-precipitin reactions and has been quantitated using the Raji assay and C1q-binding assays. Surprisingly, it still remains unknown what the composition of the major complexes detected by these procedures consists of. Some workers have obtained evidence for DNA complexes, but these do not appear to account for the major reactivity. One of the problems in studying circulating serum immune complexes is the probability that at least some of them represent complexes that are not removed and therefore are less important in tissue deposition.

This leads us to a consideration of the renal lesion in SLE, a consideration that is perhaps best begun by discussing complement depression in SLE. Hypocomplementemia may result from increased utilization in immune complex formation, reduced synthesis, or a combination of the two. In SLE, the mechanism of increased utilization is indicated by a number of findings. These include significant depression of early complement components in hypocomplementemic SLE sera, identification of early complement components in renal lesions, a high incidence of complement-fixing antinuclear antibodies (ANA) in SLE patients with active nephritis, Raji-cell binding and C1q-precipitin reactions in SLE sera, and increased anti-NDNA serum activity following DNAase treatment to free complexed antibody.

As that list suggests, there is much evidence for complement activation via the classic pathway in SLE. It should be noted, however, that a number of studies have revealed depression of serum C3 proactivator (factor B) and properdin in patients with the disease, and others have demonstrated the presence of properdin in glomerular deposits; hence, both the classic and alternative (properdin) pathways of complement activation may operate in SLE, with the former (judging from current assay techniques) more actively utilized.

As mentioned earlier, immunofluorescence studies indicate that the capillary tufts of renal glomeruli in patients with lupus nephritis contain deposits of immunoglobulin in association with complement. Similar deposits have been noted in SLE patients at the dermal-epidermal junction of both inflamed and normal sites. The resemblance of the renal deposits in SLE to those seen in experimental serum sickness, produced by repeated injection of antigen, has long been recognized; the same is true of spontaneous glomerulonephritis in NZB/W(F_1) mice, which has been shown to develop soon after the appearance of circulating ANA and to involve glomerular localization of immune complexes. Generally speaking, immune complex-type renal lesions show granular deposits in early disease and coarser, more lumpy (and more widespread) deposits in advanced disease.

In both NZB/W(F_1) mice and patients with lupus nephritis, circulating NDNA antibodies are present. These are usually 7S IgG, mostly identifiable as IgG_1 and IgG_3. These are the dominant complement-fixing IgG subclasses in man, and they are noteworthy for the ability to fix complement in tissues, in contrast to the antinucleoprotein type of ANA (which fixes complement poorly) that is typical of drug-induced lupus-like syndromes, in which nephritis is rare.

It has been noted that C1q is particularly prominent in the renal deposits of patients with lupus nephritis, and that this prominence might reflect the component's affinity for DNA in glomerular immune complexes. But what direct evidence exists for the presence of DNA complexes in the glomeruli? The best evidence yet uncovered comes from the work of D. Koffler and his associates from immunochemical analysis of eluates of glomeruli isolated from severely diseased kidneys. Treatment of the eluates with acid buffer and deoxyribonuclease indicates the frequent presence of antibodies reactive with both NDNA and SDNA; to a lesser extent, antibodies reactive with ribonucleoprotein are also present, while those reactive with double-stranded RNA are not demonstrable. Moreover, the DNA antibodies that are present in many, but not all, glomerular eluates from patients with lupus nephritis are in markedly enriched concentration (per milligram of gamma globulin), compared with serum levels—sometimes as much as a thousandfold richer. That immune complex deposition accounts for these findings is supported by the demonstration of DNA itself, distributed in a pattern similar to that of gamma globulin and complement, in glomeruli of kidneys from which DNA antibodies have been eluted; this requires pretreatment of the tissue with high-molarity salt solution and acid buffer, which allows subsequent challenge with highly purified fluorescein-labeled DNA antibodies.

Thus, there is compelling evidence that DNA immune complex systems participate in SLE—indeed, it might be said that the evidence regarding DNA complexes constitutes the cornerstone of the generally accepted view that SLE is the prototype of human immune complex disease. But, as might be expected from the variety of antibodies produced in SLE, there is also evidence that a variety of other immune complex systems participate as well. We have already alluded to cryoglobulins in SLE sera. It has long been recognized that sera from patients with active disease sometimes show a precipitate when placed in the cold, which itself is suggestive of immune complexes, because these tend to be less soluble at low temperature. Clinically, cryoglobulinemia has been correlated with active SLE in a number of patients, especially those with nephritis. Immunochemical analysis also has established that cryoglobulins *are* mainly composed of immune complexes, the most prominent of which appear to be IgG-anti-IgG complexes involving mixed 19S and 7S antibody; other antibodies selectively concentrated in cryoglobulins are similar to those found in glomerular eluates, mainly anti-NDNA and anti-SDNA, but occasionally antinuclear ribonucleoprotein antibody.

In addition, studies with C1q suggest a relationship between cryoglobulins and this molecule, which, of course, is the initiating component in complement fixation. Both cryoglobulin and C1q-reactive globulins usually appear in SLE sera during rises in anti-DNA titers. Specifically, it has been found that high molecular weight complexes containing IgM antibodies are present in cryoglobulins. This is paralleled by the finding of significant glomerular deposition of IgM in renal biopsies from SLE patients with circulating cryoglobulins. In several of these biopsies, moreover, IgM rheumatoid factor (RF) activity was demonstrable in the deposits; in one case, identical RF antigen was demonstrated in a patient's circulating cryoglobulin and in glomerular deposits via fluorescein-labeled

antibody with idiotypic specificity. C1q-reactive globulin studies also have demonstrated low molecular weight material in SLE sera that is associated with hypocomplementemia and disease activity. Current evidence indicates that these are special 7S gamma globulins that specifically activate the complement system. However, the possibility that they represent complexes of gamma globulin and small antigens has not been ruled out. Certain patients with a lupus-like syndrome (Agnello syndrome) have high concentrations of these C1q-reactive substances that appear to cause the complement depletion in vivo.

As for other immune complex systems implicated in SLE, there is a certain amount of overlap with our previous comments. For instance, antilymphocyte antibody has been found in selective high concentration in certain cryoglobu-

lins, and the same is true, in a few instances, of antiribonucleoprotein antibody. Regarding the latter, however, it should also be noted that in some serial studies most patients either have constantly elevated antiribonucleoprotein titers throughout their clinical course or show no titers at all, although a few do show peaks of activity. In addition, antiribonucleoprotein antibodies, but not the antigen, have been demonstrated in a few glomerular eluates in severe lupus nephritis. Finally, antiribosomal antibodies appear in increased incidence (25% to 50% in various studies) in the sera of SLE patients, and precipitating antibodies are prevalent in those with severe renal disease; the major antigenic determinant is ribosomal RNA.

Although there is abundant evidence for heterogeneous immune complex localization in renal glomeruli of patients with SLE, the mechanism(s) by which tissue injury is thereby produced remains unknown; it is not entirely clear whether circulating immune complexes are deposited directly in the glomeruli (the most widely accepted hypothesis), whether complex formation takes place in situ, or whether both processes may sometimes obtain. Clinically, however, the renal lesion has been classified into fairly distinct and generally accepted histologic types that are useful in assessing prognosis (see **Figure 1, page 248**). Mesangial deposition, for example, is associated with mild disease or the absence of renal disease, as is a less common pattern of linear deposition; the mesangium of the glomerulus is noteworthy for its ability to clear macromolecular substances from the blood and would thus appear to be the kidney's primary defense against circulating immune complexes. Somewhat more serious is focal proliferative deposition, in which less than 50% of glomeruli have mesangial and segmental endothelial-cell proliferation, irregular capillary-loop thickening, and varying numbers of active lesions; although its prognosis is variable, focal disease usually does not progress and generally responds to therapy

Table 1. Humoral Antibodies in SLE	
Of Diagnostic Importance	
Anti-native DNA	Most widely used for diagnosis and assessing disease activity
Anti-deoxyribonucleoprotein	Responsible for the production of LE cells in vitro; occurs in drug-induced LE
Anti-Sm	Highly specific for SLE; poor correlation with disease activity
Anti-nuclear ribonucleoprotein	Found in a variety of rheumatoid diseases; in high titer in overlap syndrome
Anti-cardiolipins	Biologic false-positive test for syphilis has been useful as a screening test for detecting patients with asymptomatic SLE
Immune Complex Formation Has Been Suggested	
Anti-native DNA Anti-single-stranded DNA Anti-nuclear ribonucleoprotein	Selective concentration in glomerular eluates and cryoglobulins has been observed; DNA antigens in serum and glomerular lesions
Anti-gamma globulin, 7S and 19S (rheumatoid factors)	Associated with cryoglobulinemia; correlated with disease activity in certain patients; demonstrated in glomerular deposits in certain cases
Anti-ribosome	Increased incidence in severe renal disease
Anti-lymphocyte	Selective concentration in certain cryoglobulins
Antibodies That Combine With In Situ Antigens and May Exert Direct Cytotoxic Effects	
Anti-red cell surface antigens	Associated with hemolytic anemia
Anti-lymphocyte	Associated with lymphopenia
Anti-platelet	Associated with thrombocytopenia
Anti-coagulant	Associated with hemostatic disorders

Figure 2

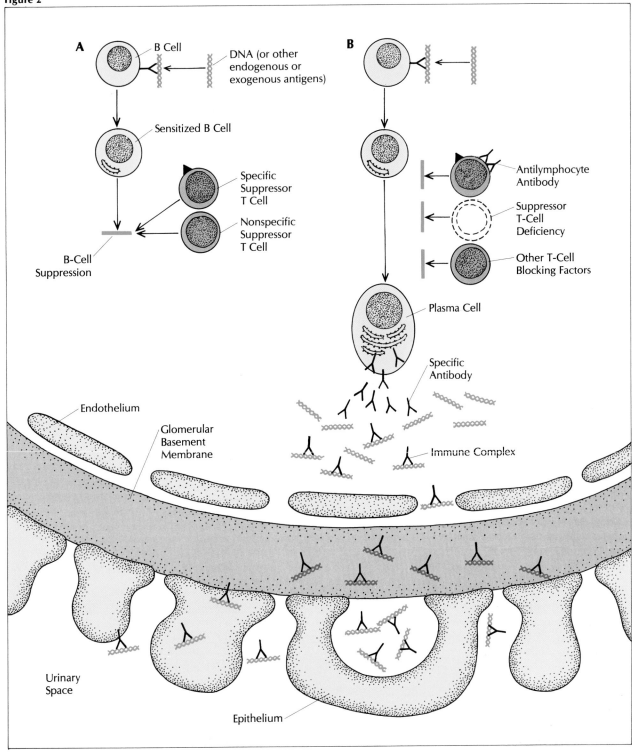

Immunopathologically, SLE is characterized by the formation and deposition of immune (antigen-antibody) complexes in target tissues, such as the glomerular basement membrane (GBM). One hypothesis implicates hypoactivity of the suppressor T cells as the underlying "lesion." The suggestion is that in the normal individual (A), immunoglobulin-secreting B cells are frequently sensitized by DNA or by other circulating antigens, but their differentiation to secretory plasma cells is interrupted by interaction with suppressor T cells that may be either antigen-specific or -nonspecific. In the SLE patient (B), differentiation and antibody secretion occur because the suppressor T cells fail to act. Such failure could be accounted for by the presence of antilymphocyte antibodies directed against the suppressor cells, by a quantitative or qualitative deficiency in their population, or by a number of other blocking factors. At any rate, the immunized B cell goes on to produce, for example, anti-DNA antibodies that combine with DNA in the circulation to form immune complexes that are trapped or deposited in GBM.

Figure 3

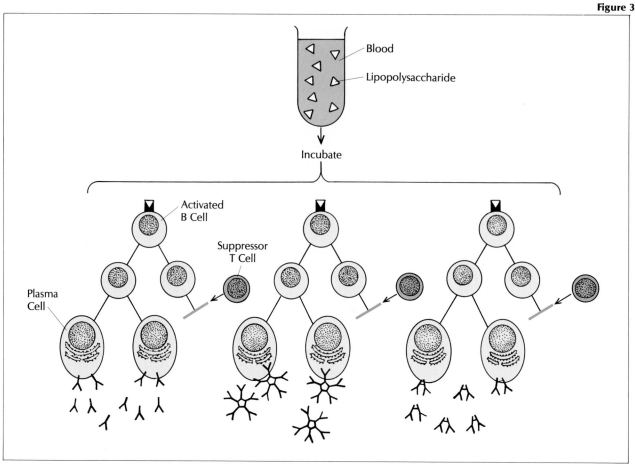

The concept of polyclonal B-cell activation is derived from experiments, graphically summarized above, that have demonstrated that when such substances as lipopolysaccharide (LPS) are incubated with blood from normal individuals, B lymphocytes will be activated to produce a wide range of antibodies of different types, including autoantibodies. Theoretically, such activation could occur in vivo in SLE with endogenous cell-membrane LPS or viral or bacterial LPS polyclonally activating B cells. Even if the suppressor T-cell function were normal, it might be quantitatively inadequate to cope with the enhanced population of activated B cells; if the suppressor T-cell population were deficient, the excess of antibodies would be exacerbated. This excess would, in turn, lead to the immune complex formation and deposition characteristic of the pathology seen in patients with SLE. The figure shows three types of antibodies produced in the polyclonal activation.

(five-year survival is about 75%), particularly with early diagnosis.

In contrast, diffuse proliferative disease (greater than 50% of glomeruli affected) is associated with a mortality of up to 50% within the first two years of diagnosis and typically establishes itself rapidly within the first year of SLE onset; it is characterized by coarse, massive deposition of Ig and complement that predominates in subendothelial sites along capillary loops. Finally, about 10% to 15% of patients with lupus nephritis have a membranous lesion in which there is a diffuse thickening of the basement membrane (but little other distortion of renal architecture) and wide-spread granular deposition, typically in subepithelial sites; nephrotic syndrome is associated with this lesion, but progression to renal failure is usually slow, and with therapy the five-year survival approaches 70%.

Although in occasional patients there may be some overlap of histologic types and although the mesangial lesion is considered by some investigators to be the lowest common denominator of lupus nephritis, these categories are generally regarded as discrete. In particular, the distinction between membranous and diffuse proliferative disease seems quite valid, but the former has presented some problems for investigators wishing to account for the development of its deposition pattern. Essentially, the question is this: If circulating immune complexes are localized in the basement membrane of renal glomeruli, does membranous deposition occur after subendothelial sites are involved, with the immune complexes somehow penetrating and migrating across the membrane to lodge on the subepithelial side? If so, then why the virtual lack of clinical overlap between membranous and proliferative disease? In animals injected with immune complexes, the proliferative type of glomerulonephritis has predominated, and in some studies subepithelial deposition has failed to develop at all; but recently, injection of immune complexes composed of low-avidity antibodies has consistently produced membranous lesions simulating those in man, apparently upholding the distinction between membranous and proliferative lupus nephritis.

Our discussion thus far has emphasized the kidney in SLE because that is where the disease poses its greatest threat. Other organ systems, of course, may be involved, ranging from the joints and muscles, the hematopoietic system, the pleura, and the eyes (all of which are frequently affected) to the lungs, heart, and GI system (which are uncommonly affected).

One other manifestation of SLE that is increasingly being seen and deserves more than passing mention is central nervous system involvement. This covers a broad range of problems, poorly understood and generally developing later than renal disease; patients with long-standing SLE predominate and will probably do so to an even greater extent as survival in SLE continues to improve.

The signs and symptoms are variable—in some patients relentlessly progressive in nature and in others, perhaps the majority, episodic—but the major manifestations include seizures, focal neurologic deficits, organic mental syndromes, and nonorganic mental syndromes. When organic mental syndromes and focal neurologic deficits are present, the prognosis appears to be poorer than when seizures and nonorganic mental syndromes are present. Microscopically, the CNS lesion seems to involve small vessels and spare the large ones. Perivascular gliosis, hemorrhage, and micro- or macroinfarcts are frequent findings; fibrinoid necrosis and vasculitis are infrequent. The vascular changes, however, do not account for many of the CNS manifestations, and other mechanisms, such as direct action of autoantibodies, have been considered.

One major question, of course, is whether immune complexes are responsible for central nervous sys-

tem damage in SLE. Some immunofluorescence studies indicate granular deposits of immunoglobulin and complement in the choroid plexus and few or no deposits in the parenchyma; the pathologic significance of these deposits is obscure, and they have been noted in SLE patients with and without overt neurologic disease. Analysis of cerebrospinal fluid has yet to produce cogent evidence of immune complexes in SLE; cerebrospinal fluid levels of C4 may be depressed, but this has not been correlated with the clinical activity of the central nervous system lesion. Recent interest has centered on specific antibodies that react with nervous tissue cells in culture. Some of these are specific for these tissues, but most also react with other cells. Special interest has centered on elevated relative levels of certain of these antibodies in the spinal fluid.

Having considered at some length two of the most salient immunologic features of SLE—generalized enhancement of autoantibody production and the evidence that the renal lesion in the disease entails immune complexes—let us now turn to the question of what may be responsible for the hyperactivity of B cells responsible for producing these antibodies. The answer is far from clear, but one possible clue lies in a type of antibody activity that has been barely mentioned thus far—that of antilymphocyte antibodies. These antibodies are frequently present in the sera of SLE patients and of NZB/W(F_1) mice, and in both cases their presence has been correlated with reduced counts of peripheral lymphocytes. In some studies, a "predominant specificity" for T-cell lymphocytes has been indicated, but it is now clear that both T and B cells may be targets for these antibodies. It is more widely accepted, however, that patients with SLE do frequently manifest depression of T-lymphocyte function, as evidenced by impaired delayed hypersensitivity reactions and decreased response to mitogens. Although it remains to be shown whether these abnormalities reflect a primary or secondary im-

munopathologic mechanism in SLE, the findings have generated interest in the hypothesis that the disease might involve a loss of T-cell suppressor activity (see Figure 2, page 251).

According to this hypothesis, antilymphocyte antibody activity in SLE depletes the population of suppressor T cells, subverting the mechanism that ordinarily blocks the development of autoantibodies and autoimmune disease. There is a fairly substantial body of data that tends to support this view. In murine models of SLE, for example, antibody responses that are under suppressor T-cell limitation (e.g., those against pneumococcal polysaccharide, poly I-C, and PVP) have been found to increase with age, correlatively with the age-related development of autoimmune disease; the ability of spleen cells from NZB/W(F_1) mice to mediate graft-versus-host reactions has also been found to be enhanced with age. Concanavalin A stimulation of suppressor activity in vitro has been noted as lower than normal in sera from patients with SLE, and in NZB/W(F_1) mice similar findings have been attributed in one study to a defect at the T-cell level. Finally, deficient functioning of an Ly123 T-cell subset (the phenotype to which suppressor T cells belong) has been found in two different mouse strains with spontaneous autoimmune disease. However, the evidence in humans is very tentative, primarily because no adequate methodology is available as yet to quantitate suppressor cells. The Con A generated system has been widely criticized.

Loss of T-cell suppressor activity in SLE is an appealing hypothesis, but it should be acknowledged that there is also a fairly substantial body of data that argues against this view. With age, for instance, the spleens of NZB/W(F_1) mice have been reported to have increased rather than decreased numbers of suppressor cells; similarly, thymocyte-mediated nonspecific antigen suppression has been found not to wane with age in hereditarily asplenic or immunologically normal

NZB/W(F_1) mice. Moreover, in the presence of virally infected cells, cytotoxic T-cell responses in NZB/W(F_1) mice have been reported to be normal, and a recent study of three autoimmune murine strains showed normal antigen-specific B- and T-cell functions (the latter including both helper and suppressor types) in old and young animals.

More recently, the possible role of polyclonal B-cell activators in SLE has aroused a good deal of interest. Experimentally, it has been shown that injection of such substances as lipopolysaccharide stimulates production of a wide variety of antibodies similar to some of those found in SLE (see Figure 3, page 252). The source(s) of polyclonal B-cell activators may be endogenous (e.g., certain nucleic acids and steroid hormones) or exogenous (e.g., viruses, bacteria, and protozoa). Possible support for this concept is seen in studies of Ig synthesis of lupus B lymphocytes. Even though these cells are less responsive than normal cells to B-cell mitogens, they show increased spontaneous Ig synthesis. This suggests that there is a natural stimulus present in the SLE patients. The exact relevance of this phenomenon has yet to be determined, but it would appear to be intimately related to concepts of

suppressor function in the disease. Specifically, it has been suggested that polyclonal B-cell activation may contribute to an overwhelming of an already taxed or deficient suppressor T-cell function and perhaps transform inactive disease into active SLE.

Although most interest today focuses on the question of B-lymphocyte activation and suppressor activity in SLE, other hypotheses—in varying degrees also supported by one set of findings on the one hand and refuted by another set on the other—have been proposed to explain autoantibody production in the disease. For example, there is Burnet's forbidden clone theory, which proposes that autoimmune responses are derived from lymphocyte clones sensitized to antigens that have somehow emerged from sequestration. This theory has fallen out of favor with the increased evidence for low levels of many autoantibodies in normal individuals and the production of autoantibodies in culture systems of normals free of suppressor influences.

Since the functioning of the immune system is in part genetically determined, one notable gap in our discussion thus far concerns evidence for a genetic component in SLE. As is well known, the disease

occurs more frequently in close relatives of SLE patients. Although environmental factors may play a role in familial clustering, recent studies indicate that SLE frequently is associated with certain allelic forms of B-cell histocompatibility antigens and that the presence of these antigens may reflect an increased susceptibility to SLE. Specifically, B-cell alloantigens of the HLA-D region (with biologic and chemical homologies with antigens of the I region of the major histocompatibility locus in the mouse) have been implicated by A. Gibofsky and R. Winchester in recently developed complement-dependent cytotoxicity assays using human pregnancy sera having no reactivity with HLA-A, HLA-B, or HLA-C antigens. Two HLA-DR antigens, DR2 and DR3, have each been observed in approximately 2:1 frequency in SLE, compared with normal controls; it is of interest that this pattern is distinct from that found in patients with rheumatoid arthritis, which has been associated with an increased frequency of HLA-DR4. In addition, J. L. Reinertsen and coworkers have reported that a single B-cell alloantiserum, Ia-715, which cross-reacts with DR2 and other HLA-DR types, frequently reacts with B lymphocytes from SLE patients. These investigators have calculated that reactivity with HLA-DR2 or HLA-DR3 confers a relative risk of SLE of about 3, that the risk is almost doubled (5.8) when reactivity with *both* antigens is taken into account, and that reactivity with Ia-715 serum further increases the risk, to about 15. Although not conclusive, such findings suggest that coinheritance of two or more B-cell alloantigens may influence susceptibility to SLE, a view supported by similar findings in the NZB/W(F_1) model. But much work remains to be done in this regard. In one study, for example, HLA-DR2 was noted in a majority of patients with rare homozygous C2 deficiency and a lupuslike (but typically nonrenal) syndrome. HLA-DR3 has been associated with another rheumatoid disease, Sjögren's syndrome, and the antigen is believed to be in

Figure 4

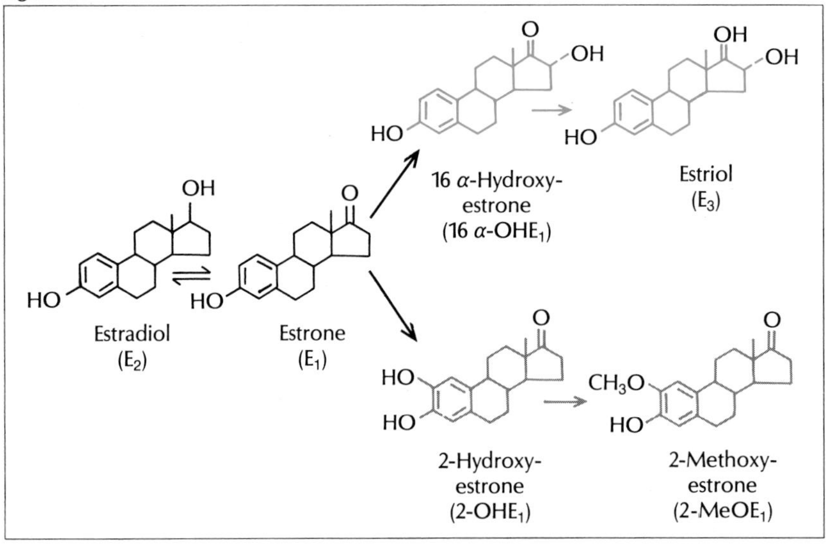

16 α-Hydroxy-estrone
(16 α-OHE$_1$)

Estriol
(E$_3$)

Estradiol
(E$_2$)

Estrone
(E$_1$)

2-Hydroxy-estrone
(2-OHE$_1$)

2-Methoxy-estrone
(2-MeOE$_1$)

The two metabolic pathways of estradiol are schematized above. It is noteworthy that the upper pathway (to estriol) is increased in SLE and that the hormonal metabolites of this pathway are more potently feminizing than those of the lower pathway.

linkage disequilibrium with HLA-A1-B8, which in turn has been associated with other such presumed autoimmune diseases as chronic active hepatitis, dermatitis herpetiformis, and myasthenia gravis. The recent finding of an association between HLA-DR3 and anti-DNA antibodies in SLE seems of special interest.

Sex hormones constitute another factor that appears to be important in the pathogenesis of SLE, as well as of other rheumatoid and non-rheumatoid diseases. As is well known, about 80% of SLE patients are female, and exacerbation is sometimes seen during pregnancy; conversely, the incidence of the disease is relatively low in prepubertal and postmenopausal females. In NZB/W(F$_1$) mice, autoimmune renal disease is more severe, with higher titers of DNA antibodies and shorter survival, in female than in male animals. The work of N. Talal and associates has shown that after castration or oophorectomy, moreover, administration of exogenous androgens has tended to suppress disease and exogenous estrogens to exacerbate it. Clinically, a few males with SLE have been found to have Klinefelter's syndrome, with an XXY karyotype and increased serum levels of estrogenic activity.

As yet, no correlation has been made between SLE and serum estrogen levels in women, but recent studies at this center indicate that SLE patients of both sexes do indeed have altered estrogen metabolism (see Figure 4, page 254). R. G. Lahita and associates noted elevated urinary concentrations of 16 alpha-hydroxyestrone and estriol, compounds with potent estrogenic activity. In a more recent study, these previous findings were confirmed through intravenous administration of estradiol radiolabeled at the C-16 alpha position. Both males and females with SLE had markedly enhanced hydroxylation of estradiol, and although no correlation with clinical activity (or steroid therapy) could be made, these findings suggested that abnormalities of estrogen metabolism in SLE are not due to excretory or conjugative distur-

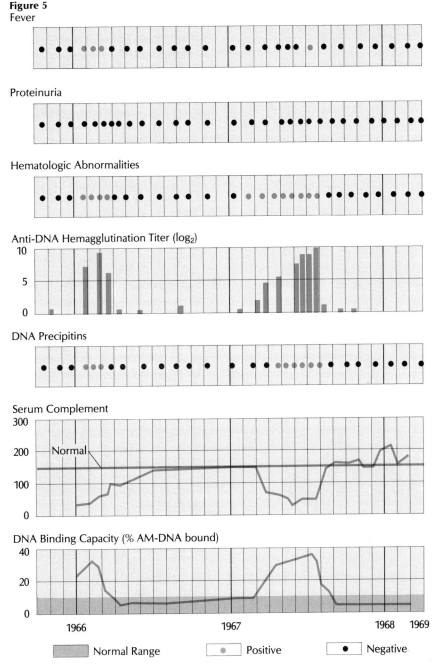

Figure 5

During a 31-month period, this woman in her twenties had two SLE exacerbations marked by fever, hematologic abnormalities, and a variety of symptoms. Immunologic activity was evident during both "flares," with simultaneous rise in anti-DNA antibodies and fall in serum complement. (D. Koffler: Annu Rev Med 25:149, 1974)

bances. In short, there is impressive evidence that female sex hormones may participate in the pathogenesis of SLE, and most physicians accordingly believe that oral contraceptives are contraindicated in females with the disease. Evidence is also coming in indicating alterations in androgenic steroids in SLE.

The mechanism by which sex hormone metabolism may influence immunologic phenomena in SLE is unknown, but the question deserves further study, particularly since it also appears to be pertinent to a spectrum of other immunologic diseases with a high female incidence, e.g., Sjögren's syndrome, hyperglobulinemic purpura, primary biliary cirrhosis, and rheumatoid arthritis.

To what extent are the immunopathologic concepts we have discussed reflected in conventional or investigative treatment of SLE? First, it must be acknowledged that this protean disease has a notoriously variable course, ranging from mild involvement of one or only a few organ systems to fulminant, life-threatening disease; hence, appropriate therapy may be minimal (aspirin when arthritis is the predominant manifestation, topical steroids or low-dose antimalarials when the skin or mucosa is primarily involved) or intensive (systemic steroids in severe forms of renal disease or, if that proves unavailing or results in serious side effects, cytotoxic drugs on an investigational basis).

One of the best therapeutic approaches appears to be the use of steroid therapy with a preventive objective primarily in mind. Since SLE is usually a chronic disease typified by remissions and relapses, every effort should be made to detect a relapse very early and initiate therapy before the relapse produces its effect on the kidney. Serial studies of antibody levels and, especially, complement levels are essential for the recognition of these exacerbations of the disease. A fall in serum complement frequently heralds such an event prior to clinical symptoms (see Figure 5, page 255), and more intensive steroid therapy at this point appears of special value.

The efficacy of intensive therapy has often been difficult to evaluate, because spontaneous remissions do occur and because ethical considerations have inhibited the design of controlled trials. Nevertheless, systemic corticosteroids are generally recognized as capable of suppressing disease activity and prolonging life, and they remain the

mainstay of intensive therapy. As for possible modes of action against the disease, both the anti-inflammatory and immunosuppressive properties of steroids have been cited. Regarding the latter, for example, high-dose daily prednisone has been associated with decreases in gamma globulin levels and in DNA antibody titers, plus normalization of serum complement, and these changes have sometimes closely correlated with clinical improvement.

Given widespread acceptance of the concepts of the immunopathogenesis of the renal lesion in SLE, and given the evidence that steroids in nephritic SLE patients act at least in part by immunosuppression, it has been reasoned that more potent immunosuppressive (and cytotoxic) agents might achieve even better results. This possibility has been investigated experimentally and clinically for the past 10 years or so. In mice, such agents as cyclophosphamide and azathioprine have been reported to retard the progression of autoimmune renal disease. In patients, the results of various reported trials are not so easily interpreted, owing to differences in disease status and patient selection, trial protocol and drug administration, and length of follow-up. Generally, however, it has not yet been shown convincingly that antimetabolites or alkylating agents reduce mortality or prevent renal failure to a significantly greater degree than do corticosteroids. On the other hand, recent studies by J. H. Klippel and co-workers at NIAMDD have shown favorable results in patients treated with intermittent intravenous cyclophosphamide or the combination of oral cyclophosphamide and oral azathioprine. After about two years, only three of the 27 patients in these two treatment groups had reductions in renal function, and

none developed renal failure. Although these results are encouraging, further studies, involving more patients and longer follow-up, are needed, in view of the potential (and potent) toxicity of these drugs.

A more recent therapeutic approach to SLE that also draws upon concepts of the immunopathogenesis of the disease is plasmapheresis. Still investigational, this approach seeks simply to remove circulating immune complexes intermittently from the nephritic SLE patient. It should be noted that there is as yet no clear-cut correlation between levels of circulating immune complexes and disease activity. Nevertheless, a number of programs evaluating plasmapheresis are currently under way. Preliminary results suggest some benefit, but it is too early to say whether the modality will assume a useful role in management.

In conclusion, we still have much to learn about the etiology of SLE, but in recent years a number of promising avenues have been opened along which the course of future investigation will undoubtedly continue. Among these are further identification of antigen-antibody components in renal and other deposits, delineation of the mechanism(s) responsible for deposition, exploration of lymphocyte suppressor function and polyclonal B-cell activation (and a possible relationship between the two), clarification of the roles that sex hormones and histocompatibility determinants may play in predisposing patients to the disease, and (particularly in regard to murine models) determining what contribution infectious or other exogenous agents may make to SLE pathogenesis. The more we learn about such factors, the better our understanding of how the disease occurs—and the better our ability to control or prevent it—will be.

The Immunopathology Of Amyloid Diseases

EDWARD C. FRANKLIN   *New York University*

Amyloidosis is actually a group of diseases, all characterized by the deposition of a proteinaceous infiltrate in a variety of tissues. It most often occurs as a primary disease or in association with plasma cell dyscrasias or chronic infectious or inflammatory diseases. Occasionally, it can be inherited or develop as a concomitant of aging. In the primary, secondary, and some of the familial amyloidosis syndromes, tissue infiltration is systemic, but amyloidosis also occurs as localized deposits involving specific tissues or organs. Amyloid deposition and tissue infiltration cause tissue destruction by compression. Except in some of the localized forms, the process is relentless, leading ultimately to death by destruction of vital organs.

R. Virchow, who discovered the tissue infiltrate in 1854, called it amyloid because of its amorphous, starchlike appearance. However, the morphologic uniformity of amyloid is an artifact of the poor resolving power of the microscope. Even when viewed in the electron microscope, all amyloid consists of fibrils about 10 nm in diameter that are composed of two longitudinal filaments separated by a clear space. The fibrils are long and twisting and tend to polymerize into bundles (see Figure 1, page 258). Since amyloid fibrils are nonimmunogenic and resist phagocytosis and proteolysis, normal host defense mechanisms are generally ineffective in removing the tissue deposits, and this probably accounts for the relentless nature of the disease process.

Although the amyloid deposits in each of the recognized clinical syndromes are identical in light and electron microscopic appearance and in staining characteristics, recent biochemical and immunologic studies have shown that there exist several different types of amyloid, each distinguished by a unique protein component. At the present time, chemical data characterizing the amyloid fiber proteins in individual cases are insufficient to justify a definitive classification of the amyloid diseases according to the protein component of the amyloid. Nevertheless, a look at the table on page 258 shows that close correlation can be demonstrated between the clinical syndromes and the protein component of the infiltrate in each and suggests that the system of classification recently proposed at the Third International Symposium on Amyloidosis will ultimately prove useful. The discovery that there are different types of amyloid strongly suggests that the pathogenesis also differs among the different amyloid diseases. Therefore, it may be useful to review the amyloidoses and to relate the new biochemical findings to potential pathogenetic mechanisms.

Amyloid deposition may be a function of aging, and asymptomatic amyloid deposits are found in the brain, the heart, and other organs in many people dying of other causes at an advanced age. Symptomatic amyloidosis occurs when unusual amounts of amyloid accumulate. The clinical manifestations relate to the organs in which the infiltrate accumulates and most often consist of heart failure if there is cardiac involvement. CNS deposits are associated with mental deterioration.

Primary amyloidosis and myeloma-associated and macroglobulinemia-associated amyloidoses have be-

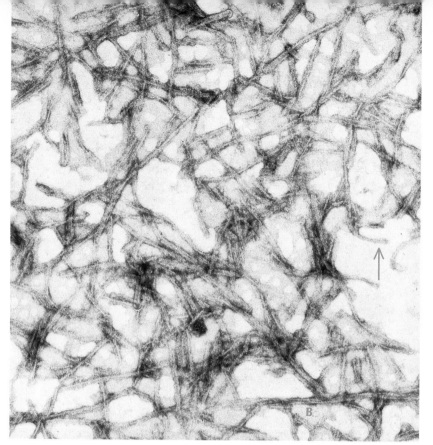

B.

EM shows isolated purified amyloid negatively stained with phosphotungstic acid. Arrow indicates single filament. Most of these end together (half circles). B is a thicker bundle of intertwined filaments (× 96,000). (Courtesy D. Zucker-Franklin; from E. C. Franklin, D. Zucker-Franklin: Adv Immunol 15:268, 1972)

The Amyloidoses

Type	Associated Diseases	Protein Type*
Primary and myeloma-associated	Myeloma, macroglobulinemia, monoclonal gammopathy, related plasma cell neoplasms	AL (lambda or kappa)
Secondary	Chronic infections, inflammatory conditions, Hodgkin's disease, etc	AA
Hereditary – many types		AF
FMF		AA
Portuguese		AF$_p$ – prealbumin
Localized Endocrine organs		AE
	Medullary carcinoma of the thyroid	AE$_t$ – thyrocalcitonin
	Diabetes	AE$_?$ – insulin?, glucagon?
	Others	AE$_?$ – other hormones?
Senile		AS
Cardiac		AS$_c$
Brain, etc	.	AS$_b$
Cutaneous	Localized amyloid	AD
Others		?

*Names agreed upon at Third International Symposium on Amyloidosis, Portugal, 1979: AL = Amyloid Light Chain, AA = Amyloid A, AF = Amyloid Familial, AE = Amyloid Endocrine, AS = Amyloid Senile, AD = Amyloid Dermatologic

Figure 1

come the most common types encountered clinically. These conditions will be discussed together because they have the same clinical characteristics and organ distribution and, as will be described later, the same amyloid protein component. Furthermore, many patients with primary amyloidosis eventually develop a true plasma cell dyscrasia, manifest by the appearance of homogenous immunoglobulins, especially Bence Jones proteins, in the serum, urine, or both and by plasmacytosis in the marrow. It seems probable that a majority would develop a full-blown plasma cell disease if they survived long enough. By the same token, about 10% of patients with myeloma have amyloidosis.

In primary and immunoglobulin-associated amyloidosis, the amyloid infiltrates are found mainly in the tongue, heart, kidney, skeletal muscle, skin, ligaments, and gastrointestinal tract but also in the liver and spleen. About 50% of patients with this type of amyloidosis develop renal disease that evolves into the nephrotic syndrome. The nephrotic syndrome is the major cause of signs and symptoms as well as of death, but patients may present with manifestations referable to involvement of other systems. They may seek medical help because of problems in speaking or swallowing due to macroglossia, because of joint pain or stiffness due to amyloid infiltration of periarticular or synovial structures, or because of the carpal tunnel syndrome associated with median nerve compression. Sensory disturbances or weakness due to peripheral neuropathy and postural hypotension due to autonomic nerve dysfunction are also seen with some degree of frequency. Gastrointestinal involvement may be manifest by intestinal obstruction, hemorrhage, diarrhea, malabsorption, protein-losing enteropathy, or disturbances in intestinal motility. Involvement of the adrenal or other endocrine glands may lead to end-organ insufficiency. Infiltration of the respiratory tract may cause pulmonary, bronchial, laryngeal, or tracheal symptoms or

Figure 2

result in respiratory failure or ventilatory obstruction. Amyloid infiltration of the small vessels of the skin and subcutaneous tissues may cause purpura and ecchymoses in the absence of trauma. The bleeding tendency in many of these patients is accentuated by a deficiency of the procoagulant factor X, which is apparently the result of complexing and accelerated removal of factor X from the circulation. Infiltration of the skin may simulate myxedema or scleroderma.

Many patients with primary or immunoglobulin-related amyloidosis manifest cardiac involvement, but amyloid infiltration of the heart is extremely difficult to diagnose clinically. The onset of cardiac failure is insidious, and the ECG changes (low voltage and a high frequency of conduction defects) are far from specific. The heart failure caused by amyloidosis is refractory to treatment, and many patients with primary or immunoglobulin-related amyloidosis die suddenly or unexpectedly of arrhythmia or cardiac arrest. In a substantial number of these cases, death occurs within hours of digitalis therapy. Failure to respond to digitalis is a characteristic of cardiac amyloidosis, and it should be used with great care in these cases.

Secondary amyloidosis was formerly associated with osteomyelitis, tuberculosis, bronchiectasis, and syphilis. With the decline in the incidence of these chronic suppurative infections, secondary amyloidosis today is more likely to be found in paraplegics and in patients with neurologic diseases, chronic pyelonephritis, Hodgkin's disease, renal cell carcinoma, leprosy, regional ileitis, or rheumatoid or other forms of inflammatory arthritis. Recently, we have seen it frequently in drug addicts using intravenous medication.

Secondary amyloidosis tends to become manifest only when the underlying disease is of long standing and severe. Amyloid infiltration occurs primarily in the kidney, spleen, liver, and adrenals and rarely in the cardiac or musculoskeletal tissues or gastrointestinal tract. A

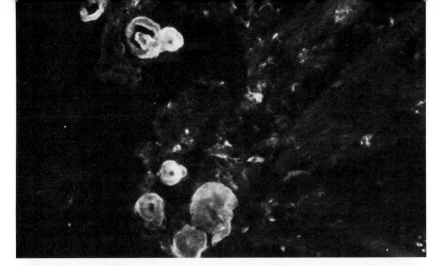
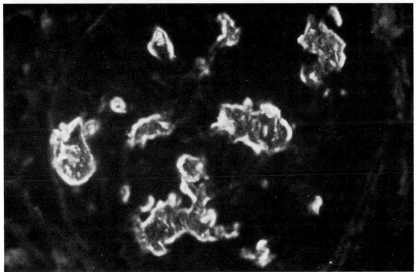

Photomicrographs show immunofluorescence-stained amyloid. At top is ileum amyloid stained with antibodies to human AA protein and fluorescent rabbit anti-IgG. Bottom photo is amyloid in glomerulus stained with anti-AA.

majority of patients with secondary amyloidosis eventually develop the nephrotic syndrome. The first symptoms of kidney involvement are usually weakness, proteinuria, and hematuria. The earliest renal lesion is usually a nodular or diffuse thickening of the glomerular basement membrane with amyloid material (see C. B. Wilson and F. J. Dixon, "Immunologic Mechanisms in Nephritogenesis"). The lesion may then progress to massive infiltration, with obliteration of the glomerular bed or with glomerular atrophy. Occasionally, amyloid is deposited in medullary areas, causing nephrogenic diabetes insipidus, but hypertension seldom develops in uncomplicated renal amyloidosis. If the nephrotic syndrome progresses, hemodialysis or kidney

transplantation may be required. At least 35 patients have had renal transplants, with survival ranging up to 10 years. Recurrences of amyloid deposits in the transplanted kidneys have been reported in a few instances. Without hemodialysis or transplantation, death usually occurs within two years of the onset of severe renal failure.

Macroglossia, purpura, and peripheral neuropathy are rarely encountered in secondary amyloidosis. Amyloid infiltration of the gastrointestinal tract, while generally asymptomatic, may contribute to the malnutrition and anemia often seen.

Several hereditary forms of amyloidosis are recognized. The most prevalent are familial Mediterranean fever and the Portuguese type of

Figure 3

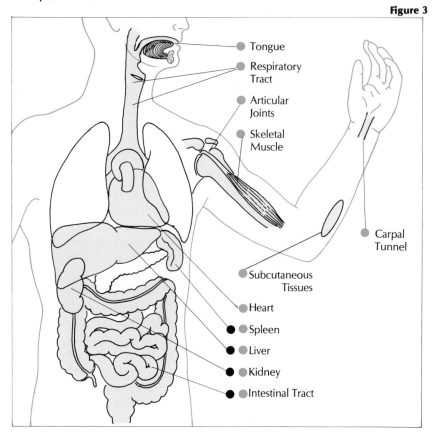

- Tongue
- Respiratory Tract
- Articular Joints
- Skeletal Muscle
- Carpal Tunnel
- Subcutaneous Tissues
- Heart
- Spleen
- Liver
- Kidney
- Intestinal Tract

Body map indicates more common sites of amyloid deposition. Colored bullets desig-nate organs and structures in which the AL protein of primary amyloidosis is likely to be found. Black bullets identify sites of AA protein in secondary amyloidosis. The AA amyloid disease of the gastrointestinal tract is generally subclinical.

lower-limb neuropathy. Familial Mediterranean fever has a recessive mode of inheritance and occurs among people of eastern Mediterranean extraction, particularly Jews, Lebanese and Syrian Arabs, Armenians, and, less frequently, Maltese, Greeks, and Italians (see S. M. Wolff, "Familial Mediterranean Fever: A Status Report," Hosp Pract, November 1978). Except in Armenians, it is commonly accompanied by amyloidosis resembling the secondary type both clinically and biochemically. The Portuguese type of lower-limb neuropathy is inherited as a mendelian-dominant characteristic among people of Portuguese extraction and is manifest by marked peripheral nerve involvement. Many other forms of familial amyloidosis have been reported. They are usually restricted to a specific and limited geographic location, and the amyloid deposits are organ specific rather than diffuse.

Localized amyloidosis is a form in which the accumulations of amyloid occur in specific organs, usually the larynx, lung, and skin. Localized accumulations in the skin produce lichen amyloidosis. Another form of amyloidosis is associated with certain tumors of neuroectodermal origin and with diabetes mellitus. The tumors include medullary carcinoma of the thyroid, pheochromocytoma, bronchial carcinoid, insulinoma, and carotid body tumors. The amyloid accumulating adjacent to these sites is distinguishable histologically from the amyloid of primary and secondary amyloidosis, according to A. G. E. Pearse.

Finally, a given patient may have more than one form of amyloidosis. For example, an elderly patient may have amyloidosis of the kidney secondary to long-standing rheumatoid arthritis and may also have senile amyloid deposits in the brain, aorta,

or heart. Thus, the amyloidogenic stimuli of chronic inflammation and of aging appear to operate independently.

Amyloidosis should be suspected in patients with unexplained congestive heart failure or renal disease, especially in those with the nephrotic syndrome; in patients with hepatosplenomegaly associated with chronic inflammatory disease or hepatomegaly without signs of liver failure; and in patients with the malabsorption syndrome, the carpal tunnel syndrome, unexplained neuromuscular disease, or purpura.

In patients suspected of having primary or immunoglobulin-related amyloidosis, the evaluation should include examination of the serum and urine for the presence of homogenous immunoglobulin-related proteins. At least 90% of patients with this type of amyloidosis have Bence Jones proteins, either alone or in association with a myeloma protein. The finding of immunoglobulin-related proteins in the secondary and familial forms of amyloidosis is unusual.

The diagnosis of amyloidosis always requires histologic confirmation. Amyloid is metachromatic with several dyes, including toluidine blue and crystal violet, but the most frequently used stain for demonstrating amyloid is Congo red. When a histologic section containing amyloid is stained with Congo red and examined under polarized light, the amyloid deposits exhibit a typical green birefringence. With the availability of antisera to several of the amyloid proteins, it has been possible to precisely classify the type of amyloid deposit by immunofluorescence or immunoperoxidase microscopy (see Figure 2, page 259). The practice of injecting Congo red in an attempt to demonstrate increased retention of the dye has been abandoned due to a high incidence of complications.

When primary or immunoglobulin-related amyloidosis is suspected, bone marrow biopsy examination is indicated to establish the presence of a plasma cell neoplasm. If bone marrow examination provides

Figure 4

histologic evidence of amyloid infiltrates in the marrow, additional biopsies are not necessary. In patients with other systemic forms of amyloidosis, renal and small-bowel biopsies usually provide positive material for histologic examination. Liver biopsy is contraindicated because of the increased risk of severe bleeding or rupture in patients with amyloidosis. If biopsy of the involved tissue is not possible, a rectal or gingival biopsy may be helpful, since it provides histologic evidence in over 90% of patients with the common systemic forms of amyloidosis. A small blood vessel should be included in the rectal biopsy specimen, because in many cases of systemic amyloidosis, involvement is confined to blood vessels only.

The most important advance in our understanding of amyloidosis in the past decade was the discovery that different types of amyloid differ in their protein constituents and that these differences correlate to a high degree with the clinical classification of the amyloid diseases (see Figure 3, page 260). The biochemical and immunologic identification of the amyloid proteins became possible with the development of techniques for the isolation of the amyloid fibrils. The fibrils account for 70% to 80% of the amyloid substance. Because they are insoluble in salt-containing solvents, they can be isolated by repeated extraction with physiologic saline, which removes contaminating proteins. The fibrils are then obtained as a colloidal suspension by extraction with distilled water.

The composition of the fibrils obtained in the water extract differs according to the type of amyloid from which the fibrils were obtained. In primary and myeloma-associated amyloidosis, the fibrils consist of immunoglobulin light chains or fragments of light chains. The molecular weight of an immunoglobulin light chain is about 25,000. The molecular weight of the protein subunits in amyloid ranges between 5,000 and 25,000. It always contains the variable region of the light chain and part or all of the constant region. This group of pro-

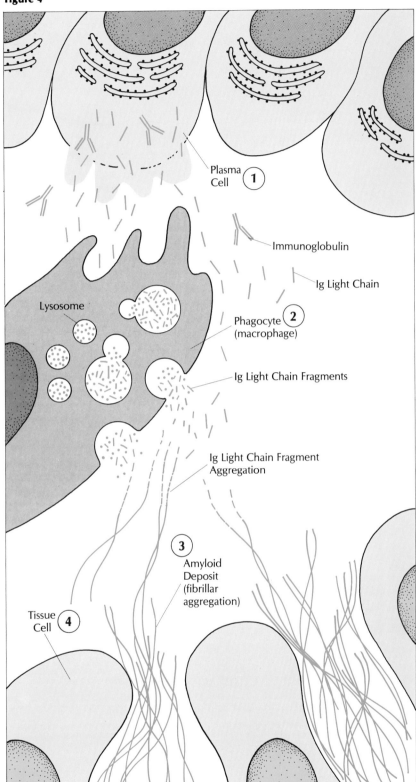

Diagram traces synthesis and deposition of amyloid composed of AL protein derived from immunoglobulin light chains. As exemplified here, an underlying plasma cell malignancy (1) results in excessive secretion of Ig light chains. Some of the light chains are incompletely digested by phagocytes (2), and the resultant light chain fragments are incorporated along with whole light chains that have bypassed degradation into amyloid fibrils (3). Fibrils, singly and in aggregates, are deposited between tissue cells (4).

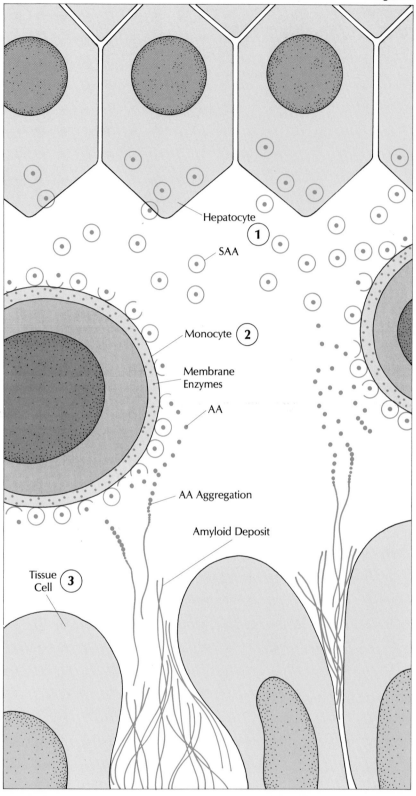

Hepatocyte ①

SAA

Monocyte ②

Membrane Enzymes

AA

AA Aggregation

Amyloid Deposit

Tissue Cell ③

AA amyloid is characteristic of secondary amyloidosis. The AA protein is derived from serum AA (SAA), secreted by hepatocytes (1). SAA is enzymatically cleaved on the surface of monocytes (2) to the AA protein, which in turn aggregates into fibrils and is deposited between affected tissue cells (3). A number of proteins, such as thyrocalcitonin, prealbumin, and other peptide hormones, can also form amyloid. Two requirements have been identified—excess production and beta-pleated-sheet structure.

teins is called AL (amyloid light chain) protein (Figure 4, page 261).

It seems highly probable that the AL proteins represent degradation products of fully synthesized immunoglobulin light chains. This view is supported by G. G. Glenner's demonstration that the amino acid sequence of the amino terminal regions of the AL proteins is identical to that of the kappa or lambda light chain variable regions. The concept is further strengthened by the finding that fibrils with the appearance of amyloid can be created in vitro by the proteolytic digestion of some Bence Jones proteins, especially those belonging to certain lambda subclasses, and by the demonstration of cross-reactivity between amyloid subunits and kappa and lambda light chains.

The immunoglobulin-related amyloid proteins or their precursors are synthesized by lymphocytes or plasma cells and are deposited either locally or at distant sites. The reason why some intact proteins and protein fragments form amyloid fibrils is not known. The tendency to form fibrils may be a consequence of some inherent structural property of the protein. There are only two kinds of immunoglobulin light chains, lambda and kappa, although each has several subclasses. Normally, two thirds of immunoglobulin molecules contain kappa and one third, lambda light chains. In contrast, in AL protein fibrils and in sera and urine of patients with primary amyloidosis, lambda chain proteins are twice as frequent as those with kappa chains, and certain lambda proteins, those belonging to the lambda VI subclass, almost always seem to be associated with amyloid deposits. It seems possible that certain types of light chains are more readily converted to amyloid fibrils by several proteolytic enzymes, including those from renal lysosomes, or that the degradative processes that function to eliminate excess free immunoglobulin light chains may be abnormal in some individuals.

The amyloid substance in the secondary type of amyloidosis, in certain of the familial forms (such as familial Mediterranean fever), and in animals (whether naturally occurring or experimentally induced) consists primarily of a protein known as amyloid A (AA) protein (see Figure 5, page 262). It has a molecular weight of 8,500, and its amino acid sequence is highly conserved in all species studied. The function of AA protein is not known. The AA protein is related to a serum component called serum AA (SAA) protein. SAA is a normal 11,000-dalton serum component and exists complexed to other proteins, such as high-density lipoproteins or albumin. Since SAA is identical to AA for the first 76 residues, it seems likely that SAA is a circulating precursor whose carboxy terminal fragment is cleaved by proteolysis in the process of AA formation. Comparison of several human AA proteins that have been sequenced and partial sequences of SAA show some amino acid variations, suggesting the existence of structural polymorphisms. AA protein has no homology to any previously recognized protein.

The function of SAA is not known. Its concentration in the serum is very low, less than 200 µg/ml, during the first five decades of life; it appears to increase in a significant number of individuals over the age of 60. SAA behaves as an acute-phase reactant; its concentration increases markedly in many acute and chronic diseases, including all types of amyloidosis, cancer, infections, rheumatoid arthritis, multiple myeloma, macroglobulinemia, lymphomas, and a variety of other disorders, and in pregnancy as well. Thus, SAA levels are of no value in the diagnosis of secondary amyloidosis. Though SAA levels tend to return to normal as the illness resolves, it seems likely that during many chronic diseases the prolonged liberation of SAA may exceed the body's capacity to degrade it, resulting in the deposition of AA fibrils.

In localized amyloidosis involving certain endocrine glands, the major protein component of the fibrils may be made up of peptide hormones. This has been shown for thyrocalcitonin in the amyloid seen in medullary carcinoma of the thyroid. It seems possible that either insulin or glucagon contributes to the amyloidosis involving the pancreas, since it has been demonstrated experimentally that proteolytic digestion of these hormones produces fibrils that look like amyloid. Nothing is known about the chemical nature of the protein in other localized forms of amyloidosis or other familial types, except in Portuguese-type neuropathy, which appears to contain prealbumin.

It is of interest that in all types of amyloid the saline supernatant contains, among many different substances, a protein known as the "P" component or, because of its shape, the "doughnut" component (see Figure 6 on this page). This molecule, whose function or role in amyloid deposition remains to be elucidated, is structurally closely related to C-reactive protein. In the presence of calcium, it interacts with a variety of cells and proteins and behaves in certain species as an acute-phase reactant. Perhaps it serves as the anchor for or the scaffold upon which the fibrils are deposited.

The pathogenesis of amyloidosis is not known, although experimental work has produced a great many clues. Both primary and secondary amyloidosis occur in situations in which the immune system may be overwhelmed by an antigenic load or has undergone neoplastic transformation, making it perhaps functionally deficient. Nevertheless, despite many attempts, a specific immunologic defect has not been found. Studies by M. A. Scheinberg and E. Cathcart and associates and many others suggest that the deposition of amyloid may be accompanied by depressed T-cell function and augmented B-cell function and that augmentation of T-cell function by thymic hormone can prevent the development of experimental amyloidosis. G. Telium had earlier shown that experimentally induced amyloid deposition could be accelerated by immunosuppressive agents and that it often accompanies immunodeficiency states. However, a majority of studies of B- and T-cell

Figure 6

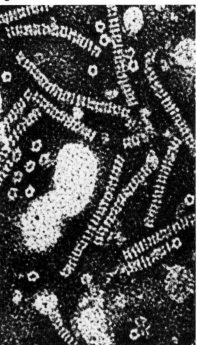

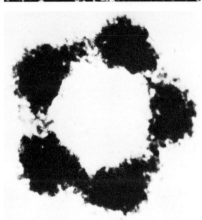

EMs show P component, which makes up about 5% of amyloid protein. Upper picture shows long-chain structure. Higher-power EM (bottom) clearly depicts pentameric structure of the P component in cross section. (EM courtesy R. Painter; from Can J Biochem 57:729, 1972)

function in amyloidosis have produced contradictory results and are, therefore, difficult to interpret. Furthermore, there is no evidence that the immune system is involved in the amyloidosis associated with the endocrine organs or with aging.

Amyloid deposits appear to occur when there is overproduction of one of several precursors that can then be processed by proteolytic enzymes to produce the characteristic fibrils.

This mechanism is most clearly evident in the light chain–related plasma cell dyscrasias associated with systemic AL protein (primary and myeloma-associated amyloidoses). In the case of AA amyloidosis, overproduction of the soluble precursor SAA also seems likely.

Overproduction of a precursor probably is not the sole factor in the development of amyloidosis because only a small fraction—10% to 20%—of individuals at risk actually develop amyloidosis. Hence, to explain the sporadic occurrence of amyloidosis in individuals exposed to a stimulus that causes overproduction of a precursor, whether it is immunoglobulin light chains, AA protein, or some other protein, an additional defect must exist. One possibility is that certain proteins are amyloidogenic, i.e., easily converted to amyloid fibrils, while others are more resistant. This appears to be clearly applicable to certain lambda light chains and perhaps also to some of the forms of SAA. Another possibility is that amyloidosis occurs as a result of the overproduction of a precursor in a host who is genetically or for other reasons defective in processing either the precursor or the fibril subunit.

Our studies of the processing of SAA in vitro also suggest that a defect, possibly genetic, predisposes certain individuals to develop secondary amyloidosis. In these studies, blood monocytes were used because they are the cells commonly found around the sites of amyloid deposition. They are active in eliminating foreign material through the process of phagocytosis and degradation by lysosomes and through the secretion of proteases, such as collagenase and elastase, and plasminogen activators.

When the blood monocytes were incubated with SAA, three patterns of SAA degradation were observed. One pattern, in which SAA was completely degraded without the production of detectable intermediates, was seen in cells of eight of 20 normal individuals and none of 20 amyloidosis patients. A second pattern, in which the SAA molecule was degraded to a low-molecular-weight molecule that behaved like AA protein before being further degraded, was observed in cells of eight of the normal individuals and all 20 patients with amyloidosis. The third pattern, in which SAA was degraded to AA-like molecules that persisted for periods longer than 48 hours, was seen in cells of four normal individuals.

These results indicated that degradation of SAA by macrophages normally involves a multistep reaction in which SAA is first cleaved into an intermediate AA-like protein and then, in a series of subsequent steps, the AA-like protein is completely degraded. The degradation process is not the result of phagocytosis or pinocytosis and is only partly due to secretion of enzymes into the medium. It occurs primarily on the surface of the cells and is caused by enzymes that are apparently membrane associated. The results of subsequent experiments indicate that the enzymes belong to the class of serine esterases and have some properties of elastase.

These findings may have some relevance to the pathogenesis of amyloidosis. Since cells from 40% of normal individuals degraded SAA without the appearance of any intermediate products, whereas cells from all of the patients with amyloidosis showed the transient appearance of an AA-like protein with the molecular size and antigenic properties of AA protein, it seems possible that a quantitative or qualitative deficiency in the second degradative step may predispose certain individuals to develop amyloidosis, provided they are subjected to an appropriate stimulus. During prolonged inflammation, when SAA levels are elevated, partial degradation of SAA may result in the accumulation of large amounts of AA protein intermediates in the serum, and further degradation may be incomplete. The undegraded AA protein may then polymerize and form amyloid fibrils. Because our results suggested that differences in patterns of proteolysis may play a role in the predisposition to amyloidosis, we are now trying to determine if the pattern of SAA proteolysis is inherited.

There is at present no treatment for amyloidosis. Colchicine prevents the febrile attacks of familial Mediterranean fever and the progression of amyloidosis in that condition but has not been very effective in other types of amyloidosis. The treatment of primary and myeloma-associated amyloidosis with melphalan, cyclophosphamide, and similar agents is the same as that of multiple myeloma and may at times arrest the progress of the disease or even cause regression. The use of other agents, such as DMSO, is still in a very early experimental stage and is not yet of proved value in patient management.

Neuroimmunologic Disease: Experimental and Clinical Aspects

PHILIP Y. PATERSON *and* EUGENE D. DAY   *Northwestern University* and *Duke University*

Two animal models of autoimmune disease—experimental allergic encephalomyelitis (EAE) and experimental autoimmune thyroiditis(EAT)—were cited to explain different mechanisms by which immunologic tolerance may break down (see W.O. Weigle, "Immunologic Tolerance and Immunopathology"). In this discussion we explore EAE in detail, with specific focus on mechanisms that modulate host immune responses to central nervous system (CNS) neuroantigens in rats. Special emphasis will be given to recent observations that implicate such modulating activity in clinically well human beings as well as in patients with the prototypical demyelinating disease, multiple sclerosis (MS). In both the experimental animal disease and its counterpart disorder in man, disruption in host regulatory control over immune responses to neuroautoantigens appears to be an important factor, one that helps set the stage for the manifestations of neuroimmunologic injury and disease.

To begin, it will be recalled that, aside from unresponsive states known to be under genetic control, the induction of immunologic tolerance requires previous contact with a specific antigen. It is easier to induce tolerance in T cells than B cells: the former require contact with much smaller doses of antigen and maintain unresponsiveness for longer periods of time. These points suggest that, for a given self-antigen present in minute quantities, the normal lymphocyte profile is likely to be characterized by responsive B cells and tolerant T cells. Autoimmunity will develop only when something intervenes to break T-cell tolerance, permitting T- and B-cell interaction, B-cell antibody production, and disease.

In the experimental form of neuroautoimmune disease, EAE, a single injection into a rat of CNS nervous tissue combined with complete Freund's adjuvant (CFA) is fol-

lowed in approximately two weeks by the appearance of hind-leg weakness or paralysis, together with evidence of urinary incontinence, a reflection of neurogenic bladder dysfunction. These clinical signs are accompanied by characteristic immunohistopathologic changes (see Figure 1): focal perivascular deposits with fibrin, best detected by immunofluorescence; perivascular accumulations of inflammatory cells, with histiocytes being numerically the most

Figure 1

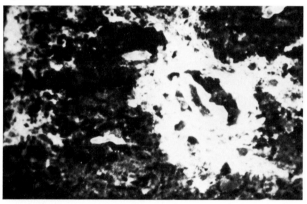

When EAE is induced in the Lewis rat by sensitization with guinea pig spinal cord in CFA, perivascular fibrin deposits (above) in the nervous system can be detected by direct immunofluorescence with rabbit antirat fibrinogen FITC-IgG conjugate. Perivascular inflammatory cells (below) are mostly histiocytes with a few lymphocytes and plasma cells.

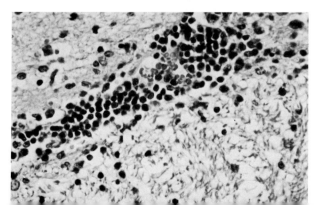

Figure 2

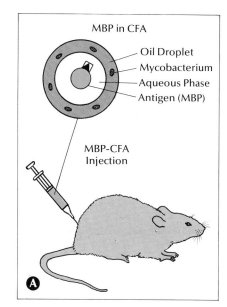

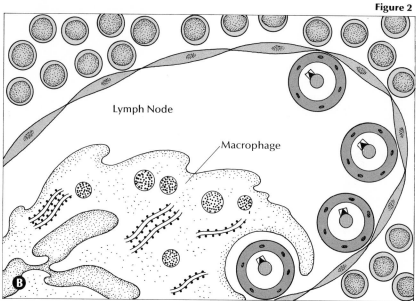

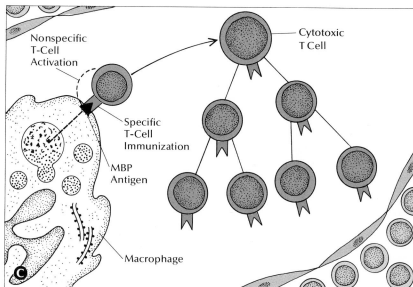

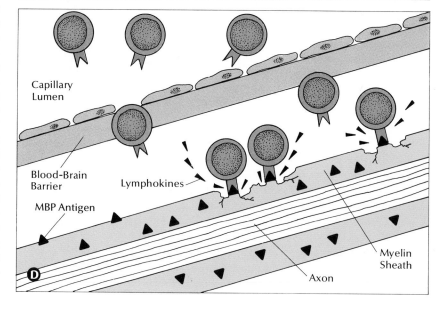

The hypothesized pathogenesis of experimental allergic encephalomyelitis is represented schematically, starting (A) with the injection into a rat of myelin basic protein (MBP) in complete Freund's adjuvant (CFA). One role of the adjuvant appears to be mobilization or activation of macrophages. As a result, the MBP-CFA is phagocytized (B). The macrophage processes the antigen, enhancing its antigenicity. Processed antigen is then presented on the macrophage surface to circulating lymphocytes (C). There it can sensitize T cells. A second nonspecific signal is also thought to be given to the now-sensitized T lymphocytes causing them to proliferate. Thus, clones of specific anti-MBP cytotoxic T cells are elaborated. These cells cross the blood-brain barrier (D) and complex with the myelin basic protein determinants in the CNS, triggering inflammatory mediators (e.g., lymphokines). Host inflammatory cells, particularly macrophages, induce demyelinization.

important cells; and varying degrees of associated demyelination. Such focal areas of inflammation and injury are often disseminated throughout the brain and spinal cord. EAE can be induced by an injection of xenogeneic, allogeneic, or syngeneic (equivalent to autologous) CNS tissue. More important, the disease can be induced by injection of myelin basic protein (MBP), a major protein constituent of myelinated nerve fibers (see Figure 2, page 266). It is noteworthy that the form of EAE elicited by MBP sensitization, in contrast to that induced by whole CNS tissues (see Figure 3, page 268), tends to be characterized by milder, usually transitory clinical neurologic signs, markedly less fibrin deposition in the neuraxis, and much less or no demyelination. Less severe disease is especially evident in guinea pigs and rats sensitized to MBP. In both of these species, the response is totally without complement-dependent cytotoxic antiglial-cell demyelinating circulating antibody. These observations, together with other preliminary data, suggest that neuroantigens in addition to MBP contribute significantly to the overall immunogenic activity of CNS tissue, including its capacity to elicit EAE. An important point to keep in mind about experimental allergic encephalomyelitis is that it is *not* monophasic, as was previously believed. When animals sensitized to whole CNS tissue are allowed to recover from the initial attack of acute EAE, a high proportion subsequently exhibit spontaneous relapses of the disease.

The view that EAE is predominantly a T cell–mediated disease is supported by several lines of evidence. EAE has been produced in agammaglobulinemic chickens, bursectomized and treated with cyclophosphamide at hatching, and then, when fully mature, sensitized to CNS tissue adjuvant. In rats and other mammals, experiments of different designs have shown that T lymphocytes are essential for development of EAE, whereas B cells do not appear to be of comparable importance. Most compelling is the finding, first established in the laboratory of one of the authors (P.Y.P.), that whereas suspensions of dissociated cells derived from lymph nodes that

drain sites where neuroantigen adjuvant was injected can transfer EAE with relative ease to normal animals, the disease cannot be transferred regularly, if at all, with systemic administration of immune serum. It should be noted, however, that transfer of donor-sensitized lymph node cells results in variable levels of circulating brain antibodies in the recipient animals. Furthermore, lesions closely resembling those of EAE, and sometimes accompanied by clinical neurologic abnormalities, have been reported by three different laboratories following infusion or multiple injections of EAE-immune serum into the ventricular cavity or lumbosacral subarachnoid space of guinea pigs, rabbits, or rats. It is not unreasonable to believe that at least one reason why antibody has not been more strongly implicated in the pathogenesis of EAE, in contrast to other analogous experimental autoimmune disorders of other organ systems, is the extraordinary capacity of the cerebrovasculature to restrict passive diffusion of antibody molecules into the CNS compartment. Delivery of antibody intraventricularly or via the spinal cord subarachnoid space would bypass this blood-brain-vascular barrier and allow antibody to interact directly with host CNS neuroantigen.

Although the weight of the evidence thus far indicates that B cells and MBP antibodies are not essential effectors of tissue damage in EAE, the possibility does exist that MBP antibodies may alter the kinetic balance in a manner that would provide effector cytolytic T cells greater access to CNS target tissue. Nor can we discount the suggestion that antibodies might be instrumental in augmenting the disease process after it has gotten under way. Alternatively, and as shown in our laboratory some years ago, immune serum can exert an impressive inhibitory effect on development of EAE in actively sensitized animals. This serum inhibitory effect, originally discovered in rats, was thought to be mediated by complement-fixing antibrain antibodies that were blocking interaction of sensitized cytotoxic T lymphocytes with neuroantigen in the CNS target tissue of the sensitized host. Our recent findings (to be discussed later)

suggest that the serum-mediated transfer of inhibition of EAE may, at least in part, be due to a high content of circulating endogenous MBP neurotolerogen.

To recapitulate, the weight of evidence suggests that mammalian B lymphoid cells exhibit little or no tolerance to neuroantigens such as MBP. MBP-binding lymphoid cells, in all probability B cells, have been demonstrated in fair numbers in the blood and/or peripheral lymphoid tissues of guinea pigs, rats, and man. Such cells, with the potential for producing antibody reactive with MBP, are, however, of little consequence, insofar as neuroimmunologic injury is concerned, since antibodies directed against CNS tissue do not appear to play a major or even significant role in effecting neuroautoimmunologic injury. In direct contrast, the relatively weak level of tolerance of T cells to neuroantigens can be easily disrupted, allowing sensitized T cells to become the effector agents of the immunologic injury that characterizes EAE. T-cell tolerance for MBP, and, presumably, other neuroantigens as well, must be marginal. The relative ease of producing EAE in most mammalian animal species undoubtedly reflects this fact. From these observations, two main questions immediately arise. First, if virtually all animals, including man, are immunologically poised to react to their own CNS antigens, what normally prevents them from doing so, thereby accounting for the comparative infrequency of neuroautoimmunologic disease? Second, what is the exact sequence of events that result in breakdown of this protective mechanism, weak as it is, thereby allowing EAE and analogous human neurologic disorders to develop?

As yet, the answer to the first question is by no means clear, but at least two points can be made with confidence. First, lack of appreciable tolerance to neuroantigens and rarity of neuroimmunologic disorders were originally believed to result from the sequestration of neuroantigen(s) within CNS; presumably they never were able to gain access to peripheral lymphoid tissues and there activate clones of potentially destructive autoreactive cells. Advances in radioimmunoassay

Figure 3

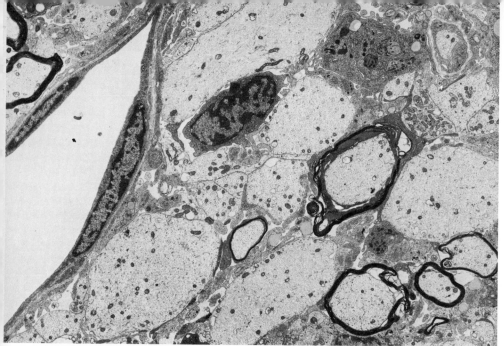

EM of neural tissue of Lewis rat with induced EAE by guinea pig spinal cord-CFA shows severe lesions with majority of axons stripped of myelin lamellae. (Prepared by Dr. M.C. Dal Canto, Department of Pathology, Northwestern University.)

technology, which have allowed detection of extraordinarily small amounts of antigen in host body fluids, have shown MBP or its fragments to be regularly present in the cerebrospinal fluid (CSF) and the blood of normal rats and rats developing EAE as well as of clinically well human beings and patients with multiple sclerosis or other neurologic diseases. Endogenous MBP, at least, clearly does circulate and therefore does impinge upon host immunocompetent lymphoid tissues. In this sense it is in a position to act as either immunogen or tolerogen. Second, as will be spelled out in greater detail later, MBP appears to circulate in the form of fragments of the whole molecule, each of which bears different immunodeterminants reactive with different subpopulations of MBP antibodies. In turn, the antibody subpopulations are characterized by different degrees of affinity binding for the corresponding (respective) immunodeterminants. The fragments of MBP that are reactive with high-affinity antibodies would be especially effective as specific neurotolerogens for T cells.

As for the question of how protection against CNS autoimmune disease may break down, let us approach the answer by considering exactly what is immunogenic about a mixture of MBP and CFA (see Figure 2).

First, the very act of homogenizing CNS tissue as a first step in extracting pure MBP is thought to alter the antigen physically. Biochemical changes in MBP may occur as a result of exposure to acid proteinases during the extraction procedure. But probably more important is the role played by CFA. This mixture of paraffin oil, suspended killed mycobacteria, and emulsifying agent is well known for its ability to augment immune responses. In addition to eliciting a powerful granulomatous response, CFA promotes macrophage infiltration. Macrophages, it has been found, are essential for the induction of an immune response to MBP. In the Lewis rat, for example, macrophages have recently been implicated to explain why suckling, as opposed to adult, animals of this strain are relatively insusceptible to EAE after MBP-CFA injection: the immature rats show deficient macrophage mobilization at inoculation sites. Interestingly, however, when suckling Lewis rats sensitized to rat MBP-CFA are given a macrophage-rich suspension of adult rat peritoneal exudate cells, they are just as susceptible to EAE as adult animals. Perhaps, therefore, the macrophages process the MBP in a way that in-

creases the likelihood of the host's mounting an immune response against MBP present in CNS tissues.

Age-related differences in susceptibility to EAE have also played an important role in the recent discovery of a serum factor that may regulate host response to EAE, account for the pattern of acute disease followed by remission, and even, perhaps, hold the key to effective therapy for CNS autoimmune diseases (see Figure 4, page 269). The prime tool in the identification of this serum factor was a highly sensitive and reliable radioimmunoassay developed by one of us (E.D.D.) at Duke. With the use of this assay, both the serum and plasma of the suckling rat were found to contain relatively large quantities of a substance that interacted with highly purified, monospecific anti-MBP antibody. Indeed, in its ability to inhibit the binding of ^{125}I-labeled (and unlabeled) MBP by anti-MBP antibody, the substance was immunologically indistinguishable from MBP itself. Second, the substance, which we originally elected to designate "MBP serum factor," or "MBP-SF," reached micromolar peak levels when rats were 11 to 20 days old, but by eight weeks had dropped to less than 0.1 μM and was virtually undetectable (see Figure 5, page 270). Third, an inverse relationship was demonstrable between MBP-SF levels and EAE susceptibility in maturing rats. Moreover, consistent with basic concepts concerning termination of immunologic tolerance to self-antigens, this age-dependent relationship could be overridden if the rats were sensitized with whole guinea pig spinal cord or guinea pig MBP. Fourth, among adult Lewis rats developing EAE, some were found to have clearly elevated levels of MBP-SF.

Meanwhile, we began to address the question whether normal adult Lewis rats could also generate MBP-SF, albeit at a much lower level. We increased the sensitivity of the inhibition radioimmunoassays, carried out the tests with more dilute antibody reagents and labeled antigen, and obtained an affirmative answer. During the development of that much more sensitive radioimmunoassay, we necessarily had to conduct our studies at a number of dilutions of antigen and antibody, a process that led us up against the dual-dilution phenomenon – the loss in measurable antigenic binding capacity (after correction for the dilution factor), as both antigen and antibody are similarly diluted before reaction with each other. (The phenomenon is a consequence of the principle: the more dilute the dual system, the more dominant high-binding affinity becomes and the greater the loss in measurable low-affinity binding.)

To our surprise we found that by measuring the same serum sample for its ability to inhibit at different dual dilutions of a standard reagent antigen-antibody system, we could detect separate inhibitors. Rarely did we find samples that would inhibit at all levels of dilution as whole MBP would do but more often noticed a dominance at a particular dilution, i.e., at a particular limited range of affinity. Moreover, we found that any one of these MBP serum factors, now collectively designated MBP-SFs and all immunochemically related to MBP, could exist in the free state in the same serum as antibody against any of the other factors. We were led by these results to the current concepts: 1) that MBP-SFs are small fragments of the MBP molecule, each fragment with a different dominant determinant or epitope of MBP; 2) that the antibodies raised against each separate determinant are relatively restricted with respect to affinity but considerably heterogeneous overall (commensurate with current immunochemical concepts of proteins as antigens developed by Dr. Morris Reichlin and others); 3) that each inhibitor and its respective antibody are mutually antagonistic but that each inhibitor is unaffected by the presence of antibodies against the other inhibitors; 4) that high-affinity MBP-SF and low-affinity anti-MBP are probably more frequent companions in a normal rat than vice versa; and 5) that MBP-SFs probably function as nonimmunogenic autoneurotolerogens in the normal adult rat.

The fragment hypothesis has been reinforced recently by passive transfer studies carried out with our colleague, Vincent Varitek. Antibodies to MBP, when transferred to normal adult Lewis rats, exhibit an anomalous behavior that can best be explained by interaction with endogenous factors resembling small fragments of MBP that appear and disappear at times independent of each other (see Figure 6, page 271). The result is a strikingly different decay pattern for high-affinity antibody activity than for low-affinity antibody, both of which are yet considerably different than the decay of passively transferred control antisera against bovine serum albumin. The fragment hypothesis would also explain why it has been so difficult to isolate and characterize MBP-SF in a direct way: the fragments apparently are so small and so heterogeneous that they have escaped previous attempts at systematic isolation and alternate nonimmunochemical methods of detection. Although the fragment hypothesis seems to be consistent with all our experimental findings and the relative importance of high-affinity fragments to be apropos, we do not yet know whether a fragment that is characterized by high affinity in one animal is necessarily of high affinity in another, or whether the autoimmune anti-MBP response with respect to affinity is genetically uncontrolled. If a particular immunodeterminant of MBP were to be found to raise uniformly high-affinity antibodies, then immune response genes would probably be found to be responsible.

There are at least two different mechanisms that could lead to circulating fragments of whole MBP. Since MBP is readily degraded by the proteinases that characterize CNS tissue, fragments may arise from proteolysis of newly synthesized MBP, not yet intercalated into myelinated nerve fibers of adult CNS tissue. In the case

Figure 4

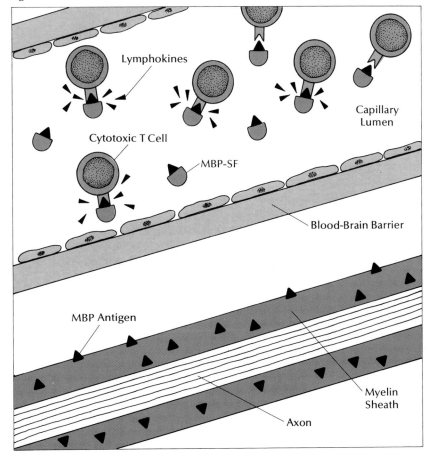

The protective function of MBP-SF is suggested schematically in this diagram. This fragment of myelin basic protein is thought to have specific surface receptors able to interact with anti-MBP cytotoxic T cells. As a result, inflammatory events that would otherwise cause demyelinization in the brain are abrogated.

Figure 5

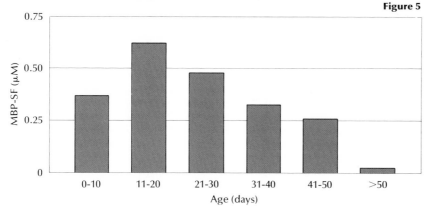

Graph above shows mean values of MBP-SF in suckling and adult Lewis rats. That below documents the inverse relationship between levels of MBP-SF and incidence of EAE in suckling rats sensitized to rat MBP in CFA.

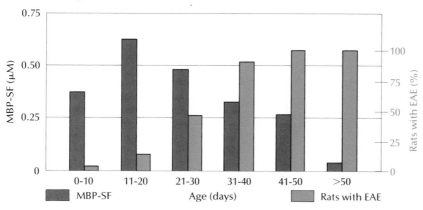

of suckling rats with minimally myelinated CNS, the amount of MBP not intercalated into neural tissue, and therefore vulnerable to proteolysis, would be far larger. Fragments of varying size resulting from such proteolysis can be visualized as leaving the neuraxis and quickly entering the systemic vascular compartment.

Alternatively, whole MBP might enter the vascular system directly and in the systemic circulation be degraded by blood proteinases of varying types. For example, it is known that when MBP is allowed to incubate in serum, enzyme activity degrades it to the extent that its encephalitogenic potential is lost; in contrast, such degradation is less pronounced when plasma is the incubation medium and is almost totally absent when phosphate-buffered saline is used. When MBP is incubated in serum that contains any of several trypsin inhibitors, little loss of EAE-inducing activity is observed. One possibility that these observations suggest is that proteases associated with the clotting cascade (plasmin being per-

haps the most prominent candidate) are responsible for degrading MBP into nonencephalitogenic fragments. It should be recalled that perivascular deposits of fibrin within the CNS are an important and early characteristic feature of the inflammatory response of EAE. Activation of the clotting cascade at sites of development of neuroimmunologic injury might well result in degradation of considerable amounts of MBP released from injured myelinated nerve fibers, with shedding of proteolytic breakdown fragments into the bloodstream.

What significance does MBP inhibitor have for development of EAE in rats? More importantly, can anything be said about MBP inhibitor in patients with MS, the prototypical demyelinating disease of humans that bears (as we shall see) many clinical pathologic and immunologic similarities to EAE? Obviously, a great deal of work is still required to answer either question, but if we work with the data in hand so far, we can provide at least tentative responses.

Let us start with the rat EAE model system and the already noted fact that it is harder to produce EAE in suckling than in adult Lewis rats using MBP as a sensitizing neuroantigen. In fact, suckling rats are virtually totally resistant to EAE if sensitized with syngeneic Lewis rat MBP. Since tolerance (or responsiveness) to a given self-antigen depends upon the concentration of that antigen relative to the number of specific receptors on T and B cells, and since it is easier to quench responsive T cells because they have fewer receptors than B cells, one would expect that, for a certain critically low concentration of self-antigen, B cells would normally be responsive while T cells would be tolerant. However, if circulating antigen is further reduced, it would be incapable of tolerizing the T cells (as well as the B cells). This would seem to be the state in which adult rats find themselves with respect to myelin basic protein. Thus, when exogenous MBP is introduced in sufficient quantity to activate a T-cell response, the result is T- and B-cell interaction and the full-blown immune response that ultimately involves endogenous MBP. Alternatively, if the number of responsive T cells is suddenly increased, as seems to happen when pure MBP is injected with CFA, CNS autoimmune disease would also result.

In suckling rats, however, high circulating concentrations of cross-reactive MBP-SF may serve to overwhelm otherwise responsive cells, muting host response either by tolerizing both T- and B-cell populations or by acting as an MBP-specific barrier between responsive T cells and the CNS target tissue (see Figure 4). Of special interest in this regard is a recent finding that draws upon the previously established point that EAE-inducing activity in the rat can be consistently transferred only after nine days have elapsed following immunization. We now know that in rats, the ninth day after sensitization is marked by a precipitous drop in MBP-SF in association with increasing concentrations of anti-MBP antibody. It is possible that this may reflect a tipping of the kinetic balance resulting from the consumption of all available MBP-SF. Theoretically, this might give sensitized T cells

Figure 6

unimpeded access to antigenic determinants on the CNS target tissue. Should subsequent antibody production, particularly of the high-affinity kind, play any regulatory role that would inhibit clonal expansion or cause shutdown, then the peak time for unimpeded T-cell interaction with host CNS antigen(s) would be sandwiched between the fall of MBP-SF and the rise of anti-MBP occurring on or around the ninth day.

As mentioned above, high-affinity MBP-SF and low-affinity anti-MBP appear to be more frequent companions in a normal (clinically well) rat than vice versa, but in the limited number of clinically well humans that have been observed, low-affinity anti-MBP circulates without an accompanying high-affinity MBP-SF (see Table 1, on page 272). In rats developing acute manifestations of EAE, the inhibitor levels eventually disappear with the rise of anti-MBP levels at all affinities (low-affinity antibodies increasing first, followed by the appearance of higher-affinity antibodies), and midway there may be (but there is not always time for it) a temporary explosion of inhibitors at all levels and particularly at the higher affinities. Our limited studies of patients with active MS to date reveal that in humans, as in rats, the various MBP-serum factors (MBP-SFs) show independence from one another and in the manner of putative fragments. In time-course studies, the affinity profile of a given patient, with respect to MBP-SFs and their complementary antibodies, may fluctuate widely, even alternating back and forth from inhibitor to antibody, a very good indication of an active and unstable process involving neuroantigens and the autoimmune responses they engender. Whether this instability of profile relates to the chronic nature of MS and its exacerbations, whether a quiescent and fixed pattern will characterize a state of remission, and whether a single profile or a number of possible patterns will characterize the clinically well individual are questions now under investigation.

The concept that MBP-SFs protect suckling rats from EAE is supported by evidence indicating that the whole, or undegraded, MBP molecule

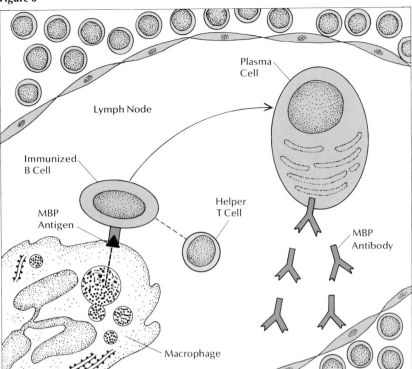

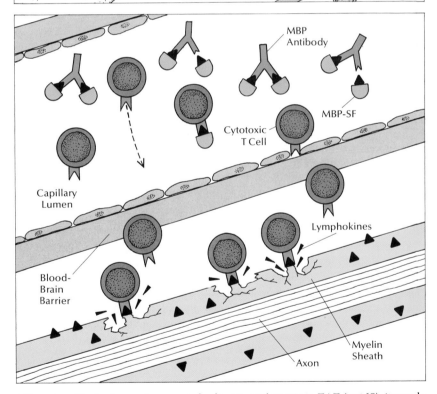

Although antibody does not appear to be directly pathogenic in EAE (or MS), it may be facilitatory. The schemes above suggest that like T cells, B lymphocytes may encounter MBP in draining lymph nodes, with resulting differentiation and anti-MBP antibody production (top). This antibody could then complex with MBP-SF in the circulation (bottom), thus denying cytotoxic T cells access to the protective SF. These T cells now have an unimpeded route to and through the blood-brain barrier. On reaching nervous system target tissue, the T lymphocytes will attack the specific MBP antigenic determinants located on the surface of the myelin sheath.

Table 1. Serum Levels of MBP-SF and Anti-MBP Antibody – Normal and Disease-Associated

Serum Donor		Number of Standard Deviations from Neutrality*					
		Inhibitor Affinity			Antibody Affinity		
Status	Species	High	Medium	Low	High	Medium	Low
Clinically well	rats:						
	1	8	<2	<3	<1	<1	10
	2	<2	>3	<2	<1	<1	<0
	3	<3	<2	<1	<1	<1	<3
	4	<1	<1	<1	<1	4	<0
	human subjects:						
	Ku	<1	<1	<3	<0	<1	6
	Wa	<1	<1	<1	<1	<0	13
	Ia	<1	<1	<1	<0	<3	10
Experimental allergic encephalomyelitis (EAE), acute phase	rats:						
	947	<1	<1	<1	20	5	17
	948	<2	<2	<2	5	<3	26
	949	<1	<1	<3	<1	>3	19
	953	<1	<1	<1	<1	5	13
Multiple sclerosis (MS), exacerbation	patients:						
	Or	<1	<1	<0	3	<0	11
	Ra-1	<2	<1	<2	<0	<0	4
	Ra-2	>3	<1	<1	<3	3	<2
	Go	<2	<2	17	<2	<0	<1
MS, chronic progressive	patients:						
	Mar	18	<2	<1	<0	<1	15
	Ga	<1	<1	<0	<0	<1	<0
	Ny	<2	<1	<0	4	<1	4
	Ak	<1	<1	<1	<1	<3	7

*Neutrality was defined in terms of a standard dual-dilution binding curve. High-, medium-, and low-affinity levels were at 0.6, 5.7, and 66 nM ^{125}I-MBP respectively. One standard deviation of inhibitor at these levels was ±0.82, ±0.62, and ±0.18 µM, respectively. One standard deviation of antibody (in terms of its antigenic binding capacity) at these levels was ±0.012, ±0.010, and ±0.008 µM, respectively. *Values were not considered significant unless at least 3 standard deviations (99%) removed from neutrality.* The term <0 indicates a negative deviation; in no case did such deviations achieve significance.

is composed of distinctly separate EAE-inducing and EAE-inhibiting fragments. For a number of years, it has been known that guinea pigs pretreated with MBP in aqueous solution or with incomplete Freund's adjuvant (IFA), lacking killed mycobacteria, do not readily succumb to EAE when subsequently sensitized with MBP and CFA. More recently, it has been found that different amino acid sequences of a given MBP molecule are recognized as the major encephalitogenic determinant by different species of animals. For example, the only tryptophan residue in MBP is known to be the major EAE determinant for the guinea pig but this residue has little or no EAE-inducing activity in rabbits, rats, or monkeys. Studies by R.H. Swanborg at Wayne State University have shown, however, that MBP can be rendered nonencephalitogenic for guinea pigs by blocking this critical tryptophan residue with 2-hydroxyl-5-nitrobenzyl bromide treatment. More important, this blocking of EAE-inducing activity does *not* affect the ability of the MBP molecule to inhibit EAE induction when it is subsequently given in aqueous solution or IFA. Moreover, G.A. Hashim at St. Luke's Hospital (Columbia) in New York has shown that the reason why bovine MBP is so much less encephalitogenic in the Lewis rat, compared with MBP of guinea pig or rat origin, is because the key encephalitogenic region on the bovine molecule is sequestered and blocked by the action of nearby amino acids. Studies using MBP obtained from rats have pinpointed another difference between EAE-inducing and EAE-inhibiting capacities of MBP. In fact, rats have two forms of MBP, the 170-residue molecule seen in other animals and a smaller molecule that lacks an essential portion of the amino acid sequence that is encephalitogenic in guinea pigs. It has

been shown that the small rat MBP molecule confers significant protection against EAE in guinea pigs. In rats, there also is increasing evidence that different amino acid sequences of the whole MBP molecule are responsible for EAE production on the one hand and for EAE inhibition on the other. At Northwestern University, one of us (P.Y.P.) has shown that guinea pig or rat MBP undergoes extensive proteolysis after incubation in normal Lewis rat serum at 37° C for eight or more hours. The degradation products are devoid of any EAE-inducing activity when mixed with Freund's adjuvant and injected into Lewis rats or guinea pigs. Such degradation products, however, still retain the capacity to inhibit EAE when mixed with IFA and injected in large amounts into Lewis rats for two weeks before such pretreated animals are challenged with MBP emulsified in CFA. In other words, the degradation of MBP by serum proteolysis destroys the immunodeterminant that produces EAE but leaves intact the immunodeterminant that inhibits the disease. Furthermore, such degradation improves the manner in which pretreatment and challenge elicits strong anti-MBP antibody responses.

What may be the relevance of all this to MS? Table 2, below, lists some of the parallels between the human and experimental diseases. First, both are characterized by remissions. Second, during acute attacks, the initial lesions of both MS and EAE are inflammatory. Early descriptions of little or no inflammation in MS were based on studies made in patients long after the acute phase of illness. Third, myelin-destructive, complement-dependent serum factors are found in MS patients; similarly, when animals are sensitized with whole nervous tissue antigen (not just purified MBP), the same is also true in EAE. Fourth, circulating lymphoid cells that proliferate in response to MBP and produce migration-inhibitory factor are found both in the animal model and in MS. Fifth, MBP is now known to be present in cerebrospinal fluid during acute attacks both in EAE and in MS. In the experimental disease, however, it may be bound to antibody, while in MS it can be found free. Sixth, in about three fourths of MS patients, enormous concentrations of IgG, plus IgG-secreting B cells, have been found in the sclerotic plaques; rats with EAE have IgG present around brain and spinal cord vessels. Finally, cells exerting an immunosuppressive effect are diminished during active disease and increased during clinical remissions.

The major discordance between MS and EAE is that evidence of T-cell sensitization to MBP (e.g., skin reactivity) is either absent in multiple sclerosis or far less pronounced than in EAE. But this difference is explicable. In EAE, the neuroantigen, plus adjuvant, is introduced at the periphery, virtually assuring an intense, *systemic* cell-mediated immune response; in MS, the absence of such a strong and generalized response could be explained by *confinement to the CNS* of some or even all of the major immunopathologic events culminating in neuroimmunologic disease.

As to how such localized sensitization to neuroantigen might be initiated in MS, EAE provides its only clue in CFA, the indispensible ingredient for disease induction when pure MBP is used as antigen. What might be the biologic equivalent of CFA in naturally occurring CNS autoimmune disease? Perhaps the foremost candidate, especially in a disease characterized by remissions and relapses, is a chronic viral infection, specifically a persistent type of infection of the CNS due to a paramyxovirus such as measles or parainfluenza virus. It must be admitted, however, that the evidence supporting this view is not particularly strong. For example, measles antibody titers have been reported to be higher in MS patients than in the general population. But when environmental, familial, and specific genetic determinants (such as HLA haplotypes) known to be associated with the MS process are taken into consideration, the differences in measles antibody titers between MS patients and matched control subjects become increasingly less marked. One group of investigators has reported isolation of parainfluenza virus from brain tissue of two patients with MS. But to date this finding has not been duplicated by the same investigative team in continued efforts along the same line, nor has it been confirmed by other research groups. Similarly, a more recent claim that a replicating agent can be isolated from bone marrow of MS patients awaits independent confirmation. To be sure, viruslike particles have been reported to be present in MS plaques, but in no case have the particles been shown to possess antigens reactive with specific antibodies directed against known virus antigens; indeed, in some cases, the structures have been shown to be artifacts.

Although the measles "case" is weak in evidence, it nonetheless remains theoretically attractive. Measles and other paramyxoviruses are notable for their capacity to persist by inserting virus-specified antigenic constituents into the membranes of infected host cells, making a self-plus-virus complex that would be expected to induce an immune response. Alternatively, this class of viruses might also be capable of making subtle alterations in self-antigens sufficient to render them effectively "foreign" by themselves. Whichever (if either) mechanism may be relevant to CNS autoimmune disease, it is worth noting that weanling hamsters chronically infected by intracerebral injection of measles virus (a defective strain isolated from a patient with subacute sclerosing panencephalitis) have been found to have a striking increase in susceptibility to EAE following sensitization by neuroantigen-CFA.

To date, MS patients have been treated with steroids, azathioprine, antilymphocyte globulin, and ACTH, and with each agent there was either no improvement or only temporary improvement. Despite this generally unimpressive record, immunosuppressive therapy, in one form or another, still retains some promise of efficacy for MS patients. For example,

Table 2. Concordance of Events in EAE and MS		
Characteristic Event	EAE (rats)	MS (patients)
Gene-determined susceptibility	+	+
Multifocal CNS signs; remittent course	+	++
Perivascular inflammation and demyelination	++	++
IgG deposits within active lesions	±	++
Cerebrospinal fluid contains: Neuroantigenic fragments	++	++
Selective increase in IgG	++	++
Peripheral blood and lymphoid tissues contain: Antimyelin cytotoxic antibodies	++	+
Lymphocytes sensitized to neuroantigen	++	+
Cells with suppressor activity	+	++

the group at Harrow, England, working under P. B. Medawar, has reported encouraging results of a uniquely controlled, double-blind study of an immunosuppressive regimen consisting initially of high-dose azathioprine and prednisolone in conjunction with antilymphocyte or antithymocyte globulin for one month, followed by tapering doses of the steroid and azathioprine over the subsequent 14 months.

Of course, two of the most specific and effective immunosuppressive reagents available are antigen and antibody. If using the EAE model one views MS as fundamentally a problem of loss of T-cell tolerance to neuroantigen, then, theoretically, one approach to therapy would be to give the MS patient large enough quantities of MBP to reinstitute tolerance through antigen excess and T-cell receptor saturation. In fact, this approach has been used clinically in two trials (the results showed neither harm nor benefit) and is currently being used or contemplated in at least two more trials, one each in the United States and Canada. In view of the ideas expressed in this account, one should imagine that use of nonencephalitogenic MBP fragments might well be more efficacious than use of the whole molecule.

Two important, and largely unanswered, questions must be posed concerning therapeutic use of MBP or any of its fragments. The first is to what extent the whole MBP molecule might be encephalitogenic in man, and the second, to what extent neuroantigens other than MBP might also be involved in the pathogenesis of MS (or, for that matter, EAE). While animal studies indicate that neither allogeneic nor xenogeneic MBP has EAE-inducing activity for rats or guinea pigs when injected in aqueous solution, there is very clear evidence that this neuroantigen can induce unmistakable EAE in these hosts when they are injected with MBP combined with a relatively weak immunopotentiating agent, such as synthetic ribonucleotides or IFA. The EAE-producing potential of the whole MBP molecule, therefore, requires very little help in order to become manifest. As for the second question, we have already noted that neuroantigen(s) other than MBP may be implicated in the immunopathogenesis of EAE, and, by analogy, the same may be true for MS. For example, complement-dependent cytotoxic IgG antibodies causing injury to glial cells and giving rise to demyelination in organotypic brain cultures have been reported in animals sensitized to cerebroside or galactocerebroside plus adjuvant. Cerebroside-reactive antibodies also have been reported to be present in normal subjects and patients with MS. Thus, the possibility exists that cerebrosides may also participate in CNS autoimmune disease. If so, therapeutic inhibition of T-cell responsiveness to MBP might serve to shut down only part of the disease mechanism.

Clearly, more studies are needed to elucidate the possible role of antibody response in EAE and MS. Just as clearly, studies of the possible efficacy of MBP-SF are also needed. If evidence can be secured that MBP degraded in serum deletes EAE-inducing determinants but leaves EAE-inhibiting determinants, then perhaps the most logical approach would be to give MS patients MBP that has been incubated in their own serum. Preliminary observations suggest that sera from MS patients and control subjects do not appreciably differ in their capacity to generate immunoinhibitory MBP fragments.

If such an approach does ultimately prove effective, it would offer an explanation for the alternating relapses and remissions characteristic of MS, one that would return us to the concept of loss of immunologic tolerance as exemplified in EAE. The critical factor regulating the clinical status of the MS patient (or EAE animal) would be the level of circulating self-antigen (MBP) relative to the level of specifically responsive lymphoid cells. A relapse would occur when the levels of self-antigen are low and insufficient to suppress the expanding clone. Administration of nonencephalitogenic but cross-reactive MBP would thus serve to suppress the host's immune response, quench the offending clone, reinstitute tolerance, and maintain remission of disease.

Autoimmune Antireceptor Diseases

JOHN D. STOBO   *University of California, San Francisco*

Many varieties of intercellular communication, including communication between adjacent cells and distant ones, are mediated by receptors. These receptors are information-rich macromolecules that confer on a cell the ability to respond to a particular molecular signal coming from without. They do this by binding specifically (i.e., recognizing) the molecule whose presence is meaningful to the cell. In the case of neuroendocrine receptors, this binding results in some biochemical activity on the part of the receptor that sets in motion an appropriate response by the receiving cell.

During the last decade, as the concept of receptors has become a familiar one, we have become aware of the existence of antireceptor diseases. These are autoimmune disorders in which a receptor becomes the target of an immune response. The receptor under attack in each of the disorders now recognized as an antireceptor disease is crucially important in mediating the physiologic function of the tissue on which it resides, and each antireceptor disease is manifest, therefore, as dysfunction of its respective tissue.

This article will discuss three antireceptor diseases: myasthenia gravis, in which the receptor in question is the acetylcholine receptor at the neuromuscular junction; Graves' disease, caused by antibodies to the thyroid-cell receptors for thyroid-stimulating hormone; and a type of insulin-resistant diabetes mellitus that results from the production of antibodies to the insulin receptor. I shall also mention a subset of allergic rhinitis and asthma that may be caused by antibodies to beta-2-adrenergic receptors.

These diseases are particularly interesting to the immunologist because they present multiple questions—not just what happens when antireceptor antibodies interact with receptors but how the disease-causing antibodies come to be produced. The loss of tolerance in antireceptor diseases can be part of a more widespread autoimmune disorder or can be highly specific, and there are suggestive parallels between these neuroendocrine receptors and the antigen receptors on lymphocytes that might also serve as targets for inappropriate immune activity.

The antireceptor disease best characterized at present is myasthenia gravis, which, as its name implies, is a disease of severe muscle weakness. It is caused, we now know, by antibodies (predominantly IgG) directed against the acetylcholine receptor at the neuromuscular junction. Acetylcholine is the neurotransmitter that carries the signal for muscular contraction across the synaptic cleft from the nerve terminal to the muscle cell. In myasthenia gravis, that signal is transmitted but not perceived. To review briefly, neuromuscular transmission is a complex process involving the synthesis of acetylcholine, the packaging of the neurotransmitter into vesicles, the release of acetylcholine at the appropriate time, its diffusion across the synapse and interaction with acetylcholine receptors, and the subsequent change in permeability of the postsynaptic membrane. Some 150 to 200 transmitter-containing vesicles are released each time the nerve terminal is depolarized by the arrival of a physiologic impulse, but the spontaneous release of even a single vesicle results in end-plate depolarization great enough to be detected experimentally as a "miniature end-plate potential."

In patients with myasthenia gravis, the miniature end-plate potentials are abnormally small in amplitude. Initially, it was presumed that this represented a diminution in available acetylcholine. It was only in the early 1970s that this finding was correctly accounted for, when D. B. Drachman and his colleagues showed with radiolabeled alpha-bungarotoxin, a snake venom toxin that binds to acetylcholine receptors, that the number of acetylcholine receptors functionally available at each neuromuscular junction is reduced in myasthenic patients to 10% to 30% of normal. The amount of neurotransmitter released by a presynaptic depolarization, therefore, may not result in a sufficient number of transmitter–receptor interactions to achieve threshold depolarization of the postsynaptic membrane.

Long before it was possible to assay acetylcholine receptors, myasthenia gravis was thought to involve autoimmunity, on the basis of the frequency (75%) of associated thymic abnormalities and its association with other diseases thought to be autoimmune in nature, such as lupus erythematosus and Hashimoto's thyroiditis. This line of thinking became firmly established with the discovery by J. Patrick and J. Lindstrom that rabbits develop a syndrome very similar to myasthenia gravis when they are immunized with purified acetylcholine receptors from electric eels. Soon antireceptor antibody was demonstrated in the blood of myasthenics; with the best current assay techniques, antibody to acetylcholine receptors can be documented in about 90% of all patients with clinical myasthenia.

The presence of antibodies in patients with a disease does not establish, of course, that they cause the disease or even that they are related to its etiology. The causative role played by antibody to the acetylcholine receptor in myasthenia gravis is firmly supported by a number of different lines of evidence. One is the development, noted previously, of a disease very similar clinically and electrophysiologically to myasthenia gravis in animals immunized against the receptors. It is also possible to induce in mice "clinical" myasthenia, reduction in the number of acetylcholine receptor sites at the neuromuscular junctions, and reduction in the amplitude of miniature endplate potentials by injecting IgG from myasthenic patients for several consecutive days. The same sort of transfer phenomenon is seen in neonates born to mothers with myasthenia gravis. In about one sixth of these infants, symptoms of myasthenia are transiently present for a few weeks after birth, and antiacetylcholine receptor antibodies, presumably transferred transplacentally, have been found in the affected babies.

One might suppose that antireceptor antibody causes the disease by "blocking" the receptor and preventing access by the acetylcholine molecule to its binding site. Blockade would be consistent with the observed decline in receptor number because the receptors can be assayed only with snake venom toxins that bind at the acetylcholine binding site and, therefore, would fail to mark a blocked receptor. In fact, however, blockade probably plays a small, if any, role in myasthenia gravis. Re-

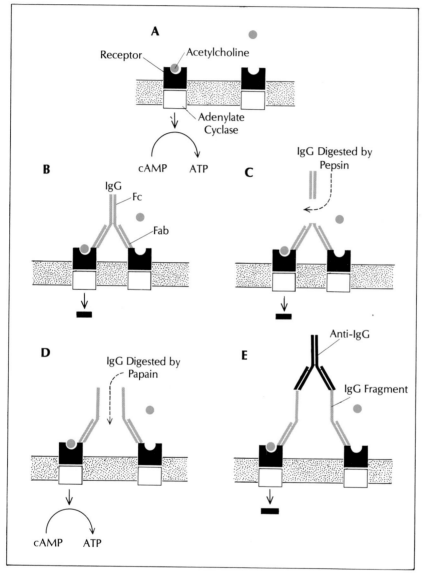

Normally, binding of hormone to neuroendocrine receptor initiates sequence of events leading to a physiologic response (A). In antireceptor disease, e.g., myasthenia gravis, functioning is prevented by accelerated receptor degradation initiated by cross-linking of receptors by divalent IgG (B). Interaction with hormone is not prevented, but transmission of signal across cell membrane is. When Fc portion of IgG molecule is digested away by pepsin (C), cross-linkage by divalent F(ab')$_2$ fragments still prevents transmission of signal. Papain digestion splits IgG into monovalent fragments, destroying cross-linkage and permitting normal transmission (D). Cross-linking with divalent anti-IgG again blocks transmission across cell membrane (E).

ceptor saturated with antibody continues to bind the neurotransmitter. The mechanism of the disease appears, instead, to involve increased destruction by the muscle cell of receptors bound by antibody. This was shown by Drachman in a tissue culture system by using radiolabeled alpha-bungarotoxin; when the toxin is attached to the receptors, it is metabolized, and the label is released into the culture medium only when the receptor itself is degraded. In the presence of myasthenic immunoglobulin, muscle cells degrade their acetylcholine receptors more than twice as fast as they do when exposed to control immunoglobulin.

It remains to be established just what happens to the receptors, but Drachman's experiments went on to show that the accelerated degradation of receptors requires that they be cross-linked, which occurs when a divalent antibody binds to two adjacent receptors. For example, one can digest antireceptor IgG with pepsin to produce the divalent antigen-binding fragment F(ab')$_2$, which lacks the Fc portion often viewed as the "effector" portion of the IgG molecule; the F(ab')$_2$ fragment is just as active as native myasthenic IgG is in accelerating receptor degradation. This is not the case with the monovalent Fab fragments produced by papain digestion of IgG. Fab fragments continue to bind to individual receptors, but they do not affect receptor degradation. One subsequently can add intact antibody directed against monovalent Fab fragments to cross-link the receptor-bound Fab, and again, increased receptor degradation results.

It is not at all obvious why cross-linking acetylcholine receptors with antibody should cause their degradation, but the phenomenon observed in myasthenic muscle cells has been noted to be analogous to "capping" in lymphocytes. Under appropriate conditions, divalent antibodies directed against membrane determinants, including receptors, on the surfaces of lymphocytes cause all or most of the receptors on a given cell to aggregate at one pole as a "cap," a mat of receptors cross-linked by antibodies. Then part of the cap is

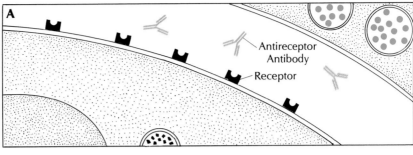

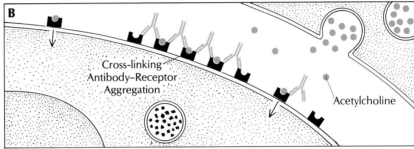

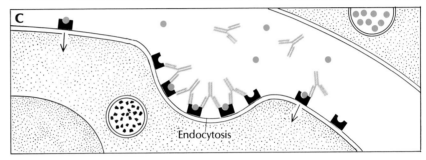

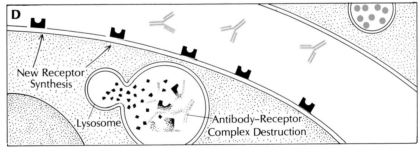

Receptors in myasthenia gravis are normal, but presence of antireceptor antibody is abnormal (A). Antibody-induced receptor degradation is thought to be analogous to "capping" in lymphocytes. Receptors aggregate as they are cross-linked by antibody (B). Areas of cross-linked antibody-receptor aggregates are then endocytosed (C) and destroyed by lysosomal enzymes. New receptor forms on the cell surface to be, in turn, cross-linked, endocytosed, and destroyed (D).

endocytosed, that is, disappears into the interior of the cell, where it is destroyed, while another portion simply falls off. This results in a decrease in the number of receptors against which the divalent antibody was directed. One can easily suppose that a continual process of receptor aggregation and endocytosis occurs on the muscle cells of myasthenic patients as new acetylcholine receptors are synthesized and bound together by antibody. This process ultimately may affect the capacity of the cell to manufacture new receptors because some patients with long-standing disease fail to improve even if the antibodies are therapeutically removed.

Degradation is not necessarily the

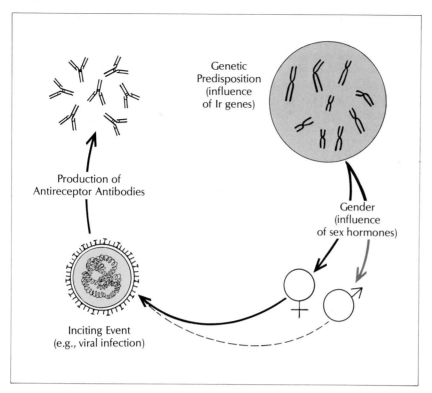

The multifactorial pathogenesis of antireceptor disease is conceptualized as starting with genetic predisposition, strengthened by female sex hormones, with an inciting event, such as viral infection, triggering an effective antibody response.

fate of every cellular receptor to which antibody binds. The outcome of interactions between receptors and antireceptor antibodies is quite different in Graves' disease. There the antibody binding on or near the receptor for thyroid-stimulating hormone (TSH) has a stimulatory effect on the thyroid cell similar to that mediated by TSH itself. The disease results from excessive production of thyroid hormones. It is not known just why, in the presence of antibody, TSH receptors continue to function vigorously while acetylcholine receptors undergo net degradation, but we do know some interesting details about the antibody–receptor relationship in Graves' disease.

The pathogenic agent in Graves' disease is an immunoglobulin, occasionally an IgM but usually an IgG, that binds as mentioned to the TSH receptors on thyroid cells. One might presume, since the antibody mimics the physiologic effects of TSH, that it binds at the TSH binding site, but in reality the situation, as worked out by R. Volpé and his colleagues at the University of Toronto, is a bit more complicated. Immunoglobulin from patients with Graves' disease, adsorbed on thyroid cell membranes, inhibits the binding of radiolabeled TSH, but so does immunoglobulin from normals. Graves' IgG has more activity by this assay, in general, but not uniformly so—IgG from about a quarter of all Graves' patients fall within the normal range. The ability of antibody to stimulate the thyroid, therefore, does not require an exceptional affinity for the TSH binding site. The converse is also true; that is, some antibodies—notably from patients with other thyroid diseases, such as Hashimoto's thyroiditis, subacute thyroiditis, and thyroid carcinoma—can strongly inhibit TSH binding and yet have no thyroid stimulatory activity. When Graves' immunoglobulin is tested for ability to stimulate human thyroid, it is almost uniformly (93%) active, and this activity is highly specific for Graves' disease.

It should be noted that similar observations have been made with regard to myasthenia gravis: 90% of myasthenic patients have antiacetylcholine receptor antibody, and this antibody will cause disease in experimental animals; but when monoclonal antibodies, selected for antiacetylcholine receptor specificity, are produced by human-mouse hybridoma clones, some but not all of these antibodies are capable of producing disease.

Curiously enough, monovalent Fab fragments of thyroid-stimulating IgG are not active. Here, too, divalence seems to be a prerequisite for the antireceptor antibodies to have their biologic effect.

Graves' disease and myasthenia gravis are, to the best of our knowledge, diseases caused exclusively by antireceptor antibodies. Antireceptor antibodies are also known to cause a small subset of diabetes mellitus (see J. Roth, "Insulin Receptors in Diabetes," Hosp Pract, May 1980). These antibodies to the insulin receptor were described first by J. S. Flier in 1975, and only about 20 to 30 cases have been detected since. The resulting disease is severe, insulin-resistant diabetes; usually the patient is a middle-aged non-Caucasian woman with the skin disorder acanthosis nigricans and some other signs or symptoms of autoimmune disease. It has been called the syndrome of insulin-resistant diabetes with acanthosis nigricans (the association with acanthosis nigricans remains unexplained) or type B insulin-resistant diabetes, in order to distinguish it from another subtype that is apparently caused by an inborn defect of the receptor system.

The initial observation in this disease was of a profound reduction in insulin affinity of normally receptive tissues, a reduction that could be reproduced in vitro with the patients' serum. Details have been added since by Flier and his colleagues C. R. Kahn, J. Roth, R. Bar, and others at the NIH. The active compound is usually IgG antibody (although IgM has been found, too—notably, in patients with ataxia-telangiectasia) that competes with insulin for binding sites on cell surfaces. Here again, however, the mechanism by which the antibodies produce disease is more complicated than simple receptor blockade. When anti-insulin receptor antibodies are added to insulin-sensitive cells in vitro, they have the same effects as insulin itself. In other words, they stimulate the receptors. The stimulated state is short-lived, however, and in a matter of hours is replaced by an extreme insulin-resistant state. Just what happens to the receptors in the interim is not known; they may be degraded. Alternatively, recent studies suggest that interactions between the insulin receptor and antireceptor antibody do not decrease the number of insulin receptors. Instead, they initiate an intracellular, postreceptor event that prevents transmission of signals from the receptor to appropriate intracellular machinery. In either case, the net effect is insulin resistance.

Whatever the antibodies may do to the insulin receptors, it requires polyvalence. Bivalent F(ab')$_2$ fragments have the same effect as native IgG, but Fab fragments bind to receptors and inhibit insulin binding, without any insulinlike activity. Once cells have been treated with Fab, however, addition of bivalent anti-Fab IgG elicits the insulinlike effect.

We know of one additional example of antireceptor antibodies associated with disease. These are IgG antibodies directed against beta-2-adrenergic receptors. Only preliminary data about these antibodies and their relationship to disease are available. They were described in 1980 by J. Venter and C. Fraser at SUNY, Buffalo, and by L. Harrison at the NIH. They examined serum from 10 atopic patients and found antireceptor antibodies in three: two patients with asthma and one with allergic rhinitis. The antibodies block binding of a beta-antagonist to lung but not heart beta-adrenergic receptors; that is, they have beta-2 specificity. This is far from proving that the antibodies cause disease, of course, but the potential significance of circulating anti-beta-2 substances in asthma is obvious; in the absence of beta-2-adrenergic input, disease might result from unopposed alpha-adrenergic, histaminergic, cholinergic, or prosta-

glandin effects. It remains to be seen what happens to receptors on living cells when they are exposed to the antibody (whether the antibody can cause disease) and just what fraction of patients with asthma and allergic rhinitis actually have this antireceptor antibody.

Now we can confront the question of how these pathogenic autoantibodies arise. Suspicion turns naturally toward the receptors themselves, and we may ask whether some change in the receptors or in their immediate environment causes them abruptly to become immunogenic, whether there is any common denominator at the level of the receptors. The answer is that there is no evidence whatever for any alteration in the receptors. Receptors are, by definition, complex molecules that are capable of antigenicity, but the normal situation is tolerance. The common denominator when this tolerance is lost is change, not in the receptor but at the level of the immune response.

Evidence for derangement in the

regulation of the immune system is found in the high frequency with which antireceptor diseases are associated with other autoimmune phenomena. From here on, I shall speak only about myasthenia gravis, Graves' disease, and autoimmune diabetes mellitus, since the data on anti-beta-2-receptor antibodies are too scanty to permit discussion. In this form of diabetes, generalized autoimmunity is most striking; it is found in virtually all patients. About one third of them have a recognizable autoimmune syndrome, such as systemic lupus erythematosus, scleroderma, or Sjögren's syndrome; the rest have laboratory abnormalities, such as antinuclear or antimitochondrial antibodies. As for Graves' disease and myasthenia gravis, there are a significant number of cases in which antireceptor antibodies are the only detectable immune abnormality, but in general, the presence of other autoimmune phenomena, either clinical or detectable only in the laboratory, is the rule rather than the exception.

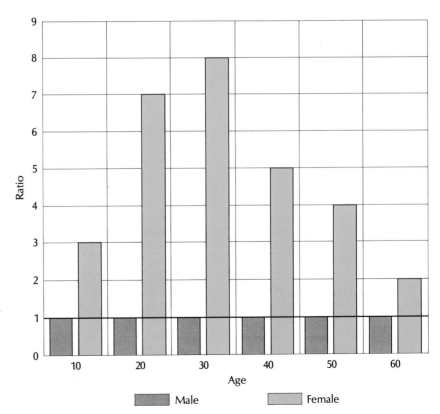

Striking predilection of autoimmune disease for females is apparent from adolescence. It peaks in the fourth decade and begins to diminish as menopause approaches.

General Features of Antireceptor Diseases

	Myasthenia Gravis	Graves' Disease	Insulin-Resistant Diabetes	Allergic Rhinitis and Asthma
Specificity of antibody	ACH receptor	TSH receptor	Insulin receptor	Beta-adrenergic receptor in lung
Incidence of antibody in disease	80%–90%	90%	Type B (small subset)	Three out of 10 patients with atopy
Biologic consequence	Muscle weakness	Hyperthyroidism	Diabetes mellitus	Allergic rhinitis, asthma
Mechanism by which antibody may cause disease	↑ Degradation of receptors	Stimulated production of thyroid hormones	↑ Degradation of receptor, postreceptor events	Unopposed effect of alpha-receptor agonists
Genetic predisposition	HLA-B8, HLA-DRw3	HLA-B8, HLA-DRw3	?	?
Associated with other autoimmune phenomena	Yes	Yes	Yes	?

One thing is certain about the development of antireceptor antibodies: It is multifactorially determined. If there is an event that results abruptly in the production of the autoantibodies, it results in disease only if a number of other factors that might be termed "permissive influences" are already present.

Sex is clearly one of those permissive influences. Women are more frequently afflicted with antireceptor diseases than men are, just as they are more susceptible to autoimmune disease in general. The ratio of female to male patients is on the order of six to one, a striking asymmetry. There have been some interesting studies that implicate hormonal influences in the development of autoimmunity. In the murine model of lupus, for example, females of the susceptible strain develop the disease earlier than males do, but this difference can be diminished by administering androgens to the females or estrogens to the males. Further evidence that hormones play a role in the development of autoimmunity comes from work done by H. G. Kunkel's group in New York; they have shown that women with

lupus erythematosus have in their urine a very potently estrogenic compound that is not found in the urine of women without the disease (see H. G. Kunkel, "The Immunopathology of SLE").

Genetic predisposition also plays a part in the development of at least some antireceptor diseases. Both Graves' disease and myasthenia gravis occur with exceptional frequency in patients bearing HLA types B8 and DRw3. We have no good data yet on HLA associations with autoimmune diabetes mellitus since so few patients have been identified. There is, however, an identical disease in mice that clearly is genetically determined. It occurs in the NZO strain, a mouse closely related to the NZB mouse that develops lupuslike autoimmune diseases.

The association of these diseases with HLA-DR determinants is highly significant in our thinking about their genesis because the HLA-D locus appears to represent the equivalent of the immune response (Ir) locus in the H-2 complex of mice. That is, we believe that immune response genes (genes that determine the antigens to which an organism

can or cannot generate an immune response) are associated with the segment of genome that encodes the HLA-DR determinants, just as in the mouse they are located in the region encoding the immune response–associated (Ia) determinants. This presumption is supported by multiple lines of evidence. First, the tissue distribution of the HLA-DR antigens is very similar to the distribution of Ia antigens in mice. Second, the fine molecular structure of the HLA-DR antigenic determinants is very similar, in terms of amino acid sequence, to the structure of the murine Ia determinants. Third, the HLA-D gene products serve as stimulating determinants in the mixed lymphocyte reaction (MLR), just as Ir gene products determine the MLR in mice.

A fourth line of evidence (indirect) lies in the association of particular HLA-DR types with diseases known to be caused by inappropriate immune responses. Graves' disease and myasthenia gravis are examples of this kind of association; another is Goodpasture's syndrome, in which there is production of antibody to basement membrane. Here the association is with HLA-DRw2.

Finally, it has been possible to show directly in humans that the ability or inability to respond to particular antigens is predictable from the HLA-DR type. T. Sasazuki's group in Japan and that of G. Fathman at the Mayo Clinic have both done this, and in my own laboratory we have recently shown that the immune response to collagen in man is controlled by genes linked to those that code for HLA-DRw4. That is, we not only know that rheumatoid arthritis, in which an immune reaction to collagen is seen, is associated with HLA-DRw4, but among normal blood donors free of disease, every individual tested who was HLA-DRw4-positive did, in fact, respond to collagen.

We are left, however, with the fact that not every individual in whom these permissive influences are present ever develops disease. Only a minority do. Thus, there must be other factors involved in pathogenesis. Viral infection is suspected as a precipitating influence. There is very little in the way of evidence to implicate viruses in antireceptor diseases; we simply have not been able to devise a more likely explanation for why a 30-year-old woman who is otherwise in good health should suddenly begin producing antibodies to antigenic determinants that she has tolerated since before birth. We suppose that in a permissive hormonal milieu—in the presence of a particular set of immune response genes and, possibly, other genetic or environmental influences that have yet to be defined—a viral infection sets off the immune reaction that culminates in antireceptor disease.

Recognition of the autoimmune nature of these diseases is obviously meaningful from the standpoint of treatment. If the pathogenesis of a disease is one of autoimmunity, then we would like to direct our treatment at the level of the immune response. Up to the present time, unfortunately, we have been limited to rather coarse and nonspecific intervention in the immune process. Plasmapheresis may remove antireceptor antibodies, but of course, it removes all the other antibodies as well. Glucocorticoids and immunosuppressive agents, such as azathioprine or cy-

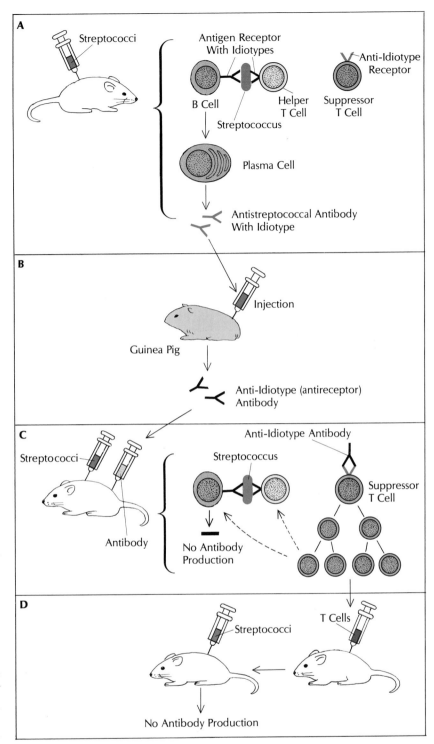

Drawings hypothesize the role of anti-idiotype antibodies in altering immunologic response, using experiments of K. Eichmann as an example. When streptococcal antigens are injected into animals (A), they interact with antigen receptors on helper T cells and B cells, and antistreptococcal antibodies are secreted. If these antibodies are injected into another species (B), antibodies directed against idiotypic determinants can be produced. Infusion of these anti-idiotype antibodies into mice can interact preferentially, under appropriate conditions, with idiotypes displayed by antigen receptors on suppressor T cells and induce their clonal expansion (C). This inhibits the production of streptococcal antibodies bearing those idiotypes. This antigen-specific unresponsiveness can be transferred with T cells (D).

clophosphamide, can suppress production of the offending antibodies, but only by subjecting the patient to the risks of generalized immunosuppression. Immunosuppressive measures are used with good results, particularly in myasthenia gravis and with preliminary reports of benefit in autoimmune diabetes mellitus. They are generally reserved, however, for cases in which nonimmunologic treatment measures have failed. In myasthenia gravis, the mainstay of treatment is anticholinesterase therapy; in Graves' disease, it is antithyroid medication.

In the near future, we shall be able to manipulate specific immune responses, and the chances are good, for example, that we shall be able to modulate the production of antibody to the acetylcholine receptor without interfering with the production of other antibodies that may be necessary in host defense. Antireceptor diseases are ideal candidates for this type of specific immunomodulation, which has already been accomplished in animal models by using foreign, exogenous antigens. Interestingly enough, it involves antibody directed against cell surface receptors—in this case, receptors on the surfaces of lymphocytes.

These lymphocyte surface receptors are receptors not for hormones or neurotransmitters but for antigen, and their specificity is responsible for the specificity of the immune response. The receptors on B lymphocytes appear to be classical immunoglobulin molecules; the determinants we find exposed on T cells are those of the portions of immunoglobulin heavy chains involved in antibody binding. On both types of cells we still find exposed the so-called idiotypic determinants. The term idiotype refers to the antigenic determinant dictated by the structure on the antibody that gives it its antigen-binding specificity. Idiotypic determinants inherent in anti-body, B-cell receptors, and T-cell receptors with specificity for one antigen are different from idiotypic determinants inherent in corresponding recognition units with specificity for another antigen.

We know that net immune reactivity reflects a complex series of interactions between distinct populations of lymphocytes. The function of some of these cells is to mediate immune reactivity; others function to control it. In other words, the immune system not only is required to react quickly and aggressively to foreign antigens but also must regulate its own reactivity. This necessitates some language through which the various populations of cells that participate in the immune response can communicate, and this communication should occur only among cells reacting to a particular antigen. N. K. Jerne has postulated (and his theory is supported by experimental data) that idiotypes serve as the language for this communication. Indeed, the immune system can be thought of as a network linked by communication occurring between idiotypes and their complement, e.g., anti-idiotypes. This network theory predicts that it should be possible to modulate immune reactivity, in an antigen-specific fashion, by interrupting the idiotype–anti-idiotype network.

In fact, this is the case. For example, Klaus Eichmann found that by administering antibodies directed against idiotypic determinants inherent in antibody to one antigen (streptococci), he could blunt the response to streptococci without impairing the animal's ability to respond to other antigens. Baruj Benacerraf and his colleagues similarly have suppressed immune reactivity to a specific antigen (azobenzene arsonate, or ABA). However, instead of injecting anti-idiotype antibodies, they isolated anti-ABA antibodies, bound them artificially to the surfaces of cells to render them immunogenic, and gave these cells back to the animal so it would generate its own anti-idiotype response.

In these models, it is apparent that the suppression of reactivity does not merely represent a blockade of cell receptors. The antigen-specific, immunologic unresponsiveness can be transferred from animal to animal by T cells. Thus, interference with the idiotype–anti-idiotype communication results in a predominance of suppressive T cells. It should be emphasized that under certain experimental conditions, interference with idiotype–anti-idiotype communication can result in enhancement, not suppression, of immune reactivity. This emphasizes the dynamic nature of the idiotype network.

These experiments point up the remarkable amount of communication that must go on in the generation of an immune response to foreign antigens. More importantly, they suggest that similar communication may be required to maintain tolerance to certain self-antigens, including neuroendocrine receptors. There is an apparent paradox in this concept for it implies that autoimmunity both represents immunologic aggression against some self-determinants and results from a defect in the immunologic recognition of others. For example, production of antibodies to acetylcholine receptors might stem from a defect in recognition of idiotypes, which normally serves to prevent such reactivity.

To an immunologist, the neuroendocrine receptor diseases are prototypes; the analogy between neuroendocrine receptors and lymphocyte antigen receptors helps to account for the possibility that spectacular and specific immunologic derangements may result when antibodies against lymphocyte receptors for antigen (i.e., anti-idiotypes) are produced.

Immunopathology of Persistent Viral Infection

MICHAEL B. A. OLDSTONE *Research Institute of the Scripps Clinic*

A very familiar scenario for the interaction between a virus and a cell ends in destruction of the cell, either by the virus or by the host's immune system. For a long time, however, it has been known that viruses are capable of persisting in eukaryotic cells in vivo for long periods without killing the host cell or provoking an immunologic attack that would do so. What has been much less clear is whether these prolonged infections cause disease and, if so, how they cause it. We are beginning to have a better understanding of the factors that enable viruses to maintain an infection for years despite a vigorous antiviral immune response by the host. It is also becoming increasingly clear that persistent viral infections do cause disease; they may do so, in fact, without causing any readily apparent damage to the cells they infect, by way of relatively subtle derangements of cellular function (Figures 1 and 2, page 284). What we know about the way in which these infections disrupt homeostatic physiologic balance raises the likelihood that persistent viral infections may cause a variety of human diseases, the characteristics of which will be described later.

Most of our knowledge of how viruses cause disease is focused on acute viral infection. This emphasis results in large part from a practical difficulty of working with viruses in the laboratory. Many of our analytical methods require quantities of virus that are more difficult to obtain with less virulent viruses. Usually, lytic viruses that grow to extremely high titers will yield enough viral products for productive biochemical studies. Our thinking about disease during viral infection, therefore, has long been dominated by the idea of cytopathology—cellular destruction caused either directly or indirectly by the virus—as it occurs in acute viral infections.

Consequently, we can construct a fairly extensive list of the means whereby viruses destroy host cells. They may disrupt the cell's plasma membrane completely or alter its permeability enough to preclude the possibility of the cell's effective regulation of its contents. They may disrupt the membranes of structures entirely within the cell, such as lysosomal vacuoles, to release lethal digestive enzymes. Viral products may block enzymes necessary for intermediary metabolism or replication. Viral proteins can alter the plasma membrane, causing cells to fuse with one another and form syncytial giant cells that are no longer capable of functioning.

Another category of cellular injury is that inflicted by the immune system on cells acutely infected with virus. Viral components that are exposed on the surface of the infected cell tend to be recognized by the immune system as foreign, and the cell can subsequently be destroyed by any of several immunologic mechanisms. Cytotoxic lymphocytes or antibody-plus-complement cytolysis play important roles, depending upon the conditions. Although immune surveillance destroys cells, it can be seen, of course, as adaptive, in that by sacrificing infected cells prior to release of progeny virus, the organism has a better opportunity to limit the spread of virus and thus to enhance its survival.

Nevertheless, the immune response to viral infections does not always work to the benefit of the host. For example, lymphocytic choriomeningitis virus

Figure 1

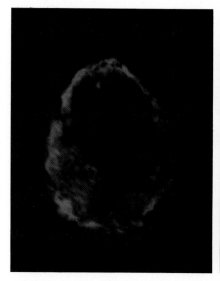
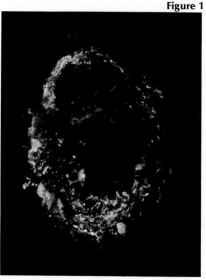

A role for persistent viral infection in vascular immune complex disease is supported by fluorescent microphotography of small artery in patient with polyarteritis nodosa. Both hepatitis B antigen (left) and specific immunoglobulin (right) are visualized. (Photomicrographs courtesy Dr. Adam Nowoslawski)

(LCMV), which will be described in considerably more detail, is a relatively noncytopathic virus, and cultured cells infected experimentally with the virus will appear normal and even grow normally as long as the culture system is free of immune effector reagents. If antiviral antibody and complement or cytotoxic T lymphocytes primed to viral glycoprotein are added to the culture when viral antigens are expressed on the surfaces of those apparently healthy infected cells, however, those cells will be killed (Figure 3, page 286). Results in vivo parallel those in vitro: Normal adult mice infected with the virus die rapidly of meningochoroidoencephalitis, but if the host animal is immunosuppressed by any of a variety of manipulations, such as thymectomy or pharmacologic means, it will survive without any dramatic disease.

From a virologic point of view, then, an acute viral infection results in the destruction of infected cells, either directly or by way of immune intervention. When these events at the cellular level are translated to the level of the individual, it is easy to see that the loss of cells can translate into some degree of disease for the host. The nature and severity of the disease that results will be a function of the particular group of cells, as well as the number, that happens to have been lost. Loss of insulin-producing cells, for example, will result in insulin-dependent diabetes mellitus. There is still no way to know just how many cases of that disease are the result of viral infection, but it is becoming clear that there are viruses that can specifically destroy enough pancreatic beta cells to cause clinical diabetes. In this event, histopathologic examination will show abnormalities that correlate with the disease: Insulin-secreting cells may simply be reduced or absent from the islets of Langerhans if they have been the victims of a lytic virus. Participation of the immune system at the appropriate time would show an inflammatory infiltrate. Similarly, lysis of cells in the central nervous system will cause neurologic disease, the loss of cardiac muscle cells may cause heart disease, and so on. I describe this almost self-evident state of affairs in some detail in order to contrast with it the events that occur in certain persistent viral infections.

One of the most remarkable facts about persistent viral infections is that they persist at all, i.e., that they escape immune surveillance so that the infected cells are not destroyed. The example I shall use to introduce this discussion of how viruses persist is, again, lymphocytic choriomeningitis virus, a virus that has been the object of a tremendous amount of research on the immune system and viral mechanisms of disease. Lympho-

Figure 2

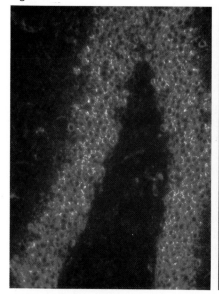
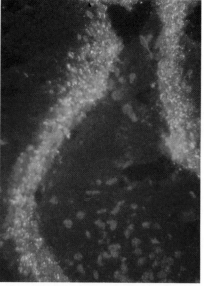

Persistent LCMV infection produced strongly positive staining with two different monoclonal antibodies directed against viral nucleoprotein of neurons in the dentate tract. At the same time, staining for surface glycoprotein was negative.

cytic choriomeningitis virus is particularly interesting since it can cause either acute or chronic disease, depending on the circumstances of the infection. Although humans can suffer from LCMV disease, it is chiefly a virus of rodents and is endemic in both wild and some laboratory populations, and most cases in humans represent zoonotic infection of persons exposed to wild or domestic mice and hamsters. LCMV is a negative-stranded RNA virus of the arenavirus group. Other arenaviruses, such as Lassa fever, Argentine hemorrhagic fever, and Bolivian hemorrhagic fever viruses, can cause severe human disease, so that laboratory work with them is restricted to high-containment areas.

Lymphocytic choriomeningitis virus, as noted, causes a fatal acute disease in adult mice. If mice are injected with the virus at birth, however, no acute disease occurs. They usually grow to adulthood more or less normally. When these adult mice are sacrificed, however, neurons in the central nervous system are found to be filled with viral antigens. For some reason, the mice do not mount a sufficient immune attack to clear the virus-infected cells.

This state of affairs has been known for a long time; in fact, the persistence of LCMV infection after neonatal inoculation is one of the models on which the idea of specific immune tolerance was originally based by Macfarlane Burnet. Since then, my colleagues and I have demonstrated that the persistently infected mice, in fact, are not tolerant to the virus; they make considerable amounts of antibody to viral proteins. This antibody is usually not found free in circulating blood, however, since there is a large excess of viral antigen and the antiviral antibody combines with viral antigens in the circulation to form immune complexes (Figure 1). These immune complexes, which may constitute the only manifestation of disease in the persistently infected animals, lead to the development of glomerulonephritis, choroiditis, and vasculitis (see C. B.

Wilson and F. J. Dixon, "Immunologic Mechanisms in Nephritogenesis").

Although antibodies to all the LCMV polypeptides can be detected in circulating and tissue-trapped immune complexes, the mice do not clear the infection. Quantitatively viewed, the amount of antibody present establishes that the mice are actually hyperimmune to the virus. It is more difficult to demonstrate the presence of cytotoxic T lymphocytes, and one might hypothesize that these cells are not present, or are being turned off or blocked, or are themselves being infected and put out of commission by the virus. One of my colleagues, Rafi Ahmed, has recently shown that LCMV can suppress a variety of immune responses in a dose-related manner, including cytotoxic T-cell responses. This viral immunosuppression, however, occurs only at titers of infection higher than those present in persistently infected animals. In general, the persistently infected mice are immunocompetent to a wide variety of antigens but show a somewhat decreased efficiency in generating cytotoxic T lymphocytes to several viruses.

At this point, it is useful to consider systematically the various mechanisms whereby a virus might plausibly escape from immune surveillance during a persistent infection. A virus might be, first of all, simply nonimmunogenic. Examples of nonimmunogenic viruses are rare—if they exist at all—but the agents of the spongiform encephalopathies (i.e., kuru, scrapie, and Creutzfeldt-Jakob disease)—if they are in fact viruses—may have this property, inasmuch as they have not evoked any demonstrable immune response. Alternatively, the virus might infect and kill or render dysfunctional the cells involved in the immune response: lymphocytes and macrophages. In this event, the immune dysfunction should be experimentally verifiable. Viruses also might be able to interfere with the immune system by other means. Blocking factors, due to either antigen per se or immune

complexes, could obstruct the function of immunologic killing mechanisms. Further, they might presumably be able to activate certain cells, and if these were suppressor cells or were capable of fabricating interferon or other interfering substances, an effective immune response could be hampered or prevented.

Modulation or stripping of viral antigens from the surface of an infected cell might permit the cell to stay one step ahead of the immune system. Good examples of this type of evasion are chronic measles virus infection (which will be discussed later) and trypanosomiasis, a parasitic disease in which the parasites, owing to immune selection, change their surface antigens as fast as antibody reponses develop.

The modulation of viral antigens from the cell surface can be done by antibody (as for measles virus and Trypanosoma infection), by genetic mutation, by genetic reassortment, or by deletion of the viral gene(s) coding for viral glycoprotein expressed on the cell surface. The end results of these different modalities are products that lose susceptibility to recognition by the immune system.

The loss of viral antigens from exposed sites on infected cells is implicated by our investigations of persistent LCMV infection. When cells in tissue culture are initially infected with LCMV, the virus rapidly establishes itself in the cultured cells. Within a few days, viral antigens are found both on the surfaces of the infected cells and within the cytoplasm, and if cytotoxic T cells or antiviral antibody plus complement are added to the supernatant, the infected cells lyse. Shortly thereafter, the amount of viral glycoprotein on the cell surfaces declines and then goes through a cyclic series of diminutions and augmentations. During the lows in this oscillation, the cells are less susceptible to immunologic killing by antiviral humoral or cell-mediated action. Along with this oscillation there is an overall decline in surface viral antigen until, ultimately, it nearly disappears altogether and the cells become resistant to lysis by immune reagents directed against the virus, even though the cells continue to carry viral gene products internally. Specific immunofluorescent labeling techniques using monoclonal antibodies have confirmed that various viral glycoproteins, which can initially be detected on the cell surface are no longer present after prolonged culture of infected cells, whereas viral nucleoprotein in the cytoplasm is still present in abundance. Another experiment showed that a defective interfering form of LCMV is invariably generated during persistent infection of cultured cells; this defective virus is capable of blocking infection with wild-type LCMV and may be responsible for the change in antigenic expression.

Using similar monoclonal antibody probes, we have been able to establish that the same phenomenon takes place during persistent in vivo infection. In the acutely infected adult mouse, both viral glycoprotein and nucleoprotein are easily demonstrable on and within cells of the choroid plexus and meninges. In persistently infected animals, i.e., those inoculated as neonates and sacrificed in adulthood, the nucleoprotein is still found in great quantity within the cytoplasm of infected cells, but the amount of viral glycoprotein on the cell surfaces is dramatically reduced (Figure 2). There is a tenfold to fiftyfold diminution in viral glycoprotein on infected cells, relative to the acute infection. The explanation for the host's failure to mount an immune attack on the persistently infected cells, then, is not necessarily inactivity of the immune system but perhaps the fact that infected cells may not express a sufficient amount of viral antigen on their surfaces to permit cytolysis by immune mechanisms (Figure 4, page 288).

There remain, nevertheless, many unanswered questions about this model of persistent infection. A prominent one is just how and why the modulation of antigen expression occurs. Perhaps this takes place via the same defective interfering virus that is seen in vitro, although the defective virus has not yet been demonstrated directly in vivo. Our thinking about the generation of this defective mutant is at present mostly speculative and based on what is known about other negative-stranded viruses, such as the vesicular stomatitis virus, a usually highly cytolytic virus that grows to very high concentrations, thereby allowing more detailed biochemical analysis. A model for vesicular stomatitis virus proposed by J. J. Holland, based on the work of his group as well as several other laboratories, explains how deletion mutants may be generated (Figure 5, page 289). We now have biochemical studies under way to determine whether the defective interfering LCMVs are uniform with respect to the deletion and whether the genes for the viral glycoproteins are deleted.

We have intensively studied the mechanisms of persistence of measles virus, which, like LCMV, can

Figure 3

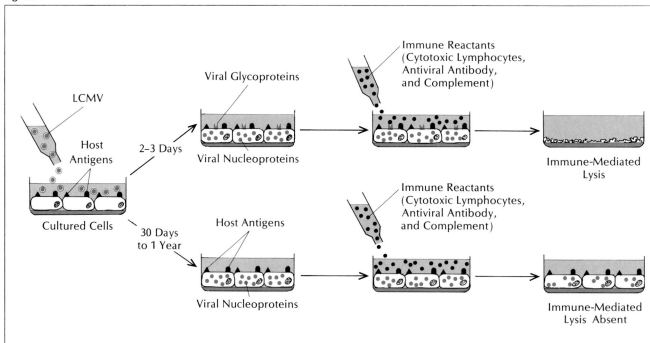

For LCMV to produce lytic disease, two conditions must pertain: 1) Infected cells must express viral antigens on their surface, and 2) immune reactants must be present in the milieu. These requirements can be demonstrated by in vitro studies with cultured cells. If cultured cells are infected with the virus and immune reactants are added within two or three days of infection, the cells will be lysed (above, top). However, if one waits 30 days or more, surface viral proteins will be either removed or internalized, and the addition of immune reactants will not cause lysis (above, bottom). An in vivo

cause both acute and persistent infections in the same host species. Measles is a human disease in both its acute and chronic forms. Some suggestive evidence raises the question of whether persistent measles virus infection may be involved in the pathogenesis of certain chronic diseases, such as multiple sclerosis. All things considered, association of those diseases with unusual titers of antimeasles antibodies seems more likely to be a reflection of underlying immune abnormalities than an indication that the virus is directly involved in causing the illnesses. There is no longer any reasonable doubt, though, that measles virus is the causative agent in subacute sclerosing panencephalitis (SSPE). This is a disease in children that, as its name suggests, runs an insidious, degenerative course of months or even years, resulting in death. It probably results from measles virus infection acquired years earlier, which for some reason the host was unable to clear. The virus itself is a negative-stranded RNA virus, like LCMV and vesicular stomatitis virus.

When researchers first addressed the question of how this virus is able to persist in an immunocompetent host and to cause disease years after the initial infection, the thinking was, as with LCMV, that the host must develop a specific immune tolerance for the virus as a result of genetic predisposition or conditions prevailing at the time of the acute infection, or both. In this case, though, it was even easier to show that the host is not tolerant of the virus in the immunologic sense. In fact, a vigorous antimeasles virus immune response is invariably present in SSPE. Sera from these patients contain cytotoxic antibody and sufficient complement to kill cultured cells infected with virus, and their lymphocytes similarly lyse virus-infected cells. Nevertheless, infection persists in spite of good immune function and a state of antibody excess. Antibody excess, it should be noted, is usually associated with persistent infections in humans—in herpesvirus, cytomegalovirus, as well as measles virus infections.

Study of biopsy material from SSPE patients provides part of the explanation of viral persistence: The surfaces of cells from infected tissues are largely free of viral antigen or budding virus, whereas in contrast, abundant and excessive viral polypeptides are found in the cytoplasm. Electron microscopy, in fact, shows viral nucleocapsids packed under the plasma membrane in a state of disarray. Like LCMV, then, measles virus persists despite immune surveillance, and its antigens, usually expressed on the surface of infected cells, are kept off the surface, where they would be subject to immune recognition and attack. There is a very important difference in the mechanism of persistence of these two viruses, however: The antigen modulation in persistent LCMV infections seems to be an intrinsic property of the virus; in measles infections, it is induced by antibody.

The viral proteins that are expressed on the cell surface in a measles virus infection have been characterized. Only two are normally expressed on the plasma membrane: the hemagglutinin (HA) and fusion glycoproteins. The hemagglutinin molecule is present as a 160,000 molecular weight dimer and is important in permitting adsorption of the virus to the cell surface. The fusion protein (F0) has a molecular weight of 67,000 and is comprised of a 46,000 nonglycosylated (F1) and a 21,000 glycosylated (F2) fragment. When inserted into the cell membrane, the F1 polypeptide causes the cell to adhere and to fuse to nearby cells, forming giant multinucleated syncytia. It is this tendency to fusion that makes the measles virus acutely cytopathic, and the giant cells are a prominent feature of the histopathology of acute measles infections. When cells in culture are infected with measles virus, their protein synthesis is not impaired, but they fuse and die.

Adding antimeasles virus anti-

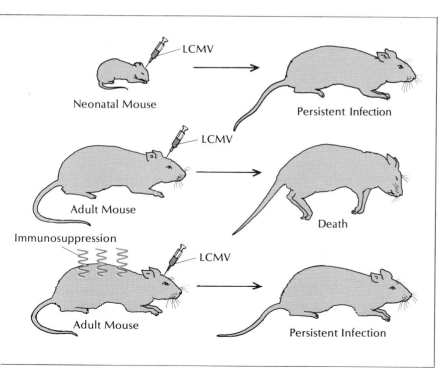

correlate experiment involves infection of newborn mice, adult mice, or immuno-suppressed adult mice. Only the nonsuppressed adult animals will develop fatal cytolytic disease. Both groups of persistently infected animals will remain apparently healthy, although it can be shown that they continuously harbor virus and develop manifestations of immune complex disease.

Figure 4

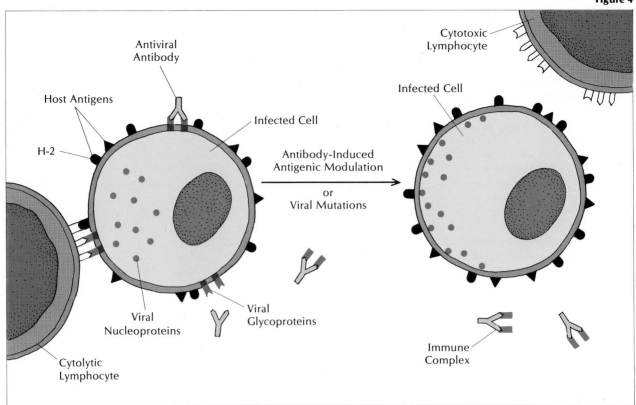

How may viral infections persist despite a vigorous host immune response? Two different, but not mutually exclusive, hypotheses are schematized above. One involves viral mutation, which could result, for example, in deletion of the part of the viral genome that codes for the viral glycoproteins that are expressed as foreign antigens on the infected cell's surface. The second hypothesis is that after initial infection, antibody strips the surface viral antigens from the cell. The infection persists and viral nucleoproteins remain in the cytoplasm, but the infected cell lacks surface antigens needed for immune recognition. Although CTLs and antibody both recognize the viral glycoproteins, they may not see the same site on the molecules.

body to the culture completely changes the aspect of the infection. Immunofluorescent and electron microscopic methods show that when polyclonal antibody or monoclonal antibody to the measles virus glycoproteins is added, the viral products coalesce into a mass at one pole of the cell, in the process known as capping (Figure 6, page 290), and then disappear from the cell surface. Analysis of the cell culture fluids reveals that the bulk of the antigen is not internalized but is shed from the cell in the form of immune complexes. As a result of this antibody-induced shedding of viral glycoproteins, the infected cultured cells no longer have F1 protein on their surfaces, do not fuse, and in fact grow and replicate as well as uninfected cells. They nevertheless continue to bear the internal viral antigens in their cy-

toplasm, and electron microscopy shows masses of disarrayed nucleocapsids under the plasma membrane exactly as seen in biopsies from patients with SSPE. These cells, denuded of both HA and F viral antigens on their surface, are no longer susceptible to killing by complement and antimeasles virus antibody or by measles-primed cytotoxic lymphocytes.

The antibody-induced modulation of viral antigen expression in this disease is more complex than simple shedding of viral glycoproteins, however. Robert S. Fujinami and I have established that the binding of antibody molecules to viral glycoproteins on the cell surface somehow causes the transmission of a signal across the cell membrane that changes the synthesis of intracellular gene products of measles virus. This effect is spe-

cific for the viral glycoproteins; antibodies to host glycoproteins, such as the HLA determinants, do not reproduce it. Furthermore, using monoclonal antibodies, we have established that antibody binding to the HA protein alone is sufficient to induce the change. One of the intracellular proteins that is altered is the viral M polypeptide, which serves to orient the nucleocapsids under the plasma membrane in preparation for their assembly into virions and subsequent release. The M protein normally is synthesized in a heavily phosphorylated form and subsequently is dephosphorylated when it is packaged into the virion. Under the influence of antibody binding to measles virus glycoproteins on the cell surface, the number of residues in the M protein that label with sulfur-35 is decreased, and the number of phosphorylated groups is increased. These changes probably relate to the ensuing failure to release infectious virus and the observed buildup of disorganized nucleocapsids.

Antibody binding causes even more dramatic changes in the production of the viral P polypeptide, which makes up part of the replicative complex of the virus along with the L and NC polypeptides. Synthesis of P protein as determined by sulfur-35 and phosphorus-32 labeling experiments drops by 80% to 90% within six to 12 hours after an infected cell is exposed to antibodies to measles virus, including monoclonal antibody to measles virus HA. We hope to characterize these biochemical events in the near future by defining the nature of the transmembrane signal and site of interference with viral protein synthesis. A similar phenomenon has been observed recently with influenza virus. A monoclonal antibody to influenza hemagglutinin modifies a viral replicase inside the host cell. Together these observations add a new dimension to our concepts of factors influencing viral replication and initiating viral persistence.

Quantitation of the amount of antibody required to bring about these changes reveals an interest-

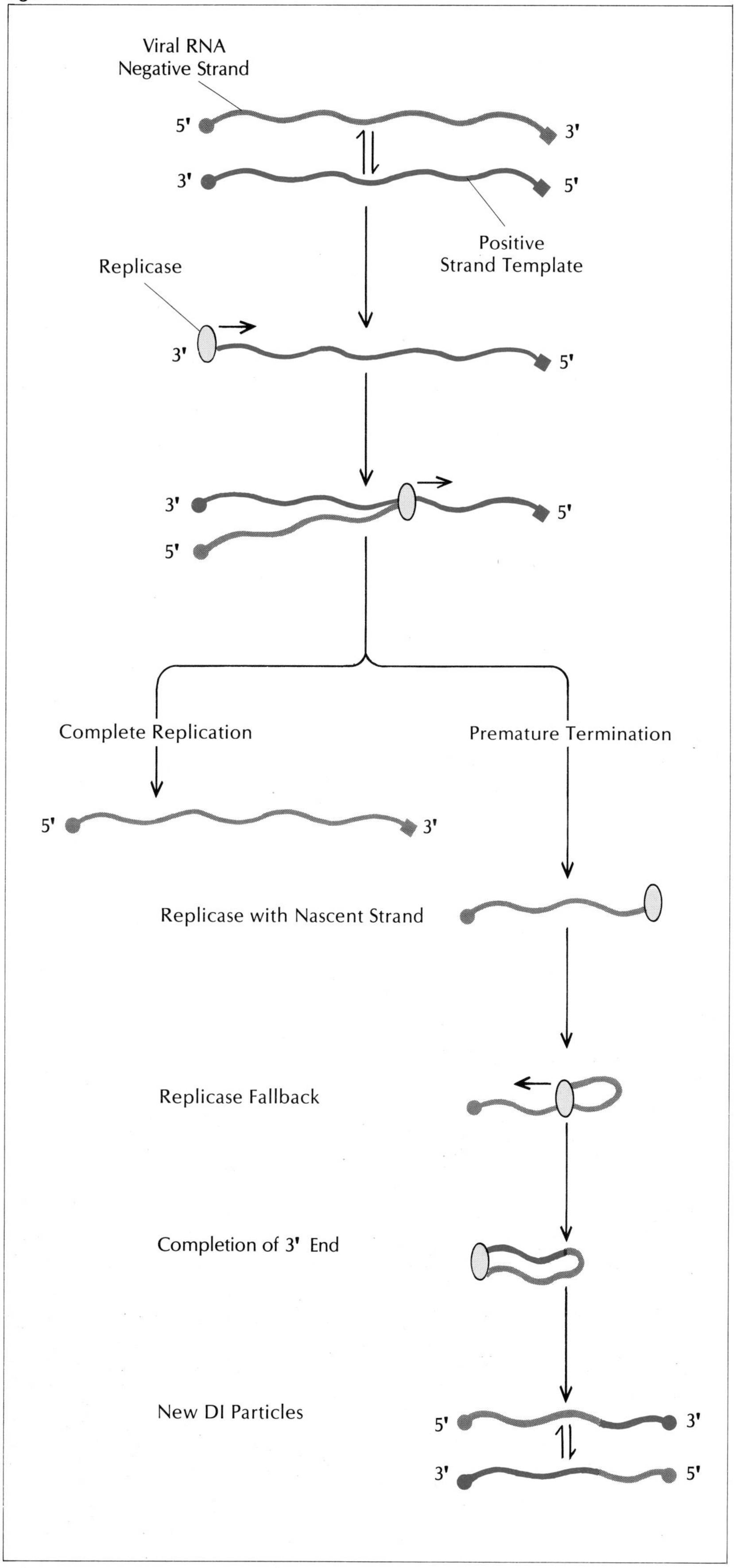

J. Holland provided this schematic, based on experimental work from his and several other laboratories, to explain the generation of mutant viruses. Perhaps the gene needed for expression of virus glycoprotein antigens on the surface of infected cells is deleted. The model might be applicable to LCMV, a negative (−) stranded RNA virus. At the top of the diagram, a "minus" RNA strand is depicted along with its "plus" RNA template. The −RNA is a template for mRNA synthesis. Synthesis of either + or − strands requires RNA replicase activity on complementary strand. If replication is complete, a "normal" RNA strand will be produced. However, if replication terminates prematurely, replicase "fallback" will result in RNA strands that are half + and half −. These are the so-called defective interfering (DI) virus particles, lacking some of the genetic information in the parent virus. DI may also arise by other means, e.g., internal deletions of virion RNA.

Figure 5

Figure 6

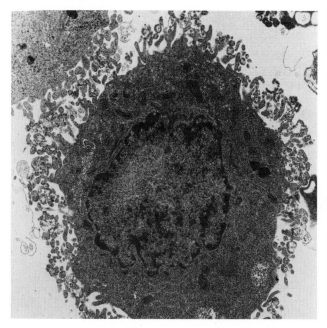

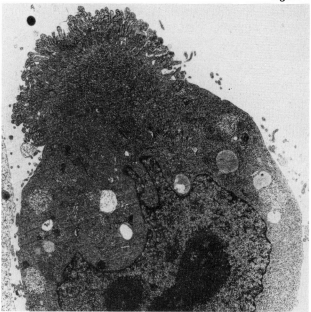

Transmission (above) and scanning (below) EMs show capping of HeLa cells after infection with measles virus (Edmonston strain). Photos at left show random circumferential distribution of viral antigens along cell surface. After incubation with

antimeasles virus antibody at 37° C, measles virus antigens demonstrate capping phenomenon, i.e., unipolar redistribution on infected cell (right, above and below). (From M. B. A. Oldstone and R. S. Fujinami)

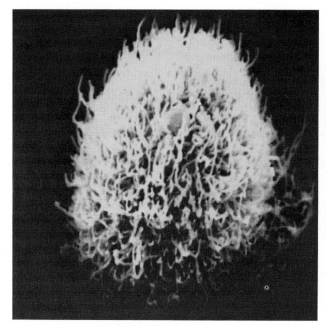

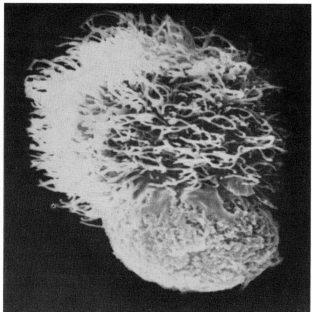

ing relationship. The amount of antibody needed to remove viral antigens from the cell surface is about 10⁵ molecules per cell, or about one fiftieth the amount of antibody needed to permit complement-mediated cytolysis and about one fifth of the amount necessary for lysis through antibody-dependent cytotoxic lymphocytes. The ob-

vious implication of this fact is that certain conditions in the host—in terms of antibody availability, antigen-antibody balance, kinetics of the immune response, or availability of effector mechanisms (i.e., complement)—will tend to promote viral persistence rather than eradication. For example, cerebrospinal fluid from patients with

SSPE has high titers of antiviral antibody but no complement activity. Thus, cerebrospinal fluid favors modulation. Sera from SSPE patients do contain functional complement activity. However, during acute measles virus infection, the normal amount of complement lytic units present is significantly reduced. The role of antimeasles virus antibody in initiating a persistent infection in vivo can be seen in animal experiments. In monkeys, measles runs a course resulting rapidly in either death or full recovery with clearance of the virus. If the animals are passively immunized with antimeasles virus antibody at the time they are inoculated with virus, however, a subacute to persistent measles infection can occur. In neonatal hamsters, measles infection is usually fatal. If the hamsters suckle a measles-immune mother at the time of measles inoculation, a persistent infection results. A similar observation is made in mice given monoclonal antibody to measles virus HA along with the virus inoculum. Thus, in all three in vivo experimental systems, correct antibody timing is important in establishing virus persistence. Furthermore, there has been a case report suggesting that a similar event may occur in humans: A child exposed to measles and treated prophylactically with gamma globulin containing antimeasles antibody subsequently developed an SSPE-like illness instead of acute measles.

These experimental and clinical observations do not provide a complete explanation for the development of SSPE. Nevertheless, many individuals who are immune to measles (passively, through their mother) and have titers of antimeasles antibody do not develop SSPE when they are exposed early in life to measles virus. On the other hand, there is accumulating evidence that several viruses, including measles, may persist in cells of the central nervous system following typical childhood illness. The evidence comes from detection of measles virus genome in neurons of adults dying of nonneurologic causes, by using in situ nucleic acid hybridization techniques, and from the realization that involvement of the central nervous system may be common with acute measles virus infection, as assessed by electroencephalography and clinical symptoms.

Another aspect of persistent viral infections that is not clearly under-

stood is tropism, i.e., the tendency of particular viruses to infect and persist in certain types of cells. In addition to its affinity for neurons, measles virus has another interesting tropism: It infects lymphocytes both acutely and persistently. On examining the lymph nodes histologically during an acute measles infection, one finds evidence of fusion and giant cell formation indicative of acute cytopathic infection of lymphocytes by measles virus. It is possible, by using cocultivation techniques, to isolate measles virus from peripheral blood lymphocytes and lymph nodes of patients with SSPE. By infecting a variety of lymphoblastoid cell lines in culture with measles virus, Fujinami and I found a possible explanation for this persistence. As noted, the measles virus fusion protein is not initially synthesized in its active form but rather as a precursor (F0), which needs to be cleaved to the F1 fragment by a host proteolytic enzyme before it can promote cell fusion or permit the release of infectious virus. Certain lymphoblastoid cell lines do not synthesize the proteolytic enzyme needed to cleave the F protein; these cells can persistently harbor the virus and release noninfectious rather than infectious virus particles. These infected cells will release infectious virus, however, if the missing proteolytic enzyme is replaced, either by fusing them with cells that synthesize the enzyme or by adding an appropriate enzyme, such as trypsin, to the culture medium. This fact leads us to hypothesize that a persistently infected lymphoid cell or its progeny might harbor virus for years, until exposed to high concentrations of proteolytic enzymes in an area of inflammation, resulting in a localized release of infectious virus particles many years after the initial infection.

Recently, Paulo Casali, working here, demonstrated another pattern of persistent infection of lymphocytes by measles virus. When cultured human peripheral blood lymphocytes are experimentally infected with measles virus, they do not

express viral antigens either on their surfaces or internally and are morphologically normal. When one subsequently stimulates those lymphocytes to divide rapidly with a plant mitogen, virtually 100% of the cells manufacture measles virus antigens. Along with Fujinami, Casali postulated that the block in expression of viral antigens and formation of infectious virus is at the level of RNA synthesis. Casali then asked whether these infected lymphocytes were capable of carrying out their immunologic functions normally. The only functions completely tested thus far are antibody-dependent, cell-mediated lysis and lysis induced by natural killer cells. In both assays, these immune functions were severely impaired.

If this functional incompetence proves to be generalized to other immune activities, it may well provide an explanation for the von Pirquet phenomenon. Von Pirquet noted that positive tuberculin skin test reactors frequently became nonreactive during the course of an acute measles infection. Skin

Figure 7

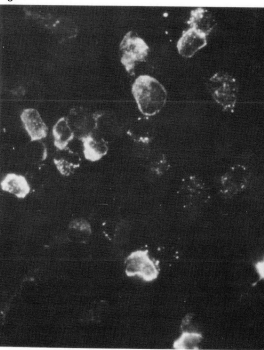

Hybridoma cells 15 months after infection with LCMV express nucleocapsid antigens in the cytoplasm but are devoid of glycoprotein antigens on their surface.

Figure 8

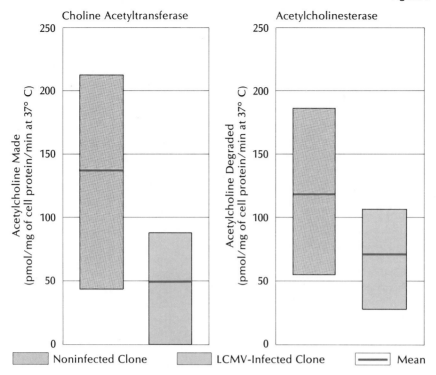

Cell clones derived from neuroblastoma culture line after 12 months of persistent infection with LCMV show levels of both acetylcholine synthesis and degradation markedly reduced from control levels. The reductions reflect respective diminution of choline acetyltransferase and acetylcholinesterase activities, "luxury" functions.

test reactivity returned after the viral infection had resolved. The same phenomenon has been noted since then with influenza and a variety of other viruses. This temporary loss of delayed hypersensitivity now seems likely to be a result of the block in lymphocyte function caused by infection of those cells by virus.

These observations are particularly interesting inasmuch as they raise the larger question of the effects viral infections might have on the functioning of the infected cells. As I have stressed, persistent viral infections, by definition, are noncytopathic—they do not destroy the infected cells. This implies that the cells are still able to perform the metabolic tasks necessary to keep them alive. We nevertheless have accumulated a considerable body of data to support the notion that persistent viral infections can and do, to varying degrees, impair the ability of cells to carry out the specialized physiologic functions that comprise their contribution to the

homeostasis and health of the host organism. These functions can be referred to as "differentiated," "specialized," or "luxury" functions, in contradistinction to the "vital" functions necessary to keep a cell alive, which presumably are disrupted by an acute viral infection. These luxury functions may still be quite vital to the host, however.

A relatively simple example of a persistent viral infection that affects the host cells' differentiated function without damaging the cells' viability is provided by the infection of monoclonal-antibody-producing mouse hybridoma cells with LCMV. When hybridoma cells are infected by LCMV in vitro, the infection follows the persistent course described previously: The virus replicates, and viral antigens are expressed both on the surface and in the cytoplasm of the infected cells, making them susceptible to killing by the appropriate antiviral immune reagents. With time, the viral glycoproteins disappear from the cell surface, but viral nucleopro-

teins remain present within the cell in large quantities. The growth rate and cloning efficiency of these cells are perfectly normal; nevertheless, the amount of monoclonal antibody produced is substantially less than that produced by uninfected cells.

Just how this infection impairs the cell's ability to synthesize antibody is not known. The tremendous concentration of viral antigen packed into the cytoplasm makes it tempting to draw an analogy to metabolic storage diseases and to consider this a kind of "viral storage disease" (Figure 7, page 291). The mechanism whereby a virus shuts down the differentiated function of a cell selectively is unknown but may relate to at least three possibilities: First, a cell's capacity for membrane translocation and synthesis may be limited, so that production of viral gene products competes with manufacture of a luxury function, thereby overloading the system. Second, virus may induce a specific alteration in an enzyme or transport system needed for the production and release of the luxury product. Alternatively, since synthesis of the luxury product may be a small fraction of the cells' total synthetic output, partial suppression of total cell synthesis capacity may impair differentiated function without affecting vital function.

The hybridoma model also illustrates the fact that all persistent viral infections do not *necessarily* interfere with cells' luxury or differentiated function. Hybridoma cell lines are persistently infected with mouse retroviruses and shed viruses continually without any known adverse effect on their antibody production

One can perform a similar experiment with LCMV by using cultured neuroblastoma cells, which retain the specialized neuronal functions of synthesis and degradation of acetylcholine. After persistent infection is established, the neuroblastoma cells maintain rates of growth and synthesis of protein and RNA that are normal with respect to uninfected cells. A variety of enzymes whose functions are essential to the survival of the cells are present in normal concentration, but the specialized enzymes choline acetyltransferase and acetylcholinesterase are significantly diminished in the infected cells (Figure 8, at left).

In cultured neuroblastoma cells, defects in the handling of acetylcholine are not of vital importance. In living neurons, however, it is clear that faulty neurotransmitter metabolism may very well correspond to faulty neurotransmission and, consequently, to disease. Similarly, defective antibody production by persistently infected hybridoma cells is of great interest because of the implication that a similar infec-

tion in vivo could cause significant immunodeficiency.

We have recently been able to characterize a disorder of hormonal regulation in the mouse that is associated with persistent LCMV infection of the anterior pituitary gland (M. B. A. Oldstone: *Science*, 218:1125, 1982). Infected animals were consistently dwarfed and were deficient in growth hormone, in the absence of morphologic changes in the hormone-secreting cells.

Although the mechanism whereby LCMV infection inhibits growth hormone production is not yet understood, this condition is a fascinating one, because it is the first instance in which persistent viral infection has been documented to

cause disease in vivo by impairing the specialized or luxury functions of a cell without visibly damaging it. One of the most intriguing aspects of this disease is that we are able to document the existence of the infection mainly because we infected the mice experimentally and thus know exactly which antibody probe to use to demonstrate the presence of the virus. If, on the other hand, we were performing histopathologic examination of the presumably hypofunctional pituitary tissues of a dwarf mouse in an attempt to explain the mouse's condition, we would probably have to conclude that the appearance of the gland did not provide an explanation for growth retardation. It

Figure 9

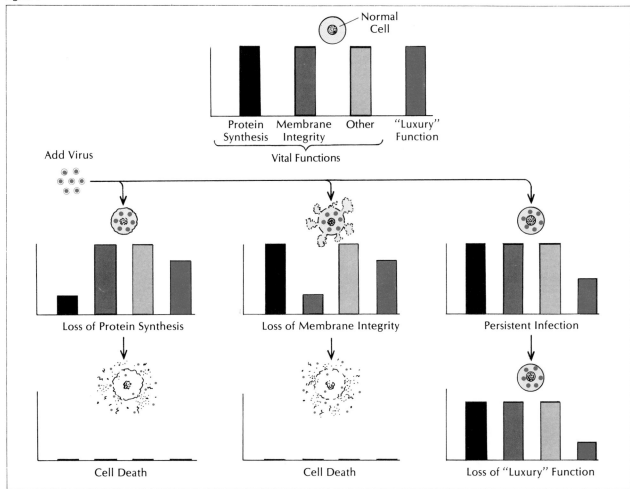

Three hypothetical viruses are depicted in the context of their effects on cellular survival and function. Viruses that cause loss of protein synthetic capacity or disruption of membrane integrity would induce cell death. Although a persistent viral

infection may permit cell survival without morphologic abnormalities, its effect may be deletion of a "luxury" function required by the organism for homeostasis. Such deletions therefore can cause disease without detectable viral lesions.

would appear, in short, that there was idiopathic dysfunction of the growth-hormone-producing cells.

If we consider the enormous variety of human diseases whose etiologies are still unknown, it is intriguing to speculate how many of these could be caused by failure of the specialized functions of specialized cells without the death of these cells (Figure 9, page 293). Consequently, one of the principal directions of our future research will be to determine whether persistent viral infections similar to this one might exist in chronic human diseases—with particular attention to failure of hormone secretion by several endocrine glands, dysfunction of neurons and oligodendrocytes in chronic degenerative and demyelinating diseases of the central nervous system, and disorders of the immune system that might be manifest either as hyperactivity or hypoactivity, depending on whether the lymphocyte subsets involved had effector or suppressor activity. One can imagine an almost endless list of diseases of various organ systems—from the heart out to the skin—whose etiologies are unknown and that could potentially be caused by mechanisms related to the one described.

Our current thinking about persistent viral infections and how they cause disease, then, is based on the idea that the organ systems of the body are made up primarily of highly differentiated, specialized cells that perform specialized functions and that the outcome on the organismal level represents the integration of this array of finely directed operations. If all these specialized tissues fulfill their roles successfully, the readout will be health; if not, it will be disease. At the same time, each of these cell types uses a unique combination of special enzymes, surface receptors, and microenvironment to enable it to carry out its appropriate function, and this unique combination may make it permissive for some particular type of viral infection.

A number of basic principles of persistent viral infection can now be stated: A persistent virus, clearly, is a relatively noncytopathic virus, whether it is an inherently noncytopathic strain or a variant of a usually lytic virus. A common thread in the ability of several viruses to persist over long periods seems to be the elimination of viral antigens from the surfaces of infected cells, enabling them to escape the host's immune surveillance. This may occur by any of several known mechanisms: A defective mutant may simply fail to express the surface viral antigens, or antibody may cause shedding of the viral protein from the plasma membrane or changes in viral gene expression. The net result is that infection can persist in spite of a vigorous host immune response, in some cases actually leading to immune complex disease. Indeed, signs and symptoms of immune complex disease may be valuable clues in showing which human diseases are the most likely prospects for documentation of a persistent viral etiology. Although persistent viral infections do not necessarily cause disease, they have the potential to do so by interfering with specialized functions of cells—functions whose loss does not cause death of the host cell. From the standpoint of the host organism, nevertheless, the impact of this loss of function is the same as if the infected cells had been killed outright: disease corresponding to the specialized function that has been lost.

27

Senescence of the Immune System

MARC E. WEKSLER   *Cornell University Medical College*

In all mammalian species studied, including the human, there is a progressive involution of the thymus after sexual maturation. This organ plays a major role in the development of the immune response. Thymic involution has been a recognized biologic phenomenon for nearly a half century, and throughout this time investigators have speculated on the effects of this phenomenon upon immunologic competence. In recent years, however, there has been a considerable change not only in the focus of these speculations but more importantly in the experimental approaches used to test them.

Whereas, formerly, investigators generally worked within a context that simply related reduction in thymic function with immunodeficiency, we have recently been more and more able, as our understanding of the complexity of T-lymphocyte differentiation has increased, to appreciate the possibilities of perturbation of immunologic regulation. The elucidation of the suppressor function of a subpopulation of T lymphocytes, for example, has made a major contribution to this expansion of context.

It now appears plausible to think of immune senescence as contributing not only to age-correlated enhancement of susceptibility to infections and to autoimmune diseases, but also to the rising incidence of neoplastic diseases and to pathology associated with chronic low-grade tissue damage, including atherosclerotic vascular disease. We may be approaching a unitary immunologic theory of aging encompassing the hypothesis that the programmed decline in physiologic competence, which we know as aging, is in fact a concomitant of changes primarily manifested in the immune system.

The collection of alterations in immune function that develop with aging has been described as an immunodeficiency state. As such, it has a certain set of characteristic laboratory features and identifiable sequelae on a clinical level. However, immune senescence is distinct in several respects from other defined states of immunodeficiency. The most obvious of these differences is its prevalence. Virtually every human being surviving into adulthood expresses it to some extent. It also has a greater degree of variability than most defined states of immunodeficiency. For most of the parameters of immune function, the variability from individual to individual increases progressively with increasing age.

Complexity, too, distinguishes immune senescence from other immunodeficiency states. Complexity, indeed, is one of the most remarkable aspects of immune senescence. Aging is associated with diverse deficits in immune function, the interrelationships of which are unclear. These include flaws in both cell-mediated and antibody-mediated effector functions, a rise in autoantibody production, and increases in other products of dysregulation, such as immune complexes and monoclonal gammopathies. Faced with this array of potentially independent, potentially interrelated immune defects, we cannot be certain whether a single primary change in some element of the immune system causes all the others or the inciting influences are multiple. Given that each component of the immune system can affect the others through its network of regulatory processes, it is quite plausible that there is a single primary alteration.

What, then, is the evidence that the involution of the thymus after sexual maturity plays a critical role in the senescence of the immune system and, arguably, in the senescence of the whole organism?

The central role played by the thymus in the immune system has long been firmly established (see Figure 1), although the details of that role are still being elucidated. It is essential to the differentiation of the thymic-derived, or T, lymphocytes. T lymphocytes are now known, of course, to include a number of subpopulations of cells with a wide range of functions in the regulatory and effector aspects of immunity. The T cells spend time within the thymus itself, en route from their origin in the bone marrow to the peripheral lymphoid organs where they will act or from which they will be mobilized. The thymic microenvironment seems to be essential to their differentiation. There is increasing evidence, too, that hormones produced by the thymus are important in permitting

Figure 1

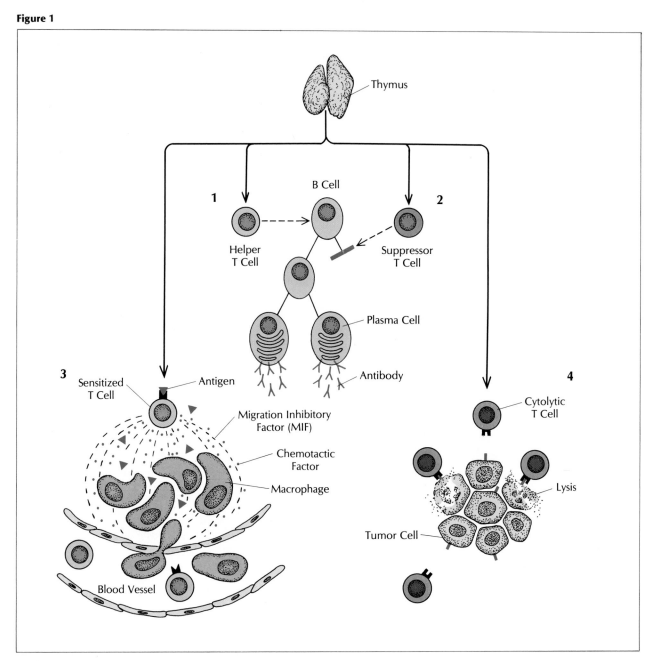

One approach to analyzing the role of the thymus in immunologic responses is the study of either congenitally athymic mice or neonatally thymectomized animals. It has been found that both types of animals are deficient in all four T-lymphocyte functions schematized above: (1) helper T-cell activity required for thymus-dependent antibody production; (2) suppressor T-cell function involved in "down regulation" of immune responses; (3) T cells that mediate delayed hypersensitivity reactions; and (4) cytolytic T cells necessary for cell-mediated immunity.

the T-lymphocyte branches of the immune system to reach normal function.

When the thymus is absent, either congenitally or because of early thymectomy, profound defects can be measured in those parameters of immune function that depend on T-lymphocyte function: delayed hypersensitivity, T-cell helper and suppressor function, and T-cell cytotoxicity. In normal human aging, of course, thymic degeneration occurs more gradually. The mass of the gland begins to decline shortly after sexual maturity, and by age 50 it has usually diminished to 15% or less of its maximum.

The aged thymus is not merely small; it is in fact functionally deficient. This was demonstrated by experiments in genetically identical inbred mice who freely accept organ transplants from mice of the same strain (see Figure 2). Young mice were thymectomized and given thymus transplants from donors of different ages. In this system, thymuses transplanted from very young mice effectively restored the T-lymphocyte population and T-cell functions of the hosts, while thymuses from older animals did not. The extent of the resulting immune defects increased with increasing age of the thymus donor, beyond about the first three months. The ability of a transplanted thymus to permit normal immune function in an animal deprived of its original thymus thus reflects the global competence of the gland, and these experiments reveal progressive loss of that competence with age, even early on in the three-year life span of these animals.

In other experiments, different components of the thymus gland's complex contributions to immunity have been isolated. One test for the presence of mature (post-thymic) human T lymphocytes is sheep red blood cell (SRBC) rosette formation (see Figure 3). Mature T cells, but not other lymphocytes, have surface receptors that bind sheep erythrocytes, so that when the two types of cells are incubated together, they **form rosettes with multiple erythrocytes surrounding a lymphocyte.**

Figure 2

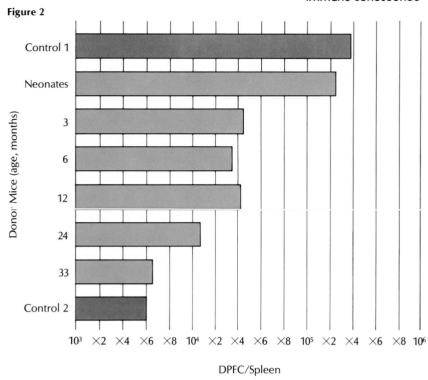

DPFC/Spleen

In the experiment, the results of which are presented graphically, K. Hirokawa and T. Makinodan sought to determine the capacity of thymic transplants from donor animals of different ages to reconstitute the antibody response in thymectomized and lethally irradiated young mice. Neonatal thymus grafts proved most effective, as measured by the direct plaque-forming-cell assay (DPFC). The capacity dropped off sharply after the neonatal period and again when donors were more than 12 months old. Two control groups were used: control 1, sham thymectomized; control 2, thymectomized but not reconstituted. Antigen was sheep erythrocytes.

Figure 3

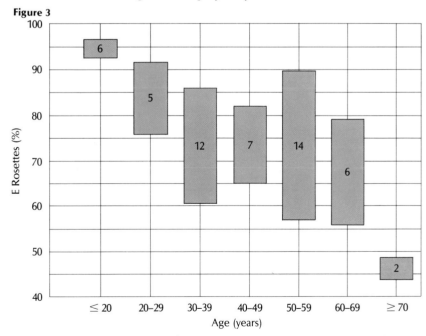

The ability of human T lymphocytes to form rosettes with sheep erythrocytes (E rosettes) is a measure of the lymphocytes' functional maturity. J. Singh and A. K. Singh (Clin Exp Immunol 37:507, 1979) demonstrated that the percentage of thymocytes able to form E rosettes declines markedly with age. The numbers in the bars indicate the number of individuals in each age group.

Some 85% of the lymphocytes present in the thymus of a 20-year-old person form rosettes in this test, but the number of rosette-forming thymocytes declines steadily with advancing age. In the 80-year-old, only half the lymphocytes isolated from the thymus gland itself are capable of SRBC rosetting, suggesting that the gland does not stimulate T-cell maturation in old individuals as effectively as in the young.

We now know that the contributions of the thymus to the immune system go beyond its serving as the site of T-cell differentiation. In the last 10 years, for example, a number of thymic hormones have been described, isolated, and characterized to some extent. These include thymopoietin, thymosin, and facteur thymique sérique (FTS). They are thought to act systemically (as well as locally), and, in humans, serum concentrations of all three decline with age. Thymopoietin begins its decline at about age 30, some years after the thymus begins to shrink, and by age 60 is undetectable in serum (see Figure 4). Thymosin and FTS start to disappear at an earlier age.

Recently, it has become possible to identify a role played by the thymus in the final differentiation of B lymphocytes, which do not share with T cells a period of residence within the gland. Until a few years ago, the differentiation of B cells was thought to occur independently of the thymus, although their function was known to involve complex interrelationships with several kinds of T cells. It is now known that some stage in the maturation of B cells requires the presence of functioning thymocytes. This was shown in cell transfer experiments, again with syngeneic mice. In the absence of thymocytes, immature B cells will not differentiate sufficiently to be capable of a normal heterogeneous high-affinity antibody response; that differentiation is permitted by the presence of thymocytes from young mice. Optimal function results when thymocytes from four- to eight-week-old donors are used; progressively greater impairment results when the donor is older, and thymocytes from a donor six months of age or older have very little activity in this assay.

All of the experiments discussed above document age-related changes in the immune system that are clearly linked to the involution of the thymus. There are many other age-related changes in immune function for which relationships to changes in the thymus are conjectural. Two pieces of circumstantial evidence support the notion that thymic atrophy may precipitate these other changes as well. One is the fact that, temporally, thymic involution is the first age-related defect in the immune system to develop. The other is the exceptional invariability of thymic changes between individuals. While other aspects of immune senescence are, as mentioned, highly variable, the diminution of the mass of the thymus and of the concentrations of thymic hormones in the blood occurs with great consistency.

The functional interrelationships between observed immune defects are potentially complex and still largely hypothetical. For the sake of clarity, this paper will first present a discussion of changes manifest in a less effective response to foreign antigens, then a discussion of those related to diminished tolerance of autologous antigens.

Old people are more susceptible to infectious disease than young adults. That this susceptibility is a reflection of impaired immune responsivity has been established in a number of studies. This relationship between clinical disease resistance and immune function is apparent, for example, in the case of delayed hypersensitivity, a phenomenon mediated by helper T cells. The tuberculin skin test is a measure of delayed hypersensitivity to proteins of *Mycobacterium tuberculosis*. Reactivity to the skin test reagent declines in patients after the age of 70, the same group in which the reactivation of tuberculosis is most common. As reactivity is impaired toward antigens to which hypersensitivity has been established, so is there impairment of the ability to develop a new hypersensitivity response. Dinitrochlorobenzene is a chemical that usually sensitizes the individual on first contact, so that at subsequent challenge 95% of subjects younger than 70 years old will show a contact

Figure 4

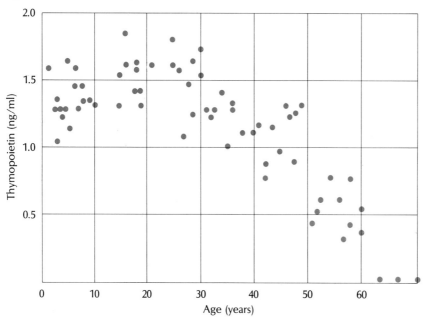

Bioassays in 67 subjects showed a decline in serum thymopoietin levels with age. The reduction in circulating thymic hormone accelerated, starting in the fourth decade and reached undetectable levels beyond age 60.

sensitivity reaction. In subjects older than 70, only about 70% react after experimental immunization.

Antibody responses, too, are known to be impaired in older individuals. This has been studied using Salmonella flagellin as an antigen. The titer of antibody developed in the serum was shown to decrease as a function of increasing age. Humoral immunity, in fact, was the first subdivision of immune activity in which age-related impairment was noted. Titers of antibodies to AB blood group antigens are lower in old people, as some of the early blood group investigators observed in 1929.

These basic facts about immune deficits of aging have been elaborated upon by in vitro and animal experiments. An immune response in an intact organism is the product of an extremely complex series of interactions, but by evaluating the functions of isolated lymphocytes (either alone or in cell transfer experiments in which a functional immune system is reconstituted using cells from different sources), the functional aberrations of the aging immune system can be dissected with greater resolution.

In vitro experimentation was applied to the problem of tuberculin reactivity, for example, to answer the question whether the diminished responsiveness seen in old people results from a defect of the lymphocytes themselves or some aspect of the internal environment of older individuals interferes with lymphocyte function. When lymphocytes isolated from peripheral blood are incubated with an antigen to which the donor has been exposed, they respond by multiplying. This proliferative response can be quantified by measuring the incorporation of tritiated thymidine into cellular DNA. Lymphocytes from subjects exposed to the tubercle bacillus proliferate when incubated in vitro with tuberculin purified protein derivative (PPD). The strength of the proliferative response in vitro is found to correlate inversely with age (see Figure 5). The diminished responsiveness of lymphocytes from old persons even in a standardized

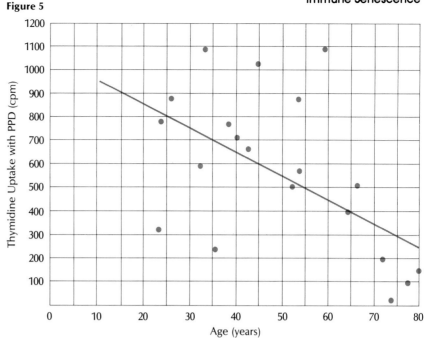

Figure 5

Evidence that age-related functional T-cell defects are intrinsic was obtained in studies reported by B. S. Nilsson (Scand J Respir Dis 52:45, 1971). Lymphocytes from tuberculous patients were incubated with PPD, and their proliferative response determined by measuring tritiated thymidine uptake. It fell linearly with age.

in vitro environment implies a functional defect intrinsic to the cells. This conclusion has been corroborated by a number of other studies.

The stimuli to which T lymphocytes respond in vitro include lymphocytes from different individuals, which can be recognized as antigenically foreign—the mixed lymphocyte culture (MLC) reaction—and natural plant mitogens. Lymphocytes from old human donors are less reactive to the MLC as well as to the pokeweed mitogen and phytohemagglutinin (PHA).

The PHA response has been studied in detail in my laboratory. The first stage in the response of lymphocytes to PHA is binding, and we determined that both the percentage of cells binding PHA and the affinity with which they bind it are the same in lymphocyte preparations from young and old persons. The percentage of T lymphocytes that respond to PHA, however, is only about half as great in cells from the old as it is in the young. Among those cell lines that do proliferate, furthermore, the number of divisions each cell undergoes de-

clines with age (see Figure 6, page **300**). A similar limitation in the ability to divide repeatedly in vitro has been observed in several different types of nonlymphoid cells from old individuals since Leonard Hayflick first noted it in fibroblasts.

Similar experiments with murine lymphocytes showed that their response to plant mitogens also declines with age and that the deficit also involves a decrease in number of cells responding and in divisions per responding cell. In mixed lymphocyte culture, cell preparations from old mice show not only less proliferation as measured by thymidine incorporation but also a decline in the generation of cytotoxic T lymphocytes, which comprise an important part of the effector arm of the immune system.

Looking further into the defective proliferative response of lymphocytes from old people, we studied the role of a substance called T-cell growth factor (TCGF), or interleukin-2, which seems to be necessary for T-cell proliferation; it is secreted by T cells themselves. Relative to cells from young subjects, T cells from old subjects when tested in vi-

Figure 6

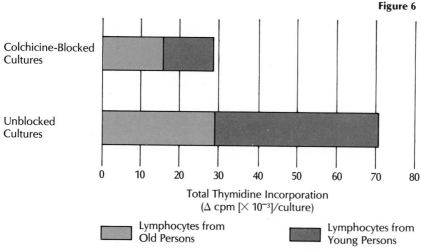

Total Thymidine Incorporation
(Δ cpm [$\times$ 10^{-3}]/culture)

Lymphocytes from Old Persons

Lymphocytes from Young Persons

T lymphocytes from young (20–30 years) and elderly (65–97 years) persons were stimulated in culture with phytohemagglutinin (PHA) and their proliferative response measured (as thymidine incorporation). In some of the cultures, mitotic division was blocked by colchicine so that measurements essentially relevant only to a single division could be made. In the colchicine-blocked cultures, the young lymphocytes had a proliferative response to the PHA more than half again as great as the old cells. In the unblocked cultures, the young-cell response was almost threefold greater.

tro are deficient both in the production of TCGF and in their ability to bind and respond to the factor.

Before going on to discuss the antibody response in aging subjects, I will summarize the available data on macrophage function. Macrophages have a number of important roles in the activity of the immune system, but most of these are still difficult to quantify. As phagocytes, they are important in disposal of immunologically undesirable material; this is their well-known effector function. They also act in the afferent portion of the immune response by ingesting antigen, processing it in some way, and presenting it to lymphocytes so as to elicit an appropriate response. Finally, they generate a number of humoral factors that influence the activities of lymphocytes. Phagocytic and antigenic-presentation functions have not yet been measured well enough for us to know if they are altered in the process of aging, but we have assayed one of the third group of functions. In the presence of lipopolysaccharide, human macrophages secrete a factor called T-cell replacing factor that can substitute for the presence of mouse T cells in the in vitro primary antibody response of mouse B cells

to sheep erythrocytes. Human macrophages from old and young individuals are no different in their ability to secrete this factor. From our studies and other reports, we can conclude that there is little evidence that macrophage function is impaired in old age.

The antibody response represents the outcome of a complex interaction of lymphocytes from different classes and subclasses. That interaction has been explored with respect to its B-cell and T-cell components, both in vivo and in vitro, in humans and mice. One of the most useful systems for measuring the antibody response is the plaque-forming cell (PFC) assay, in which plaques of sheep erythrocyte lysis (in the presence of complement) are the quantified endpoint. When formalinized staphylococci are used as an antigenic stimulus for isolated human lymphocytes in vitro, the number of plaque-forming cells (i.e., the antibody response) declines as the age of the donor increases, indicating an age-associated defect in antibody production. This observation, in unfractionated lymphocyte preparations, confirms in vivo observations, showing impairment of humoral immunity in aged individuals. Impairment is found in

both T-dependent and T-independent antibody responses.

When preparations of purified B lymphocytes are tested in the same assay system, however, no age-associated decline in plaque forming cells is detectable. Indeed, the contribution of non-B cells to the response is very different for young and old individuals. In young individuals, a preparation of unfractionated lymphocytes gives a more vigorous plaque formation response than one of purified B cells. When an old donor's cells are used, the response of unfractionated cells is considerably weaker than that of pure B cells. This implies that the diminished antibody response in aging results from changes in the T-cell rather than B-cell population. In young persons, the net T-cell contribution to the antibody response is stimulation, whereas in old persons, it seems to be suppression. The literature on immune senescence contains a number of conflicting conclusions on changes in B-cell function with aging, perhaps because of a failure to eliminate or isolate the effects of T cells on the assay system. However, it now appears that the function of B lymphocytes, if altered with age, is impaired to a lesser extent than is that of T lymphocytes. Furthermore, it is possible that B-cell changes may be secondary to age-associated changes in T-cell function.

The experiments just described were done with human peripheral blood lymphocytes; parallel (but not totally similar) data have come from in vitro work with mouse lymphocytes, usually spleen cells. In unfractionated lymphocyte preparations, results depend on whether one uses T-independent antigens, the response to which is independent of T-cell function, or T-dependent antigens, the response to which requires T-cell help. When sheep erythrocytes, which act as a T-dependent antigen, are used, the magnitude of plaque formation by cells from 18-month-old mice is only about 5% of that seen when cells from three- to six-month-old mice are used. Failure of T-cell help provides a ready explanation for this decline, but there is also evidence for an increase in suppressor-cell activity and, in the mouse at least, an intrinsic B-cell defect. A smaller age-related decline is found in the response to T-independent antigens.

The data for a defect in murine B lymphocytes come from observation of the plaque-forming response of mouse spleen cells to the T-independent antigen, dinitrophenyl (DNP)-polyacrylamide beads. An age-associated diminution in the PFC anti-DNP antibody response is seen even when comparing cell preparations carefully depleted of T cells. The role played by the thymus in mediating the differentiation of B cells has already been discussed. Thus, the decline in thymic function with age may contribute to this B-cell defect, as may other unknown factors.

To delineate the role of suppressor cells in the senescence of the immune system, experiments were performed to measure the function of old lymphocytes in young mice. In these studies, young mice were lethally irradiated, thymectomized, and their immune systems reconstituted by the transfer of spleen cells from healthy donors of various ages (see Figure 7, page 302). When spleen cells from old and young donors were mixed in this system, the vigor of the immune response in reconstituted hosts was markedly suppressed. That is, when cells from older animals were transferred together with those of young animals, the response of the host was inhibited by as much as 90% relative to that in animals given cells from young animals only. The interpretation of these results is that the cells from old donors have a net suppressor activity in this system that can be distinguished from any deficiency in helper activity.

The antibody response in aged mice is qualitatively as well as quantitatively defective. There is, in the response to T-dependent antigens, a preferential loss of high-affinity antibody and of IgG antibody, in addition to the globally diminished antibody production. The loss of the high-affinity antibody re-

sponse probably has implications for the efficacy of immunity that are as great as those of the decline in total antibody. The cause of this defect is uncertain. It is known that the normal high-affinity antibody response and shift from IgM to IgG antibody production depend on helper T-cell function. One can postulate that thymic involution may indirectly lead to loss of the high-affinity response through loss of an effective helper-cell population. One fact supporting this theory is that the high-affinity antibody response is lost at an earlier age in thymectomized animals.

Cell transfer studies further clarify the circumstances surrounding the loss of high-affinity antibodies. First, the defect is intrinsic to the peripheral lymphocyte population rather than the internal environment of old individuals. This was documented by challenging lymphocytes from old donors in a young irradiated host and showing that the defect remained. Next, it was shown that loss of the high-affinity response is not caused by suppressor cells. In experiments with the transfer of old and young lymphocytes into the same animal, the old lymphocytes caused suppression of antibody production overall, but without any preferential inhibition of the high-affinity response.

Another series of cell transfer experiments carried out in my laboratory strongly implicated thymic involution as contributing to the age-related loss of the high-affinity antibody response. When spleen cells from old donor animals are transferred to a young irradiated host with an intact thymus, the defects in high-affinity and IgG antibody production by the donor cells are reversed over the course of about eight weeks. This restoration of function is prevented by thymectomizing the host animal, but cells from young donors transferred at the same time as the old animal cells can still correct the defect. Still another measure found to restore the ability of old lymphocytes to produce high-affinity and IgG antibodies is incubation of the donor cells with thymopoietin before

transferring them to the host. When spleen cells from old mice are treated with exogenous thymopoietin, furthermore, the high-affinity response is restored. This, of course, may have therapeutic implications.

One can easily hypothesize that the loss of high-affinity antibody responses increases an elderly individual's susceptibility to infectious disease. High-affinity antibody is probably more effective in combating infection than low-affinity antibody. If the same shift to low-affinity receptors occurs among cell surface receptors, the immune response would be delayed; it is likely that a certain number of surface receptors must bind antigen in order for a lymphocyte to be activated, and if those receptors are of low affinity, then a higher concentration of antigen would be required to elicit a response. In the case of infectious disease, this would correspond to more advanced disease. In support of this notion is the observation that the maximal antibody response of an old animal is elicited by a higher dose of antigen than is required to elicit the maximal response from a young one.

We can summarize the basic facts about age-related changes in the response to foreign antigens briefly before going on to discuss autoimmunity and immune dysregulation in old age. In elderly animals, humans included, there is a generalized decline in the ability to respond, and, in fact, the decline of many functions begins before the animal reaches the midpoint of its usual life span. Defects can be measured in delayed hypersensitivity, mitogen response, cytotoxic T-cell generation, secretion of and response to humoral regulatory factors, and the quantity and quality of the antibody response. These defects seem to reside in the lymphocytes themselves even when functioning in vitro or in a young syngeneic host, and although defective function can be localized to B lymphocytes in a mouse system, most of the immune defect, especially in humans, is ascribed on the basis of available data to T cells. Both failure of T-cell help and an increase in

Figure 7

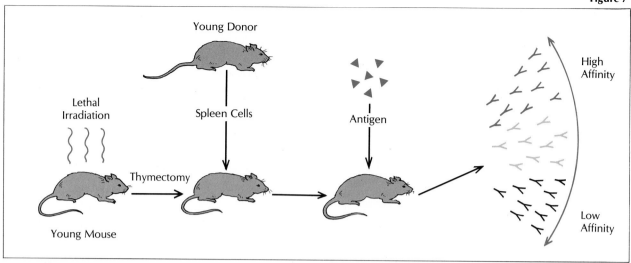

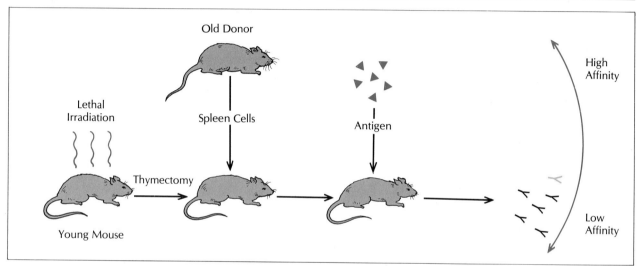

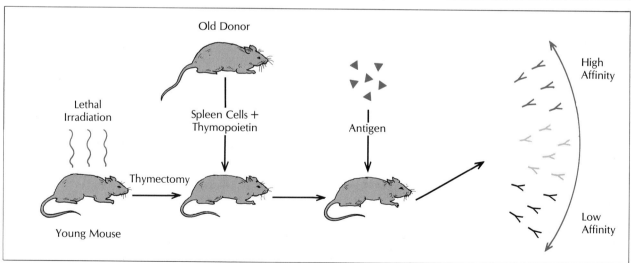

Cell transfer experiments in mice have delineated the differential effects reconstituting recipients with spleen cells from young and old donor animals. The recipients are first lethally irradiated and then thymectomized. When the spleen cell donors are young, the subjects will respond to antigenic challenge with an essentially normal array of antibodies. When the do-nors are old, not only is the total antibody response reduced but there is a more profound loss of high-affinity antibodies. However, if the old spleen cells have been treated with thymo-poietin, the cell transfer essentially reconstitutes the antibody response, both quantitatively and qualitatively. The effect is like that achieved with splenic tissue from young donors.

suppressor T-cell activity probably contribute to the waning of the antibody response.

The enigma of the immunodeficiency of aging lies in the simultaneous occurrence of diminished responses to foreign antigens and an overall increase in phenomena of autoimmunity. As will be discussed in more detail below, one can hypothesize either that these two kinds of immune defect occur independently or that one follows from the other.

An increase in the incidence of autoantibodies is one of the more striking changes in the immune system that regularly occur with aging (see Figure 8). There is, for example, a six- to eight-fold increase in the incidence of antithyroglobulin, anti-DNA, and antihuman immunoglobulin antibodies in 80-year-olds relative to 40-year-olds. There is a comparable rise in the prevalence of high titers of circulating immune complexes. Another sign of dysfunction of the aging immune system is an increasing incidence of benign monoclonal gammopathies. Their frequency increases with age in both humans and animals, and the frequency increases further after thymectomy.

These phenomena, interestingly enough, do not have quite the same implications for health in old populations as in young. Circulating immune complexes and autoantibodies occur in healthy old people without the disease manifestations with which they are associated in younger adults. Their role may nevertheless be less than benign. Autoantibodies, themselves, and immune complexes might cause slowly progressive low-grade tissue damage and in this manner cause or contribute to the degenerative physical changes of aging, perhaps including atherosclerotic cardiovascular disease (see Figure 9, page 304). An immunologic theory of aging, first proposed by R. L. Walford in 1969, hypothesizes that this sort of autoimmune tissue damage is of major importance in the aging process. Further investigations in this area will be of major importance, particularly to delineate the role of

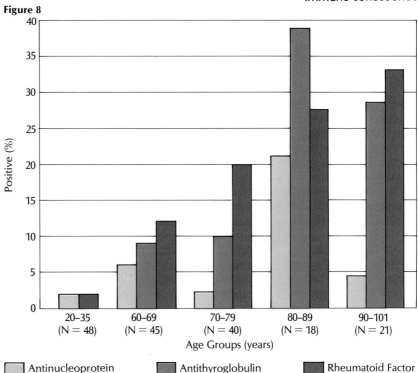

Figure 8

Studies of three circulating autoimmune antibodies—antinucleoprotein, antithyroglobulin antibody, and rheumatoid factor—show that all increase with age. The reversal of the trend in the very old could, of course, reflect selection by survival.

circulating immune complexes and to correlate their presence with diseases of aging.

At this point it is worthwhile to review briefly what is known about the mechanisms that prevent the normal immune system from producing antibodies to autologous antigens. There appear to exist mechanisms of tolerance mediated by B cells only, by helper T cells, and by suppressor T cells. There are also suppression mechanisms other than those mediated directly by T cells. It appears likely that a specific tolerance intrinsic to the B-cell population is responsible for tolerance toward autologous antigens present at high concentration. Tolerance toward many other autologous antigens seems to be a function of helper T cells, and the activation of autoreactive B-cell clones usually requires helper T-cell participation representing a failure of T-cell tolerance. The physiologic role of suppressor T cells is probably as a backup system to limit autoimmune activity that bypasses the two tolerance systems described

above. Age-associated changes have been documented in each of these systems for maintenance of self-tolerance.

B-lymphocyte tolerance is tested using a mouse system with a DNP hapten as the antigen. By prior administration of the synthetic peptide antigen, DNP-D-GL, one can cause a great reduction in the magnitude of the antibody response to DNP-bovine gamma globulin (DNP-BGG) on subsequent immunization, in young mice. In older mice, there is a manyfold increase in the dose of the DNP-D-GL tolerogen needed to bring about a comparable reduction in the immune response. By means of cell transfer experiments we showed that the property of resistance to tolerance induction is intrinsic to the B-cell population in old mice. It is possible to speculate on the mechanistic relationship of this tolerogen resistance to the change in antibody affinity with aging that has been discussed in the preceding paragraphs. It has been established that B-cell tolerance in this system is

Figure 9

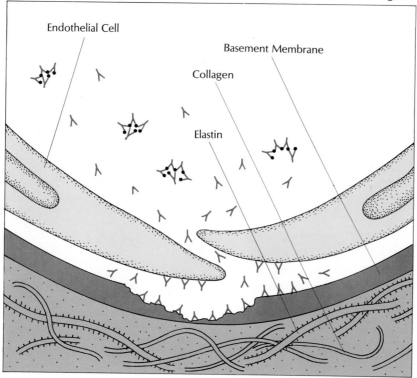

The enhancement of autoimmune phenomena with aging suggests a possible etiologic role for immune senescence in coronary atherogenesis. Antibodies directed against intracoronary structures or immune complexes could initiate the progressive endothelial and basement membrane damage that facilitates the process of arterial thrombosis.

induce a given degree of tolerance than in young mice. The role of affinity changes in this phenomenon is unknown because a change in binding affinity of *helper* T cells with age has never been measured. However, there is some evidence that *cytotoxic* T cells from older animals bind their targets with reduced avidity.

Suppressor function is another area in which major changes occur in the course of immune senescence. It is increasingly apparent that suppressor activity is of major importance in immunoregulation in health and disease. Excessive suppressor activity has been associated with diseases of immunodeficiency, and deficient suppressor activity has been found in autoimmune diseases. The state of immune senescence is remarkable for having characteristics of both these conditions. The response to foreign antigens is diminished, while the level of autoimmune activity is augmented.

How are these changes linked to suppressor activity? There is in old age an increasingly active population of suppressor T lymphocytes. The in vitro and cell transfer experiments proving this were presented in the earlier discussion of diminished antibody responses. There are at least two other different kinds of immunosuppressive activity that are probably involved in immunoregulation. One involves macrophages that may modulate the immune response via prostaglandin mediators. In culture, they produce E-series prostaglandins that inhibit the proliferative response to T lymphocytes. Macrophages from old people secrete greater amounts of PGEs than those from the young, and T cells from the old are inhibited to a greater extent by equimolar amounts. Furthermore, indomethacin, which inhibits prostaglandin synthesis by blocking the enzyme cyclo-oxygenase, partially corrects diminished lymphocyte proliferative responses in cell preparations from old donors.

The other major mechanism now known to have a role in down-regulating the immune response in-

induced more easily in cells bearing high-affinity antibodies than in cells with immunoglobulins with low affinity. This phenomenon may be the result of a requirement for a certain number of sites to bind antigen before a critical cell activation, or inactivation, can occur. As noted, binding by low-affinity antibody requires a higher concentration of antigen to achieve comparable saturation of binding sites. Thus, the difficulty in inducing tolerance in B cells from aged mice may result from the lower affinity of their antibodies. Another possibly contributory age-related change in B-cell function relates to handling bound antigen; B cells from old rats have a defect in the capping of surface immunoglobulin when treated with antiimmunoglobulin antibodies, relative to cells from young mice.

Not only is the induction of new B-cell tolerance more difficult in older animals, there also seems to be an increased prevalence of competent B lymphocytes bearing spec-

ificity for self antigens. This is demonstrated by the use of lipopolysaccharide stimulation. Lipopolysaccharide directly activates B cells and incites them to produce antibody, independently of antigen exposure or T-cell help. The polyclonal antibodies thus produced are thought to represent the range of specificities carried by the B-cell population tested. There is some evidence that autoreactive clones make up a greater fraction of the B-lymphocyte population with increasing age.

A tolerance induction system used to study helper T-cell mediated tolerance is similar to the B-cell tolerance induction system described above. The tolerogen used is ultracentrifuged bovine gamma globulin. In subsequent challenge with DNP-BGG, the animal's anti-DNP response is feeble relative to that of naive animals. This is referred to as "carrier-specific unresponsiveness." In old mice, a higher dose of tolerogen is necessary to

Figure 10

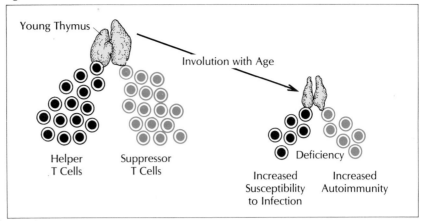

volves a set of autoantibodies descriptively called auto-anti-idiotype antibodies. The idiotype of an antibody molecule is simply the antigen-binding site in the context of its behavior as an antigenic determinant. An anti-idiotype antibody, then, is an antibody directed against the binding site of another antibody.

In a normal immune response, auto-anti-idiotype antibodies are produced along with antibody specific for the foreign antigen in question. It is becoming increasingly clear that this auto-anti-idiotype response is part of the immunoregulatory process. The different components of the immune system recognize and communicate with each other via idiotype and anti-idiotype pairs; this is an essential part of the network theory of the regulation of the immune system elaborated by N. K. Jerne in 1974. Under experimental conditions anti-idiotype antibodies can either suppress or stimulate an antibody response. On the whole, their effect seems to be suppressive. In vivo they can turn off an ongoing antibody response, and in vitro they can specifically inhibit secretion of antibody by B lymphocytes on whose surfaces they bind the appropriate idiotypes. In mice, greater amounts of auto-anti-idiotype antibody are produced with increasing age. This, too, probably has a net immunosuppressive influence.

We must explain, then, the simultaneous augmentation of autoantibody production and of multiple mechanisms of immunosuppression underlying the simultaneously increasing autoimmune activity and decreasing immune reactivity to foreign antigens associated with aging. It has been suggested that there may be two separate sets of immunosuppressive mechanisms and two different populations of suppressor lymphocytes, one involved in the response to foreign antigens and the other regulating activity toward autologous antigens. If that were the case, one could suppose that the former set becomes hyperactive with age and causes the immunosuppressive

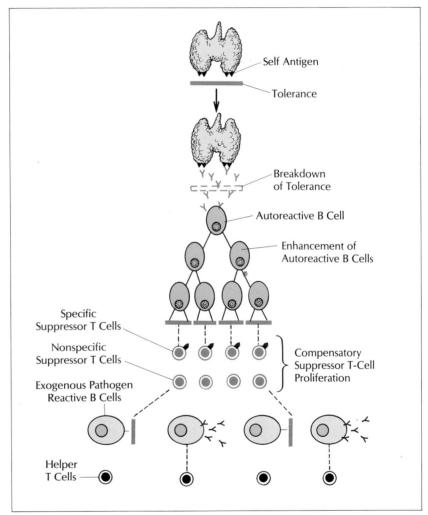

The increased susceptibility to infection and to autoimmune diseases that accompanies aging has been explained on the basis of a general deficiency of T lymphocytes (top panel), with the lack of helper T cells enhancing infections, and the lack of suppressor T cells accounting for the rise in autoimmune diseases. However, Siskind and Weksler have hypothesized a different concept in which the initiating event for both types of susceptibility is a breakdown of tolerance to self antigens. This results in clonal expansion of autoreactive B lymphocytes, with a compensatory increase in suppressor T cells, both specific and nonspecific. The specific T cells will be mobilized to cope with the autoreactive B cells, while nonspecific T suppressors will reduce antibody response to bacteria and other exogenous pathogens.

phenomena that have been described, while the cells responsible for suppressing autoimmunity selectively fail in old age. Some evidence presented by Walford and his collaborators suggests that this is the case. However, the precise regulation of multiple suppressor systems raises other conceptual questions.

Another hypothesis considered by Gregory Siskind and me is that an increasing production of autoantibodies is the event initiating the series of changes (see Figure 10, page 305). The augmentation of processes that down-regulate the immune response, such as suppressor T-cell activity and auto-anti-idiotype antibody production, represents a corresponding physiologic change that serves to compensate partially for increased autoreactivity. Suppression of the immune response to foreign antigens, then, would be an unavoidable side effect of processes whose primary effect is to limit autoimmunity.

We can relate many of our other observations on immune senescence to this hypothetical chain of events, according to the causal relationships tentatively postulated. Impairment of tolerance induction mechanisms could lead to autoantibody manufacture via a progressive increase in autoreactive B-cell clones. The defect in tolerance induction that occurs with aging might, as pointed out, be a consequence of the progressive loss of high-affinity antibody. This change in affinity, as cell transfer experiments have shown, is closely connected with the loss of thymic function.

This line of reasoning makes it seem feasible that most of the age-related changes in immune function stem from the series of events precipitated by involution of the thymus. But that hypothesis remains quite tentative. Prolonged exposure to autologous antigens may, for example, play a role, and it is easy to speculate that thymic atrophy is programmed because it compensates adaptively for some independently occurring phenomenon.

The elucidation of the interrelationships and actual consequences of the age-associated changes of immune function is of potentially great significance. The importance of immune senescence in the rising susceptibility of the elderly to infection is obvious, and it is clear enough that the senescence might also contribute to the age-related rise in cancer. It has been suggested, though, that in addition to the permissive role played by immune senescence in diseases causing premature death, these changes in immune function could actually establish the maximum life span of species.

One line of reasoning lending support to this concept is the previously discussed hypothesis that chronic low-grade tissue damage by autoantibodies and immune complexes is responsible in whole or in part for the physical degeneration of the aging individual. There are several strands of other evidence supporting a connection between immune senescence and maximum life span. One is that genetic control of life span in inbred strains of mice can be localized to the same portion of the genome, the major histocompatibility complex, that seems to control, among other aspects of immune function, the rate of immune senescence. Attempts to alter the life span of species experimentally are also suggestive; two measures, undernutrition and hypothermia, which regularly increase life span in cold-blooded animals, also induce profound changes in their immune system. Conversely, changes in the immune system have been linked with reduced longevity in humans. High titers of autoantibodies, low suppressor activity, and severe impairment of cutaneous hypersensitivity all correlate with increased mortality.

The experiment that establishes as fact a role for immune senescence in causing human senescence and death would be one in which an intervention restoring normal immune function could be shown to prolong life. Before attempting therapeutic intervention, however, more sophisticated understanding of the interrelationships of age-related changes in immunity is necessary. One possible therapeutic measure, for example, might involve treatment with thymic hormones, intended to maintain or replace one function of the thymus. If, however, thymic involution serves a physiologic compensatory role in protecting against autoimmune disease or otherwise keeping the immune system in check, such measures could even accelerate the aging process via autoimmune reactions. Ongoing investigation of this area should shed further light on this question and could have great clinical impact in the long run.

Section IV
IMMUNOLOGIC DIAGNOSIS, PROPHYLAXIS, AND THERAPY

Detection of Immune Complexes: Techniques and Implications

ARGYRIOS N. THEOFILOPOULOS *and* FRANK J. DIXON   *Research Institute of the Scripps Clinic*

The formation of antigen-antibody complexes, which are then phagocytized, is, of course, a crucial component in the normal defense against pathogens and other foreign substances. Physiologic immune responses are designed to eliminate or neutralize antigens and thus protect the host. Under some circumstances, however, immune complexes become pathogenic, causing injury to the host (see C. B. Wilson and F. J. Dixon, "Immunologic Mechanisms in Nephritogenesis"). In this particular role, immune complexes may induce inappropriate activation or inactivation of either humoral or cellular immunologic effectors. The humoral mechanism most often involved in immune complex pathogenicity is the complement system. The cells that usually mediate immune-complex-induced injury are the polymorphonuclear cells and macrophages, which interact with the immune complex, resulting in the release of hydrolytic and lysosomal enzymes that produce inflammation and tissue injury.

The harmful effects of immune complexes were first suggested by von Pirquet, who proposed that serum sickness was due to toxic factors produced by the interaction of host antibody and antigen. F. G. Germuth and F. J. Dixon identified the toxic factors as immune complexes in the 1950s. The same group then demonstrated that the appearance of immune complexes in the circulation and the simultaneous decrease, through consumption, of serum complement activity coincided with the onset of generalized vasculitis and glomerulonephritis in experimental serum sickness.

Immune complexes have been associated with glomerulonephritis and vasculitis in a wide range of disease states, including bacterial, viral, and parasitic infections, as well as autoimmune diseases, such as rheumatoid arthritis and systemic lupus erythematosus. Immune complexes consisting of tumor antigens and antibodies have also been identified in the sera and glomeruli of patients with various malignancies, including leukemia, lymphoma, Hodgkin's disease, colon carcinoma, melanoma, and lung carcinoma.

Endogenous as well as exogenous antigens can trigger immune complex formation. Antibody can react with structural antigens that form part of the cell surface membrane or with intracellular structures. Basement membrane, for example, contains a structural antigen that provokes an autoimmune response leading to a variety of anti-basement membrane diseases, including anti-glomerular basement membrane glomerulonephritis and Goodpasture's syndrome. Antibody also can react with antigens secreted or injected locally. The classic example of the latter is the Arthus reaction, caused by the interaction between the injected antigen and antibodies in and about the blood vessels that carry the antibodies to the site of injection (see Figure 1, page 310). Finally, antibody can interact with soluble antigens in the circulation; the immune complexes thus formed may then deposit in various organs. The clinical expression of the resulting disease depends on the site where immune complexes deposit. Circulating immune complexes lodge on any vascular basement membrane but most frequently on that of the glomerulus, skin, uveal tract, and synovium. This review will discuss primarily circulating immune complexes.

Figure 1

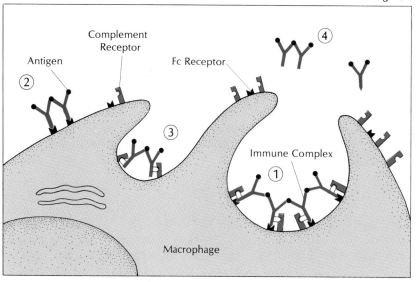

Because complement facilitates the attachment of immune complexes to macrophages, and therefore phagocytosis, ICs that include complement and appropriate Fc receptors (IgG_1, IgG_3) (1) are likely to be phagocytized better than those that bind only through Fc receptors (IgG_4) (2) or those that bind only through C receptors (IgM) (3). ICs that neither bind to Fc receptors nor fix complement because of size or of Ig class are likely to remain in the circulation for prolonged periods (4).

A number of factors have been identified as contributing to the pathogenicity of circulating immune complexes. Chronicity of immune complex formation appears to be a major one. As noted previously, immune complexes are usually rapidly sequestered by the host's phagocytic system. In experimental "one-shot" serum sickness, for example, more than 90% are eliminated by the Kupffer cells of the liver. Antigen exposure in this model is of limited duration, and tissue injury and clinical effects are transient. If antigen exposure is protracted, continuing immune complex formation may lead to chronic disease, as in "chronic" experimental serum sickness.

The nature of the antigen and the antibody strongly influences the disposition of the resulting immune complex. Potent antigens usually evoke a strong antibody response followed by rapid elimination of the antigen from the circulation, but poorly antigenic substances may stimulate smaller quantities of antibody of weak affinity, resulting in immune complexes that continue circulating for long periods. Moreover, certain antigens, such as DNA

and lectins, have affinity for basement membranes, thereby providing a mechanism for in situ immune complex disease. Important features of the antibody are its immunoglobulin class, which determines its ability to bind to cellular Fc receptors and to activate complement, and its affinity for the specific antigen. Attachment of immune complexes to macrophages is promoted by complement, but both complement activation and phagocytosis require an intact Fc region of the IgG in the complex. If the antibody in the complex does not fix complement or does not interact with cellular Fc receptors, immune complexes may circulate for prolonged periods.

The fate of circulating immune complexes is also determined by the quantitative relationship between antigen and antibody (see Figure 2, page 311). A balanced antigen-antibody relationship, or one with a slight excess of antigen, results in sizable soluble immune complexes that are capable of fixing complement, that are not completely phagocytized, and that tend to lodge in filtering structures. Immune complexes formed with a large amount of antibody and a small amount of

antigen (antibody excess) are large but not pathogenic because they are rapidly phagocytized. Interactions between a small amount of antibody and a large amount of antigen (antigen excess) form small immune complexes because the capacity of one antibody molecule to interact with the antigen is limited. These complexes are too small to lodge in filtering structures and to fix complement, and they tend to remain in the circulation.

Because of their role in normal as well as pathologic immune responses, it may be useful to take a closer look at the function of immune complexes. When they deposit on tissues, immune complexes activate the complement system through both the classic and alternative pathways. Activation of complement generates biologic activities that contribute to injury, including immune adherence, leukocyte chemotaxis, neutrophil exocytosis, anaphylatoxin activity, and cell lysis.

In addition, immune complexes activate the cellular immune system by interacting with cell surface receptors on a variety of cells. Lymphocytes of both the B- and T-cell lines, as well as unclassified lymphocytes known as K cells, bind immune complexes via Fc and complement receptors. This binding is critical in the B-T interactions, both with respect to helper and suppressor functions. Thus, T cells with IgM Fc receptors are helper cells in B-cell differentiation to plasma cells. On the other hand, T cells with IgG Fc receptors are suppressors of B-cell differentiation to antibody-secreting plasma cells. B cells have high-affinity receptors for C3b and C3d but low-affinity receptors for IgG Fc. Eosinophils, which mediate antibody-dependent cellular cytotoxicity against certain parasites, have receptors for IgG Fc, C3b, and C3d, as do mononuclear cells. Binding of immune complexes through these receptors leads to phagocytosis and release of proteolytic enzymes. Thus, immune complexes may modify the immune response by enhancing or suppressing lymphocyte activation, inhibiting T cell–mediated cytolysis, and inducing or inhibiting antibody-dependent cellular cytotoxicity. In fact, activation or suppression of lymphocyte functions may be the most important effects of immune **complexes in some diseases (see Figure 3, page 312).**

The role of immune complexes in cancer is of particular interest because tumors express antigens that elicit both humoral and cellular immune responses. It has been suggested that tumorigenesis represents an escape from the normal immune surveillance system, and several theories have been proposed to explain how this occurs. One involves the blocking factors originally identified by I. and K. E. Hellström in **sera of cancer patients. Blocking factors interact with either a target** cell (tumor cell) or an effector cell (lymphocyte) and block or inhibit the lymphocyte functions that would normally destroy the tumor cell. Although it has not been shown conclusively that blocking factors are immune complexes, there is convincing evidence that tumor antigen-antibody complexes can deny access of lymphocytes and other immunocompetent cells to tumor cells.

For instance, eluates from tumor cells or from lymphocytes of animals with tumors contain factors that block the cytolysis of the tumor cells by lymphocytes. These factors have been separated into high molecular weight and low molecular weight components. Separately, neither component has a blocking effect, but when recombined, they again block cytolysis. The view that these components represent antigen (light) and antibody (heavy) is supported by evidence that synthetic immune complexes, made with purified tumor antigens and antibodies, inhibit the cytolysis of tumor cells by sensitized lymphocytes. It also has been shown that sera from cancer patients in remission that contain antitumor antibodies, when added to sera from cancer patients that contain blocking factor, will inhibit the blocking effect. It is believed that the "unblocking" effect is due to alterations in the antigen-antibody complex caused by the excess of antibody in the remission serum. Numerous studies have shown that blocking factor in the sera of cancer patients correlates with the size of the tumor and indicates a poor prognosis.

The manner in which immune complexes may block cellular defenses is not clear, but several **mechanisms have been suggested (see Figure 4, page 313). If the immune complex is in antibody excess and is also bound to the tumor cell** surface, it may mask the tumor antigens and thus prevent attack by sensitized lymphocytes; or by interacting with the tumor antigens, it may induce shedding of the antigens from the cell surface, again preventing attack by sensitized lymphocytes. If the immune complex is in antigen excess, it may interact with receptor sites on lymphocytes by an antibody-mediated cross-linking of antigen, resulting in a specific blockade of the lymphocytes. Alternatively, immune complexes, by binding to lymphocyte Fc receptors, may initiate complement fixation and lysis of the lymphocyte, activate suppressor T cells, block activated T cells, inhibit the proliferative response of effector cells to tumor antigens, or alter the traffic patterns of lymphocytes. However, it should be noted that these actions of immune complexes may be positive as well as negative. Immune complexes in antibody excess,

Figure 2

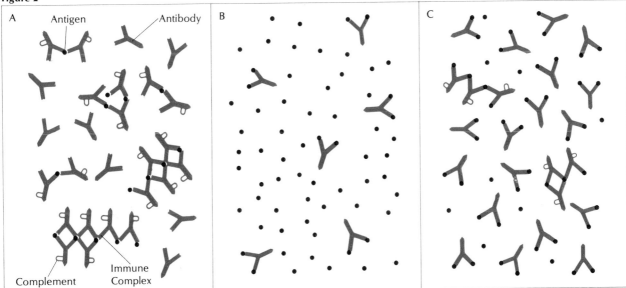

The ratio of antigen to antibody is the most important factor in determining the fate and biologic activities of ICs. Complexes formed when there is a very large excess of antibody (A) are large, fix complement, and have phlogogenicity. However, since they are phagocytized and catabolized rapidly, their phlogogenic potential is limited. ICs formed at large antigen excess (B)

do not fix complement and by and large cannot initiate inflammation. The greatest pathologic potential seems to lie between the two extremes of complex size, i.e., for ICs formed when antigen excess is modest (C). These complexes are soluble, they disseminate as they circulate, they fix complement, and they are not rapidly phagocytized.

Figure 3

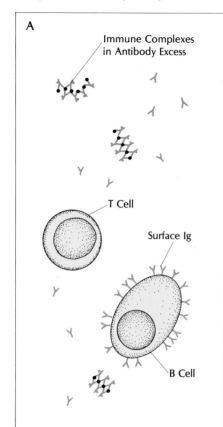

A

Immune Complexes
in Antibody Excess

T Cell

Surface Ig

B Cell

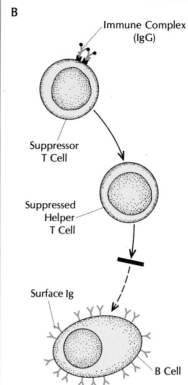

B

Immune Complex
(IgG)

Suppressor
T Cell

Suppressed
Helper
T Cell

Surface Ig

B Cell

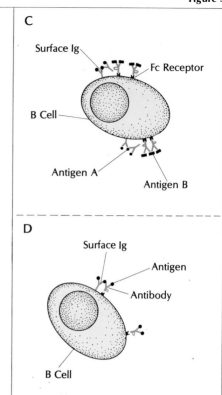

C

Surface Ig

Fc Receptor

B Cell

Antigen A

Antigen B

D

Surface Ig

Antigen

Antibody

B Cell

ICs may suppress or augment immune responses depending on the molar ratio of antibody to antigen, antibody mass, class, affinity, ability to fix complement, etc. Suggested mechanisms for IC-mediated suppression of humoral immune responses are depicted above: (A) antigen shielding or masking by antibody (blockade of antigen recognition by antigen-receptor-bearing B and T cells); (B) activation of IgG Fc-receptor-bearing suppressor T cells with release of factors that suppress helper T cells; (C) antigen-non-specific inhibition by unrelated ICs that occupy Fc receptors on the B cell; (D) antigen-specific inhibition at the B-cell level, in which antigen reacts with B-cell-surface Ig and then antibody from the circulation combines with that Ig and adjacent Fc receptors, thereby transmitting inhibitory signals to B cells. IC suppression could also involve inhibition of plasma-cell antibody secretion, binding to Fc receptors on B cells and subsequent release of suppressor factors, binding to soluble factors from helper T cells, and inhibition of T-B-macrophage interactions. (E) shows mechanisms of IC enhancement of humoral responses. Macrophages may process ICs and release Fc subfragments that stimulate helper T and B cells; or IgM-containing ICs may react with IgM Fc-receptor-bearing helper T cells to induce release of helper factors.

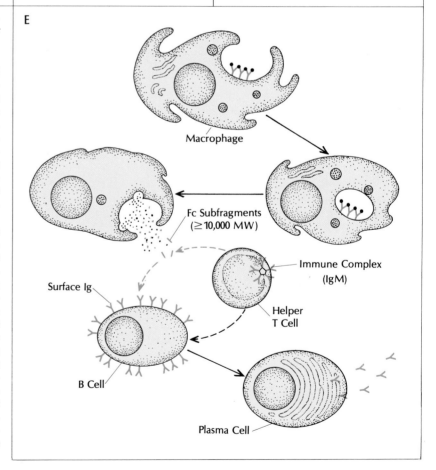

E

Macrophage

Fc Subfragments
(≥10,000 MW)

Immune Complex
(IgM)

Surface Ig

Helper
T Cell

B Cell

Plasma Cell

for example, may induce antibody-dependent cellular cytotoxicity rather than induce blocking.

The profound effects of immune complexes in immune responses and human diseases imply that it would be clinically useful to detect circulating immune complexes. The detection of immune complexes in tissue generally is performed satisfactorily by using immunofluorescence and other standard techniques. Immune complexes in tissue can be eluted and separated into their antigen and antibody components. Immune complexes in biologic fluids can be detected when the antigen is known. The ideal procedure for detecting circulating immune complexes of unknown antigenic composition has not been discovered, but detection techniques are evolving rapidly. Procedures for detecting immune complexes containing unknown antigen in biologic fluids are based on physical properties, such as changes in the size of antibody when it combines with antigen.

Methods used to detect such changes in physical properties include analytic and sucrose gradient ultracentrifugation, polyethylene glycol precipitation, and cryoprecipitation. Changes in activity can be demonstrated in systems employing serum proteins – notably, complement, conglutinin, and rheumatoid factors – or by cellular techniques. The cellular techniques include platelet aggregation, inhibition of phagocytosis by peritoneal macrophages, and the Raji cell assay (see Figure 5, page 315).

A brief description of these tests will indicate the different types of information they provide. The complement-consumption assays are based on the observation that serum containing immune complexes, when added to a standard amount of complement, will consume some of the complement. The decrease in complement activity can be detected by adding sensitized erythrocytes. Less lysis will occur than would be expected if the complement had not interacted with the immune complex–containing serum. Another type of complement assay involves the interaction of immune complexes

Figure 4

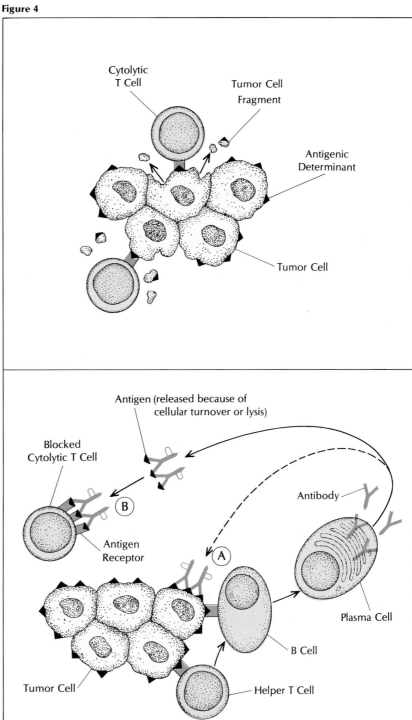

Hypothetically, immune complexes may serve as "blocking factors" that impede an effective immune response to tumors in several ways. The premise is that such a response requires access of cytolytic T cells to antigenic determinants on the tumor cell surface (top). However, stimulation of humoral immune responses via antigen sensitization of antigen-receptor-bearing helper T and B cells will also result in anti-tumor antibodies (bottom). These antibodies, although usually beneficial to the host, may sometimes block anti-tumor cellular responses by combining directly with antigen on the tumor cell surface, thereby rendering it inaccessible to cytolytic T cells (A), or they may combine with tumor antigens (released or shed after tumor cell lysis) in the circulation, form complexes, and then bind to antigen-receptor-bearing cytolytic T cells, thus blocking them from access to and direct interaction with tumor cell determinants (B).

with C1q, which recognizes antibody and fixes to Fc receptors on the antibody. H. G. Kunkel's group showed that serum containing immune complexes will interact with C1q and form a precipitin line. Several variations on the C1q assay are used, including inhibition of C1q binding to sensitized erythrocytes or to other particles in the presence of serum containing immune complexes.

The conglutinin assay, a solid-phase radioimmunoassay for the detection of complement-fixing immune complexes, was developed in this laboratory. Conglutinin is an unusual protein that occurs naturally in the serum of cattle but is not an immunoglobulin. It produces strong agglutination of sheep erythrocytes coated with antibody and complement and has been used for years in various serologic tests. It has a high affinity for immune complex-fixed C3. The binding of conglutinin to immune complexes appears to be specific for a fragment of the activated form of the third component of complement, C3bi. Theoretically, the conglutinin assay should detect only large complexes that have fixed C3 without interference by other serum factors, such as DNA, antibodies directed toward cellular components, or aggregated IgG. On the other hand, this assay does not detect complexes that lack C3bi. Thus conglutinin has preferential reactivity with large immune complexes and detects only a portion of the complement-fixing immune complexes. The chief advantages of the conglutinin assay are its specificity and relatively simple technology. The sensitivity of the assay is on the order of 5 to 10 μg of aggregated human gamma globulin (AHG)/ml.

A solid-phase F(ab')$_2$ anti-C3 assay has also been developed in our laboratory. In this assay complement-fixing immune complexes that bind to anti-C3 are quantitated with radiolabeled or enzyme-linked anti-IgG or radiolabeled staphylococcal protein A. This assay is simple, sensitive, and specific, and it correlates well with the Raji cell assay. The specificity of this assay has been substantially improved by the use of currently available monoclonal antibodies that recognize the subfragments C3b, C3bi, and C3d but not the native noncomplex-fixed C3 molecule.

Rheumatoid factors are IgG or IgM antibodies directed against IgG. Monoclonal rheumatoid factors found in the sera of patients with Waldenström's macroglobulinemia and lymphoproliferative disorders have a higher affinity for immune-complexed IgG than polyclonal rheumatoid factors. Monoclonal rheumatoid factors are used in several ways for detecting immune complexes in sera. One is the precipitin test developed by R. J. Winchester, Kunkel, and associates; others are based on the competitive inhibition of binding of AHG. Rheumatoid-factor radioimmunoassays are very sensitive – on the order of 1 to 25 μg AHG/ml. They detect IgG complexes as small as 8S, and they are independent of the complement-fixing properties of the immune complexes. However, these assays detect only complexes with IgG, and the results may be influenced by high concentrations of monomeric Ig or of intrinsic rheumatoid factors in the serum sample.

The cellular techniques detect measurable changes in the activity of various cell types after they have interacted with immune complexes. The platelet aggregation test, for example, is based on the observation that platelets aggregate after their surface Fc receptors interact with IgG-type immune complexes. The method is sensitive, but a number of other serum factors, such as antiplatelet antibodies, myxoviruses, and enzymes, also induce aggregation, while still others, such as rheumatoid factors and immune complexes with fixed complement, inhibit platelet aggregation.

The inhibition of phagocytosis by peritoneal macrophages is a competitive assay in which immune complexes in a serum sample compete with radiolabeled aggregated immunoglobulins for binding to Fc receptor sites on guinea pig peritoneal macrophages. If immune com-

plexes are present in the sample, they will inhibit the phagocytosis of radiolabeled aggregated gamma globulin added to the macrophages. Antibody-dependent cellular cytotoxicity is another competitive assay. If immune complexes are present in the serum sample, they will interact with Fc receptors on the effector cell and inhibit antibody-dependent lysis of a target cell. Similarly, the presence of immune complexes will induce phagocytosis and intracytoplasmic Ig inclusions by polymorphonuclear cells.

Finally, we have the Raji cell assay, a cellular technique developed in this laboratory that is based on the interaction of complement-fixing immune complexes with complement receptors on the Raji cell surface (see Figure 6, page 316). The Raji cell is a lymphoblastoid cell with B-cell characteristics, which was derived from a patient named Raji who had Burkitt's lymphoma. In common with B cells, the Raji cell has low-affinity Fc receptors for binding immunoglobulin and high-affinity receptors for binding complement, but uncommonly it lacks surface Ig. Therefore, any IgG bound to the Raji cell is due to interaction with immune complexes.

In testing human serum for immune complexes, the Raji cells are incubated with the serum and then reacted with rabbit anti-human ^{125}I-IgG. The amount of radioactivity is then determined, and the amount of immune complexes present in the serum is derived from a standard based on anti-human IgG uptake by cells incubated with normal human serum containing various amounts of AHG (see Figure 7, page 318). The sensitivity of the assay is about 6 μg AHG/ml.

The technique is reproducible, is easy to perform, and requires only small amounts of serum. It detects complexes of various sizes but, preferentially, larger ones. It can also be used to identify antigens on the cell-bound immune complexes by using fluorescein or radiolabeled antisera. All cellular techniques, including the Raji cell assay, have one potential disadvantage, which is interference by IgG-type anticellular antibodies with allospecificity.

None of the methods described above can be reliably applied to the measurement of all types of circulating immune complexes. However, these assays have been used to assess the incidence and levels of circulating immune complexes in patients with autoimmune disorders, infectious diseases, and various types of malignancies. Our studies with the Raji cell assay have shown that only 3% of normal individuals have values exceeding 12 μg AHG Eq/ml serum, whereas the mean value of complexes or like materials detected in patients with various diseases has ranged from 100 to 300 μg AHG Eq/ml. The percentage of patients with positive results varies from 40% to 90%, depending on the type of disease. In patients with autoimmune diseases, such as systemic lupus erythematosus and vasculitis, mean values of 100 to 300 μg AHG Eq/ml have been found. In patients with bacterial endocarditis and in patients with viral diseases,

such as hepatitis, cytomegalovirus infections, subacute sclerosing panencephalitis, and dengue hemorrhagic fever, values have been intermediate. In patients with malignancies, values of 50 to 100 μg AHG Eq/ml have been found.

In general, there is a good correlation between levels of circulating immune complexes and disease activity. For example, in patients with systemic lupus erythematosus, several investigators using different techniques have found a close relationship between immune complex levels and antibodies to DNA, low complement levels, and clinical manifestations. Furthermore, immune complexes have been shown to disappear with remission. In both acute and chronic hepatitis, the Raji cell technique has been used to detect immune complexes, and the hepatitis surface antigen has been demonstrated in the complexes. In patients with bacterial endocarditis, an excellent correlation has been found between circulating immune complex levels, duration of disease,

and extravalvular manifestations. Immune complex levels returned toward normal after appropriate treatment or valvulectomy. In addition, it has been possible to differentiate septicemia associated with bacterial endocarditis from septicemia without endocarditis because high levels of immune complexes are found in the former but not in the latter. In idiopathic interstitial pneumonia, high levels of immune complexes are associated with the cellular form but not with the diffuse fibrosis form. The response to corticosteroid therapy is better in patients with elevated immune complexes, and the elevated levels return to normal after treatment. However, in patients with neurologic diseases, we have not found a good correlation between circulating immune complexes and clinical state.

The Raji cell assay was used in an extensive study of over 500 patients with various types of malignancies. The results indicate that immune complex levels may provide a means of monitoring the response to treat-

Figure 5

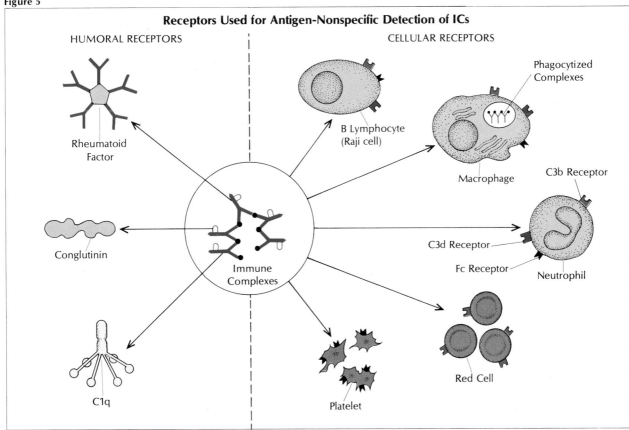

Receptors Used for Antigen-Nonspecific Detection of ICs

HUMORAL RECEPTORS

CELLULAR RECEPTORS

Rheumatoid Factor

Conglutinin

Immune Complexes

C1q

Platelet

B Lymphocyte (Raji cell)

Phagocytized Complexes

Macrophage

C3b Receptor

C3d Receptor

Fc Receptor

Neutrophil

Red Cell

ment and of making a prognosis in some types of malignancy. Patients with active disease tend to have higher levels of immune complexes than patients with no clinical evidence of disease. From 16% to 52% of patients were positive for immune complexes, depending on the type of malignancy. The incidence of immune complexes was significantly greater in patients with malignant melanoma, colon carcinoma, osteogenic sarcoma, breast carcinoma, and esophageal carcinoma than in patients with prostate, pancreatic, or lung cancer or lymphoma. In general, large tumors and metastatic disease were associated with high levels of circulating complexes.

In patients with malignant melanoma, tumor mass also appeared to influence the incidence of immune complexes. In addition, patients who had surgery and were considered cured had a much lower incidence of immune complexes than those who were subjected to surgery but not considered cured because of metastases. However, patients who had received melanoma vaccine plus BCG showed an enhanced level of immune complexes, possibly indicating that the vaccine boosted antibody production, resulting in the formation of immune complexes. This observation suggests that monitoring immune complex levels could serve as an indication to intensify vaccination procedures so as to produce more antibody until an antibody excess is achieved. Presumably, antibody that forms immune complexes is not available to attack tumor cells, but antibody in excess, stimulated by the vaccine, would be free to do so.

Other investigators have used different techniques to detect immune complexes in cancer sera with notable success. P. H. Lambert of the World Health Organization in Geneva used a C1q-binding assay and found evidence of immune complexes in some patients with acute myeloid leukemia and acute lymphatic leukemia and in patients with blastic crisis of chronic myeloid leukemia. The median survival times of patients who did not have immune complexes were more than 18

Figure 6

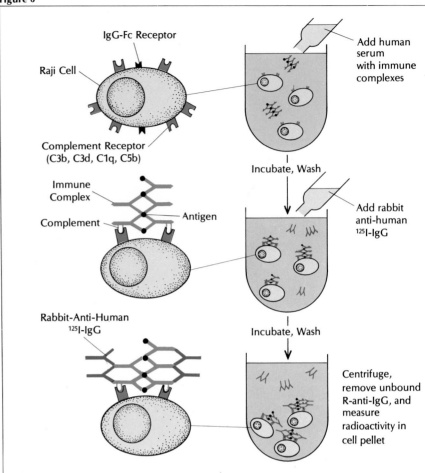

Schematized are steps in the Raji cell radioimmunoassay (left) and in the solid-phase conglutinin and F(ab')₂ anti-C3 solid-phase assays (right). The Raji cell is a lymphoblastoid cell of B-lymphocyte derivation, having many receptors for complement and few for IgG Fc. Because it lacks surface Ig, any Ig on the Raji cell surface after it binds immune complexes will be derived from the complexes. One can measure the com-

months in acute myeloid leukemia, 18 months in acute lymphatic leukemia, and more than eight and a half months in patients in blastic crisis of chronic myeloid leukemia, whereas the corresponding median survival times of the patients who had elevated immune complex levels were 64, 135, and 90 days, respectively. In the same study, Lambert noted a good correlation between the results of the C1q-binding assay and the Raji cell assay, which he used for some of the patients.

Studies by R. W. Baldwin in England showed that patients with breast cancer identified as having a good prognosis had normal immune complex levels in serum, while those

who had detectable metastases at the time of diagnosis or who died within 22 months after mastectomy had significantly elevated immune complex levels. N. K. Day and associates at the Sloan-Kettering Institute for Cancer Research in New York have reported a close correlation between high levels of circulating immune complexes and poor prognosis in patients with neuroblastoma. R. D. Rossen in Houston has found a relationship between high levels of circulating immune complexes and a poor prognosis in patients with lung cancer. Others have established an association between immune complex levels and stages of Hodgkin's disease. Thus, with the

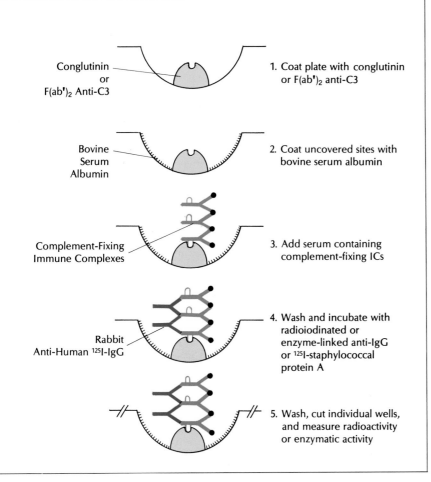

Conglutinin
or
F(ab')₂ Anti-C3

1. Coat plate with conglutinin or F(ab')₂ anti-C3

Bovine Serum Albumin

2. Coat uncovered sites with bovine serum albumin

Complement-Fixing Immune Complexes

3. Add serum containing complement-fixing ICs

Rabbit Anti-Human ¹²⁵I-IgG

4. Wash and incubate with radioiodinated or enzyme-linked anti-IgG or ¹²⁵I-staphylococcal protein A

5. Wash, cut individual wells, and measure radioactivity or enzymatic activity

plexes by incubating the cells with serum containing ICs, adding radiolabeled anti-human IgG antibody, and then quantifying the surface radioactivity of the Raji cells. Complement-fixing ICs can also be detected by either conglutinin or anti-C3 bound to a solid matrix. The bound ICs are then "counted" with radioiodinated or enzyme-linked anti-Ig or with labeled staphylococcal protein A.

limited studies cited above, it appears that detecting immune complexes in the sera of patients with various malignancies has prognostic value. In some instances, it may be useful as a means of monitoring the effectiveness of therapy. It is hoped that routine availability of these assays in many institutions and further application will establish the degree to which immune complex measurement is useful in clinical oncology.

The World Health Organization recently sponsored a study comparing the methods described above for detecting immune complexes in serum. Investigators from 10 laboratories around the world participated in the study in which coded sera from patients with idiopathic inflammatory diseases, cancer, and tropical diseases were tested. The results indicated that because of the idiosyncrasies and specificities of the different tests, certain immune complexes may react preferentially with one test reagent but not with others. No universal and absolutely specific reagent is yet available. The ideal test would be specific, sensitive, and easily reproducible and would detect immune complexes of all Ig classes, both complement fixing and noncomplement fixing, and of all sizes, but particularly small, soluble immune complexes that can persist in the circulation. Until such a test is developed, optimal screening for immune complexes in human sera may require the use of several tests. At this stage, it would seem important to conduct studies in well-defined patient populations, using a battery of tests, including one based on the complement assay, one of the cellular techniques, and a conglutinin assay in the serial screening of sera to determine if these tests will be clinically useful. It should be emphasized that the detection of immune complexes in biologic fluids does not necessarily indicate that the pathology of the disease under study results from these complexes. A further requirement is the demonstration of immune complexes in affected tissues.

In most diseases associated with pathogenic immune responses, the nature of the antigen is unknown. One approach to the identification of the antigen would be the isolation of immune complexes. The antigen might then be identified directly or after dissociation of the antigen-antibody union and subsequent isolation of the antigenic component.

Some progress has been made in this direction by using Raji cells and other substances (C1q, staphylococcal protein A, conglutinin, concanavalin A) as in vitro concentrators of immune complexes in sera. Raji cells are suitable for this purpose because they possess large numbers of high-affinity receptors for complement and, therefore, bind sufficient quantities of complement-fixing immune complexes to allow further analysis. The complement-fixing immune complexes are separated from serum and concentrated on complement receptor–bearing Raji cells. Then the cell-bound immune complexes are radiolabeled and eluted from the intact cells or immunoprecipitated from cell lysates. The constituent antibodies and antigens are then separated by a gel electrophoresis technique. From the work reported, it appears that immune complex–binding substances, together with a variety of immunochemical and physicochemical assays, may provide the tools for immune complex isolation and characterization of their components. Another approach to identifying the antigen is the

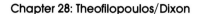

Figure 7

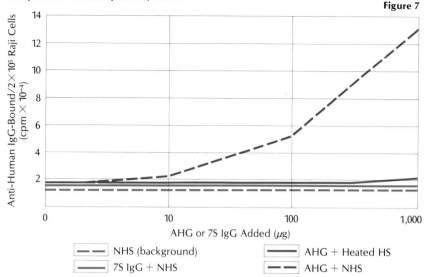

- – – – NHS (background)
- ——— 7S IgG + NHS
- ——— AHG + Heated HS
- – –– AHG + NHS

Graph is derived from experiments demonstrating the ability of complement receptors on Raji cells to detect immune complexes (aggregated human gamma globulin, or AHG) in human sera, as shown in sharply rising curve. Flatter curves show control situations in which heated serum replaced normal human serum (NHS), or noncomplement-fixing 7S IgG was used in lieu of AHG, or just NHS was tested.

production of antisera against the antigens in isolated immune complexes. We have been able to make antisera against the antigens within complexes by injecting immune complex–coated Raji cells or eluates of the cells into experimental animals, which in turn produce specific antisera against the antigens. The antisera then can be used to detect the antigen in tissue or serum, or they can be used to isolate large quantities of antigens that can in turn be studied by various biochemical or immunochemical procedures.

It is still a mystery why some individuals develop "immune complex disease" but others do not, considering that immune complex formation is a somewhat common event. Genetic factors, the nature of both antigen and antibody, and their rate of production all seem to play some role. The presence of anti-cellular antibodies with anti-Fc or anti-C3 receptor activity in sera of individuals with autoimmune diseases may also be responsible for observed defects in immune complex clearance in such patients. Moreover, certain types of immune complexes may initiate the production of anti-idiotypic antibodies, which may contribute to immune complex disease by forming complexes with the relevant idiotype and so on. The result would be a variety of persistent idiotype–anti-idiotype immune complexes, independent of the release or retention of the antigen involved in the original stimulation. Continued study of the characteristics, handling, and incidence of immune complexes should provide better understanding of immune complex–associated diseases.

Antinuclear Antibodies
In Diagnosis and Management

ENG M. TAN   *Research Institute of the Scripps Clinic*

A great deal has been learned in the past few years about the role antinuclear antibodies play in certain autoimmune diseases. To be sure, there is still much more to be learned, but we have arrived at the point where the fruits of intense basic research are being put to practical clinical use in management as well as diagnosis of these diseases.

Antinuclear antibodies are a family of circulating autoantibodies directed against components within a nucleus. One might more correctly call them autoantibodies to nuclear antigens, but they are commonly called antinuclear antibodies, or simply ANAs. They are present in a wide variety of immunologic diseases, including autoimmune thyroiditis, allergic encephalitis, and autoimmune liver disease, but not to the extent that they are found in what might be called ANA diseases—i.e., diseases in which ANAs seem to have a primary pathogenic role: systemic lupus erythematosus, Sjögren's syndrome, mixed connective tissue disease, scleroderma, polymyositis, and its variant, dermatomyositis.

Antinuclear antibodies are by no means the only autoantibodies operative in ANA diseases. There are several other types, including those against red cell, white cell, platelet, and clotting factors. There are also autoantibodies to specific organ tissues, such as thyroid, liver, stomach, and muscle. But antinuclear antibodies have received the most intensive scrutiny and can be classified in great detail. Basically, they are directed against components within the cellular nucleus: DNA, RNA, or proteins, or molecular complexes of these.

ANAs may be directed against histone and nonhistone nuclear proteins. Histones are basic, whereas most, but not all, nonhistones are acidic. The DNA antibodies may be directed against either double-stranded (native) DNA or single-stranded (denatured) DNA. The principal complexes against which ANAs are directed are deoxyribonucleoprotein (DNP) and ribonucleoprotein (RNP). DNPs consist of DNA and a histone; RNPs are made up of RNA and a nonhistone. All of the antigens are intranuclear, although some may be on the nuclear membrane. Several are within the nucleolus, and there is a distinct possibility that some may shuttle back and forth between the nucleus and nucleolus. Some may even travel between the nucleus and the cytoplasm. For the most part, antinuclear antibodies are IgG, but a small percentage are IgM and a still smaller percentage are IgA.

The pathogenesis of ANA disease is not known, but it is highly likely that several factors, acting serially or in concert, are involved. One cause may be viral; perhaps a ubiquitous virus triggers disease when there is an unusual host response. Another may be a deficiency of intracellular enzymes that normally synthesize or degrade nuclear and cytoplasmic macromolecules. Genetics also is involved, since family clustering of these diseases is present and certain HLA phenotypes may be predominant in some diseases. Environmental factors, too, are highly suspect. Exposure to sunlight has long been associated with de novo SLE as well as its exacerbation. And chemicals, including many food additives, also may be important. A number of chemicals are known to combine with and alter the structure and function of DNA. Furthermore,

ANA Profile in SLE

Antibodies to native DNA
Occur in 50%–60% of patients at significant titers

Antibodies to DNP
Occur in up to 70% of patients usually at titers of >1: 10,000 by hemagglutination

Antibodies to Sm antigen
Occur in 30% of patients usually at titers of 1 : 40–1 : 640 by hemagglutination

Antibodies to histones
Occur in up to 60% of SLE patients and 95% of drug-induced lupus patients

Antibodies to multiple other antigens, including
SS-A 30%–40%
SS-B 15%
RNP 30%–40%
PCNA . . . . <5%

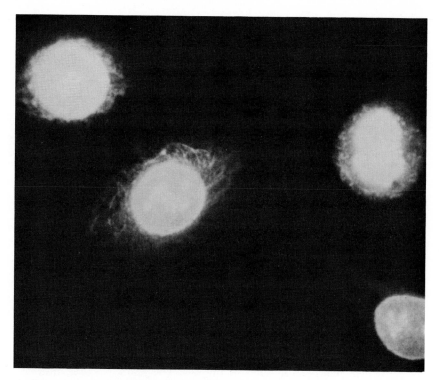

Antihistone antibody from a patient with SLE

we know that such drugs as procainamide and hydralazine can cause an SLE-like disease. Sex hormones, too, may be important since these diseases tend to be far more common in females than in males.

Even though we do not know the precise causes of ANA diseases, the primary mechanism of tissue injury is formation of antibody-antigen immune complexes. If there are no relevant antigens present in or accessible to the circulation, it is highly possible that a patient with circulating ANAs may never be sick at all; but if for some reason nuclear antigens also enter the circulation to form immune complexes, severe disease could result. Thus, although antibodies are not in themselves harmful, any patient

who harbors them has the potential of developing serious disease. Most studies of immune complexes in tissue injury have dealt with kidneys, showing a clear relationship between immune complex deposition in the renal microvasculature and the nephritides. But there also is considerable evidence that other organs, such as the heart, lungs, skin, and brain, are similarly affected. Moreover, whereas there is no definite proof that exacerbations and remissions are tied to the appearance and disappearance of immune complexes, there does seem to be some clinical correlation.

One of the most important discoveries concerning the ANA diseases is that each entity presents a rather distinct ANA profile. None of the antibodies is 100% specific for each disease, of course, but the profiles, which are characterized by the absence as well as the presence of certain antibodies and their titers, can greatly aid diagnosis. Let us start with SLE, which has a multiplicity of ANAs as well as other autoantibodies and, therefore, is considered the prototype of autoimmune diseases. About 80% of SLE

patients are women. The clinical manifestations vary with the extent of the disease and its distribution, which can affect virtually any organ system. A majority of patients have renal involvement, which may be benign and asymptomatic or progressively serious and fatal unless treated. Most SLE patients have arthralgias and arthritis of varying severity and erythematous cutaneous lesions. The disease may begin suddenly with fever, simulating an acute infection, or there may be only occasional episodes of fever. Systemic lupus may be quite difficult to differentiate clinically from other autoimmune diseases, but testing for ANAs can facilitate the diagnosis.

The first suggestion of an ANA in lupus came as a result of the discovery of the LE cell by M. M. Hargraves in the 1940s. This is a healthy polymorphonuclear leukocyte that has ingested the nuclear debris of a dead cell coated with antibody. In the mid-1950s it was shown that this antibody is directed against deoxyribonucleoprotein. In rapid succession many other antinuclear antibodies were identi-

ANA Profile in Sjögren's Syndrome

Antibodies to SS-A
Occur in 70% of patients

Antibodies to SS-B
Occur in 60% of patients

fied in SLE, many of which also appear in the other ANA diseases in varying degrees.

Until the advent of ANA tests, LE cell tests were the main laboratory indicators of lupus. Today, however, it is not necessary to get an LE cell test if ANA testing is available because the ANA test is more sensitive. In fact, in many larger hospitals and university centers LE cell tests are no longer performed. The LE cell is caused indirectly by antibody to DNP, and this antibody is detected directly on ANA tests. Both LE cells and DNP antibodies are present in up to 70% of SLE patients.

In addition to DNP antibodies, antibodies to both native and denatured DNA are frequently found in systemic lupus. Of these, native DNA (NDNA) antibodies have assumed special significance. When coupled to NDNA antigens, they form the immune complexes that are the main contributors to the kidney disease of lupus. Antibodies to NDNA occur at high titers in 50% to 60% of SLE patients. They occur very rarely, if at all, in other diseases. Antibodies to single-stranded DNA (SS-DNA) are found in many ANA diseases and in nonrheumatic diseases, particularly those characterized by chronic inflammation. Thus, SS-DNA antibodies are not particularly helpful in distinguishing one ANA disease from another, and we accord them less importance in the diagnostic profiles. However, SS-DNA antibodies can be very important pathogenically because of their participation in immune complexes.

Another very important ANA in lupus is directed against the Sm antigen, which is a nonhistone protein. This antigen was first described at The Rockefeller University in 1966 and carries the initials of the patient in whom it was identified. Since then it has become a marker for SLE, in that it is practically unseen in other autoimmune diseases. Moreover, the rare exceptions seem to be restricted to patients who have overlapping ANA diseases. The Sm antibody appears in only about 30% of SLE patients,

but when it appears, it is diagnostic. Sm antibodies are not found in discoid lupus. Other nonhistone antibodies found in SLE are directed against ribonucleoprotein and SS-A/Ro and SS-B/La antigens.

RNP antibodies are present in low titers in about 30% to 40% of SLE patients and to a lesser degree in discoid lupus, scleroderma, and rheumatoid arthritis. They are most commonly seen in mixed connective tissue disease (MCTD), where they occur in very high titers. The RNP antibody has become important in basic biology as a reagent for studying the functions and structures of the nonhistone antigens. There are indications that a part of the antigen called U-1 RNA complexed to a protein (U-1 RNP) results in a particle that may be very important in the processing of RNA. Before transcribed RNA can be transported across the nuclear membrane into the cytoplasm, it must be processed, and some molecular biologists are beginning to believe that U-1 RNA and U-1 RNP are involved in this process. The RNP moiety is immunologically identical to the Mo antigen described by T. Tomasi and colleagues.

The other nonhistone antibodies associated with SLE (SS-A and SS-B) are found more frequently in Sjögren's syndrome; indeed, SS stands for that syndrome. But 30% to 40% of SLE patients have SS-A antibodies, and 15% have SS-B antibodies. SS-A/Ro antibodies also are found in MCTD, scleroderma, polymyositis, and dermatomyositis.

An important point about nonhistone antigens is that they are remarkably soluble in physiologic buffer. This can lead to erroneous laboratory reports. For example, if tissue culture cells are rinsed in physiologic saline, they may lose significant amounts of RNP and SS antigens from the nuclei, producing false-negative antibody readings. Also, the antigenicity of nuclear antigens may be destroyed by fixatives, such as ethanol and methanol, again giving rise to false-negative ANA tests.

Antibodies to histones are present in up to 60% of SLE patients,

ANA Profile in Mixed Connective Tissue Disease

Antibodies to RNP
Occur in 95%–100% of patients

Absence of other ANAs

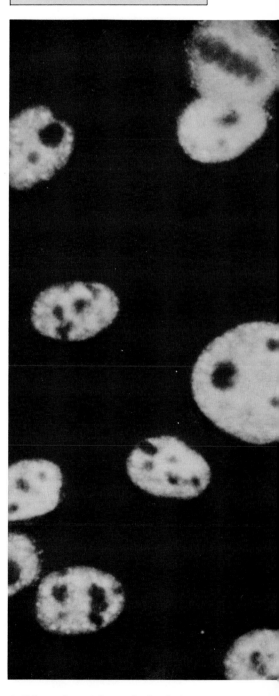

Antiribonucleoprotein antibody from a patient with MCTD

ANA Profiles in Scleroderma and CREST

Antibodies to Scl-70
Occur in 10%–20% of patients

Antibodies to nucleolar antigens
Occur in 40%–50% of patients at titers varying from 1:100 to 1:1000 by immunofluorescence

Antibodies to multiple other antigens, including RNP, SS-A, and SS-B at low titers

Antibodies to centromere antigens
The CREST variant usually contains only anticentromere antibodies, which occur in 80%–90% at titers of 1:100 to 1:1000 by immunofluorescence.

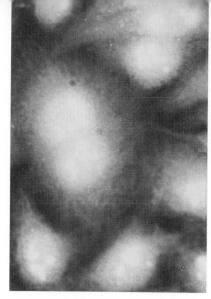

Antinucleolar antibody from a patient with scleroderma

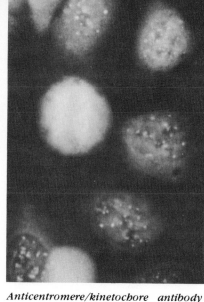

Anticentromere/kinetochore antibody from a patient with CREST

but more important diagnostically is the fact that they are present in about 95% of cases of drug-induced lupus. A number of drugs—primarily procainamide and hydralazine—can cause a lupuslike syndrome. This syndrome usually disappears after the drugs are stopped, but up to 40% of patients continue to have symptoms for extended periods. Clinically, drug-induced lupus behaves like systemic lupus, with two notable exceptions: These patients generally do not have kidney or central nervous system manifesta-

ANA Profile in Rheumatoid Arthritis

Antibodies to RANA
Occur in 85%–95% of patients at titers of ≥1:16 by immunodiffusion and 1:32 to 1:64 by immunofluorescence

Antibodies to histones
Occur in 20% of patients

ANA Profile in Polymyositis and Dermatomyositis

Antibodies to PM-1 antigen
Occur in 50% of polymyositis patients and in 10% of dermatomyositis patients at titers of 1:2 or 1:4 by immunodiffusion

Antibodies to other nuclear antigens, including Jo-1 may be present.

tions, and they do not have multiple types of ANA. Their ANAs are usually restricted to antihistones, although a small percentage of patients with drug-induced lupus have antibodies to denatured DNA. Antihistone ANAs are also present in about 20% of rheumatoid arthritis patients, but at much lower titers.

Antibody to proliferating cell nuclear antigen (PCNA) also may be present in SLE, but its occurrence is rare. Less than 5% of SLE patients have PCNA antibodies. The SLE profile, then, includes multiple ANAs, particularly to native DNA, which occur in about 60% of SLE patients; the Sm marker, which occurs in about 30%, and DNP or histone antibodies, which occur in up to 70% of patients.

Since the frequency of multiple ANAs is so high in lupus, the diagnosis should be reconsidered if the ANA test is negative. But one should not rely on a single negative test. Many negative readings subsequently prove positive when retested on different substrates. This was clearly shown in 50 SLE specimens that had tested negative in one substrate. When the same specimens were retested on tissue culture cell substrates, 30 were positive. And additional testing in more substrates increased the number of positives to 40. Some patients with SLE may have negative ANAs, as some investigators suggest, but if

so, they probably represent a very small proportion of cases.

Sjögren's syndrome, like SLE, can affect many body systems. A main feature of this disease is the so-called sicca complex, characterized by dryness of the eyes and mouth. Other important manifestations include extreme hypertrophy of the lymph nodes, enlarged parotid glands, myositis, and kidney disease. Arthritis occurs in approximately one third of the patients, with a distribution similar to that in rheumatoid arthritis. The disease occurs most commonly in women over the age of 40.

The major ANAs in Sjögren's syndrome are SS-A and SS-B, present in 70% and 60% of patients, respectively. Both antibodies occur in very high titers. Some Sjögren's patients also may have RNP antibodies, but these tend to occur in low titers. Therefore, the ANA profile in Sjögren's essentially is anti-SS-A and anti-SS-B at very high titers and perhaps some anti-RNP.

Mixed connective tissue disease was described by G. C. Sharp and colleagues in 1972. There is still some question whether this is a distinct syndrome, but most rheumatologists believe it is. Patients with MCTD have the symptoms seen in SLE, scleroderma, and dermatomyositis, yet the clinical picture is not typical of any of these. One of the major manifestations of MCTD is Raynaud's phenomenon, which occurs in almost all cases. In addition, a great many MCTD patients have a peculiar swelling of their hands, giving their fingers a sausagelike appearance. Almost all MCTD patients have polyarthralgias, and many also have esophageal abnormalities. Unlike SLE, MCTD has a relative—but not total—absence of renal disease. And although patients generally have swollen fingers, their skin is not hard and tightly bound as it is in scleroderma. The age range for MCTD is five to 80 years, with a mean of 37 years. About 80% of these patients are female.

Mixed connective tissue disease can be somewhat difficult to characterize clinically, but it is very easy to characterize immunologically. Antibody to RNP is present in very high titers in 95% or more of MCTD patients. A very few patients may have some SS-A or SS-B antibodies, and about 20% to 25% of them have antibodies to SS-DNA, which, as noted, are usually not included in the diagnostic profiles. And even though MCTD patients frequently have some of the symptoms of systemic lupus, LE cells are characteristically absent. Thus, the ANA profile in MCTD essentially is a very high titer of anti-RNP antibodies and an absence of other ANAs.

Scleroderma, or progressive systemic sclerosis, is characterized by fibrotic and degenerative changes of the skin, muscles, joints, and viscera. It occurs in two forms: 1) diffuse, in which many body systems are affected, and 2) a variant called CREST (calcinosis, Raynaud's phenomenon, esophageal dysfunction, sclerodactyly, telangiectasia) (see M. C. Hochberg, "The Spectrum of Systemic Sclerosis—Current Concepts," Hosp Pract, March 1981). CREST patients do not have the widespread involvement seen in diffuse scleroderma; skin changes are confined to the hands and face. Diffuse scleroderma is very much like SLE in that it is characterized by a multiplicity of antinuclear antibodies. In addition to antibody to scleroderma-70 (Scl-70), which occurs in 10% to 20% of scleroderma patients, many other ANAs, includ-

Disease Associations of ANAs

Antibodies to native DNA
SLE: 50%–60%

Antibodies to Sm antigen
SLE: 30% of SLE patients

Antibodies to histones
SLE: Up to 60%
Drug-induced SLE: 95%
Rheumatoid arthritis: 20%

Antibodies to SS-A
Sjögren's syndrome: 70%
SLE: 30%–40%
Scleroderma and mixed connective tissue disease:
at low frequency and low titer

Antibodies to SS-B
Sjögren's syndrome: 60%
SLE: 15%

Antibodies to RNP
Mixed connective tissue disease: 95%–100% at titers ≥ 1 : 10,000
SLE: 30% at lower titers
Scleroderma: at low frequency and low titer

Antibodies to PCNA
SLE: <5%

Antibodies to Scl-70
Scleroderma: 10%–20%

Antibodies to nucleolar antigens
Scleroderma: 40%–50%

Antibodies to centromere antigens
CREST: 80%–90%

Antibodies to RANA
Rheumatoid arthritis: 85%–95% at titers of ≥ 1 : 16 by immunodiffusion
and 1 : 32 to 1 : 64 by immunofluorescence

Antibodies to PM-1
Polymyositis: 50% at titers of 1 : 2 or 1 : 4
Dermatomyositis: 10% at titers of 1 : 2 or 1 : 4

ing those against RNP, SS-A, and SS-B antigens, may be found at low titers in this disease.

A unique feature of diffuse scleroderma is that antinucleolar antibodies—some against 4-6S RNA—are found in 40% to 50% of patients. These antibodies are rarely seen in other ANA diseases. Another unusual feature is the presence of anticentromere antibodies, which are directed against the constricted regions of chromosomes. These antibodies are seen in 80% to 90% of CREST patients. They also are seen in 10% to 15% of diffuse sclero-

derma patients who apparently do not have CREST, but it is quite possible that these patients may actually have an overlap of the variant form. Anticentromeres very rarely occur in other diseases and virtually never in the titers seen in CREST. The ANA profile for diffuse scleroderma, then, includes anti-Scl-70 antibodies, antinucleolar antibodies at varying titers, and a multiplicity of other ANAs at low titers. The CREST profile usually contains only anticentromere antibodies.

For a long time the only major autoantibody found in rheumatoid arthritis was the rheumatoid factor, but it now has been shown that some patients also have antibodies to histones. As noted in the context of drug-induced lupus, approximately 20% of rheumatoid arthritis patients have antihistone antibodies. In addition, antihistone activity is present in some rheumatoid factors. Another relatively new finding is a possible association of rheumatoid arthritis with the Epstein-Barr virus, which is found in both normal subjects and rheumatoid arthritis patients at roughly the same frequency: 85%. EB virus has the ability to induce transformation of B cells, i.e., to cause B cells to proliferate as well as to produce new types of nuclear antigens. In the normal person, EB-virus-induced B-cell changes are held in check by T cells and other cell types. Recent studies show that the rheumatoid arthritis patient has a defect in this control system, thus allowing B cells to produce new types of nuclear antigens.

In our laboratory we have discovered antibody to a rheumatoid-arthritis-associated antigen (RANA) that is found in 85% to 95% of patients with rheumatoid arthritis but in only 30% to 40% of normal subjects. RANA is one of the new nuclear antigens induced by EB virus in infected B cells. Anti-RANA titers can be determined by immunofluorescence or by immunodiffusion. With immunofluorescence, the titers are 1:32 to 1:64 in rheumatoid arthritis patients; with immunodiffusion, they are about 1:16. In normal subjects RANA titers are less than 1:8 by immunofluorescence and less than 1:4 by immunodiffusion. Therefore, aside from the RA factor, clinicians now have an ANA profile to aid in diagnosis of rheumatoid arthritis, which in

essence consists of histone antibodies in 20% of patients and RANA antibodies in 85% to 95% of patients, at titers of 1:16 on immunodiffusion or 1:32 to 1:64 on immunofluorescence.

The last autoimmune disease under discussion is polymyositis. Characterized by inflammatory and degenerative changes in muscles—with concomitant skin involvement in its other form, dermatomyositis—the disease is not rare, although it is less common than SLE. It occurs twice as frequently in women as in men, and it can present at any age but appears most commonly between 40 and 60 years. There is an important association between dermatomyositis and malignant tumors.

The ANAs in polymyositis and dermatomyositis have been discovered only recently, but it is known that they are directed against nuclear antigens. The main ANAs in these diseases are PM-1 and Jo-1. The PM-1 antibody is present in approximately 50% of polymyositis patients and in 10% of those with dermatomyositis. In both types the titers are very low, roughly 1:2 to 1:4. Tests for the ANAs in polymyositis and dermatomyositis are currently available only in some research laboratories, but we expect them to become more generally available in the not too distant future.

From a clinician's point of view, testing for ANAs can significantly aid diagnosis when the results are evaluated in conjunction with the clinical findings. Laboratories detect the presence of ANAs by various methods, including immunofluorescence, immunodiffusion, and radioimmunoassay. If a positive ANA response is obtained, it is then nec-

essary to determine what types of ANA are present to delineate the profile. For example, if there is a high titer of anti-RNP antibodies and no antibodies to native DNA or Scl-70, one can be reasonably certain that the patient has MCTD, not SLE or scleroderma.

For the most part, the initial ANA test is relatively inexpensive, but complete profiles are somewhat costly. Individual tests could be ordered on the basis of the most likely diagnosis. If the clinical picture suggests SLE, tests for native DNA are in order. If it is scleroderma, one would want to test for the antibodies to Scl-70, centromere, and nucleolar antigens. To reduce costs a number of laboratories, including ours at Scripps, are developing automated systems of ANA testing analogous to an SMA-12, which could give a rather complete profile readout at relatively little cost.

In addition to aiding diagnosis, ANA tests can be useful for monitoring the effects of therapy. One cannot depend on titers alone, of course, but periodic testing of ANA titers correlated with the clinical picture can be of considerable aid in guiding therapy. If the titer rises and there are other indications that the patient is getting worse, increased dosages or a change of medication may be needed. On the other hand, a reduced titer combined with signs of clinical improvement generally indicates that therapy is on the right track.

In conclusion, it has become clear not only that antinuclear antibodies play a very important role in autoimmune diseases but that their distinct profiles and titers in certain of these diseases make excellent diagnostic and management tools.

Hybridomas as a Source of Antibodies

MATTHEW D. SCHARFF, SUSAN ROBERTS, *and* PALLAIAH THAMMANA
Albert Einstein College of Medicine

Antibodies have been used in clinical medicine for almost a century for tissue and blood typing, for the identification of microorganisms, and for passive immunization. The development of radiolabeled and enzyme-linked immunoassays extended the usefulness of antibodies to the quantification and identification of an even wider variety of substances, including hormones, drugs, and enzymes. Immunoassays require large amounts of highly specific antisera, which are usually obtained by injecting a purified antigen into an animal and then testing to determine if its serum reacts specifically with the immunizing agent.

An animal is capable of elaborating millions of different antibody molecules that react with the many antigens present in nature. The clonal selection hypothesis developed by Burnet and his colleagues in the 1950s explains how an animal can produce antibodies capable of reacting specifically with each of this seemingly unlimited number of antigens. According to the hypothesis, each antibody-forming cell (B lymphocyte or its fully differentiated progeny, the plasma cell) is committed to the production of one type of antibody molecule that has the potential for reacting with one or, at most, a few structurally similar antigenic determinants. Only a small fraction of B cells recognize any given antigen. During the immune response, those B cells recognizing a particular antigenic determinant, in collaboration with other immunoregulatory cells, are stimulated to replicate and differentiate into antibody-secreting cells.

One must also keep in mind certain structural characteristics of the antibody molecule (see Figure 1, page 326) to understand the heterogeneity of humoral immune responses. Antibodies, or immunoglobulins, are, of course, a part of the class of serum proteins that are designated on the basis of their electrophoretic mobility as gamma globulins.

The basic immunoglobulin molecule is composed of four polypeptide chains. Two chains have a molecular weight of about 55,000 to 75,000 (depending on the subclass) and are designated as heavy chains; the other two are about MW 25,000 and are the light chains. The two identical light chains and two identical heavy chains of each antibody molecule are joined by disulfide bonds. The molecule is also divided into variable and constant regions. The 100 amino acids at the amino terminal portion of each pair constitute the variable region, and it is this region that makes contact with antigen and from which the specificity of the antibody is derived. Because it contains a great degree of amino acid sequence heterogeneity, a vast number of three-dimensional binding sites are possible, at least one of which will be complementary to a foreign antigen, thus allowing the antibody to bind to the antigen noncovalently. The amino acids of the carboxy-terminal constant region of both heavy and light chains have a limited number of sequences, with variations therein determining both chain and immunoglobulin class. In all, there are two classes of light chains and eight or nine classes of heavy chains. Different classes have different biologic activities, and some classes share biologic activities, such as complement fixation, enhancement of phagocytosis by macrophages, aggregation, or precipitation of antigens.

When an antigen is introduced into an animal, it is

processed by macrophages, interacts with thymus-derived helper and suppressor T cells, and, through a series of cellular interactions, is presented to those B cells that bear a surface antibody that reacts with the antigen. If the antigen is a complex macromolecule, such as a protein, it contains many antigenic determinants, and many B cells will be stimulated to replicate, differentiate, and generate clones of plasma cells secreting antibody. Each antigenic determinant elicits antibodies that bind specifically with it. Thus, any naturally occurring antigen elicits the responses of a large number of B cells, and a variety of antibodies differing in size, charge, and affinity appear in the serum.

That is why production of specific antisera by the classical technique is more of an art than a science. Even when a highly purified antigen is used as the immunizing agent, the resulting antiserum is a mixture of many different immunoglobulins with different antigenic specificities and biologic functions (see Figure 2, page 327). Further,

the relative amounts of particular types of antibody that make up the antiserum vary considerably from animal to animal, even from bleeding to bleeding of the same animal.

Most routine serologic assays are not affected by the heterogeneity of antisera, although they do require that the antisera be highly specific. Such antisera are usually obtained by using purified antigens and by absorbing out any nonspecific antibodies with cross-reacting macromolecules. For example, white blood cells contain many complex antigens, but antibodies specific for individual transplantation antigens can be obtained by immunizing an individual of the appropriate genetic background or by absorbing with cells that contain the other transplantation antigens. Similarly, antisera specific for individual classes or subclasses of human immunoglobulins can be generated by immunizing with purified myeloma immunoglobulins of a single class or subclass and then absorbing with myeloma proteins of the other classes or subclasses.

It is even more difficult to generate good antisera with impure or less well-defined antigens, e.g., those that distinguish between normal and malignant cells or between different subclasses of lymphocytes. If one has succeeded in obtaining an antibody that detects a tumor-cell antigen on a leukemia cell, for example, it is virtually impossible to reproduce the antisera, even in the same animal, because of the heterogeneity and unpredictability of the antibody response.

Attempts have been made to overcome these problems by generating monoclonal antibodies. Multiple myeloma provides one model for a monoclonal response. In this disease, a single antibody-forming cell undergoes malignant transformation and then proliferates in an uncontrolled fashion, producing large amounts of a single antibody. It is usually not possible to determine the antigen with which a given myeloma immunoglobulin reacts or to induce a myeloma immunoglobulin that reacts with the immunizing agent. Of thousands of human and mouse myeloma tumors examined, only a few have produced antibodies that react with known antigens, and these were identified only by screening against a large battery of potential antigens. Another approach has been to transform heterogeneous populations of human, murine, or rabbit lymphoid cells with Epstein-Barr, Abelson, or SV40 virus, respectively. This has been successful in a few instances, resulting in production of monoclonal antibodies against some red-cell and transplantation antigens.

A method for routinely producing monoclonal antibodies in quantity was discovered by G. Köhler and C. Milstein at the Medical Research Council Laboratory in Cambridge, England, in 1975. This method involved the fusion or hybridization of antibody-secreting plasma cells and myeloma cells. In the fused product ("hybridoma"), the plasma cell contributes the capacity to produce specific antibody; the myeloma cell, the longevity in culture and ability to form tumors in animals.

The development of the hybrido-

Figure 1

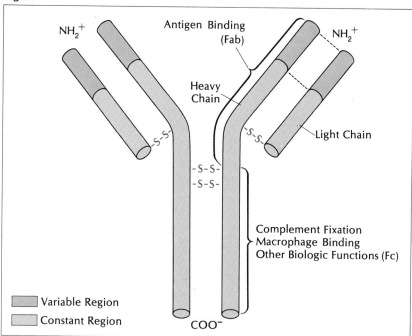

Prototypic structure of an antibody molecule consists of two identical light chains and two identical heavy chains joined by disulfide bonds. The variable region in the so-called Fab portion of the molecule provides antigen specificity and binding capability, while the Fc portion has a constant amino acid sequence within an immunoglobulin class (e.g., IgG) and provides such biologic functions as complement fixation.

ma actually evolved out of studies of the genetic control of antibody expression. For the purposes of these studies, which need not be detailed here, Milstein's group fused rat myeloma and mouse myeloma cells and showed that the fused cells continued to secrete both rat and mouse immunoglobulins. Encouraged by these results, Köhler and Milstein fused a plasma cell with a myeloma cell in the hope that the hybrid cell would secrete antibody of the plasma-cell specificity.

For this experiment, they immunized mice with sheep red blood cells (SRBC) because these cells are powerful immunogens and antibody against them is easily assayed. Spleen cells from the immunized mice were then fused with myeloma cells in tissue culture. The successfully fused cells were isolated and cultured; then those cells that secreted antibody against SRBC were selected and cloned to produce continuous cultures of hybridomas that secreted a single type of antibody of predefined specificity.

Although Köhler and Milstein were doing basic experiments on the genetics of immunoglobulin synthesis in mouse myeloma cells, the hybridoma technology they developed has revolutionized immunology and serology in the clinic as well as in the research laboratory. To understand why, it is important to realize that the essential difference between the classical and hybridoma methods of producing antisera is that in the former, one has to absorb out all of the unwanted antibodies, whereas in the latter, one selects for the clone of cells producing only the antibody that is wanted. Because the hybridoma technique clones an individual antibody-forming cell from among all others present in the spleen of the immunized animal, cells reacting to other antigens are eliminated.

The method of producing hybridomas in most laboratories is essentially that of Köhler and Milstein (see Figure 3, page 328).

Mouse spleen cells are used because they provide a convenient source of antibody-secreting plasma cells. Normal plasma cells ter-

Figure 2

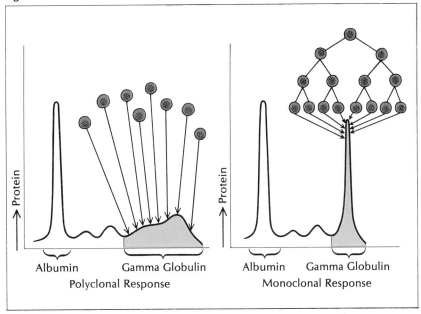

Broad distribution of gamma globulin in serum electrophoretic pattern on left indicates many different types of antibody produced by multiple plasma cell clones. Sharp peak in pattern at right reflects monoclonal antibody produced by a single plasma cell clone.

minally differentiate after a few cell divisions and die—hence, the requirement for fusion with a malignant cell. Mouse myeloma cells are used because they have a similar function, antibody secretion, and grow continuously in tissue culture. When fused with spleen cells, they confer their immortality on the progeny. The mouse myeloma cells generally used are from a cell line that has two mutations inserted into it. One results in loss of ability to produce the myeloma immunoglobulins. This is important because fusion of an immunoglobulin-producing myeloma cell and an immunoglobulin-producing spleen cell would result in antibody consisting of various combinations of the polypeptide chains of both parent cells and, possibly, of unpredictable specificities. The nonimmunoglobulin-producing myeloma cells do not affect immunoglobulin synthesis by the spleen cell; thus, the fused cells produce only spleen cell antibody. The second mutation involves loss of the enzyme hypoxanthine phosphoribosyl transferase (HPRT), and its significance will be described.

The spleen cells are obtained from mice that have been immunized and then boosted. The spleens of those animals that produce the highest antibody titer to the immunogen are removed two to four days after the boost. The nucleated cells from each spleen are mixed separately with myeloma cells in a ratio of 5:1 and exposed to an agent that promotes cell fusion, such as polyethylene glycol (PEG), for eight minutes. The cell mixture is resuspended in a growth medium containing hypoxanthine, aminopterin, and thymidine (HAT). Because only about one out of every 200,000 spleen cells actually forms a viable hybrid with a myeloma cell, the unfused cells and the myeloma-myeloma hybrids must be eliminated, and this is done by the selective HAT medium. The myeloma cells, which lack HPRT, cannot use exogenous hypoxanthine to synthesize purines, and when grown in the presence of aminopterin, which blocks endogenous synthesis of purines, these cells die. Only myeloma cells that have fused to spleen cells containing HPRT are able to use the hypoxanthine and thymidine in the HAT medium and, therefore, survive. There is no need to select for unfused spleen cells because they die out in culture and also are rapidly overgrown by the hybrids,

Figure 3

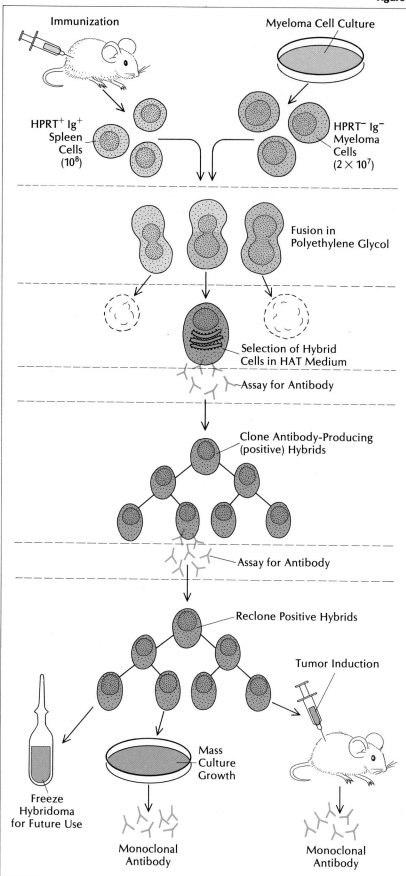

Immunization

Myeloma Cell Culture

HPRT⁺ Ig⁺
Spleen
Cells
(10^8)

HPRT⁻ Ig⁻
Myeloma
Cells
(2×10^7)

Fusion in
Polyethylene Glycol

Selection of Hybrid
Cells in HAT Medium

Assay for Antibody

Clone Antibody-Producing
(positive) Hybrids

Assay for Antibody

Reclone Positive Hybrids

Tumor Induction

Freeze
Hybridoma
for Future Use

Mass
Culture
Growth

Monoclonal
Antibody

Monoclonal
Antibody

which double every 17 to 18 hours.

Hybrids begin to appear one week after fusion. They have the same morphology as the parent myeloma cell. After two to six weeks in HAT medium, between 150 and 500 hybrid clones are present. The medium is removed from each well containing a hybrid and screened, by a quick, simple immunoassay, for the presence of antibody against the immunogen. As many as 50 hybrids producing significant amounts of antibody may be found if a potent immunogen, such as SRBC, has been used. On the other hand, if the immunogen was weak or the animals responded poorly to immunization, no antibody-producing hybrids may be found.

When the positive hybrids have been identified, they are grown and cloned on an appropriate medium as quickly as possible. Recloning is necessary because variants arise that may overgrow the antibody-producing clones. The subclones are screened again for antibody. Some 10% to 20% of the hybridomas that were initially positive continue to make specific antibody. The best clones produce up to 100

Hybridoma production begins by immunizing a mouse with a selected antigen. The animal's spleen cells are harvested and mixed with mouse myeloma cells and briefly incubated with polyethylene glycol to promote fusion. Cells are transferred to a growth medium containing hypoxanthine, aminopterin, and thymidine (HAT). Unfused myeloma cells and myeloma-myeloma hybrids, which lack the enzyme HPRT, cannot survive in the HAT medium. Unfused spleen cells and spleen-spleen hybrids die naturally after a few replications. The remaining spleen cell–myeloma hybrids are assayed for antibody production against the immunogen, and positive hybrids are cloned. Later, they are again assayed for antibody production, and the positives recloned. At this point, the hybridomas can be frozen and stored. To amplify antibody production, hybridomas are injected into mice, in which they produce ascites tumors that generate large amounts of monoclonal antibody. In the case of human spleen cell–human myeloma hybridomas, amplification would be done by growing the cells in mass culture or in immunosuppressed animals.

μg/ml of specific antibody in the culture fluid. They can be frozen and stored until needed.

Once a hybridoma has been developed, it provides a source of specific antibody indefinitely. When antibody is needed, it can be obtained from the tissue culture medium or prepared by injecting the hybridoma cells into mice. The cells form ascites tumors, and very large amounts of antibody accumulate in the ascites fluid. From 10 to 15 milliliters of fluid can be obtained from each mouse, and the titer of antibody in that fluid is often 100 to 1,000 times higher than can be obtained from the serum of an immunized animal. Thus, a single mouse can produce as much monoclonal antibody as a well-immunized rabbit, and the antibody produced in the mouse is more concentrated and more easily purified than the polyclonal antibody generated in the larger animal. Because the hybridoma cells can be frozen and recovered later, the supply of a particular antibody can be renewed whenever needed, and laboratories all over the world can use the identical reagent.

A major benefit of hybridoma technology is the ability to obtain a pure antibody from an impure antigen. Thus, it now will be possible to identify and purify substances with rare specificities, such as tumor antigens and hormone receptors. For example, R. Levy and his colleagues at Stanford have generated two hybridomas that produce antibody that distinguished malignant from normal cells in the peripheral blood and bone marrow of patients with acute lymphocytic leukemia (ALL). The antigen detected by these monoclonals apparently is not a true tumor antigen because the antibodies also react with normal lymphocytes in the cortex of the thymus. However, since these cells are not present in peripheral blood, the hybridoma antibody should be useful in the diagnosis and monitoring of treatment of patients with ALL.

Differentiation antigens that identify functional subsets of human T lymphocytes have been identified by S. F. Schlossman and associates at Harvard and by G. Goldstein and colleagues at Ortho. These monoclonals differentiate subclasses of T cells in the peripheral blood from other lymphocytes. One identifies the cytotoxic/suppressor T cells, one distinguishes T helper cells, and one identifies all thymus-derived lymphocytes. These reagents are now available commercially. They are being used to study the role of T cells in many immunologic diseases. It is likely that they will be used eventually in the diagnosis and, possibly, the treatment of immunologic diseases.

In the field of virology, the use of monoclonal antibodies has made it possible to identify new substrains of many viruses and to make distinctions between isolates from different parts of the world, in situations not possible with conventional antisera. The influenza virus has been studied intensively by W. Gerhard and H. Koprowski and their associates at the Wistar Institute and by R. Webster at St. Jude Hospital using monoclonal antibodies. The antigenic instability of the influenza hemagglutinin and, to a lesser extent, its neuraminidase is thought to be responsible for the frequent appearance of new strains of the virus. These workers have used monoclonal antibodies to select variants that arise in tissue culture. Their studies have shown that antigenic differences result from single amino acid substitutions in the hemagglutinin. They also have demonstrated a previously unrecognized antigenic difference between influenza virus strains circulating in England and those isolated in the United States and Australia during the 1968 pandemic. In the future, the use of monoclonal antibodies should make it possible to identify changes in the virus in nature that permit escape from immunologic surveillance and cause pandemics, to refine epidemiologic studies, and to make more effective influenza vaccines.

Other studies by investigators at the Wistar Institute, using monoclonals generated against the rabies virus, have shown that this presumably stable virus is as antigenically unstable in tissue culture as is the influenza virus. T. J. Wiktor and Koprowski defined several different serotypes in the laboratory and street isolates from all over the world. These serologic differences may account for occasional vaccine failures. Conventional antisera usually do not reveal differences be-

---

Applications of Monoclonal Antibodies

Reported to Date
    Routine diagnostic and investigative serology and tissue typing
    Identification and epidemiology of infectious agents
        Viruses
            Influenza: Monoclonal antibodies create genetic drift in vitro; map antigenic
                domains on hemagglutinin; compare in vitro mutants and in vivo variants;
                refine epidemiology
            Rabies: Monoclonal antibodies reveal antigenic instability; reveal serologic
                subtypes in street virus; refine epidemiology
        Bacteria
        Parasites
    Identification of tumor antigens; classification of leukemias and lymphomas
    Identification of functional subpopulations of lymphoid cells

Anticipated in Man
    Passive immunization against
        Infectious agents
        Drug toxicity
    Provision of graft protection
    Potentiation of tumor rejection
    Manipulation of the immune response
    Targeting of diagnostic or therapeutic agents in vivo for
        Detection of metastases
        Delivery of cytotoxic agents to tumor cells

tween laboratory and street strains of the rabies virus isolated from patients and animals; therefore, it is generally assumed that vaccine strains, most of which are derived from the original Pasteur strain, are universally protective. The ability to identify distinct serotypes of the virus should lead to further refinements in its epidemiology as well as in rabies vaccines.

Similarly, the diagnosis and epidemiology of many other viral diseases and of rickettsial, parasitic, and bacterial diseases will be greatly facilitated by the use of monoclonal antibodies. Monoclonals against structural proteins of herpes simplex types 1 and 2, murine leukemia, dengue, and measles viruses and against the surface antigens of the malaria sporozoite have been generated. In the case of parasites, monoclonals could be used to purify a surface antigen that conferred protection against infection, and that antigen could then be used to produce a vaccine. Alternatively, when human monoclonals of the right specificity become available, it may be possible to intervene in the life cycle of the parasitic organism by passive immunization.

Passive immunization in cases of drug overdose is another potential clinical use for hybridoma-generated monoclonal antibodies. For instance, a monoclonal antibody that bound digitalis specifically would form, when injected, an antigen-antibody complex and rapidly remove the drug from the circulation. Another application would be the use of monoclonal antibodies as vehicles to deliver diagnostic or therapeutic agents in vivo. In the case of myocardial infarction, a radiolabeled monoclonal antibody could be used to identify the damaged part of the heart muscle and to quantify the percentage of muscle damaged. Similarly, in malignant diseases, it may be possible to use radiolabeled monoclonal antibodies to locate metastases. In both examples, a radiolabeled antibody would be injected, and an external scanning method would be used to locate and quantify the radioactivity. Preliminary experiments in mice have shown that radiolabeled monoclonal antibodies can be used to locate tumors of a reasonable size. Finally, in this category of applications is the potential for delivering cytotoxic agents to tumor cells. It may be possible to kill tumor cells by raising a monoclonal antibody against a tumor antigen, then attaching a toxic agent, such as diphtheria toxin, to the antibody and injecting the composite. As the antibody reacted with its antigen, it would deliver the toxin to the tumor cell.

At the present time, two major obstacles stand in the way of such clinical applications. One is the lack of suitable human monoclonal antibodies. Monoclonal antibodies produced by mouse- or rat-cell hybridomas are quite useful for in vitro studies, such as routine serology and tissue typing, but they would cause acute or chronic allergic reactions if injected repeatedly into a human. A human spleen cell-human myeloma cell hybridoma that produces human antibodies against a given antigen has been produced by H. Kaplan and L. Olsson at Stanford. Their system provides a model for developing other human monoclonal antibodies.

The second obstacle may be more difficult to overcome: The monoclonal antibodies produced by hybridomas are the products of malignant cells. It may be difficult to be certain that the antibody is free of all virus particles. The potential in vivo applications in human disease, therefore, may be limited to life-threatening conditions.

The essential value of hybridoma technology is the ability to produce a stable, well-defined chemical reagent against virtually any antigen and to produce it in large quantities and whenever needed. The initial investment is considerable—it takes about four months to generate a hybridoma—but in the long run, the availability of tailor-made monoclonal antibodies will improve the reliability and reduce the cost of immunoassays. Hybridomas producing antibodies against many human serum components, blood group and transplantation antigens, hormone receptors and neurotransmitters, carcinoembryonic antigens, and many microorganisms have already been developed. Those that are useful for routine diagnostic tests probably will be made available by commercial firms that manufacture serologic reagents. Others, mainly of interest to researchers, are available already from cell banks funded by the National Institute of Allergy and Infectious Diseases and the National Cancer Institute.

The Development of Synthetic Vaccines

RICHARD A. LERNER, NICOLA GREEN, ARTHUR OLSON, THOMAS SHINNICK, *and* J. G. SUTCLIFFE
Research Institute of the Scripps Clinic

If one accepts the premise that synthesis is a goal in medical science, then it becomes apparent that with respect to vaccines, achievement of this goal has taken a long time—nearly 200 years since Jenner first injected cowpox virus into a child to protect him against smallpox in 1796. This time span can be compared with the bare quarter century between Fleming's discovery and the first successful semisynthetic penicillins.

However, as with any scientific accomplishment, the reality had to wait for the development of a pertinent body of prerequisite knowledge. For vaccine synthesis, this meant 1) recognition of the DNA character of genes; 2) conception and working out of the genetic code so that the relationships between DNA nucleotides and the amino acids they code for could be delineated; 3) ability to sequence both genes and peptides; 4) sufficient understanding of protein molecular structure so that starting from a determined DNA nucleotide sequence, it is possible to predict what "pieces" of the viral protein are most likely to act as antigens; and 5) ability to synthesize peptides.

This article will be devoted in the main to the sequential application of this conceptual and technical knowledge to the synthesis of small immunogenic peptide fragments that elicit antibodies to hepatitis B, influenza, rabies, mouse leukemia, and hoof-and-mouth disease viruses. Before embarking, however, let me first try to answer the question, Why should the physician want to use synthetic vaccines?

A good starting point for answering this question is a brief summary of current approaches to immunization, starting with natural infection—sometimes abetted, as with the time-honored practice of deliberately exposing a young boy to mumps. The first medically systematic technique (that of Jenner) was the use of a cross-reactive virus, presumably of low human pathogenicity, to immunize against a virus of known high pathogenicity. More recently, we have employed attenuated live viruses, agents retaining their immunogenicity and their capacity to replicate but, again presumably, not their pathogenicity. An alternative approach has been to use killed and therefore nonreplicating virus for immunization. More recently, starting from the premise that immunologic responses are directed against surface determinants, so that in this context the interior of the virus is unnecessary, vaccines have been made from only such surface components. Capsular-antigen vaccines exemplify this concept.

Obviously, one cannot gainsay the immense progress inherent in this formidable array of immunization approaches and their applications to both viral and bacterial diseases. At the same time, it must be recognized that vaccine safety remains one of the primary incompletely solved problems of medicine. Some of the difficulties are readily apparent, for example, the Guillain-Barré "epidemic" in the wake of mass influenza immunization, the SV-40 contamination of poliovirus vaccines, etc. However, prudence dictates that we regard these dramatic problems as only surface manifestations of a basic question. The fact is that when we inoculate whole virus (live or dead), or substantial portions thereof, into a patient, we are burdening that patient with a great deal of largely unknown and often

Figure 1

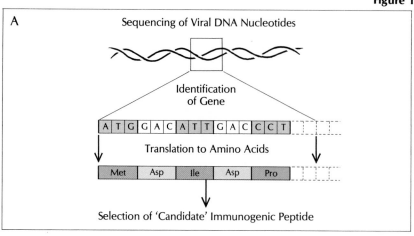

A

Sequencing of Viral DNA Nucleotides

Identification of Gene

| A | T | G | G | A | C | A | T | T | G | A | C | C | C | T |

Translation to Amino Acids

| Met | Asp | Ile | Asp | Pro |

Selection of 'Candidate' Immunogenic Peptide

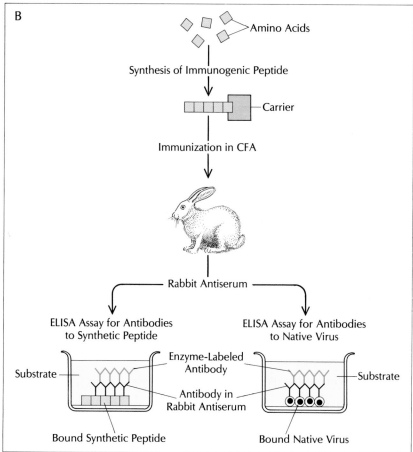

B

Amino Acids

Synthesis of Immunogenic Peptide

Carrier

Immunization in CFA

Rabbit Antiserum

ELISA Assay for Antibodies to Synthetic Peptide

ELISA Assay for Antibodies to Native Virus

Substrate — Enzyme-Labeled Antibody — Substrate

Antibody in Rabbit Antiserum

Bound Synthetic Peptide

Bound Native Virus

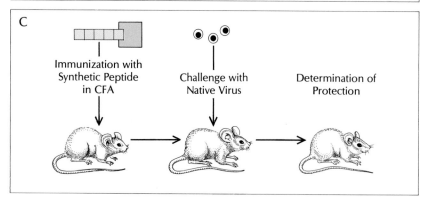

C

Immunization with Synthetic Peptide in CFA

Challenge with Native Virus

Determination of Protection

highly mutable biologic material. If the virus has been grown in tissue culture, it is impossible to guarantee the absence of biologic contamination. The more we learn about virus mutability and virus latency, the more we have to wonder about long-term effects. Along with the immunologic determinants we need for protection against disease, we are unquestionably introducing "irrelevant" immunogenic molecules, which may well elicit antibodies capable of participating in the formation of pathogenic immune complexes. Can we really be sure that the increasing numbers of cases of malignant disease, and of nonmalignant degenerative disease occurring in our aging population, do not have their etiologic origins in immunizations that antedate the diseases by decades?

It is in this context that synthetic vaccines promise truly definitive solutions. Their outstanding characteristic is that their content is completely known. Moreover, synthetic vaccines are, by definition, uniquely specific and totally uniform. One can add to this roster of advantages the fact that synthetic vaccines are cheap. The prepara-

The various steps in preparing a synthetic antiviral vaccine and assaying both its immunogenicity and protective efficacy are schematized in diagrams at left. As shown in panel A, the initial step requires knowledge of the nucleotide sequence of the viral DNA or of a surface antigenic component (e.g., hepatitis B surface antigen or the influenza hemagglutinins). From this knowledge, one can deduce the amino acid sequence of the protein, and by studying that primary structure, predict the peptide sequences most likely to be located on the surface of the virus. It is these sequences that are synthesized (panel B), coupled to carriers and injected in complete Freund's adjuvant (CFA) into rabbits to raise an antiserum. This antiserum is then assayed for antibody against both the immunogenic peptide and the native virus. Those synthetic peptides that demonstrate adequate antibody titers against both are then used as vaccines in test animals (panel C). After vaccination, the animals are challenged with native virus to evaluate protectivity.

Figure 2

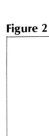

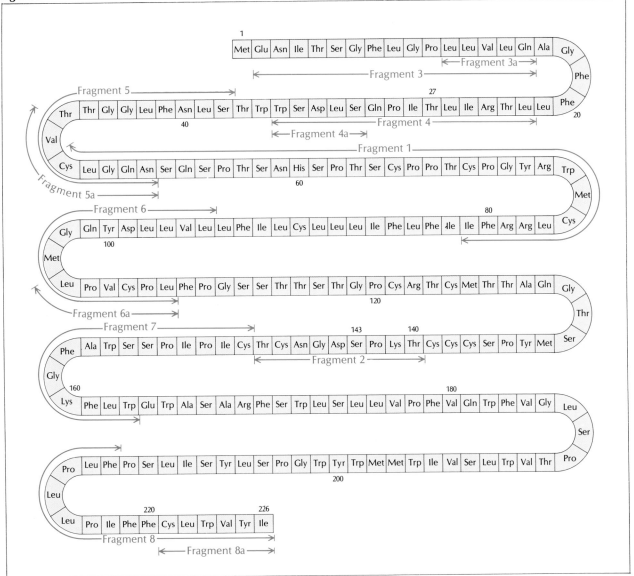

The amino acid sequence of hepatitis B surface antigen as translated by M. Pasek et al (Nature 282:575, 1979) is shown *above. The sequences selected for immunogenicity testing are indicated (see Figure 3, page 334 for testing procedure).*

tion of natural virus vaccines requires the obtaining of the virus from human or animal sources, the maintenance of the virus in tissue culture, and the various procedures that attenuate or inactivate. Obviously, this is far more costly than simple synthesis.

Having cited some advantages of synthetic vaccines, along with the rationale for developing them, let's turn now to the question of what a synthetic virus vaccine is and how one might make it (see Figure 1, page 332). The approach we have taken demands first knowledge of

the DNA sequence of the virus. Such sequences are now known for many viruses, and DNA sequencing of viruses is proceeding very rapidly in many laboratories. With the knowledge of the DNA sequence of the four bases, or nucleotides—adenine, thymine, guanine, and cytosine (A, T, G, and C, respectively)—one can, of course, deduce the amino acids being transcribed from the triplet combinations of the genetic code—e.g., TTG is the triplet codon for leucine, AGC for serine, GAC for aspartic acid, etc. Moreover, we are now able to recognize those

segments of a DNA strand that are likely to function as actual genes. It has been observed that in DNA there is a stop codon (a triplet, such as TAG, that directs the transcribing machinery to stop) at about every 21 1/3 triplets, or at about every 64 bases. However, within the DNA one will also find so-called open reading frames, in which no stop codons are found over a stretch much longer than the 21 1/3 triplets. We now know that when an open reading frame extends to about 500 bases, it can be predictively assumed to contain a gene

Figure 3

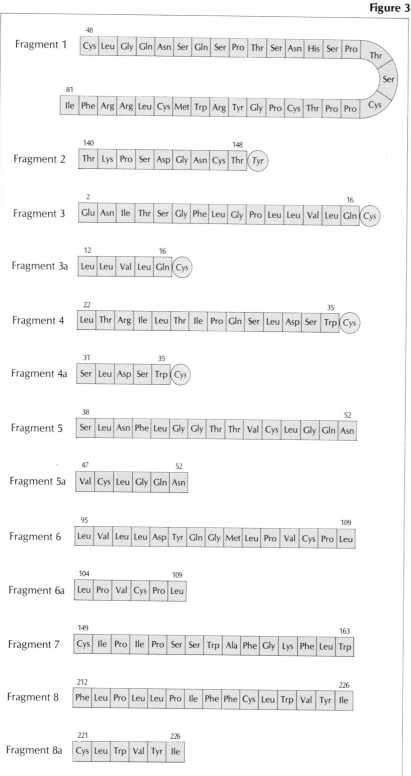

Fragment 1 — 48: Cys Leu Gly Gln Asn Ser Gln Ser Pro Thr Ser Asn His Ser Pro Thr Ser Cys
81: Ile Phe Arg Arg Leu Cys Met Trp Arg Tyr Gly Pro Cys Thr Pro Pro Cys

Fragment 2 — 140: Thr Lys Pro Ser Asp Gly Asn Cys 148: Thr (Tyr)

Fragment 3 — 2: Glu Asn Ile Thr Ser Gly Phe Leu Gly Pro Leu Leu Val Leu Gln 16: (Cys)

Fragment 3a — 12: Leu Leu Val Leu 16: Gln (Cys)

Fragment 4 — 22: Leu Thr Arg Ile Leu Thr Ile Pro Gln Ser Leu Asp Ser Trp 35: (Cys)

Fragment 4a — 31: Ser Leu Asp Ser Trp 35: (Cys)

Fragment 5 — 38: Ser Leu Asn Phe Leu Gly Gly Thr Thr Val Cys Leu Gly Gln 52: Asn

Fragment 5a — 47: Val Cys Leu Gly Gln 52: Asn

Fragment 6 — 95: Leu Val Leu Leu Asp Tyr Gln Gly Met Leu Pro Val Cys Pro 109: Leu

Fragment 6a — 104: Leu Pro Val Cys Pro 109: Leu

Fragment 7 — 149: Cys Ile Pro Ile Pro Ser Ser Trp Ala Phe Gly Lys Phe Leu 163: Trp

Fragment 8 — 212: Phe Leu Pro Leu Leu Pro Ile Phe Phe Cys Leu Trp Val Tyr 226: Ile

Fragment 8a — 221: Cys Leu Trp Val Tyr 226: Ile

As depicted above, 13 linear amino acid sequences were selected and synthesized for use as immunogens. The antibody titers elicited both against themselves and against native hepatitis B virus envelope are shown in Table 1. Note that in a number of peptides either cystine or tyrosine was added to the natural sequence to facilitate bonding to the carrier protein, KLH, or radioiodination. (Figure and table adapted from Lerner et al, Proc Natl Acad Sci 78:3405, 1981.)

coding for a protein.

With the DNA base sequence of the gene obtained, the next step is to deduce the primary structure of the protein that is the gene product. And, as has been noted, this is done by the straightforward use of the genetic triplet code. In this way the amino acid sequence of the protein can be set down, and one can then begin to work out the problem of determining the best candidate immunogens. Enough is known about protein structure so that we can establish criteria. We know, of course, that we are interested in peptides that reside on the surface of the virus; therefore, we focus on the hydrophilic amino acids. We also know from bonding characteristics and relationships to the amino and carboxyl terminals what the folding characteristics, and therefore the three-dimensional character, of the peptide chain will be; again, this knowledge bears on the objective of making sure that the peptides we synthesize relate to the viral structures that present to the circulation and function as immunologic determinants.

Keeping these principles in mind, we can now review their application to the synthesis of one of the four viruses cited earlier, hepatitis B. The DNA base sequence of the hepatitis B surface antigens (HB_sAg) gene had been worked out by investigators at Harvard, at the University of California, San Francisco, and at the Hôpital Saint-Louis, Paris. The 226–amino acid sequence of the HB_sAg polypeptide had been deduced by M. Pasek et al at Harvard, as shown in Figure 2, page 333. This polypeptide is particularly challenging not only because of its size but because it is extremely hydrophobic, and as noted above, to synthesize a vaccine one needs a hydrophilic and, therefore, soluble peptide sequence. However, from a medical point of view, the importance of hepatitis B is obvious, and from an investigational point of view, we were able to operate from the premise that techniques and concepts derived from vaccine-synthesis work with such a "hostile" virus could be expected to have general application.

A study of the molecule reveals certain relevant characteristics. In general, it can be divided into five regions, or domains. Three are extremely hydrophobic—one each near the amino and carboxyl terminals and one occupying a large part of the chain between residues 80 and 110. This last is flanked by the two relatively hydrophilic regions, residues 45 to 80 and 110 to 150. One can also note that the cysteines are largely clustered in the two hydrophilic domains (suggesting that these are the sites of disulfide bonding) and that the molecule is rich in proline peptides. One of the basic tenets of protein structure is that peptide chains will bend at prolines.

We selected 13 peptide fragments for chemical synthesis. These fragments in position on the whole polypeptide chain are depicted in Figure 3, page 334, along with the code numbers assigned to them (1 to 8 and 3a to 8a). In this selection we chose a number of peptides from the more hydrophilic or soluble portions of the chain, as well as peptides containing cysteine to facilitate coupling to a carrier protein (in some cases we added a cysteine or a tyrosine to the C terminal, where none was predicted by the nucleotide codons). Peptides corresponding to the portions of the chain nearest to the amino and carboxyl terminals were also used because of previous experiments showing that these locations provided a high probability of immunogenicity. Finally, we chose sequences encompassing proline-containing junctions between hydrophilic and hydrophobic domains because we believed these to be sites at which the molecule might be expected to turn and expose "corners."

After making these choices, we proceeded to synthesize the peptide fragments, using Merrifield synthetic techniques and amino acids obtained from commercial sources. The process is, of course, automated; more important, it has the advantage of utilizing reagents (the amino acids) that have no history of contact with the viruses against

which the resulting vaccines are intended to provide protection.

The synthetic peptides were then injected into rabbits, and antibody responses were assayed by the ELISA system. The column headed "Peptide" in Table 1, below, shows the response to the various radioiodinated fragments. Seven of the 11 tested peptides (two proved insoluble and were not tested) demonstrated some degree of immunogenicity when coupled with a carrier protein (keyhole limpet hemocyanin, or KLH). One other showed only marginal immunogenicity (peptide 2); on the other hand, there was a good antibody response to peptide 1 even without coupling to a carrier. It should be noted parenthetically that the immunizations were done with complete Freund's adjuvant, a problem that will be discussed later.

The next set of experiments were in a very real sense designed to test what may be fairly described as the most crucial question in synthetic vaccine research and development: Will antibody to the individual peptides recognize the whole virus?

To determine whether the antibodies to the individual peptides would react with the HB$_s$Ag, we tested the antibodies' ability to immunoprecipitate the intact radioiodinated surface antigen derived from hepatitis B Dane particles. Antibodies to a number of the peptides did in fact react with the HB$_s$Ag, as can be seen from the data presented in the last two columns of Table 1.

Obviously, in a study as complex as this one, there are many technical considerations of importance mainly to workers in the field. How-

Table 1. Reactivity of Antipeptide Sera

| Peptide | Antibody Titer | | | |
| | Versus Peptide | | Versus Viral Envelope | |
	4 weeks	15 weeks	4 weeks	15 weeks
1*	6.4	8.4	8.3	13.4
1*	8.6	7.6	28.0	52.0
1†	3.7	—	1.0	—
2	2.1	1.3	2.4	1.0
2	2.7	1.7	1.1	0.9
3	1.6	20.0	2.0	5.8
3	5.2	15.8	14.0	36.0
3a	Insoluble			
4	7.9	7.5	32.5	92.0
4	4.8	6.1	7.2	71.0
4a	1.0	—	1.0	—
4a	1.0	—	1.0	—
5	8.5	—	1.0	—
5	5.9	—	1.0	—
5a	5.3	—	1.0	—
5a	5.8	—	1.0	—
6	51.0	85.0	75.6	113.0
6	17.7	83.0	9.5	37.0
6a	12.3	—	1.0	—
6a	11.0	25.0	1.0	1.0
7	Insoluble			
8	1.0	—	1.0	—
8	1.0	—	1.0	—
8a	1.0	—	1.0	—
8a	1.0	—	1.0	—

*Injected at pH 5.3
†Injected at pH 8.5
Antibody titer is expressed as radioactivity (cpm) precipitated by test serum divided by radioactivity precipitated by normal serum.

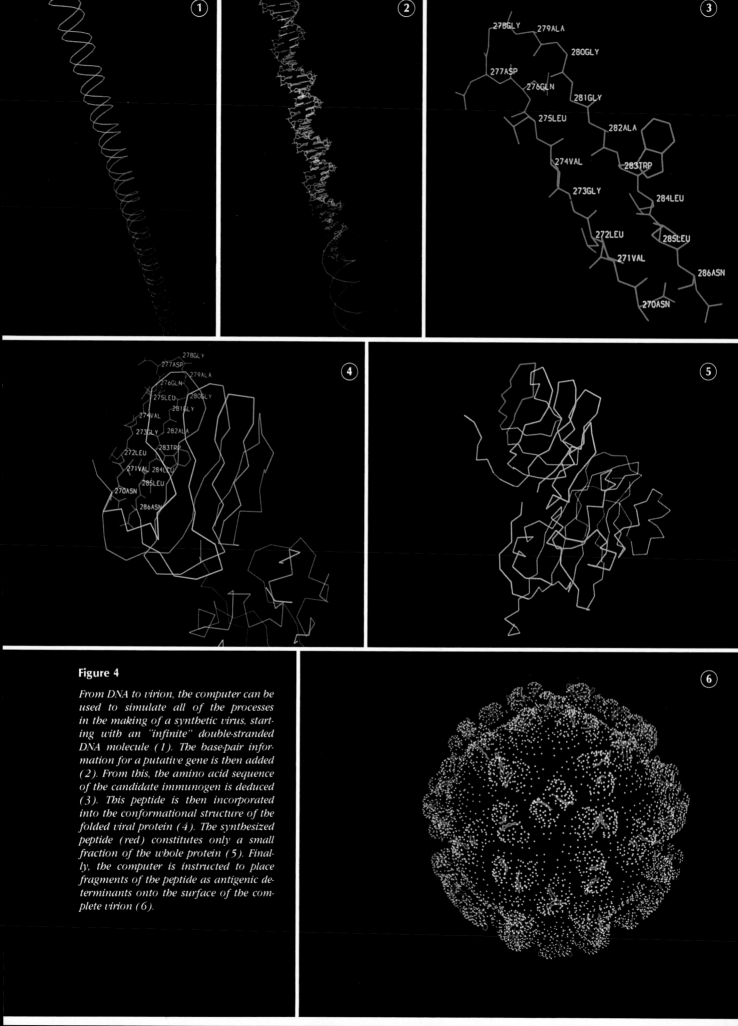

Figure 4

From DNA to virion, the computer can be used to simulate all of the processes in the making of a synthetic virus, starting with an "infinite" double-stranded DNA molecule (1). The base-pair information for a putative gene is then added (2). From this, the amino acid sequence of the candidate immunogen is deduced (3). This peptide is then incorporated into the conformational structure of the folded viral protein (4). The synthesized peptide (red) constitutes only a small fraction of the whole protein (5). Finally, the computer is instructed to place fragments of the peptide as antigenic determinants onto the surface of the complete virion (6).

ever, for the purposes of this review, certain generalizations are noteworthy. Clearly demonstrated is that one can take a given nucleotide sequence, decode it, and thereby derive the instruction necessary to synthesize polypeptides from various domains of the molecule. Some of these polypeptides will elicit antibody capable of recognizing and reacting to the native molecule. To immunologists, this has been perhaps the most surprising aspect of synthetic vaccine research. Prior to such demonstrations as the one described, few would have predicted such an outcome. It would have been reasonably argued that conformational characteristics of the native molecule were so vital to immunologic recognition that amino acid homology would be insufficient for recognition of the native molecule, unless it was also accompanied by extensive analogy in the tertiary molecular structure. We have found that whatever conformational analogy can be encompassed in a peptide chain as short as six amino acids is sufficient for the vital recognition function, provided that the synthetic peptide is soluble. It is also probably helpful if a proline is present. As previously noted, this last requirement appears consistent with the known presence of prolines in molecular structural turns.

This study can be viewed in the context of the HB_sAg studies by G. N. Vyas and colleagues at the University of California, San Francisco. Their studies suggested that the antigenicity of hepatitis B virus was completely abolished when its disulfide bonds were disrupted. It seems highly plausible to conclude that when a short linear sequence of peptides remains a part of a large denatured molecule, it will not elicit antibodies against the native molecule. However, when the same sequence is liberated from the constraints of the native molecule, it will be an effective immunogenic surrogate for the native molecule.

This interpretation finds theoretical support in the concepts advanced by D. H. Sachs and colleagues at the NIH, who have pro-

posed that a peptide in solution exists in a state of equilibrium among all possible conformations. When one injects the peptide into an intact animal, the recipient's immunologic recognition system will be presented with this full range of conformational possibilities and responds to a variety including that which corresponds to the conformation taken by the peptide sequence in the native molecule.

An important correlate of this theoretical construction bears on the clinical safety of synthetic vaccines. It should be noted that despite the lack of conformational requirements in synthesizing a short polypeptide, the antibodies to which can recognize a whole virus, conformation remains an essential restrictor of immunologic reactivity. The effective immunogen may be the peptide that "happens" to assume the conformation of its homologous amino acids on the surface of the virus. On the other hand, should the amino acids also assume the conformation of a homologous sequence in a host organ or structure, it would be prevented from autoreaction by all of the normal immunologic defenses against reactions to self.

It should be emphasized that the description of the work in hepatitis B presented in this article constitutes a review of experimentation designed to answer conceptual questions rather than an overview of the approach to making a synthetic vaccine. However, such an overview is presented in Figure 4, page 336. This figure is the product of the application of computer technology to the concept of predicting amino acid sequences from DNA nucleotide sequences, then "locating" the peptide structure on the complete protein, and finally selecting the candidate sequences most likely to be capable of recognizing the native virus.

Obviously, once this recognition function has been documented, it is still necessary to demonstrate that with this recognition goes protection. There is good preliminary evidence that synthetic vaccines do protect against influenza, and some

of this work in our laboratory has been submitted for publication. It should be pointed out, however, that we have not yet demonstrated protective antibody for hepatitis B simply because we lack a good animal model in which to do immunization experiments. We are now entering into a cooperative experiment with the National Institute of Allergy and Infectious Diseases, in which chimpanzees at the colony maintained at the NIAID will be immunized. Since chimps do get hepatitis, the protective value of the synthetic peptides can be tested in them, and of course, the biological resemblance of the animals to humans makes these experiments particularly appealing.

To date we have not been able to test the synthetic vaccines against rabies and mouse leukemia virus, largely because the work of preparing immunogenic peptides was only recently done. Nor have we taken this step with hoof-and-mouth disease, in this case because U.S. quarantine regulations pose formidable problems for experimentation.

The success that has been enjoyed in making synthetic small peptides that recognize and react with native virus, in other laboratories as well as ours, leads to confidence that the basic problem has been solved. One can reasonably predict that if synthetic vaccines can be made against a virus as large and complex as hepatitis B, they can be made against most viruses. Obviously, the value of any particular viral vaccine will depend on whether protection against disease is dependent on extracellular humoral antibody. Although we have not talked about the use of the synthetic approach to bacterial diseases, there is no reason to believe that synthetic bacterial vaccines are not equally feasible. This optimism is reinforced by the tremendous body of knowledge that bacterial geneticists have amassed about the bacterial genome.

However, to avoid giving the impression that the clinical testing and subsequent availability of synthetic vaccines are just around the corner, it would be well to take cognizance of some of the major technical problems that still require complete solution.

There are, in fact, two such problems that merit discussion. The first, and probably the one that is closer to solution, is the requirement of a carrier coupled to the synthetic immunogen. It will be recalled that we employed KLH in the experiments described. This is, of course, a very large protein molecule, so that its use to some extent defeats the purpose of using a minimal amount of protein material for immunization. However, we have identified some linear amino acid sequences that do not seem to require carriers to remain immunogenic, which are somewhat larger than the smallest effective peptides. Indeed, we have now taken such an amino acid chain (limited to seven residues) and, by extending it on either side to a total of 29 amino acids, obviated the need for a carrier. This maneuver adds somewhat to the cost of synthesis, but with currently available automated machinery, the difference is not prohibitive.

Perhaps even more promising is the approach taken by M. Sela and R. Arnon in Israel, who have synthesized not only the immunogen but also small peptide carriers—actually, amino acid copolymers, such as D-alanine. It seems likely that this will be the direction taken in solving the problems related to providing carrier molecules for synthetic vaccines.

The more formidable problem is that of adjuvant. Basic immunologic dogma is that the more potent the adjuvant, the more immunogenic the specific antigen. It was for this reason that complete Freund's adjuvant (CFA) was employed in our experiments. Obviously, however, CFA could never be employed in a vaccine designed for clinical use because it is far too toxic and far too strong as a nonspecific potentiator of a wide variety of host immunologic responses. A number of investigators are experimenting with less potent preparations, including the traditional pertussis. However, it is yet to be demonstrated that these preparations have adequate adjuvant potency to ensure sufficient immunogenicity of the synthetic vaccines.

There are some other questions that remain to be answered before we can contemplate use of synthetic vaccines in humans. An obvious one in the case of a nonreplicating material is duration of protection, which only time and further experimentation will answer. But for the present it seems justified to conclude that the most basic questions about small-polypeptide synthetic vaccines have been answered. For any virus (or bacterium) that can be neutralized by soluble circulating antibodies, we should be able to make synthetic vaccines derived from a wide variety of amino acid sequences on the surface of the pathogen, and these vaccines should be capable of recognizing the entire pathogenic molecule. These synthetic vaccines have the potential of providing us with medically ideal agents, those that constitute "perturbations that are totally known."

Therapeutic Uses of Immune Suppression and Enhancement

ROBERT S. SCHWARTZ   *Tufts University*

Manipulation of the immune system has become a cornerstone of therapy in a number of disease states. Immunosuppression is essential for the maintenance of organ transplants and is being used increasingly in the treatment of autoimmune diseases. Immune enhancement is undergoing clinical trials as an adjunctive therapy in the management of cancer and also is being recommended for the treatment of autoimmune diseases. In this context, this chapter will discuss both current methods for inducing immune suppression or immune enhancement and some of the problems associated with manipulating the immune system.

The standard immunosuppressive regimen for organ and tissue graft recipients includes prednisone and azathioprine. Cyclophosphamide also has been used in combination with corticosteroids, but its effects are more difficult to control, and it is more toxic than azathioprine in transplant recipients. When prednisone and azathioprine are used, graft survival of at least one year is achieved in a substantial proportion of cases. For HLA-identical kidney grafts, the one-year survival is about 95% and the two-year survival is about 88%. Grafts from living related donors mismatched for one or more HLA haplotypes have a two-year survival of 80%, and cadaver grafts have a two-year survival of 60% to 75%, depending on the closeness of HLA matching. A one-year survival rate of 67% has been reported for cardiac transplant recipients by Norman Shumway and his colleagues at Stanford.

In addition to the "standard" drugs, other agents are being used experimentally in the effort to make immunosuppression more effective and less toxic in the transplant patient. One such new drug, cyclosporin A (CyA), a cyclic polypeptide derived from two species of fungus, is a potent immunosuppressant. CyA blocks the receptor for a growth factor, interleukin-2, which is necessary for the proliferation of T lymphocytes. The action of the drug appears to be selective for certain subsets of T cells. Recently, N. L. Tilney at Brigham and Women's Hospital, Boston, reported that CyA acts primarily on helper T lymphocytes and spares suppressor T-cell function. This effect could be desirable because suppressor T cells modulate the residual immune response of the immunosuppressed allografted patient (see Figure 1, pages 340, 341).

CyA is currently undergoing clinical trials in several transplantation centers, and the initial reports of its efficacy are encouraging. However, a number of cases of immunoblastic sarcoma have been reported in patients treated with CyA. We shall return to this problem later.

Preparations of antilymphocyte serum (ALS) or antithymocyte globulin (ATG) have been used for more than a decade in renal transplantation. A commercial preparation of equine antithymocyte globulin has been undergoing clinical tests in kidney transplant recipients for more than eight years and is now being tried in cardiac and bone marrow transplant recipients. One-year graft survival in recipients of cadaver renal transplants treated with ATG has been about 70%. ATG therapy is usually combined with the standard azathioprine-prednisone regimen. R. H. Rubin and associates at Harvard were able to reduce the dosage of these drugs by 50% when they were given in combination with ATG, without impairing the one-year survival rate or increasing the risk of cytomegalovirus infections, in a controlled trial in kidney transplant recipients.

Immunosuppression by irradiation of all lymphoid

Figure 1

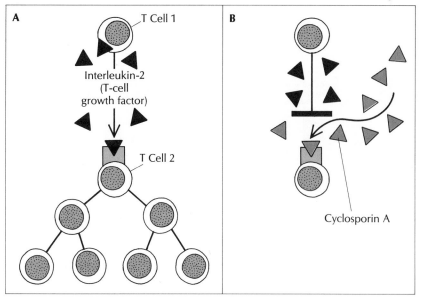

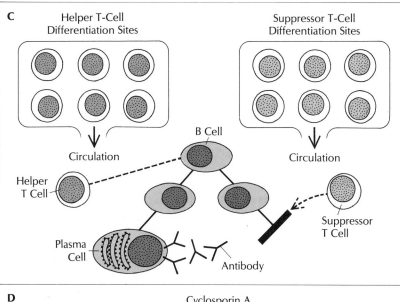

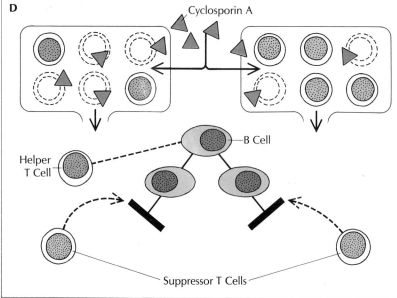

Although the mechanisms by which various immunosuppressive agents and modalities work are still not fully understood, the assumption is that they either impair the proliferation of antigen-stimulated immunocompetent cells or modulate other immunologic effectors. The schemes on the left diagram two possible modes of action for the new cyclic polypeptide immunosuppressant, cyclosporin A (CyA). As shown in panel A, there are two populations of T lymphocytes. The first, represented as T cell 1, secretes a soluble growth factor, interleukin-2, that stimulates proliferation of a second T cell, which, it is postulated, has specific receptors for interleukin-2. CyA's hypothesized action (B) is blockade of the interleukin receptor with consequent abortion of T-cell proliferation. Alternatively, or additionally, it has been suggested that CyA is more active in the physiologic sites of helper T-cell differentiation than in those of suppressor T-cell differentiation (C), thus tipping the balance between helper induction of antibody secretion and suppressor modulation in favor of latter (D). Panel E (right) postulates the mode of action of irradiation and cytotoxic drugs (e.g., cyclophosphamide) on the basis of their activity against dividing cells. A key point is that the suppressor T cell is relatively resistant to irradiation and cytotoxic drugs, possibly because these immunosuppressants are most potent against dividing cells.

tissues is a new application of total lymphoid irradiation (TLI), a technique developed by Henry Kaplan at Stanford for the treatment of Hodgkin's disease more than 15 years ago. In patients with Hodgkin's disease who received a total of 4400 rad to lymphoid tissues—including cervical, axillary, mediastinal, para-aortic, iliac, and inguinal nodes as well as the thymus and the spleen (if they had not been removed surgically)—TLI produced marked T lymphocytopenia. These effects lasted for as long as 10 years in patients who had no recurrence of the disease.

The problems of malignancy and opportunistic infection that can occur with immunosuppressive chemotherapy are uncommon with TLI, despite the intense and prolonged immunosuppression.

Samuel Strober at Stanford has investigated TLI as a means of inducing immunosuppression prior

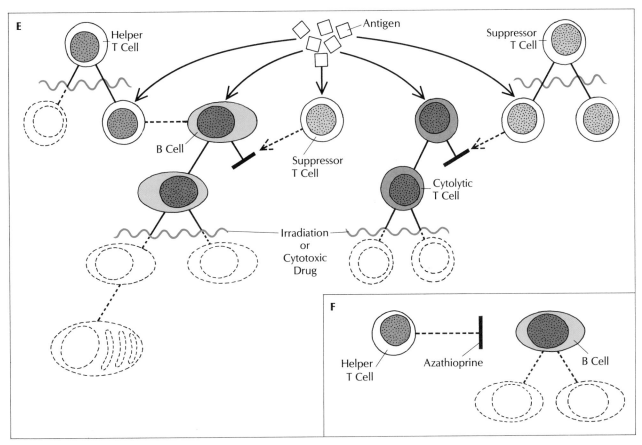

Finally, there is evidence that the drug azathioprine acts by interference with the induction stage of antibody response, here depicted as inhibition of helper T–B cell interaction (F). It should also be noted that azathioprine, like prednisone and other corticosteroids, also exerts some of its effects through its anti-inflammatory properties.

to organ grafting (see "Managing the Immune System with Total Lymphoid Irradiation"). In their experiments on allogeneic bone marrow transplantation in mice, rats, and mongrel dogs, Strober's group was able to induce, by TLI, tolerance and blood and bone marrow chimerism without evidence of graft-versus-host disease. Evidence from these experiments suggested that antigen-specific suppressor T cells were generated after TLI and allografting.

There is interest now in applying the technique to human kidney, bone marrow, and cardiac transplants. John Najarian at the University of Minnesota has used TLI in 17 patients who received second or third kidney grafts after prior grafts had been rejected. The patients were given steroids after transplantation, and two years later all except two were alive with functioning grafts; the two patients died

of unrelated causes. Despite this success, a logistic problem with TLI must be overcome. The irradiation regimen may take six weeks to complete, and organ transplantation should be done immediately upon its completion. When cadaver organs are transplanted, however, the unpredictable availability of a suitable organ renders such precise timing difficult. But if TLI is really as effective as early reports indicate, new means of storing cadaver kidneys could solve this problem.

Prolonged immunosuppression in transplant recipients has two major complications: an increased susceptibility to infection and an increased risk of cancer. Cytomegalovirus infection is commonly associated with immunosuppression. Rubin has reported that between 60% and 96% of renal transplant recipients demonstrate laboratory or clinical evidence of cytomegalovirus infection within the first year after trans-

plantation. Cytomegalovirus infection causes febrile episodes; predisposes to potentially lethal superinfection with viral, fungal, and bacterial organisms; and may contribute to graft dysfunction. Other common causes of infections in immunosuppressed transplant recipients are herpes zoster and *Pneumocystis carinii*.

The incidence of tumors in renal allograft recipients ranges from 5% to 20%. Cancers of the skin and lymphomas are the types most frequently associated with organ transplantation. Israel Penn of the Veterans Administration Medical Center, Denver, reported that the incidence of de novo tumors in renal and cardiac transplant recipients is approximately 100 times greater than that in the general population in the same age range. (see Table 1, page 343). The incidence rises with years elapsed after the transplant. A. G. R. Sheil at the

University of Sydney, Australia, found an incidence of 11% in renal transplant recipients at one year and 24% at five years. Among recipients of cardiac transplants at Stanford, the incidence of de novo tumors was 3% at one year and 25% at five years.

Sheil reviewed the cases of 389 cadaver-donor renal transplant recipients who survived for at least one year with a functioning graft and who were followed for periods of one to 10 years. Cancer developed in 76, or 20%. The majority of these 76 neoplasms (61) were skin cancers. The second most frequent malignancies were lymphomas in seven patients, followed by adenocarcinomas in six patients. Penn reported on 693 cases of malignancy in transplant recipients; the most common (after various skin cancers) were lymphomas (which occurred in 150).

The tumors that are most common in the general population—cancers of the colon and rectum, lung, and breast—occur infrequently in transplant recipients. Penn observed that their relative scarcity in transplant patients may be related to the young average age (40 years) of these patients at the time of transplant.

Skin cancers have different characteristics in transplant patients than in the general population. Squamous cell carcinomas are more common, and multiple tumors occur at twice the usual rate, in immunosuppressed graft recipients. Transplant recipients are, on the average, 30 years younger when they develop skin cancer than are persons in the general population. Most skin cancers in transplant recipients are of low-grade malignancy, but in Penn's series of 277 transplant patients who developed skin cancers, metastatic disease caused 14 deaths —eight from metastatic squamous cell carcinoma and six from melanoma. In Sheil's series, 15 of 61 patients with skin tumors had basal cell carcinoma, which was cured in all cases by local treatment, and the rest (six of whom died of the malignancy) had squamous cell carcinoma alone or in association with

basal cell carcinoma.

Another peculiarity of malignancy in transplant recipients is the short time interval between transplantation and appearance of the tumor. In renal transplant and cardiac transplant recipients who developed lymphoma, the tumors were diagnosed an average of 27 and 20 months after transplantation, respectively.

The incidence of lymphomas, especially those of the central nervous system, is disproportionately increased in transplant recipients. Lymphoma involving primarily the central nervous system is found in less than 2% of persons who develop lymphoma and who are not transplant recipients. According to Penn, of 150 kidney transplant recipients who developed lymphoma (excluding 21 with Kaposi's sarcoma), 57 had CNS lymphoma. These figures were paralleled on a much smaller scale by J. L. Anderson of Stanford, who reported the occurrence of three CNS lymphomas in seven cardiac transplant recipients who developed lymphoma.

Immunosuppressive therapy is being used increasingly in the management of immunoinflammatory conditions, including systemic lupus erythematosus, rheumatoid arthritis, Sjögren's syndrome, immune hemolytic anemia and thrombocytopenia, inflammatory bowel diseases, and a number of other nonmalignant disorders. Among 109 patients with one or another of these conditions who were treated with immunosuppressive agents, 24 developed lymphoid tumors, and 28 developed acute myeloblastic leukemia (AML). However, among 94 patients representing the same spectrum of diseases who did *not* receive immunosuppressive therapy, 42 developed lymphomas, and three developed AML. Thus, although the combined incidence of lymphoma and AML was approximately equal in immunosuppressed and nonimmunosuppressed patients, the distribution was distinctly different. With respect to the occurrence of other types of malignancies, the two groups were similar.

In the group treated with immu-

nosuppressives, the most frequent factor associated with the occurrence of AML was treatment with an alkylating agent. Unfortunately, our knowledge of the risk of neoplasms in treated versus nontreated patients with certain immunoinflammatory disease is limited, and it is therefore difficult to know whether immunosuppressive therapy influences the risk one way or another. Several studies indicate that patients with lupus erythematosus have a slightly higher incidence of malignancies than the general population, whether they receive immunosuppressive therapy or not.

In patients with cancer who have received aggressive chemotherapy or combined chemotherapy and radiotherapy (modalities which, of course, are immunosuppressive), certain types of secondary malignancies have an increased frequency. In patients treated for Hodgkin's disease, the risk of developing AML is increased 75-fold over that of the general population; in patients with multiple myeloma, it is increased 100-fold. In patients with ovarian cancer who were treated with an alkylating agent, R. R. Reimer and associates found that the risk of AML was 36 times the expected risk and increased to 170 times in those who survived for two years. Once again, however, it must be pointed out that these comparisons are with a general population, and it is therefore impossible to know whether the increases in AML after treatment with alkylating agents are due to the therapy or to the natural history of the original disease. One possible exception to this dilemma is ovarian cancer. Reimer et al did find that there was no increase in AML risk for ovarian cancer patients treated by standard irradiation methods.

The occurrence of lymphomas after chemotherapy for cancer is infrequent. J. G. Krikorian reported six cases of non-Hodgkin's lymphoma and six cases of AML in 579 patients with Hodgkin's disease treated with combined chemotherapy and radiation therapy. Sporadic case reports of non-Hodgkin's lymphoma occurring in patients treated for Hodgkin's disease have appeared in the literature, but there is not enough evidence to assert that lymphoma is increasing as a secondary tumor in treated Hodgkin's patients.

Several intriguing observations have been made about the lymphomas that arise in immunosuppressed patients. A large proportion (more than 40%) are immunoblastic sarcomas. Among allograft recipients, 70% of lymphomas are of this type, whereas Hodgkin's disease is rare.

Why do so many immunosuppressed patients develop cancers? Certainly, one factor to be considered is the mutagenic effects inherent in many immunosuppressive modalities, including irradiation and cytotoxic drugs. Beyond that, the usual explanation for the susceptibility of immunosuppressed patients to malignancies is that immunosuppression impairs a natural antitumor surveillance mechanism. An alternative explanation for the high incidence of lymphomas in the immunosuppressed patient is imbalanced immunoregulation.

A brief review of the current concepts of the normal immune response will provide a background for considering how malignant lymphoid proliferation could occur in the immunosuppressed patient. These ideas derive from Jerne's hypothesis that the immune system functions as a network of integrated signals. Some signals have a positive effect; that is, they turn on antibody production or cell-mediated immunity. Others have a negative effect and return the system to a resting state. In this scheme, the signals come from antigens and cell surface receptors on lymphocytes and macrophages. The cell surface receptors also serve as recognition units. The recognition units on B cells are immunoglobulins. Those on T cells are not so well defined, but they seem to consist of polypeptide chains that are similar to the heavy chains of the immunoglobulin molecules. Antigens and helper T cells supply the "on" signals, and suppressor T cells and

antibodies provide the "off" signals. Antibodies modulate the response by acting on antigens, suppressor T cells, or B cells. Although some of the evidence and hypotheses in this review suggest that at least one of the off signals—the suppressor T cells—are relatively less affected by immunosuppression, one cannot exclude the possibility that an impairment in the off signals could result in unrestricted B-lymphocyte proliferation, which could give rise to a malignant clone of such cells, e.g., a lymphoma.

It is believed that a disturbance anywhere in the signal network can have a "ripple" effect, causing disturbances in neighboring and even distant lymphoid structures. Evidence that the ripple effect can occur is provided by the observation that experimental hyperimmunization with a specific antigen induces not only specific antibody but large amounts of immunoglobulins that do not bind with the immunizing agent.

A situation in which hyperimmunization, or polyclonal B-cell activation, exists together with an impairment of the off signal might lead to a persistent high-grade lymphoproliferative response that could provide the setting for malignant transformation. This phenomenon has been seen in mice with a chronic graft-versus-host reaction, in which normal histocompatibility antigens drive a benign lymphoproliferative reaction into a malignant lymphoma.

Another element that requires consideration is the role of viruses in the development of lymphomas in immunosuppressed patients. Activation of latent herpes viruses occurs commonly during immunosuppression. Particularly noteworthy is the serologic and immunologic evidence that immunosuppression can activate latent infection with Epstein-Barr virus (EBV). This virus is a polyclonal stimulator of B lymphocytes, and it could thereby contribute to unchecked lymphoproliferation in chronically immunosuppressed patients. Its role in the pathogenesis of Burkitt's lymphoma is well known, but the EBV con-

Table 1. De Novo Malignancies in Organ Allograft Recipients

Type of Neoplasm	Patients	
Cancers of skin and lips	277	
Squamous cell carcinoma		147
Basal cell carcinoma		75
Squamous and basal cell carcinomas		39
Malignant melanoma		10
Unspecified		6
Solid lymphomas	150	
Reticulum cell sarcoma		93
Kaposi's sarcoma		20
Unclassified lymphoma		17
Lymphosarcoma		10
Plasma cell lymphoma		4
Hodgkin's disease		3
Lymphoreticular tumors		2
Histiocytic reticulosis		1
Carcinomas of cervix or uterus	49	
In situ		38
Invasive		7
Unspecified		4
Carcinomas of lung	36	
Head and neck carcinomas	24	
Thyroid		9
Tongue		4
Parotid		3
Floor of mouth		2
Other		6
Carcinomas of colon and rectum	21	
Metastatic carcinomas (primary site unknown)	21	
Carcinomas of breast	18	
Leukemias	17	
Carcinomas of kidney	16	
Carcinomas of urinary bladder	14	
Carcinomas of liver and bile ducts	12	
Miscellaneous cancers	78	
Total	733	

From I Penn: In *Transplantation Today*, vol 5, p 1048, 1979

tribution to the development of lymphomas in transplant recipients remains enigmatic.

In the human allograft recipient, there is a known impairment of immune regulation. The lymphoproliferative response to alloantigens in the graft proceeds unchecked because immunosuppressive therapy interferes with feedback inhibition. However, for lymphomagenesis, an-

Figure 2

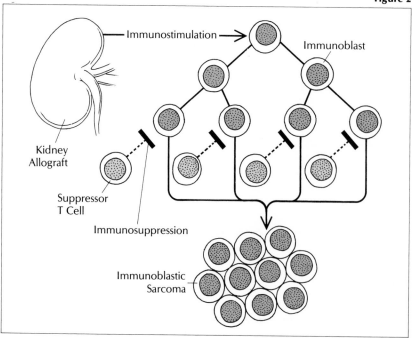

Kidney
Allograft

Immunostimulation

Immunoblast

Suppressor
T Cell

Immunosuppression

Immunoblastic
Sarcoma

A postulated tumorigenic pathway is schematized, starting with the continuous immunostimulation provided by a renal allograft. The consequence suggested is immunoblastic proliferation. Without immunosuppression, the immunoblasts might be held in check by suppressor T cells. If this barrier is deleted or weakened by immunosuppression, the conditions for consolidation into a sarcoma could exist.

other element may be required, such as a genetic predisposition interacting with physical, chemical, or viral factors.

For instance, Anderson et al found that prior cardiomyopathy and age were significant risk factors in the occurrence of lymphoma in cardiac transplant recipients. These investigators had noted previously that a defect in mononuclear suppressor cell activity was present in all patients with idiopathic cardiomyopathy but in none with coronary artery disease or in healthy controls. Lymphoma developed in seven of 37 transplant recipients who had cardiac grafts because of idiopathic cardiomyopathy and in none of 61 who had prior coronary artery or other cardiac disease. In addition, they noted that lymphoma occurred only in patients under 40 years of age. The mean age of all patients with antecedent cardiomyopathy was 37.0 years (range, 14 to 53 years), but the average age of those who developed lymphoma was 25.8 years (range, 14 to 39 years). Age, therefore, appeared to be a significant risk factor in these patients.

On the basis of these findings, they postulated a two-event model of oncogenesis. First, reduced suppressor lymphocyte activity in young (less than 40 years of age) allograft recipients with cardiomyopathy may permit abnormal lymphoid proliferation in response to the constant alloantigen stimulation associated with transplantation. The administration of a chemical agent, such as azathioprine, to prevent graft rejection may then have an additional effect in promoting malignant transformation (see Figure 2 on this page).

A positive correlation between the antecedent cause of renal failure and the subsequent risk of lymphoma in kidney transplant recipients has not been demonstrated, except possibly in the context of polycystic kidney disease. However, uremia is known to have an immunosuppressive effect that involves cell-mediated immunity in particular.

Three cases of fatal immunoblastic lymphoproliferation reported by M. S. Borzy et al are of interest because defective suppressor cell activity, similar to that described by Anderson, was demonstrated in all three. The patients were children with combined immunodeficiency who had received transplants of cultured thymus cells. A lack of concanavalin A-induced suppressor cell activity was demonstrated in all three before transplantation and in two of the three afterward.

Returning briefly to the immunoinflammatory diseases, it is noteworthy that the production of autoantibodies is a major feature of these diseases. A still unresolved question is whether autoantibody production is due to intrinsically abnormal B lymphocytes or is secondary to defects in regulatory circuits, especially those that involve suppressor cell function. There is considerable evidence in support of both points of view, and indeed, either may be operative, depending on circumstances. A defect in suppressor T-cell function is known to occur in systemic lupus erythematosus. We recently demonstrated that a concanavalin A-induced suppressor cell defect is present also in healthy relatives of patients with systemic lupus erythematosus. Why some individuals with this immunoregulatory defect develop overt disease and others do not is unclear.

When we turn from immunosuppression to immune enhancement, we move from reasonably solid ground to a much shakier area. "Enhancing" immunotherapy has been tried in the management of cancer and in the treatment of various autoimmune diseases. Its use in cancer is based on the assumption that cancer cells bear antigens potentially recognizable by the patient's immune system and that enhancing the immune response will enable the patient to destroy the tumor cells.

Among agents that have been used to activate or boost the immune system are BCG, *Corynebacterium parvum*, levamisole, and interferon. Passive immunotherapy has been attempted with infusions of autologous serum and leukocytes, normal human immune globulin, and blood or plasma from patients in whom a tumor has regressed spontaneously. Adoptive immunotherapy has been tried using normal allogeneic spleen cells; blood lymphocytes, thoracic duct lymphocytes, or blood lymphocytes from other cancer patients immunized against the patient's tumor; the patient's own lymphocytes stimulated in vitro nonspecifically with phytohemagglutinin or specifically with tumor cells; lymphocytes from pigs immunized with tumor fragments; or transfer factor and RNA from the lymphoid tissue of sheep immunized against the patient's tumor.

In general, the initial reports of trials of such immunotherapy have indicated some degree of effectiveness, but follow-up studies have been disappointing. Although many clinical trials are still in progress and the results unknown, no significant benefit has yet been achieved.

An interesting new approach to immune enhancement involves protein A, a substance produced by certain strains of *Staphylococcus aureus*, which binds avidly to the Fc portion of IgG. D. S. Terman and his colleagues at Baylor University have shown in preclinical trials in dogs with mammary carcinoma that cytotoxic activity appears in plasma that has been perfused over protein A that is attached to a solid surface. The procedure has resulted in rapid necrosis of tumor nodules. The cytotoxic activity is specific for tumor cells and appears only in treated plasma from tumor-bearing individuals. Presumably, the protein-

A treatment unblocks cytotoxic antitumor antibodies in the plasma, but this interpretation of the phenomenon remains unproved. In no case studied has the cancer regressed completely, and side effects of the technique have included hypotension and pulmonary insufficiency. Nevertheless, these early results with a novel approach to cancer therapy are promising enough to merit further intensive investigation.

As mentioned, attempts to direct the cancer patient's immune system against his own tumor cells are based on the assumptions that malignant cells bear antigens that are recognizable as such by the patient's immune system (i.e., they are autoantigenic), that these antigens can stimulate an effector humoral or cellular response, and that they can serve as a site for antibody-mediated or cell-mediated damage to the tumor cell. There is evidence that malignant cells possess such autoantigens. The development of hybridoma technology, which has made it possible to produce monoclonal antibodies against specific cell surface antigens, has made available a new approach to this problem (see M. D. Scharff, S. Roberts, P. Thammana, "Hybridomas As a Source of Antibodies"). It may be possible to produce antibodies against any antigen that is expressed in greater concentration on tumor cells than on nontumor cells. Such antibodies could be used to identify tumor cells specifically—something that is not possible now. For instance, tumor antigen–specif-

ic monoclonal antibodies could be labeled with radioactive or other substances that would render tumor cells "visible" by an appropriate diagnostic technique when the monoclonal antibodies reacted with the tumor antigen. Similarly, it may be possible to attach radiosensitive or toxic agents to tumor antigen-specific monoclonal antibodies, thus making the tumor cells more vulnerable than normal cells to irradiation or cytotoxic drugs.

As our understanding of the immune system has expanded, so has our appreciation of its complexity. The current view of the immune system as a network of highly specialized cells that function through a constant exchange of signals implies that successful manipulation of the "on" and "off" signals calls for more precise clinical approaches than have been used to date. In the area of immunosuppression, the newer treatments discussed previously (notably, CyA and total lymphoid irradiation) show promise as agents that affect specific cell-mediated and antibody functions.

In the future, even greater specificity may be achieved by applications of such molecular manipulations as hybridoma-antibody production and HLA-D gene cloning. Most attempts to amplify the immune response so far have been nonspecific; that is, they have simply been attempts to augment the general immune response of the patient. The ability to produce monoclonal antibodies against any antigen offers the potential for developing more logical approaches to immunoenhancement.

Immunologic Aspects Of Transplantation

JOHN S. NAJARIAN   *University of Minnesota*

It is scarcely more than a quarter century ago that the first tentative clinical organ-grafting experiments were performed. In the ensuing years, the surgical specialty of organ transplantation has progressed from a novelty limited to a very few pioneers grafting kidneys between identical twins to a mature and scientific technology applied at virtually every major medical center. Practitioners can now do allografts, with reasonable anticipation of success, not only of the kidney but also of the heart, liver, pancreas, lung, and—en bloc—heart and lung. Several thousand transplantations are performed annually in the United States, and of course, the procedures are by no means limited to this country.

In some measure, this progress can be attributed to the development of appropriate surgical techniques. Without question, however, most gains have been achieved by our ever-increasing ability to control and blunt what has been from the beginning the major impediment to individual-to-individual organ transplantation: immunologic rejection.

This will be the focus of my article, which will be concerned with approaches to donor selection—particularly as related to histocompatibility matching—and with the sequential improvement in methods of immunosuppression. Note will be taken of such adjunctive approaches to enhancing the chances of graft acceptance and survival as splenectomy, transfusion, and high-dose irradiation. For the most part, the discussion will be centered on renal transplantation, both because this is where most of our experience has been obtained and because one can readily extrapolate from the kidney to the other transplantable organs.

Omitted from this discussion will be bone marrow transplantation, because its problems are somewhat unique and are discussed elsewhere in this volume (see R. A. Good, "Immunologic Reconstitution: Achievements and Potentials"). Also omitted are corneal transplantation, because such grafts are essentially nonvascularized and therefore have little exposure to host immunologic responses, and skin allografts, because they are used almost exclusively as temporary biologic dressings, so that concerns about long-term survival are minimal.

Our experience with kidney transplants in which the donor is a living sibling of the recipient indicates that the probability of functioning graft survival for at least five years, and perhaps for 10 years or more, is between 90% and 95%. Even without such closeness of genetic relationship, such long-term transplant survival can be achieved in well over 70% of cases. Unquestionably, the keystone of such success rates is the ability to select the most appropriate kidney donor by matching the donor and the recipient at the major histocompatibility complex, which is designated in humans as HLA (see J. G. Schaller and J. A. Hansen, "HLA Relationships to Disease").

The HLA gene complex is located on the sixth chromosome. It contains alleles coding for a myriad of immunologic and immunologically related molecules, among them the so-called immune response genes and a variety of genes involved in cell-cell interactions. In the context of transplantation immunology, we currently classify HLA antigens into two groups: class I and class II. This differentiation is biochemical, and the numbering is based on the historical sequence of

Figure 1

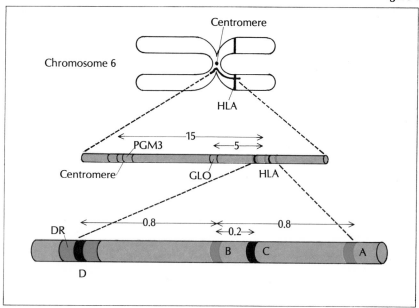

The location of the HLA major histocompatibility complex on the short arm of human chromosome 6 is mapped at the top of the figure. The first blowup (middle) relates HLA to other genes and gene complexes on the chromosomal arm. A closer-in "view" (bottom) shows specific HLA loci, with those that are serologically detected depicted in red. HLA-A and HLA-B are routinely used in transplantation matching.

their characterization rather than on their significance. Thus, those antigens coded at the A, B, and C loci of the HLA (see Figure 1 above) are class I, and those coded at the D locus, class II. Until recently, antigens that were products of genes at a fifth locus, the DR (or D-related), were believed also to be class II, but newer evidence strongly suggests that they are class I. (Figure 2 on the opposite page depicts the structural differences between class I and class II antigens.)

From the point of view of the clinical transplanter, host-recipient matching is dependent on the ability to identify two pairs of class I antigens serologically: those coded for at the A and B loci. Indeed, when one has a sibling donor who is matched with the recipient at both the HLA-A and HLA-B loci, one is virtually assured of long-term graft survival; with appropriate immunosuppression, the chances of 10-year survival are, conservatively, above the 90% level. Unfortunately, one cannot attribute the same success rates of graft survival to situations in which the

relationship between donor and recipient is not that of siblings. If one has an unrelated donor who serologically appears to be perfectly matched with the recipient for both HLA-A and HLA-B, the chances of avoiding rejection of a transplanted kidney are only in the range of 60% to 70%. The crucial question is, Where has the 20% or 30% been lost?

The best answer that can be given is that when brothers or sisters share a common heritage of HLA-A and HLA-B antigens from one of their parents, they are likely to have inherited most or all of the genes in between these two loci. When unrelated individuals seem to be identical at the A and B loci, they very likely have many genes in between that are not identical. The fact that we cannot identify these genes serologically—that we do not have defined antibodies against these genes and their products— does not preclude the presence of antigens that will be recognized immunologically by the host with consequent rejection.

Recognition that in HLA match-

ing one can look at only a few serologic markers and that these represent only a small fraction of the complete genome has helped guide the strategy of our group as it relates to the priorities in donor selection (see Figure 3, page 350). Obviously, the best and rarest donor is a monozygotic twin. The next best is a sibling who shares with the patient both HLA-A and both HLA-B antigens. Failing that, the third best choice is a sibling who has haplotype identity with the recipient, i.e., one who has two similar antigens and two dissimilar ones. One sometimes finds a sibling who is matched with the patient for only one of four HLA-A and HLA-B antigens, and there are those who maintain that this is no better than complete dissimilarity. However, we prefer the sibling who is matched for the single antigen. Indeed, our bias is in favor of any sibling donor, even one who is a complete HLA mismatch, over parent donors. This perception is based on the fact that with a parent (or a child) of the recipient, one is assured at once of haplotype matching and haplotype mismatching. With a sibling, even if all of the marker antigens are different for the two individuals, we believe there is a strong likelihood that having the same parents will provide the siblings with more relevant antigenic similarities than dissimilarities.

As implied, we choose parent or child donors if siblings are not available. After that, our choice would be a close relative. Only when the possibilities of related donors are exhausted do we turn to cadaver sources, and with cadavers, we insist on at least a two-antigen HLA match before we do a transplant. It might be noted parenthetically that despite our conservatism (or perhaps because of it), our experience with cadaver kidney transplantation has been extremely good.

At the outset of the discussion on HLA matching, it was stated that we limit the serologic compatibility studies to the A and B loci. In a routine sense this is true. However, there are special circumstances in which we also match effectively for D and even for DR. Take the situation in which the surgeon has a choice of donors, say, several siblings, all of whom are HLA-A- and HLA-B-compatible with the patient and all of whom are willing to serve as donors. From animal experiments, we have determined that the longest and most trouble-free survival is likely to be achieved when the donor's leukocytes provide the least stimulation of the recipient's leukocytes (and vice versa) in the mixed leukocyte culture (MLC) system. In an analogous clinical situation, therefore, we would elect the sibling donor with the lowest MLC reactivity with the patient. Since it has been established that MLC reactivity is controlled from the HLA-D locus, we therefore would be indirectly performing D matching in such a case.

DR matching, which is a serologic procedure, is largely reserved for cadaver transplants at our institution. Practically speaking, we cannot D-match cadaver kidneys with the patient simply because MLC takes five days and, of course, a cadaver kidney cannot be held that long and then transplanted. In such situations, we do DR, as well as A and B, matching and have found that if there is compatibility at all three loci, the prognosis is slightly better than with just A and B matches. (The difference has not been so great as we were led to expect by a number of the European workers, some of whom maintain that DR is really more significant than either A or B. However, the series on which this conclusion is based have been small.)

There is one other matching procedure that we do routinely before transplantation. Once the donor has been selected on the basis of HLA specificities, a cytotoxic cross-match test is performed. Donor lymphocytes are mixed with patient serum, and antibody actions are assayed. If the recipient has cytolytic antibodies to the donor—a positive cross-match test—transplantation is not feasible.

Such a patient then becomes a candidate for cadaver transplantation. We have a list of such patients, people whose kidneys have failed and who are on dialysis. Each person on that list is tested against a panel of cells from 20 people, and every month we test the reaction of the serum of the patients with lymphocytes from each member of the panel. In that way, the alloantibody status of the candidates can be evaluated on a percentage basis: If the serum is reactive with one of 20, the patient's antibody status can be rated at 5%; with four, at 20%; and so forth. In general, the longer the patient remains on dialysis, the more frequent the antibody response and the less likely that any cadaver kidney will be suitable. However, whenever we get a cadaver kidney, we can quickly react serum from the cadaver against members of the various patient panels until we find one that is compatible for one of the patients.

Basically, that is the matching approach, except, of course, for the need for transfusion compatibility between donor and recipient. Therefore, we do test ABO blood group status. However, we are not concerned with any of the minor blood group antigens or with Rh. We have found that such compatibilities or incompatibilities are completely irrelevant.

Before we turn to the progress in

Figure 2

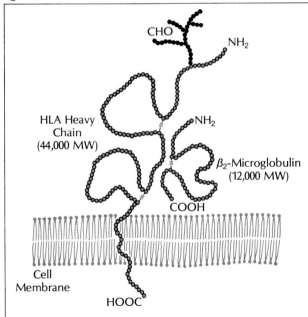 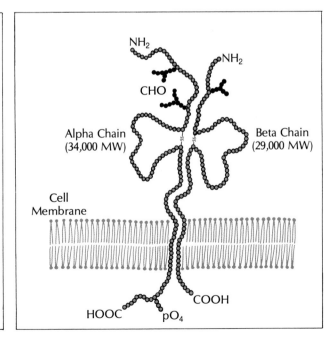

The molecular structures of HLA class I (left) and class II antigens are schematized. HLA-A, B, and C antigens have been identified as class I, and HLA-D, as class II. The weight of evidence favors classifying the DR antigens as class I.

**Priorities in
Allograft Donor Selection**

(in decreasing order of immunologic similarity)

1. Monozygotic twin
2. Dizygotic twin
3. HLA-A and HLA-B identical sibling
4. HLA one-haplotype identical sibling
5. <2 HLA-antigen-matched sibling
6. HLA one-haplotype identical child
7. HLA one-haplotype identical parent
8. First-order relatives (grandparents, uncles, aunts, cousins, etc)
9. Cadavers, ≥2 HLA antigens matched
10. Cadavers, <2 HLA antigens matched

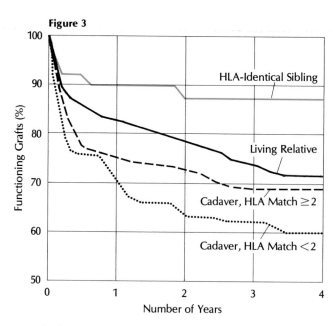

Figure 3

Table lists priorities applied to matching of organ graft donors and recipients at University of Minnesota. Accompanying

graph demonstrates relationship between selection of donor and the clinical success in maintaining functional renal graft.

immunosuppression that has been so critical in improving transplantation results, two adjunctive procedures that have proved extremely beneficial are noteworthy: pretransplantation transfusion and splenectomy.

The effects of pretransplantation transfusion (see Figure 4, opposite page) were discovered fortuitously, but the discovery has led to adoption of a routine protocol in which the prospective transplant recipient is given a series of five to 10 small transfusions (50 to 100 cc). The transfusions are of polyspecific whole blood or of red blood cells, fresh or frozen, no more than a month and no less than two or three days before transplantation. The red cells seem to be the critical element. The reason for the effectiveness of tranfusion is not understood; perhaps it is a form of nonspecific immunosuppression or an immunologic enhancement phenomenon. There appears to be some relationship to the HLA-DR locus, in the sense that it has been found that patients who are not transfused will do better if they are matched with donors for DR, but with transfusion the DR matching seems to be unnecessary.

As a modification of the transfusion protocol, which has become

almost universal, some transplant surgeons have experimented with specific transfusions of the kidney donor's blood to the patient. Significantly improved kidney transplant survival has been reported when donor-specific transfusions have been used before transplant. However, there is one formidable drawback to this approach: In something like 35% or 40% of cases, specific donor transfusions will cause the recipient to become specifically sensitized to donor tissues, so that the transplant cannot be carried out. This may be too high a price to pay for the benefits that may be derived.

Occasionally, even the polyspecific blood transfusion will produce a sensitization to donor tissues in the recipient and force us to turn to a cadaver transplant. In fact, some investigators have suggested that the real value of polyspecific transfusion is as a selection process, i.e., one that selects out in advance those hypersensitive individuals whose transplants are destined to be rejected.

Turning to the question of performing splenectomies in conjunction with transplants, one gets into an area that still must be classified as controversial—at least in the sense that some transplantation

groups do them, whereas others do not. However, on the basis of the experience at the University of Minnesota—bolstered by carefully controlled studies—the case for splenectomy seems to be strongly convincing.

The rationale for splenectomy is a simple one. The spleen is probably the first port of call for any intravascular antigen. Moreover, the organ is both the anatomic residence and the site of differentiation for a large portion of the body's immunoresponsive lymphocytes, particularly antibody-secreting B cells. Thus, extirpation of the spleen should decrease significantly the cohort of the specifically sensitized immunoresponsive cells.

On this basis and supported by our impressions of the clinical benefits, we did splenectomies routinely with our transplants between 1967 and 1977. During this period, the results in terms of graft survival at Minnesota were consistently 10% to 15% better than those in other programs not performing splenectomies. It was felt that one of the reasons was splenectomy. In order to test this, a randomized prospective trial of splenectomy was initiated in 1977. We matched by the usual criteria 150 renal transplant patients for whom splenectomies were done and 150 controls who underwent transplantation without splenectomy.

The results confirmed the clinical impression of splenectomy benefit (see Figure 5, page 352). With two-year graft survival as the end point, the 10% to 15% advantage held for splenectomized patients whose grafts were obtained from living related donors or cadavers. The only exception was the group whose donors were HLA-identical, for whom splenectomy was of little value. Of course, these patients did extremely well with or without removal of the spleen. Current policy, therefore, is to do splenectomies for all kidney recipients except those who have HLA-identical donors.

A question often asked with respect to splenectomy in patients who are going to be immunosuppressed for a number of years is whether this raises the risk of infection to the level of a significant problem. Infection, of course, has to be considered as a significant problem in any immunosuppressed individual. However, we now have splenectomized 1,700 transplant patients and have had only one case of overwhelming sepsis, which was in a patient who had discontinued antibiotic prophylaxis.

The splenectomized patients are maintained on trimethoprim, which provides good antibiotic prophylaxis against overwhelming gram-positive sepsis—the greatest risk in splenectomized patients—as well as against Nocardia and other opportunistic organisms. In addition, since the advent of effective pneumococcal vaccine, we have used it routinely.

In an immunologic context, optimal matching of donor and recipient can be considered half the battle in kidney transplantation. The other half, of course, is effective control of host immunologic responses, so as to prevent rejection or at least to control rejection episodes well enough to keep them from progressing to the loss of the transplanted kidney. For this, our weapons are immunosuppressive agents.

Historically, our current approach to pharmacologic immunosuppression dates back to the development by Robert Schwartz at Tufts University of azathioprine, an azo derivative of the antimetabolite 6-mercaptopurine. Azathioprine basically interferes with an enzyme system involved in nucleic acid synthesis; therefore, it affects all replicating cells. Obviously, when a person receives a transplant, the most actively replicating cells are those of the lymphoid systems, so that the drug preferentially inhibits lymphocyte proliferation and activity. However, azathioprine is by no means specific for lymphocytes. It also will inhibit myeloproliferative cells, gastrointestinal mucosal cells, and other rapidly dividing cell populations. Azathioprine was first shown to be effective against kidney transplant rejection in animals and humans by Roy Calne.

Prednisone was added to azathioprine in 1962 as an additional immunosuppressive agent. The mechanism of action of steroids is both different from and additive to that of azathioprine (see Figure 6, page 352). Whereas azathioprine limits lymphocyte proliferation, prednisone is lympholytic. Thus, with the combination, which is still employed, we have a two-pronged attack on immunoreactive cells.

In 1967, antilymphocyte globulin (ALG) was introduced as a third immunosuppressive agent, thereby adding an immunologic attack against lymphocytes to the chemical weapons. A number of variants of ALG are in use at different centers. Conceptually, they are basically the same and involve the raising of antisera whose antibodies recognize lymphocytes and initiate complement-dependent lysis of the target cells. At Minnesota, we make our own version of ALG, called antilymphoblast globulin. In its preparation, we use lymphocytes from a cell line maintained since 1967. These lymphocytes are injected into horses to raise an antiserum. From the antiserum, we separate out IgG antibodies. The immunoglobulin is then deaggregated, so that it will be tolerogenic rather than immunogenic, and administered intravenously to the transplant patient over a 14-day period postoperatively. This protocol protects against

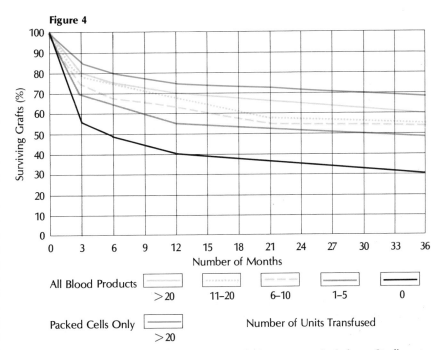

Figure 4

Surviving Grafts (%) vs. Number of Months

All Blood Products					
	>20	11–20	6–10	1–5	0

Packed Cells Only	
	>20

Number of Units Transfused

The benefits of pretransplantation blood transfusions are graphed above. Studies encompassed 3,521 patients who received first kidney transplants from cadaver donors. Except for those receiving more than 20 transfusions, there were no significant differences between the efficacy of packed red cells and that of "all blood products."

Figure 5

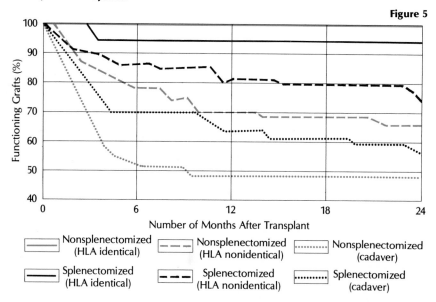

A prospective randomized study by D. S. Fryd et al demonstrated that splenectomy improved graft survival in patients undergoing kidney transplantation from all donor types except those in which the donor and recipient were completely HLA-identical.

sensitization of the patient in two ways—despite the fact that IgG is of equine origin and includes a wide range of antibody specificities other than the antilymphocyte. It has already been mentioned that the IgG is deaggregated. In addition, administering it intravenously and under a prednisone cover helps direct the material toward tolerance rather than sensitivity. Thus, our ALG can be given for as long as desired and can be used for subsequent courses either to treat a rejection episode or prophylactically for another kidney transplant in the same patient, if that becomes necessary.

The lack of specificity of ALG, coupled with the recent development of monoclonal-antibody technology, has made it natural for investigators to attempt to develop a monoclonal-antibody ALG. Theoretically, the approach is extremely tempting. Conventional animal-derived ALG antibodies are all polyclonal. With the monoclonal approach, one can obtain antibodies with unique specificities against each of the T-cell subsets: helper, suppressor, and cytolytic.

In fact, monoclonal antilymphocyte antibodies are now available commercially, and at least one major transplantation group, that at the Massachusetts General Hospital, has reported on their use. At this stage, a number of drawbacks are evident. Current monoclonal antibody cannot be given prophylactically, i.e., at the time of the transplant, as conventional ALG is used. Because it is immunogenic and not tolerogenic, it can be used for only a single and usually limited course. Thus, its use has been limited to attempts to reverse developing rejection episodes. In addition, the preparations tend to be too specific, and there is some risk that some of the antitransplant immunoreactive cells will be left behind. In addition, although rejection can be reversed in most cases, a majority (80%) will have a second rejection episode after the initial one.

It should be noted that to date monoclonal ALG has been administered without prednisone, largely because many transplant surgeons believe that eliminating cortisone, with all of its known side effects, from the immunosuppressive regimen is a highly desirable objective. Perhaps this is a case in which an attempt to kill two birds—lack of ALG specificity and cortisone side effects—with one stone has been self-defeating. At any rate, in offering the opinion that monoclonal ALG preparations have been disappointing so far, I would add that

Figure 6

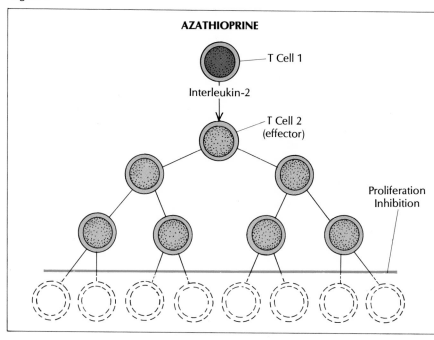

Diagrams compare the sites of action of various immunosuppressive agents. Azathioprine inhibits proliferation of effector lymphocytes; prednisone is cytolytic. Since neither is specific for the T lymphocytes most prominently involved in graft rejection, it is still too early to rule out the possibility of their future value.

In the meantime, however, another great stride has been taken in providing effective immunosuppression by more conventional means. The agent involved is cyclosporine, also introduced by Calne into transplantation management. Cyclosporine began its therapeutic life as a fungus-derived metabolite with antibiotic potential in 1972. In 1978, Calne started using the drug clinically and found it to be potently immunosuppressive.

This impression has more than been confirmed. Unfortunately, cyclosporine remains an investigational drug, so that its use has been limited to a handful of centers, including ours. The need for a controlled evaluation of cyclosporine was recognized quickly, in the interest of both Food and Drug Administration approval and our basic understanding of the drug's place in immunosuppressive regimens. We have undertaken such a randomized study in our kidney transplantation program. The investigation has been in progress for about two years, and we have

enrolled about 70 patients in the study group and an equal number in a control group. We have not included any HLA-identical cases in either group and have had to limit the program to adult (over age 18) patients because of FDA regulations. The patients have included individuals receiving grafts from related HLA-nonidentical donors and cadaver donors. The control patients have received what we consider our most effective immunosuppressive regimen, consisting of azathioprine, prednisone, and ALG. As judged by the prevention of rejection, it is our impression that cyclosporine alone is at least as good as the control regimen (see Figure 7, page 354), and there are indications that in the long run it will prove better in some ways.

With respect to side effects, cyclosporine is superior both theoretically and practically. It works very differently from azathioprine, which, it will be recalled, acts by inhibiting cellular proliferation. Azathioprine does this with respect to lymphocytes, thereby exerting its therapeutic effect; but it also inhibits myelogenous cells, causing bone

marrow toxicity and leukopenia. Cyclosporine has no myelotoxicity at all. Its mode of action appears unique and extremely specific. Although all of the details have not been worked out, it is well established that cyclosporine's site of action is related to the inhibition of action of interleukin-2, or T-cell growth factor (TCGF). Interleukin-2 is a mediator released by one subset of T lymphocytes that is required for the differentiation of other T cells, including cytotoxic T cells and helper T cells. The TCGF inhibition may involve either blockade of the mediator's receptors or, more likely, direct inhibition of its production. Either way, by preventing activation of both helper T cells and cytotoxic T cells, it suppresses both the antibody and cellular effectors of immunologic response.

In this "catalogue" of immunosuppressive modalities, some attention should be given to total lymphoid irradiation (TLI). A full description of the technique has been presented elsewhere in this volume (see S. Strober, "'Managing' the Immune System With Total Lymphoid Irradiation").

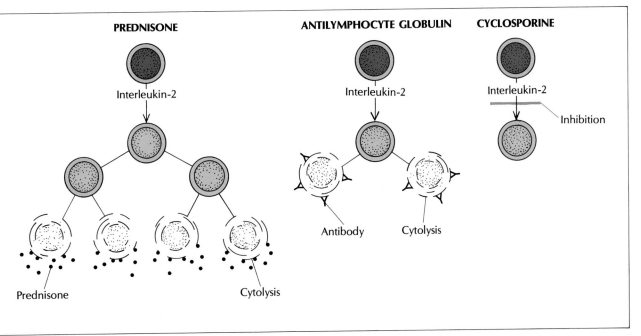

PREDNISONE   **ANTILYMPHOCYTE GLOBULIN**   **CYCLOSPORINE**

Interleukin-2   Interleukin-2   Interleukin-2

Inhibition

Antibody   Cytolysis

Prednisone   Cytolysis

their untoward effects can include bone marrow suppression and susceptibility to infection. Antilymphocyte globulin adds immunologic attack but will be directed against B as well as T cells, with consequent infection risks. Only cyclosporine is appropriately specific. By inhibiting production or activity of interleukin-2, it aborts the signal for effector T-cell proliferation.

Figure 7

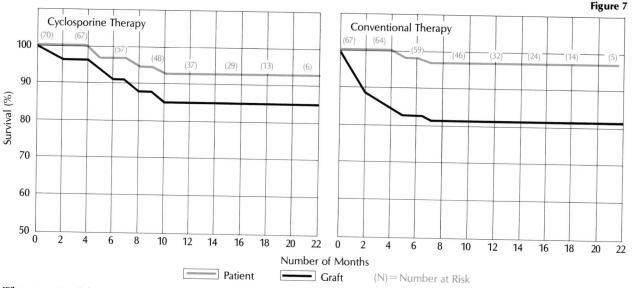

When an actuarial comparison was made between cyclosporine alone and a conventional immunosuppressive regimen consisting of azathioprine, prednisone, and antilymphocyte globulin, little difference was seen over 22 months in terms of either patient or graft survival. However, when frequency of rejection episodes and of infections, length of hospitalization, and dollar costs per patient were tabulated (right), distinct advantages accrued to the cyclosporine regimen. Table also lists the side effects of cyclosporine. Data, from a randomized prospective trial at University of Minnesota, were analyzed as of July 15, 1982.

There is no doubt that TLI is a powerful immunosuppressant, one of the most potent known. It kills lymphocytes but for some reason seems to spare suppressor T cells, at least relatively. However, for all of its efficacy, it also has serious problems. It takes six weeks to administer, and most important, it exposes the patient to very high doses of radiation. There is no way to predict what the long-range effects of that radiation will be, particularly with respect to oncogenesis. Finally, TLI is very poorly tolerated by patients, particularly by diabetics.

For these reasons, we have adopted a strategy that reserves TLI for a very difficult type of patient: the person who has already rejected one, two, or three grafts within six months after transplantation. As shown in Figure 8 on the opposite page, the prognosis for survival of a new renal transplant in such cases is relatively poor. After one rejection, there is about a 50% survival rate, and after multiple grafts, it falls to about 35%. However, when TLI is used for the multiple-rejection group, in our clinical experience with 24 transplant patients, two-year graft sur-

vival is increased to 70% or 75%— in other words, about doubled. Even at that, there is some reluctance to use TLI for the reasons stated previously, and we have recently been investigating the efficacy of cyclosporine in this high-risk group.

What of the adverse consequences of immunosuppression? Essentially, this question addresses two problems: oncogenesis and infection. The latter can be summarized quite briefly. Immunosuppression does carry with it a significant added risk of both viral (primarily herpetic) and bacterial infections. For the most part, the former are self-limiting, and the latter can be effectively managed with appropriate antibiotics. Interestingly, in our controlled study, it was found that the incidence of both viral and bacterial infections was halved by cyclosporine. The reasons for this advantage have not really been elucidated, but one can postulate that because cyclosporine acts on interleukin-2, it has little or no effect on B lymphocytes, so that the ability to mount an antibody response to at least some viral and bacterial antigens is unimpaired. In contrast, ALG is cytolytic for all

lymphocytes without any significant discrimination. Furthermore, the decrease in infection may reflect the decrease in steroids as a consequence of fewer rejection episodes in the cyclosporine group. Actually, after the first year, the patients in the cyclosporine group had received only half as much of the total dose of prednisone as the control group.

Unfortunately, the situation with regard to immunosuppression and the development of malignant disease has not undergone any parallel improvement. With any effective immunosuppressive agent, one is likely to see tumor formation at significantly elevated rates. The better the immunosuppression, the higher the cancer risk. For example, in our relatively few TLI patients, we have already had two lymphomas. Very probably, this risk could be reduced by lowering the radiation dose—which can be done without adversely affecting the results—but the problem is not likely to be eliminated. Similarly, in the early studies of cyclosporine, there were a great number of lymphomas. In our current series, we have seen only one, and this was easily

Cyclosporine vs 'Conventional' Immunosuppression

	Cyclosporine	Conventional
Rejection (%)	17	54
Average hospitalization (days)	12	21
Infections (excluding CMV)	10	20
CMV infections	2	22
Average cost per patient	$28,585	$45,129

Cyclosporine Complications

Mild hirsutism
Fine tremor
Mild reversible hepatotoxicity (4%)
Mild reversible nephrotoxicity (58%)
Lymphoma (~1%)

and successfully treated with acyclovir. Perhaps our rate is low because we have learned to regulate the dose and to adjust it on the basis of constant monitoring of blood levels of the drug. There is no doubt that some degree of malignancy is the price of too much immunosuppression, but some increase in oncogenesis is inevitable at any level of immunosuppression necessary to prevent allograft rejection. Our own overall lymphoma rate in 1,800 transplants has been brought down to 1%.

Perhaps the best statistical analysis of the relationship between immunosuppression for transplantation and cancer has been done by Israel Penn. He has maintained a clearinghouse for tumors that arise de novo after transplantation. Here are some of his exemplary figures: Of 418 renal transplant patients in one series, 26% of those who survived a year developed cancer; in another program, 252 solid lymphomas were diagnosed in 1,300 patients; skin cancers occurred in about 500 of the 1,300. Obviously, the price of immunosuppression can be a high one.

To consider the broader subject

of transplantation of various organs, perhaps it should be stressed that all transplanted organs are immunogenic. The concept, once quite widely held, that some organs would be "immunogenically privileged" is just not valid. There are some minor gradations in immunogenic degree, but they are really not very significant. It is more difficult for the host to reject a kidney, liver, or heart—all of which are vascularly anastomosed to the recipient—than a skin graft that starts out with a rather tenuous connection to the recipient. Similarly, grafts of individual cells are less protected against rejection than whole organs. This was probably the chief reason for temporary abandonment of pancreatic islet-cell transplantation.

There are, of course, great differences in the consequences of rejection of different organs. If a heart transplant is rejected, the event is most often terminal; with kidney transplant rejection, a large majority of patients can survive with dialysis and subsequently with retransplantation. However, in thinking about rejection, it is very important to differentiate between rejection that eventuates in loss of the graft and that which is reversible. Regardless of the organ in

volved, our strategy is essentially the same. With one exception, diagnosis of a rejection episode is dependent on biopsy and gross and microscopic examination of the specimen (see Figure 9, page 356). The exception is the pancreas, which rarely is biopsied.

When a rejection episode is taking place, it can be most effectively reversed, in our experience, with a combination of ALG and an increased dose of prednisone, given either orally or intravenously. Very close to 100% of rejection episodes will be reversed with this protocol. If ALG is not available, just raising the steroid levels will be adequate in a large majority of cases.

After the first such rejection episode is reversed, the patient remains at very high risk of a second episode. The magnitude of that risk is dependent on the regimen used to reverse the initial episode. Thus, with the ALG-prednisone protocol, we have found that the risk of a second rejection is about 36%. With either monoclonal-antibody ALG plus steroids or steroids alone, about two thirds to three fourths of patients have a second episode.

It has been our policy to treat two rejection episodes vigorously. Then if a third episode occurs, un

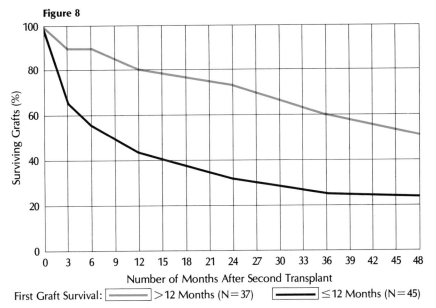

Figure 8

First Graft Survival: ▭ >12 Months (N=37)   ▬ ≤12 Months (N=45)

Study by R. R. M. Gifford et al documented adverse prognostic significance of first graft rejection, particularly rapid rejection, for survival of subsequent renal grafts.

Figure 9

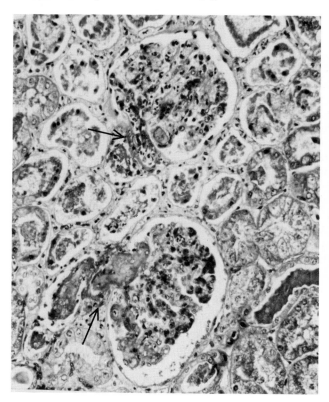

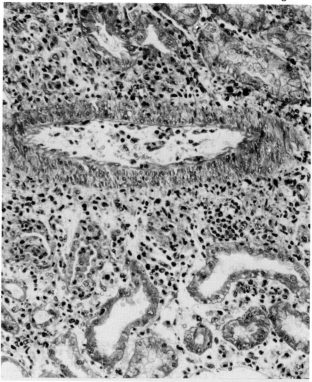

Photomicrographs illustrate histologic phenomena accompanying various types of renal transplant rejection. Hyperacute rejection (top left) is characterized by fibrin thrombi and fibrinoid necrosis of small arteries, afferent arterioles (arrows), and glomerular tufts with PMN exudaton. One sees tubular necrosis and eventually thrombogenic cortical necrosis. Acute interstitial rejection (top right) is manifested by an interstitial mononuclear cell infiltrate, edema, and hemorrhage. Tubules may be erratic, as here, or necrotic. In severe acute vascular rejection (bottom left), one sees fibrinoid necrosis and necrotizing arteritis (arrows) or vascular thrombosis, as well as mononuclear-cell disruption of vessel endothelium. Finally, in severe chronic vascular rejection (bottom right), the picture shows an interlobular artery with marked fibrointimal proliferation causing stenosis and renal ischemia. Note prominent juxtaglomerular apparatus hyperplasia (arrow).

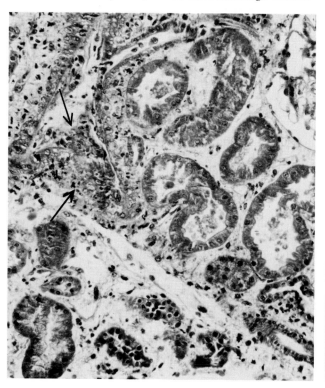

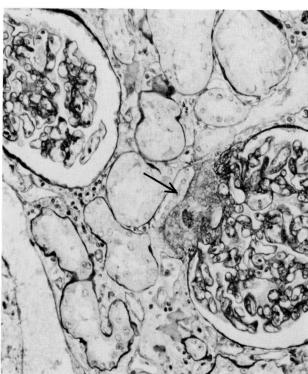

less it is relatively mild, the tendency is to accept the loss of the kidney and consequently to taper the immunosuppressive treatment gradually. Our reasoning here is dominated by fear that the excessive immunosuppression required for treatment of more than two episodes would leave the patient too vulnerable to infection and oncogenesis. Obviously, this policy applies to kidney transplants. For heart transplants, rejection is treated as long as there is any chance of saving the graft, and there is usually no second chance. Our experience with other organs is not sufficient for the enunciation of any policy beyond individualized treatment of rejection.

Heart transplantation, in terms of the number of procedures done, is now second only to kidney transplantation. Since the first heart transplant done in 1967 in South Africa, with great fanfare, it has become, after a reactive period of quiescence, a relatively common procedure. Probably close to 500 heart transplants have been done, with increasingly good results. Technically, heart transplantation is relatively easy; it requires only three vascular anastomoses. The procedure is well tolerated by the patient, and with the advent of intravascular cardiac biopsies, developed by Norman Shumway and his colleagues at Stanford, one can monitor for rejection very closely and institute treatment promptly. At the present time, the results with cadaver heart transplants are

about equal to those with cadaver renal transplants. The heart also affords us the advantage of a multitude of electrocardiographic and other techniques to monitor organ function—another asset in early detection of rejection.

Liver transplantation comes after heart in frequency of performance. Technically, it is the most difficult of all, requiring four vascular anastomoses and the construction of a biliary conduit to the intestine. The conduit has proved the most difficult part of all hepatic-transplant techniques, but this has largely been solved through the work of Thomas Starzl and Calne. They have demonstrated to virtually everyone's satisfaction that one can circumvent the difficulties seen in maintaining functioning patency of choledochocholecystocholedochal, choledochocholedochal, or choledochojejunal anastomosis. Immunologically, liver transplantation seems to present about the same type and magnitude of problems as does kidney transplantation.

Pancreatic transplantation experience by now encompasses more than 200 procedures of various types. Both whole-pancreas and islet-cell transplantation have largely been abandoned because of attendant problems, but segmental pancreatic transplants—involving all of the organ except the head—are increasing in frequency. We have done 55 segmental pancreatic transplants. Technically, they require only two vascular anastomoses, and the problems of immu-

nosuppression are very much like those seen with the kidney. In this context, we are finding the availability of cyclosporine a significant factor. The major problem has been, anatomically, how to drain exocrine secretions from the graft. We believe that either duct occlusion with silicone rubber or intestinal drainage with pancreaticojejunal anastomosis has largely solved this problem, or at least promises to do so.

Finally, lung transplants should be mentioned. The lung was one of the most difficult organs to transplant, both for technical surgical reasons and because of the significant problem of infection. The surgical problems were greatly diminished when the Stanford group developed a technique for lung transplantation employing heart-lung preparations. At this writing, they have used this technique on at least six patients, of whom four are surviving and appear to be doing well. The infection problem may be greatly reduced by cyclosporine immunosuppression, perhaps even to the point where solitary lung grafts again may be used.

From this review, it should be clear that organ transplantation has traveled a long distance from the exotic to a place as a significant, if not routine, part of the physician's healing skills. That journey has been greatly facilitated by the ever-growing understanding of the immunologic problems and the ever-improving means of coping with them.

34

Immunologic Reconstitution: Achievements and Potentials

ROBERT A. GOOD *Oklahoma Medical Research Foundation*

The immunodeficiency diseases are a group of rare genetic and congenital disorders that have been characterized as "experiments of nature." Through them has come a great deal of our current body of knowledge about the cellular components and functioning of the immune systems, and particularly about the effector limbs of those systems. There is, therefore, considerable scientific and medical satisfaction emanating from the fact that the knowledge so derived has been cycled back to provide a powerful modality for the correction of the immune deficiencies: immunologic reconstitution via transplantation of bone marrow and other hematopoietic and lymphopoietic tissues and stem-cell populations.

However, the therapeutic application of immunologic reconstitution has not been limited to the immunodeficiency diseases and syndromes. We have already seen its effective use in treatment of the leukemias, of aplastic anemia and other blood dyscrasias, and of osteopetrosis; and we have good reason to anticipate its efficacy in the lymphomas, in autoimmune mesenchymal or connective tissue diseases, and even in enzyme abnormalities. Perhaps most important, we believe that a theoretical and methodologic basis has been developed to make immunologic reconstitution a medically safe procedure, so that its uses need not be limited to patients with far-advanced disease for whom no other hope for survival remains.

How did all of this come about? Where is immunologic reconstitution going from here?

This review will, in the main, be devoted to an attempt to answer these questions. Our own imagination was awakened to the possibility of using cellular engineering to treat immunodeficiencies by work, nearly 20 years ago at the University of Minnesota, with thymectomized newborn mice. These animals, like their "natural" counterparts, congenitally athymic mice, are unable to live in a normal environment. They are runted and unable to withstand infection. They often develop autoimmunities and sometimes have horrendous skin diseases. However, we found that these animals would develop normally, and all of their diseases and disorders would resolve, if they were given thymus transplants. At first, these experiments were performed with syngeneic donors, but later we found that allogeneic transplants would also work, provided the donor and recipient were matched with respect to their major histocompatibility complexes (H-2). We also discovered a bit later with Douglas Biggar and Osias Stutman that transplantation could be achieved with just small, wet membranes of embryonic thymus—in other words, thymic tissue before it differentiates into lymphoid tissue; and we also were able to achieve reconstitution in these mice with matched peripheral lymphoid cells taken from spleen or lymph nodes. This work was done with Edmund Yunis.

With these experiments in mind, we decided to address the problem of attempting to correct clinical immunodeficiency diseases by the transplantation of matched lymphoid cells. The first step was to analyze various immunodeficiencies to identify those that might parallel the condition of thymectomized mice. As a background for this effort, we already had extensive information on the existence of the two basic components of immunity, one dependent primarily on the thymus, the other on the bursa of Fabricius or its mammalian equivalent. These are, of course, what we now know as the T-cell and B-cell systems. A great deal of this analysis had been done in Minnesota by M. D. Cooper and R. D. Peterson, building on the work of Bruce Glick and associates at Ohio State and the Australian investigators N. L. Warner and A. Szenberg.

At any rate, we identified children with the DiGeorge syndrome as the immunodeficiency patient population most closely akin to the thymectomized mice. These children clearly had a primary defect in the system that we could analogize to the thymus in mice, rats, and hamsters. They lacked T lymphocytes but had very large numbers of B cells. Clinically, their primary defect appeared to be in cell-mediated immunity, while their humoral antibody immunity was erratic, albeit also often deficient. Our conclusion was that these children had failed to develop their thymuses and that they were candidates for thymus transplants. Actually, the first such transplant in a DiGeorge patient was performed in Miami by William Cleveland, using a thymus sent to him by Humphrey Kay in England. Since then, about a dozen DiGeorge patients have been treated with thymic transplants, several with grafts consisting of bits of wet membrane from embryonic thymus. Once it was established that prelymphoid thymic membranes would develop and differentiate into functioning organs, the advantage of their use was obvious. Because the thymic anlagen lack lymphoid cells, they are not recognized as being foreign by the hosts. Because this tissue lacks immunologically competent lymphocytes, it is less likely to mount graft-versus-host (GVH) attack. Even when lymphocytes develop in residual lymphoid tissue and from these epithelial primitive precursors, they do not recognize that the host is foreign. In some as yet un-

known way, development of the repertoire of reactivity is controlled within the thymus, and after such transplants, reactivity to host antigens is excluded.

Thymic transplants have proved capable of reconstructing immunologic capacity in the majority of DiGeorge syndrome patients. They produce sustained levels of thymic hormones and effectively process T lymphocytes, so that one sees not only a repletion of T zones in the spleen and lymph modes but also a full array of T-cell immunologic functions. With the rise in T lymphocytes, there is a posttransplantation normalization of the previously elevated B-cell levels, so essentially, the patients become immunologically normal. Unfortunately, all too often, successful transplantation of thymic tissue in DiGeorge patients turns out to be a somewhat hollow victory. These patients usually have an array of other abnormalities, including cardiac outflow-tract defects, often of the truncus arteriosus type, which, of course, can be lethal.

As an intriguing aside, there is now considerable evidence that the DiGeorge syndrome can be produced in experimental animals either with maternal zinc restriction or with drugs that are zinc chelators. The implication, of course, is that the syndrome may be congenital but not genetic, sometimes resulting from a lack of maternal dietary zinc.

In retrospect, such T-cell immunodeficiencies as the DiGeorge syndrome were relatively easy to reconstitute. Basically, the etiology lay in a single structure—the thymus—and it was both plausible and realistic to expect that straightforward transplantation of that organ could correct the underlying defect. On the opposite side of the immunodeficiency coin were the B-cell agammaglobulinemias, prototypically X-linked infantile (Bruton's) agammaglobulinemia. Here one did not have any neat self-contained structure, such as the thymus, to transplant. Theoretically, one could conceive of using peripheral B cells for reconstitution. However, the use of pe-

ripheral cells could have meant infusing or injecting cells that were themselves immunologically mature and antigenic, with all of the implicit problems in circumventing both rejection and GVH. Moreover, to function immunologically the B-cell population must encompass almost an infinite array of discrete antigen-response capabilities, so it was almost impossible to imagine defining these specificities, let alone identifying and obtaining the lymphocytes capable of reacting to them. For these patients, preparations of gamma globulin for intramuscular administration (and more recently for intravenous administration) have provided a form of substitution therapy that has greatly relieved the susceptibility to bacterial infection that characterizes these children.

The problems seemed to point toward the need to use, not B cells per se, but B-cell precursors. At the same time, investigators interested in immunologic reconstitution were wrestling conceptually with a group of diseases that were far more devastating clinically than the B deficiencies, specifically the severe combined immunodeficiency (SCID). About a half dozen such syndromes have now been defined; in some, neither B nor T cells developed; in others, B cells developed and T cells did not, but functionally both systems were nonoperative.

It was already known that both lymphocyte populations differentiated from a single stem-cell line; and from work done by Malcolm Moore as well as by Stutman in our own laboratories, we knew that such stem cells could be found in both the bone marrow and the fetal liver. We therefore proposed that the solution to both B-cell deficiency and SCID might lie in bone marrow or fetal liver transplantation.

This was in 1967, and we did not have long to wait for the clinical testing of this proposition. A young child with SCID was referred to our hospital. Since this boy had no siblings, we felt that obtaining bone marrow from a histocompatibly matched donor would be a formidable problem. For this reason, a de-

Figure 1

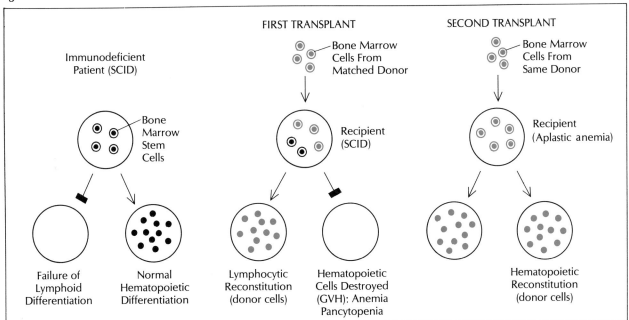

Among the first patients to be immunologically reconstituted was a child with severe combined immunodeficiency disease (SCID). He lacked both T- and B-cell immunity but was hematopoietically normal (left). Marrow transplant restored lym-

phocytic functions, but graft-versus-host disease resulted in aplastic anemia (center). Second transplant corrected the anemia, and the child became essentially healthy, with both lymphocytic and hematopoietic cells derived from donor stem cells.

Figure 2

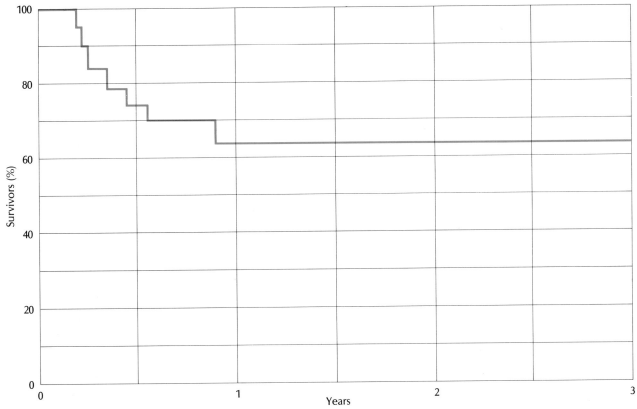

Based on experience in Seattle, E. D. Thomas and colleagues presented this graph showing estimated survival percentages of patients with acute myelocytic leukemia, acute myelomono-

cytic leukemia, and acute monocytic leukemia given bone marrow transplants during remissions of their disease (from New England Journal of Medicine 301:598, 1979).

Figure 3

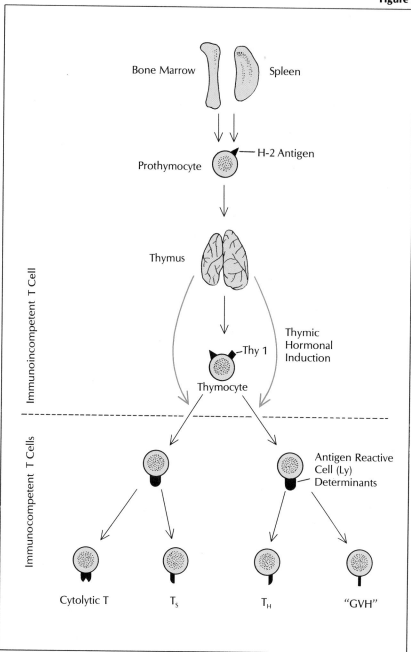

Bone Marrow   Spleen

H-2 Antigen

Prothymocyte

Immunoincompetent T Cell

Thymus

Thymic
Hormonal
Induction

Thy 1

Thymocyte

Immunocompetent T Cells

Antigen Reactive
Cell (Ly)
Determinants

Cytolytic T T_S T_H "GVH"

T-cell line derives from stem cells. After differentiation in the thymus, thymocytes have acquired Thy-1 antigens but are not yet immunocompetent. Later differentiation leads to various subpopulations of immunocompetent peripheral T cells.

During the 10 weeks the child survived, there was good evidence of immunologic reconstitution. His lymphocytes were chimeric—that is, they included cells that could be identified as originating from the donor. However, we were obviously deeply concerned about the lethal GVH disease and concluded that the next time around we would attempt reconstitution with bone marrow from a sibling member matched at the human major histocompatibility (HLA) loci. It should be noted that at the time of this case, one of those loci, the D, had not yet been identified; but the mixed leukocyte culture (MLC) and the A and B loci had. We knew from the studies of R. Ceppelini and J. Dausset, and of J. F. Bach and D. B. Amos, that if you analyzed the HLA constitution of siblings of candidates for allografts, about one in four would provide favorable matches.

A short time after we came to the conclusion that GVH reaction might be minimized or avoided altogether by transplanting the marrow from an HLA-matched sibling donor, an infant boy with a severe combined immunodeficiency was brought to us. This child's family history included 12 deaths over four generations, all from SCID and all occurring before the patients' second birthdays. The boy had four sisters, one of whom was matched, albeit not perfectly. The potential donor was matched at the MLC and B loci but mismatched at the A locus, as well as with respect to blood group antigens. However, because the patient's disease was lethal, the decision was made to proceed with the **marrow transplantation (see Figure 1, page 361).**

The first result of the transplant was complete correction of the immunologic deficiencies, both B-cell and T-cell. However, the child went on to develop two serious iatrogenic sequelae: a GVH and an aplastic anemia. From our animal experience, we felt that the GVH would not be lethal in this case and could be managed medically. Attention was therefore turned to the life-threatening anemia. This attention

cision was made to do a fetal liver transplant. The graft actually corrected both of this child's immunologic systems. However, the child did succumb to a GVH reaction. In this case, it was difficult to identify the cause of this reaction since the patient had received blood transfusions, and it had been shown that transfusions can be lethal in SCID

simply because the immunocompetent lymphocytes in the transfused blood are able to mount an unopposed immunologic attack on the host. Nevertheless, we could not exclude the transplanted fetal liver as the source of the GVH reactions. Subsequently, we have learned that one does not see GVH disease after early fetal liver transplantation.

took the form of a second marrow transplant from the same donor. We were now dealing with a patient whose own stem-cell population had been essentially wiped out and whose aplastic anemia had effectively nullified his erythrocyte antigenicity. The second transplant took, and he was completely converted cytologically from his own genetic makeup to that of his donor sister. The boy, now 14, is immunologically and hematologically completely normal; all of his cells carry an XY karyotype; his blood type, originally A, is his sister's O.

With this one case, the ability to treat effectively two different lethal diseases, a SCID and an aplastic anemia, was documented. Subsequently, the use of bone marrow transplants from matched sibling donors had proved effective in the correction of all six genetic forms of SCID, as well as in Wiskott-Aldrich syndrome, and repeatedly in aplastic anemias. It really has become an almost routine procedure to perform with immediate therapeutic results, provided you have a patient with SCID free from infection and a matched sibling donor. The latter qualification, however, is a formidable one, particularly if one keeps in mind the statistical odds against such a match and the usual family size in the populations of the United States and other advanced societies. We will return to this problem and its possible solutions a little later.

From a historical point of view, the next great stride in immunologic reconstitution came with the pioneering work of E. Donnall Thomas and his colleagues in Seattle. In 1971, these investigators first employed bone marrow transplantation from HLA-matched sibling donors for treatment of a leukemia. After an appropriate period of experimentation with dogs, Thomas et al moved into the clinic. Because of the problems with GVH, and because of the experimental nature of the approach, the first efforts were with adults with acute myeloid leukemia (AML) who had failed or ceased to respond to available chemotherapeutic agents. In

other words, their patients were essentially in the terminal phase of disease. Nevertheless, they demonstrated that withal they could achieve a 10% to 15% long-term survival rate, and this encouraged them to attempt bone marrow transplantation earlier in the course of the disease, specifically during the first remission of patients with AML, which, of course, was considered to be a cancer with a 100% fatal prognosis.

The protocol used for leukemia in Seattle, and subsequently at a number of other centers, involved, first, use of cystoreductive drugs supplemented by lethal irradiation, in order to destroy all leukemic cells. This is followed by HLA-matched bone marrow transplants. The results achieved by this means have been remarkable and have been attained not only in Seattle but in numerous other centers in **both the United States and Europe** (see Figure 2, page 361). Long-term survival was achieved in about 60% of the patients, and the criteria for cure can be expected eventually to be met in more than 50%. Importantly, the survival curves in these leukemias, as well as in the treated aplastic anemias, showed high early mortality and then a prolonged plateau period, during which there were very few additional deaths. Recurrences have proved rare. The early deaths were largely attributable to GVH disease and to infections that themselves were often concomitants of GVH. GVH disease in both leukemia and aplastic anemia tends to be much more severe and life-threatening than it is in SCID. The main exacerbating factor appears to be the use of cytotoxic drugs and irradiation in conjunction with and prior to bone marrow transplantation. In addition, as noted earlier, prior blood transfusion increases the risk of failure of the bone marrow transplant. Thus, in aplastic anemias, controlled studies have shown about a 65% cure rate in the general patient population, with up to an 85% cure rate if one selects patients without prior transfusions.

Subsequent to the early efforts

by Thomas involving patients with AML, bone marrow transplantation has been extended by the Seattle group and by others to other leukemias, including those, like acute lymphatic leukemia in its first exacerbation, that are not as relentlessly lethal as AML, or for which more effective chemotherapeutic and radiation therapy protocols are available. With our colleagues, led by Richard O'Reilly, we and others have now successfully employed marrow transplants for treatment of several forms of anemia, for severe neutrophil dysfunction, for Kostmann's agranulocytosis, for cartilage hair hyperplasia, for the immunologic and hematologic abnormalities in the Wiskott-Aldrich syndrome, and even for marble bone disease (osteopetrosis). All in all, 20 or more otherwise fatal diseases have been managed by bone marrow transplantation. The efficacy of bone marrow transplantation has been augmented by various cytoreductive and immunosuppressive regimens and, particularly in animals, by total lymphoid and total body irradiation (see S. Strober, "Managing the Immune System with Total Lymphoid Irradiation"). In general, these adjunctive modalities have been designed either to obviate graft rejection or to create noncompetitive environments for the marrow engraftment and also to facilitate complete replacement of the patient's stem-cell populations with healthy donor stem cells.

A good example of the development of bone marrow transplantation technology relates to the management of patients with Wiskott-Aldrich syndrome. One of the most significant early accomplishments of cellular engineering was the *immunologic* cure of an infant boy with Wiskott-Aldrich syndrome by Bach and M. M. Bortin in Wisconsin. Wiskott-Aldrich is characterized by a profound state of immunodeficiency involving both T and B cells, and it also includes a number of associated hematologic abnormalities, most prominently a profound thrombocytopenia. Because the immunologic deficiency in this

Figure 4

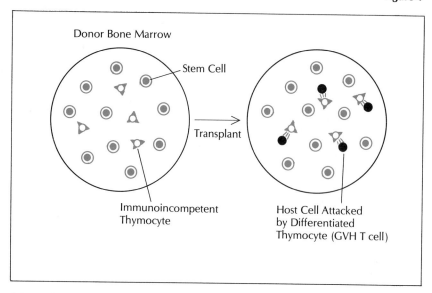

Donor Bone Marrow

Stem Cell

Transplant

Immunoincompetent
Thymocyte

Host Cell Attacked
by Differentiated
Thymocyte (GVH T cell)

Schematized is concept that GVH is mediated by immunoincompetent thymocytes capable of differentiating into competent T cells that attack host cells and tissues.

syndrome is not total, a primary concern in transplanting sibling bone marrow was graft rejection. To circumvent this, Bach and Bortin pretreated the patient with massive immunosuppressive doses of cyclophosphamide. Under this cover, the transplant was accepted and the immunologic defects completely corrected. However, the child's hematologic problems were not fully corrected, and although he survived and thrived, he continued to have bleeding problems related to his thrombocytopenia and monocyte defects.

Subsequently, Roberts, and Parkman and his colleagues in Boston, addressed Wiskott-Aldrich in a more total way. Their protocols included total body irradiation, antithymocyte globulins, and cytoreductive agents, which, in combination, completely destroyed the patients' stem-cell populations. In this way, they were able to obtain "full" bone marrow transplants and to correct platelet and monocyte abnormalities as well as the immunocyte defects. Children so treated were completely normalized. A variation on this approach was employed by our colleagues Neena Kapoor, O'Reilly, et al at Memorial Sloan-Kettering, who used busulfan to knock out stem cells and cyclo-

phosphamide for immunosuppression. With both of these protocols, a number of complete cures of Wiskott-Aldrich syndrome have been accomplished.

From the discussion thus far, one can certainly conclude that bone marrow transplantation has already assumed a significant place in the treatment of a broad spectrum of immunologic and hematologic diseases; some, such as the immunodeficiency diseases, are extremely rare; others, like the leukemias and aplastic anemias, are relatively common. All have been characterized by their overwhelmingly high mortality, and this lethality has made it acceptable for physicians to employ an approach that carries with it the burden of GVH disease. But that burden has been a heavy one. It will be recalled that for patients with AML and aplastic anemia who are managed with marrow transplantation, early mortality is—with rare exceptions—not from their original disease but from GVH. Clearly, for marrow transplantation to be assigned an expanded role as therapy for a host of diseases for which it theoretically would be appropriate, the GVH problem must be solved. Solutions do appear to be at hand.

As early as 1958, D. E. Uphoff

noted that fetal liver transplantation was not followed by GVH reactions. This observation long went unexplained until such transplants were done and analyzed by Ö. Tulunay, working with Yunis and me in Minnesota. Liver transplants did not trigger GVH, provided the tissue was obtained early enough during differentiation, so that in addition to lacking postthymic immunocompetent (T) cells, it lacked postthymic immuno*in*competent cells. It will be recalled that when lymphocytes migrate through the thymus (see Figure 3, page 362), they acquire their repertoire of surface antigens that, in turn, relate to their subsequent immunologic functions (see E. A. Boyse and H. Cantor, "Surface Characteristics of T-Lymphocyte Subpopulations"). When thymocytes first leave the thymus, they are functionally committed but not yet functionally competent. It was these postthymic cells—a few of which migrate back to the bone marrow and are lacking in fetal liver (see Figure 4, this page)—that appeared to be responsible for GVH, at least early on. A number of investigators, including O'Reilly et al, have employed fetal liver to treat children with SCID. With O'Reilly's interest, the experience we had at Memorial Sloan-Kettering with this approach to treatment of patients with SCID was especially large. In at least 25% of the cases treated, immunologic reconstitution was achieved without GVH.

However, there are significant problems with fetal liver. The tissue is difficult to obtain, and when you get it, the number of cells is often too small to provide adequate material for transplantation. The challenge was to obtain bone marrow inocula that were devoid of both immunocompetent T cells and these postthymic immunoincompetent thymocytes, which Stutman has described and defined so well. The first solution that suggested itself was immunologic, i.e., the use of antisera directed against these thymus-derived cells. Theoretically, this seemed to be attractive since, as was noted, the thymocytes have already acquired distinct surface antigenic determinants. In the mouse system, the surface marker is Thy 1.

The production of such an antiserum was not only theoretically attractive but when we approached the problem, there was evidence that one had already been produced in the rat system. W. Müller-Ruchholtz and his colleagues in Kiel, West Germany, had reported the production of an antiserum that effectively eliminated all postthymic lymphocytes from rat bone marrow, facilitating transplantation across the major histocompatibility barrier without GVH. However, a number of other workers had failed to reproduce this work, and as a result it had not been accepted.

Experiments by K. Joh in our laboratory were successful in duplicating the German studies and preparing transplantable bone marrow that was apparently free of both postthymic immunocompetent T cells and the committed immuno-incompetent precursors of T cells that might develop into functional T cells capable of initiating the GVH reaction. The recipients of such marrow transplants became stable chimeras functionally able to recognize cells and tissues from "third parties" but tolerant to both self and donor cells and tissues. From a theoretical point of view, we felt that we had solved the GVH problem and that the solution lay in destroying or eliminating all postthymic cells in the marrow graft. However, such a theoretical solution still left us a long way from the clinic. To begin with, the surface antigen characteristics of postthymic cells had been much more fully worked out in mice and rats than in humans. Added to that was the fact that even in the experimental animals, the desirable antiserum that would eliminate all of the unwanted lymphoid has proved a difficult antiserum to make. Nevertheless, a number of workers in several centers, including Boston, Seattle, Los Angeles, and New York, continue to work on antisera that will permit this approach, so

effective in animals, to be extended directly to patients (see Figure 5, page 366).

Just about that time, my attention was called, prior to its publication, to a paper prepared by Yair Reisner et al of Nathan Sharon's laboratory, in the Weizmann Institute for Science in Israel. They described the separation of all stem cells from all peripheral lymphocytes in the mouse, employing agglutination techniques. These techniques were based on using plant lectins capable of agglutinating cells on the basis of interactions of the sugar constituents of the cell surfaces and the plant sugars or glycopeptides. They used a double agglutination, employing peanut and soybean agglutinins followed in each instance by centrifugation, and with this methodology were successful in getting rid of all unwanted cells and transplanting bone marrow across the H-2 barrier in lethally irradiated recipients without inducing GVH. We found that the chimeric recipients were usually tolerant to donor and to self but completely immunologically reactive to third parties, just as are recipients in the antiserum experiments. With our young colleagues Kazunori Onoe and Gabriel Fernandes, and in separate experiments with Susan Krown and Richard Coico, we tested this method in mice. We felt transplantation of marrow across major histocompatibility barriers might be accomplished in mice because J. Sprent and his colleagues had shown that parent-to-F_1 chimeras could be achieved without apparent GVH diseases if anti-thy-1 antiserum was used to eliminate the postthymic cells from the marrow prior to transplantation. In both sets of experiments in our laboratories, treatment of bone marrow prior to transplant with anti-thy-1 antisera completely eliminated the cells that initiated GVH disease and permitted the regular establishment of long-lived chimeras without any signs of GVH reactions.

Reisner was invited to come to Memorial Sloan-Kettering to investigate the possibilities of using the

human cell surface sugar code, so that this type of methodology could be applied clinically. He accepted and joined O'Reilly, Kapoor, Marquis Hodes, and me in these experiments.

Reisner first tried to apply the peanut and soybean double agglutination approach to human cells, but it was not successful in completely separating the stem cells from the lymphocytes. He later modified the technique, using only the soybean lectin followed by rosetting with sheep erythrocytes (E rosetting). When a final separation using neuraminidase-treated sheep erythrocytes is done, the resulting separation of all postthymic cells, competent and incompetent, from the stem-cell population appears to be complete.

Again, we were in a situation in which the theoretical basis of the approach seemed solid but in which it was felt that a more comparable animal model than the mouse was needed before clinical application could be contemplated. Reisner found that the cynomolgus monkey had exactly the same sugar code on its cell surfaces as the human; therefore, he did the fractionation. Under cover of lethal irradiation, he transplanted his stem-cell fraction from monkey to monkey, and it worked. No GVH reaction was encountered, and the recipient monkeys were reconstituted hematologically.

With Reisner, Kapoor, and O'Reilly, we have now applied this technique, tested on the monkeys, in a series of some 10 clinical cases, all individuals with far-advanced and often complex diseases. Among them were patients with severe combined immunodeficiency diseases, recurrent leukemia, and other malignant and hematologic diseases. In nearly every case, the marrow transplantations free of dangerous lymphoid cells took, and in no case was there a GVH reaction.

It seems clear that with techniques either like that developed by Reisner and his colleagues or involving appropriate antibodies, the way is being opened to use

Figure 5

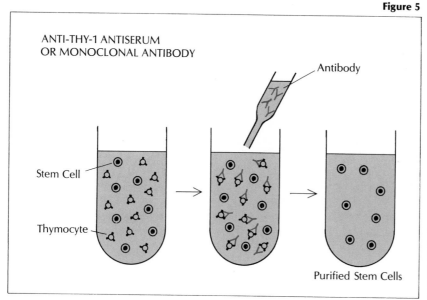

ANTI-THY-1 ANTISERUM
OR MONOCLONAL ANTIBODY

AGGLUTINATION

Antibody

Lectin

Stem Cell

Thymocyte

Purified Stem Cells

Three different approaches to the elimination of immunoin-
competent thymocytes from bone marrow stem–cell popula-
tions are depicted. Two involve specific antibody against Thy-1
determinants. The antibody could be derived either from rais-

bone marrow transplantation in the management of a much broader range of diseases. The elimination of GVH reactions would represent a major step in this direction simply by making it acceptable to use marrow transplantation in diseases that are not posing an immediate threat to the life of the patient. The full extent of the applicability, however, will not be understood until we have a greater understanding of the full functional range of bone marrow stem cells. We do know, of course, that their progeny includes all of the lymphocytic and monocytic cell lines, red blood cells, platelets, and other cellular components of the circulation. However, there is a growing body of evidence that these mesenchymal stem cells also subserve important informational functions with respect to other cells and perhaps even to epithelial organs and tissues.

For example, one of the diseases successfully treated by bone marrow transplantation is osteopetrosis. This is a condition (with both human and animal counterparts) in which the subject's osteoclasts are unable to remodel bone, so that osseous tissue progressively encroaches upon and fills the marrow cavity. As a result, the environment

for hematopoiesis is lost, and bone interrupts neural pathways, so that deafness, blindness, and eventually death result. After bone marrow transplantation in both animal subjects and human patients, bone remodeling capacity is restored and the disease is reversed.

This phenomenon can be interpreted as representing a local extension of the benefits of marrow transplantation because it is impossible to view the beneficial effects as being the by-products of improving the immediately adjacent bone marrow environment. Nevertheless, it is the functional defect of osteoclasts that seems to be corrected, suggesting that the transplanted stem cells may be fulfilling a role both in providing precursors of osteoclasts and in creating an appropriate environment for hematopoiesis.

Such a communications role is also implied in the effects of bone marrow transplantation on children with SCID. Almost without exception, these children have extremely underdeveloped thymuses, both functionally and morphologically. However, when they receive allogeneic bone marrow to correct their lymphocyte defects, there is an accompanying development of the thymic epithelial tissue, so that

the thymus is now able to secrete hormones normally. It certainly would appear that in some still undefined way, the mesenchyma is "talking" to the epithelium, directing it to develop and to subserve its endocrine functions.

These phenomena are not limited to the immunologic system. During the course of experimentation with total lymphoid irradiation by H. S. Kaplan's group at Stanford, S. Slavin gave bone marrow transplants to animals that lacked β-glucuronidase activity and discovered that the transplantation corrected that enzyme deficiency.

In this case the enzyme involved is probably produced by cells derived directly from the bone marrow, so the correction might be simply another stem-cell differentiation effect. However, observations related to another enzyme seem to suggest activity not at all linked to bone marrow in the traditional sense. The experiment was one of a series performed by H. Jyonouchi, P. W. Kincade, Fernandes, and me (see Figure 6, page 368). We studied BALB/c mice, which have high serum lipase levels, and transplanting their bone marrow into B6 mice, which have low lipase levels, and vice versa. We found that the recipient animals demonstrated low

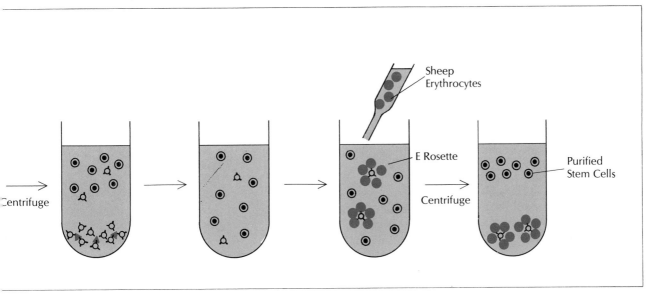

Sheep Erythrocytes

E Rosette

Purified Stem Cells

Centrifuge

Centrifuge

ing a specific antiserum or through the production of appropriate monoclonal antibodies. The third uses a double agglutina- *tion approach, in which the initial separation employs a plant (soybean) lectin, and final purification requires E rosetting.*

serum lipase levels appropriate for low lipase levels in the genetically dominant B6 mice. It should be emphasized that the lipase is produced in and secreted by the pancreas and perhaps a little bit by the liver. The secretory cells are not in any known way produced by marrow cells or cells derived from the marrow. The possibility that in some way the marrow is controlling the function of epithelial cells in the pancreas or liver must therefore be considered.

This consideration suggests a host of clinical possibilities for bone marrow transplantation. Certainly the safety that would come with definite obviation of the GVH risk would give physicians license to attempt bone marrow transplantation as treatment for such hematopoietic disease as thalassemia, and even for sickle cell disease, and for a variety of additional lymphoid and other neoplasias. But if bone marrow cells also function to control remote functions of epithelial cells, might not replacement have a therapeutic effect in enzymatic, hormonal, and even autoimmune diseases? Indeed, already evidence is at hand, from work done by Jyonouchi and Kincade in collaboration with Fernandes and me, that bone marrow transplantation from

appropriate donors resistant to autoimmune disease can correct all the known abnormalities of the autoimmunity-prone NZB mice. It seems certain that transplantation of bone marrow constitutes transplantation of significant components of the genome, and this newly introduced genetic information may be used to treat many different diseases.

This last speculation is even now not without experimental support. Let me return to the question of resistance genes mentioned previously in passing. The existence of resistance genes and susceptibility genes has long been accepted from studies done with inbred animal strains. For example, one of the characteristics of AKR mice is that they have an enormously high incidence of leukemia. CBA/H mice, on the other hand, have a low incidence of leukemia, as do C3HBi mice and C57BL/6 mice.

If one crosses AKR mice with CBA/H mice, the F_1 offspring have a low incidence of leukemia. We say this is so because the susceptibility genes possessed by the AKR mice are prevented from effective expression by resistance genes in the CBA/H mice. These resistance genes are expressed in another way. If the virus that causes leukemia is in-

jected into CBA/H mice, few of them get leukemia because they possess a resistance gene. With C57BL/6 mice, a similar capacity for resistance to leukemia can be attributed to resistance genes. Not so with C3H/Bi mice, which have low frequency of leukemia but which do not have resistance genes as demonstrated by either of the methods cited above. Indeed, the inoculation of leukemia virus into young C3H mice was the classic technique used by Ludwik Gross to produce his famous passage leukemia.

The critical question is: Can resistance genes be introduced by marrow transplantation? The answer seems to be: Yes, since bone marrow transplants to AKR mice from either CBA/H mice or C57BL/6 mice inhibit or completely prevent the development of leukemia, whereas bone marrow transplants from AKR or C3H donors do not seem to retard leukemogenesis at all, even though in each instance the recipient AKR mice are given the same irradiation treatment.

From the clinical point of view, of course, this understanding has had no impact as yet because we have no way of identifying human cancer resistance genes, assuming that

Figure 6

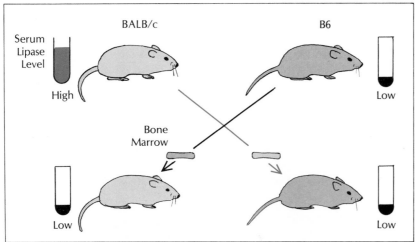

Serum lipase is produced by the liver and the pancreas, with no apparent relationship to bone marrow–derived cells. However, bone marrow transplants from B6 mice, who have low lipase levels, into BALB/c mice, with high lipase levels, will convert the BALB/c to the B6 lipase pattern. The reverse will not work, suggesting that the gene for low lipase is dominant. This and other experiments suggest the possibility of marrow-derived cells functioning in the control of enzymatic activity.

they exist. This is where the bone marrow and bone marrow transplantation come in. Many of the previously mentioned experiments by Kincade et al involved bone marrow transplantation between NZB mice and mice of other strains. The NZB mice are, of course, notorious for their susceptibility to a wide range of autoimmune diseases and malignancies. The experimenters found that by transplanting bone marrow from nonsusceptible strains into NZBs, all of the NZB abnormalities could

be inhibited from development. On the other hand, NZB marrow caused the development of the full range of abnormalities in otherwise unsusceptible animals. In this context, talk of genome transplantation does not seem at all farfetched.

This review has departed rather sharply from a basic consideration of immunologic reconstitution into much broader areas of cellular engineering. In doing so, it has frequently moved back and forth between the experimentally and clini-

cally documented aspects and the speculative aspects of the subject. However, it is my feeling that such speculation is justified by the truly dramatic enhancement of our ability to analyze and manipulate the systems that concern us. Some components of this enhancement have not even been mentioned, in part because they are covered elsewhere in this volume on immunopathology. An example is the whole subject of monoclonal antibodies (see M. D. Scharff, S. Roberts, and P. Thammana, "Hybridomas As a Source of Antibodies"), which have a huge potential for addressing such problems as GVH diseases and for analyzing the effector components of the immune system, so that the objectives of reconstitution can be ever more specifically defined and specified. In a sense, we are now at a stage comparable to that of 15 years ago when we "knew" that marrow transplantation had a role in the treatment of the congenital immunodeficiencies but could only hopefully speculate that they might play an even bigger part with respect to leukemias and other diseases. We now know that bone marrow transplantation is of value in leukemias and anemias, and in a variety of hematologic-immunologic disorders, and we can plot the pathways that may make it a safe and important approach to many seemingly unrelated diseases.

35

Managing the Immune System With Total Lymphoid Irradiation

SAMUEL STROBER   *Stanford University*

The limiting factor in our ability to replace irretrievably damaged organs and tissues by transplantation is the problem of immunologic rejection. Without treatment, the host's immune system mounts a rapidly destructive cytotoxic attack on the foreign tissues. Despite considerable research efforts aimed at this problem area, current clinical management of transplantation is almost entirely based on crude forms of immunosuppression using corticosteroids, cytotoxic drugs, and lymphocyte-depleting techniques. The agents used for immunosuppression have severe side effects, of which the most important may be nonspecific suppression of the host's defenses. Effective patient management requires an agile walking of the thin line between rejection and infection. Immunosuppressive therapy still forms the last line of attack on severe autoimmune diseases.

It is within this framework that one must place total lymphoid irradiation (TLI), a technique with potentially great clinical utility for the prevention of allograft rejection. When it is used to prepare graft recipients for transplantation, TLI seems to exact a markedly lower cost in side effects than other methods that achieve a comparable degree of immunosuppression. The greatest potential usefulness of TLI, however, stems not from its value as an immunosuppressive regimen but rather from its ability to induce specific tolerance. In animal models, TLI has permitted indefinite survival of grafted tissues while leaving the host capable of mounting an immune response against other antigens. TLI produces lasting changes in the regulation of the immune system and is clearly beneficial in

animal models of autoimmune diseases. Clinical trials now under way suggest its utility in the management of human autoimmunity.

Total lymphoid irradiation is a technique designed to deliver high doses of radiation to the lymphoid tissues while protecting radiosensitive nonlymphoid tissues. It was developed about 20 years ago by Henry Kaplan here at Stanford and soon became internationally accepted for the treatment of patients with early stages of Hodgkin's disease and certain non-Hodgkin's lymphomas. X-rays are targeted to lymph nodes in the cervical, axillary, mediastinal, para-aortic, inguinal, and iliac groups, as well as to the thymus and spleen, or splenic pedicle. Heavy lead blocks custom-tailored to the individual patient sharply delimit the radiation field in order to shield the kidneys, lungs, central nervous system, bone marrow, gonads, etc.

The total radiation dose in TLI is delivered in multiple fractions over a period of weeks. First, the target tissues above the diaphragm are irradiated. This radiation field is referred to as a "mantle" port. The usual course consists of about four fractions per week, at 150 to 250 rad per fraction, until the desired total is achieved. For Hodgkin's disease, the end point is about 4400 rad, although it appears that 2000 may suffice when the therapeutic goal is the induction of specific immunologic tolerance. Then the procedure is repeated for the target tissues below the diaphragm (a field called the "inverted-Y" port for obvious reasons) to the same total dose. This is a very substantial dose of radiation. The lethal single dose of whole-body irradiation for 50% of the human population is not much more than 400 rad. By shielding essential organs and fractionating the dose, we can deliver more than 10 times the LD_{50} to the lymphoid tissues.

Thanks to Kaplan's extensive clinical experience with TLI for treatment of Hodgkin's disease, we have excellent follow-up data on the morbidity of the procedure. We also have had abundant opportunity to follow the immune status of patients after TLI. These basic studies led to a remarkable conclusion: While the immunologic parameters we tested in irradiated Hodgkin's disease patients were as depressed as those of Stanford heart transplant recipients, who are immunosuppressed with a regimen that includes steroids, cytotoxic drugs, and antithymocyte globulin, the Hodgkin's patients had less morbidity resulting from their treatment. In particular, the incidence of severe bacterial and viral infections was much less in the Hodgkin's patients than in the transplant group. We can explain this, at least in part, by the fact that TLI has far less marrow toxicity than conventional immunosuppression, simply because it can be selectively targeted so as to spare large portions of the bone marrow.

The morbidity of TLI can be described briefly. Kaplan developed this as an outpatient procedure, and less than 1% of patients who undergo TLI for Hodgkin's disease have complications severe enough to require hospitalization. Virtually all patients have moderate constitutional symptoms, such as fatigue, anorexia, diarrhea, abdominal pain, and general malaise, during the 10- to 12-week course of radiotherapy. In women, sterility is inevitable if the ovaries are irradiated, but this can be prevented by fixing the ovaries surgically, prior to TLI, into a position where they can be shielded. Another common problem is herpes zoster. About 30% of patients get herpes zoster within two years after the completion of therapy. Disseminated zoster occurs in about 0.3% of patients; in the rest, the disease is generally limited to a single dermatome and resolves within six weeks. Many patients who have TLI for Hodgkin's disease develop ab-

normalities in thyroid function tests, and about 20% become hypothyroid. When we give TLI for nonmalignant disease, we can shield the thyroid completely, and the incidence of hypothyroidism drops to a few percent. There is also an increased risk of thyroid cancer associated with thyroid irradiation. We have seen three cases in 544 patients given TLI for Hodgkin's disease and followed for 10 years, but we expect to see considerably less with more extensive shielding of the thyroid.

There are other complications of TLI that can be quite severe but occur rarely. Bone marrow depression, particularly neutropenia or thrombocytopenia, can occur. In most cases, declining counts are detected early and the radiotherapist will avert severe marrow depression by interrupting treatment to allow a recovery interval and then resuming treatment at a lower dose per fraction. Radiation pneumonitis, carditis, or enteritis in severe enough form to require hospitalization occurs in a few tenths of a percent of TLI patients. Severe bacterial or viral infection occurs in less than 1%, and the incidence in Hodgkin's disease patients who have had TLI is not significantly greater than that attributable to splenectomy, which most of them undergo at the time of staging. Leukemia and other malignancies do not occur as complications of TLI alone, but TLI used in conjunction with chemotherapy for lymphomas does raise the risk of leukemia. The drugs that appear to interact with TLI to increase the incidence of leukemia are the alkylating agents, of which the ones most commonly used in Hodgkin's disease are nitrogen mustard and cyclophosphamide. The latter is also used as an immunosuppressive. These drugs are associated with an increased incidence of cancer when used alone, and TLI may act synergistically to amplify their carcinogenic effect.

Manifold alterations in immune function are seen in patients who have received TLI for Hodgkin's disease. By the end of the course of

TLI therapy, there is a profound depletion of lymphocytes in the peripheral blood. The lymphocyte count then rises gradually and stabilizes near the normal value about two years after treatment. There are, however, lasting changes in the lymphocyte subpopulations, since the percentage of T lymphocytes stabilizes at about half the pretreatment value and the percentage of B cells is doubled. This reversal of the usual ratio of T and B cells persists for at least 10 years after TLI. The response of peripheral blood lymphocytes to phytohemagglutinin drops after TLI and remains depressed for at least 10 years.

The mixed leukocyte reaction (MLR) is completely eliminated by TLI and remains undetectable for almost two years, but then it gradually returns to normal by about five years after treatment. Those patients capable of mounting a delayed hypersensitivity skin reaction to dinitrochlorobenzene lose their reactivity by the end of TLI. The majority then regain reactivity by one year after treatment, but about 30% remain anergic as long as they are followed. The findings noted in this paragraph led us to hope that TLI might be a practical means of immunosuppression for organ transplantation. The MLR has long been considered an in vitro counterpart of both graft rejection and graft-versus-host reactions. The other depleted immunologic functions are the main concomitants of cellular immunity, which, of course, plays a basic role in transplantation reactions.

Members of my laboratory, in collaboration with those in Kaplan's, embarked on animal studies of TLI in relationship to organ transplantation. In mice, the findings shortly after TLI are similar to those in humans. Lymphocytes virtually disappear from the peripheral blood, and the spleen, lymph nodes, and thymus shrink to about a tenth of normal size. The phytohemagglutinin response and MLR are both suppressed, but MLR returns over two to three months. B lymphocytes begin to reappear in peripheral blood during the second week, and T cells come back during the second month; as in humans, the ratio of B cells to T cells is permanently increased. Furthermore, there are changes within the T-cell subsets. A new subpopulation is found, which is identified by the presence of the thymus-leukemia (TL) antigen. This is ordinarily a surface marker for very immature T lymphocytes, and in normal animals it can be detected on T cells in the thymus but not in peripheral lymphoid tissues. Within a few days after total lymphoid irradiation is completed, one finds that about half the T lymphocytes in the spleen and lymph nodes carry the TL marker. This change persists throughout the one-year follow-up period. From surface markers alone, then, we can conclude that TLI induces long-lasting changes in the balance of the various lymphocyte subpopulations.

The results of functional studies are even more intriguing; they show the dominance of suppressor cell populations shortly after TLI. Israel Zan-Bar, who studied the antibody response in my laboratory, found both nonspecific and specific suppressor cells.

For a period of at least 100 days after TLI, mice can be specifically tolerized to bovine serum albumin (BSA) injected intraperitoneally without adjuvant. These mice fail to make an antibody response to a subsequent injection of dinitrophenylated BSA (DNP-BSA) in Freund's adjuvant. Mice treated with TLI alone can mount an antibody response to DNP-BSA, whereas the response is minimal in mice given TLI and then tolerized to BSA. The BSA-tolerized mice, however, can still respond to other antigens, such as DNP conjugated to bovine gamma globulin (DNP-BGG). Spleen cells from mice tolerized in this manner showed specific suppressing properties in what is called an adoptive transfer system.

In this system, mice were given a single dose of sublethal whole-body irradiation, and their ability to respond to DNP-BSA was artificially reconstituted by giving DNP-primed

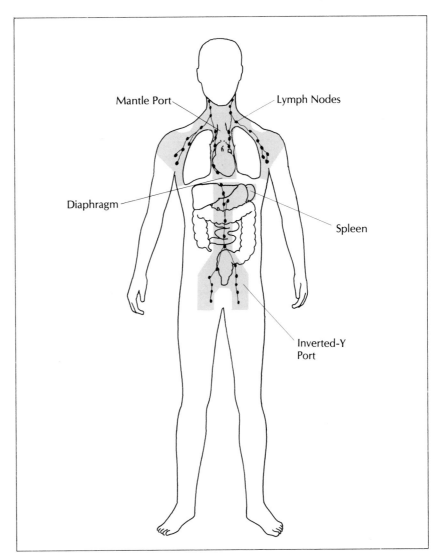

Clinically, total lymphoid irradiation (TLI) is administered to two fields. One field encompasses lymphoid tissues above the diaphragm with radiation delivered to the "mantle" port. The other involves such tissues, including the spleen, below the diaphragm via an "inverted-Y" port. By appropriate shielding, a dose approximating 10 times the human whole-body LD_{50} can be administered to lymphoid structures.

B cells and BSA-primed T cells from animals of the same strain that had been immunized with the appropriate antigens a few months earlier. The combination of primed B and T cells enabled the irradiated animals to mount a vigorous antibody response when they were challenged with DNP-BSA. Zan-Bar showed that by giving T lymphocytes from the spleens of animals tolerized to BSA, along with the primed T and B cells from normal animals, the antibody response was suppressed. When the adoptive transfer system was set up for DNP-

BGG, however, by using DNP-primed B cells, BGG-primed T cells, and a DNP-BGG challenge, spleen cells from a mouse tolerized to BSA had little effect on the antibody response. Larger doses of cells from the spleen of an animal given TLI without tolerization nonspecifically suppressed the antibody response to either DNP-BSA or DNP-BGG.

One also finds, in the period following TLI, a separate population of lymphocytes with the ability to suppress nonspecifically the mixed leukocyte reaction. These cells were characterized in my laboratory by

Donna King. As mentioned, for a period of time after TLI, the irradiated animal's spleen cells are incapable of responding in the MLR. We found, more surprisingly, that these cells are also incapable of acting as stimulator cells in the MLR with responder cells from another strain. This is due to the presence of cells with suppressor qualities rather than any loss of critical surface structures, as King showed in a series of MLR coculture experiments. Spleen cells from TLI-treated animals, when mixed with spleen cells from normal animals of the same strain, prevented the normal spleen cells from responding to foreign stimulator cells. In fact, spleen cells from TLI-treated animals prevented responder cells from virtually any strain from responding to stimulation by cells of any other strain. They not only prevented the proliferative response usually measured by tritiated thymidine uptake, they also prevented the generation of cytolytic T cells. The majority of these suppressor cells proved to be T lymphocytes, present in the spleen but not the lymph nodes. They are highly resistant to in vitro radiation; the suppressive effect is maximal at the earliest time point after TLI when one can harvest a significant number of cells, and it gradually disappears over the course of about 40 days after irradiation is stopped. Similar cells nonspecifically suppressing the MLR have been found in the blood of patients given TLI for Hodgkin's disease and rheumatoid arthritis.

King went on to look at the TL antigen and its association with these suppressor cells. To our surprise, she found that the cells that suppress the MLR—and are thus most closely related to the kind of immune response relevant to transplantation—are TL-negative. This was surprising because there is a considerable body of evidence in favor of the idea that immature T cells, when confronted with antigen, tend to become suppressors, while mature T cells should respond to antigen by turning into killer cells. The cells that suppress the development of humoral im-

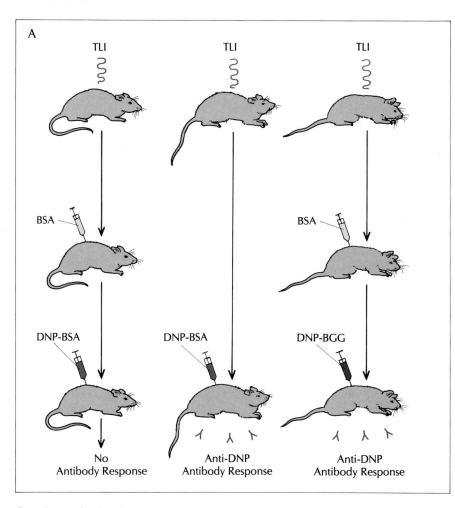

Experiments by Zan-Bar demonstrated that TLI permitted induction of both specific and nonspecific immunologic suppression, apparently mediated by separate subpopulations of suppressor T cells. First (panel A), mice were irradiated and within 100 days given bovine serum albumin (BSA) in saline. They were nonresponders to antigenic challenge with dinitrophenylated BSA (DNP-BSA) in adjuvant. Specificity was shown

munity, on the other hand, were indeed TL-positive. By performing a thymectomy on mice prior to TLI, one can prevent the development of this TL-positive population and of suppressor cells of the antibody response. The suppressors of the MLR develop despite pre-TLI thymectomy and may be relatively long lived.

As to why these suppressor cell populations dominate after TLI, we can only suppose that by virtue of differential radiosensitivity or influences on cell maturation, the balance between mutually interacting subsets of the immune system is profoundly altered. In this respect, it is well known that lymphocytes in general succumb more readily to radiation than most oth-

er cells, and it is reasonable to suppose that some kinds of lymphocytes are more, or less, radiosensitive than others. Indeed, King had shown that the splenic suppressor T cells functioning to blunt the MLR are relatively radioresistant. This kind of differential sensitivity may involve differences in the kind and amount of DNA repair enzymes the cell has at its disposal. Another factor that is probably more important for lymphocytes is the role of cell division in radiation toxicity. Cells whose function does not require cell division may continue to perform despite considerable radiation damage, whereas cells whose function involves proliferation are destroyed when they are activated

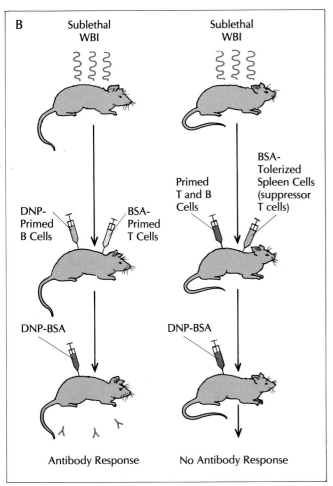

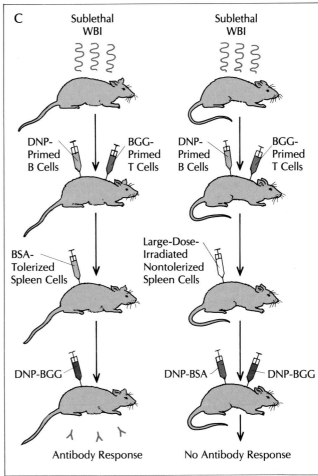

by either omitting tolerizing antigen or challenging with a different antigen, such as DNP with bovine gamma globulin (DNP-BGG). In both cases, the animals made antibody. Antibody responses could be reconstituted with specifically primed lymphocytes (panel B), and specifically tolerized suppressor T

cells again abolished the response. Finally (panel C), BSA-tolerized spleen cells left intact the response to DNP-BGG, but a large enough dose of nontolerized spleen cells apparently brought into play a nonspecific suppressor T-cell population, so that recipients were unable to respond to either DNP-BGG or DNP-BSA.

to undergo division. From a functional standpoint, the latter cell type may be inactivated even though it sustains no more molecular damage than the former. These considerations are based on cell destruction. Equally, the effects of TLI may result from influences on cell maturation and differentiation during the repopulation of lymphoid tissues rather than the cytoreductive phase. Since TLI lasts for weeks, the lymphoid tissues are exposed to radiation during repopulation after the initial reduction in cell mass. It may induce permanent changes in the lymphoid microenvironment as well, and these could affect the way lymphocytes differentiate and interact. In particular, it may alter non-

lymphoid cells that interact with lymphocytes.

In the light of our findings about the activity of suppressor cells following TLI, we concluded the procedure might have a value in transplantation far beyond that of an immunosuppressive. Other investigators have shown that the immune response in transplantation can be conceived in terms of two opposing arms. The aspect of the response that first comes to mind, of course, is the generation of cytotoxic T cells that mediate graft rejection and graft-versus-host disease. At the same time, however, the immune system generates antigen-specific suppressor T cells that down-regulate the process of

rejection. If one could find a method to block the generation of cytotoxic T cells temporarily, shut off the killer-cell arm, and at the same time leave the feedback-suppression arm intact, then one might permit the suppression arm to become predominant, with the development of a stable state of tolerance. This might be desirable in animals given a foreign bone marrow transplant. The host immune system ought to generate a population of antigen-specific suppressor T cells that would specifically prevent the host system from responding to donor antigens, while a population of donor-type suppressor cells specific for host antigens would arise to prevent transplanted lymphocytes from mounting a graft-versus-host response.

Total lymphoid irradiation appears to fulfill these needs. The TLI-treated animal has, for a limited period of time, a supply of cells that are potent nonspecific suppressors of the cytotoxic T-cell response. These cells, besides preventing the host from responding to donor antigens, can prevent donor cells from responding to the host. If the feedback-suppression arm of the immune response remains active, then TLI will permit chimerism in the host tissues, with mutual tolerance initially induced by nonspecific suppressor cells but maintained by antigen-specific suppressor cells generated during the period of "single-armed" immunologic activity.

Bone marrow transplantation experiments were performed in my laboratory by Shimon Slavin. He gave mice TLI immediately followed by bone marrow cells from a donor strain that was mismatched with the recipients at the major histocompatibility loci. The majority of the animals so treated accepted the marrow grafts and became stable chimeras, with functioning marrow of both the donor and host types. They had peripheral blood lymphocytes and erythrocytes of both host and donor types, in roughly equal amounts, 100 days after transplantation. The presence of donor cells after that interval implies that the host was tolerant to donor antigens and, indeed, we found that the chimeric mice would accept skin grafts from the donor strain indefinitely. The same mice promptly rejected skin grafts from a "third-party" strain that differed from both donor and host strains. In other words, by the end of the 100-day interval the host's tolerance of donor tissues was specific.

Equally remarkable in these experiments was the lack of graft-versus-host disease, implying that the immunologically active cells derived from the donor were tolerant of the host's antigens. In control marrow transplantation experiments, in which the recipients were prepared with lethal whole-body irradiation

instead of TLI, the host animals died within 60 days of typical graft-versus-host disease. Experiments with splenic lymphocytes, carried out by Michael Gottlieb during his stay in my laboratory, confirmed that the donor-type lymphocytes in chimeric mice are specifically tolerant of host antigenic determinants and not merely nonspecifically suppressed. Recipient mice were prepared by sublethal whole-body irradiation, then transfused with donor-type spleen cells. Spleen cells from normal donor-type mice invariably killed the hosts with graft-versus-host disease. Donor-type spleen cells from chimeric mice, however, which were purified by killing off the host-type cells with antiserum and complement, caused no graft-versus-host disease in host-type mice.

These transplantation experiments, along with in vitro experiments using lymphocytes from the chimeras, showed clearly that in mice TLI does, indeed, permit us to combine the immune systems of two animals with the development of specific mutual tolerance. We also carried out the same experiments in rats, extending them to include heart transplantation. After TLI in conjunction with marrow transplantation, we sutured a heart from a rat of the donor strain to the abdominal aorta and vena cava of the marrow recipient. In this position, the function of the grafted heart could be checked by electrocardiography and palpation. Four of five such transplanted hearts continued to function for more than 300 days.

We experimented with mongrel dogs in our next step toward clinical application. We have had uniform success in transplanting bone marrow in dogs treated with TLI. They become chimeras without any signs of graft-versus-host disease. Attempts to transplant the donor's heart along with bone marrow in collaboration with members of the heart transplantation unit at Stanford, however, were unsuccessful. The donor heart was rejected despite marrow chimerization in most cases. This may be due in part to

the dog's limited tolerance for radiation, which required us to limit the radiation dose in TLI to 1800 rad. Another possible explanation for the difficulties encountered with these large outbred animals is that they may have polymorphic organ-specific transplantation antigens, so that tolerization to bone marrow would not necessarily tolerize to heart or vascular endothelial antigens from the same donor. Our limited success using marrow transplants to tolerize dogs for organ transplants led us to try a wide variety of combination transplant regimens, using TLI to prepare the host, in conjunction with antithymocyte globulin (ATG) and immunosuppressive drugs. To our surprise, we have been able to obtain long-term graft survival with a regimen that does not involve marrow transplantation, which we originally tried as a control in a marrow tolerization experiment. Cardiac transplantation one day after TLI is followed by six doses of ATG and a three-month course of azathioprine. At the end of 90 days, all immunosuppressive therapy is discontinued. Some of these dogs have been followed for more than a year now, and in the two longest survivors, we transplanted a third-party heart into the abdomen. The dogs rejected the third heart within two weeks, while the second heart continued to function. A comparable regimen of ATG and azathioprine without TLI does not permit graft survival for more than five weeks. These experiments show that large outbred animals are different from mice in ways very important for organ-transplant tolerance, but these do not preclude the possibility of successful tolerization.

Human organ transplantation is, of course, a much more difficult area in which to experiment. One problem is the unpredictability of the exact time when a transplantable organ will become available. In mice, for example, if marrow transplantation is performed one week after the completion of TLI, only about 50% of the animals will become chimeric, as opposed to nearly 100% when the delay is a single day. The recovery of immunologic function after TLI is much faster in the mouse than in man, however, so we have no reliable estimate of the duration of TLI's effects on transplant tolerance in man. Our tentative protocols employ a compromise solution we call a "back-burner" regimen: a core dose of radiation that stops somewhere short of the target dose, followed by ongoing treatment at one or two fractions per week. This is designed to prolong the suppressor-dominated immunologic state until a donor organ becomes available.

The only published clinical trial of TLI for allograft survival in humans was carried out by J. Najarian's renal-transplant group at the University of Minnesota. They used TLI to supplement the regular immunosuppressive regimen of prednisone and azathioprine in patients who had already rejected at least one kidney allograft and, therefore, were at high risk for early rejection of another. They used a back-burner regimen with a total dose of 3000 to 4000 rad. In some patients they transplanted marrow from the same donor along with the kidney. Postoperatively, they followed the usual procedure of giving prednisone and azathioprine in initially high doses tapered to a lower level, which is maintained indefinitely.

By comparison with comparable patients treated earlier without TLI, the 23 patients in this group had substantially better graft survival. Two children suffered a very severe form of infectious mononucleosis and died. Graft rejection episodes have been rare, and most patients have not had irreversible graft rejection. We do not know whether any of these patients have become specifically tolerant to their grafts. The only way to find out would be to withdraw all nonspecific immunosuppressive therapy—a sort of trial by fire that would be difficult to justify.

A very important point is that the protocol Najarian's group used was designed around TLI as an adjunctive immunosuppressive regimen, rather than a tolerogenic one. Although there is no question that

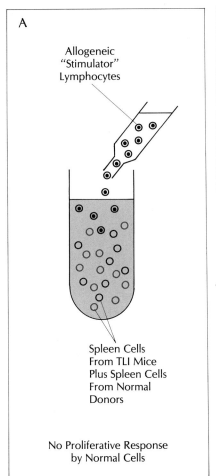

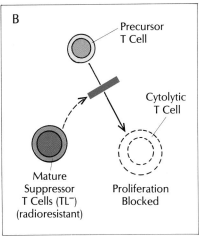

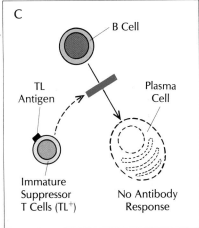

Experiments by King showed that the suppressor T cells following TLI were able to prevent stimulation of normal spleen cells by allogeneic spleen cells in mixed leukocyte reaction (MLR) cocultures (A). Further analysis showed that inhibition of T-cell proliferation was a function of mature (TL⁻) suppressors (B), while inhibition of antibody responsivity was effected by immature (TL⁺) suppressor T lymphocytes (C).

TLI is powerfully immunosuppressive and that it compares quite favorably in terms of efficacy and morbidity, both with conventional pharmacologic immunosuppression and with other experimental techniques, such as thoracic duct drainage, its greatest significance for organ transplantation lies in its potential for tolerization. This would permit one to do away with ongoing immunosuppressive therapy and leave the patient with a functional immune system. For this reason, the work with TLI in organ transplantation at Stanford is directed at tolerization. One implication of this emphasis is that we intend to apply TLI only to patients who have not been exposed to foreign anti-

gens in the form of prior rejected transplants or multiple blood and blood product transfusions. This decision stems from animal studies in which we found that an animal primed to minor antigenic determinants by blood transfusion prior to TLI can no longer be tolerized to transplanted tissues bearing those determinants.

The other major area in which TLI holds promise as a substantial improvement over currently available therapy is autoimmune disease. We have used TLI in three animal models of autoimmune disease: The lupuslike disease of NZB/NZW mice, the lymphoproliferative autoimmune disease of MRL/l mice, and adjuvant arthritis in rats. We have also used it clinically in patients with severe intractable rheumatoid arthritis. I will speculate on just why TLI has the effects we have observed in autoimmune diseases.

The autoimmune disease of NZB/NZW mice is similar to human lupus erythematosus in that the mice generate anti-DNA antibodies and develop an immune-complex glomerulonephritis. Glomerulonephritis is usually the cause of death. Brian Kotzin, in my laboratory, administered the usual mouse TLI protocol to NZB/NZW mice that had already developed proteinuria and found that the treatment could reverse proteinuria, decrease titers of anti-DNA antibodies, and markedly prolong the animals' life relative to untreated littermates. He also found that TLI prolonged the survival of mice selected for advanced disease prior to treatment. These findings are particularly significant, since most other immunosuppressive methods can prevent the disease from developing if administered before the mice become ill but have little effect once proteinuria is present.

We have experiments in progress aimed at determining just how TLI-induced changes lead to improvement in this disease. There may be an element of specific tolerization to one or more autoantigens, or the effect may depend on the persistent TL-positive cells that nonspecifically suppress the antibody response. It has been shown that these mice have deficiencies of suppressor T cells, and the disease can thus be viewed as one of immune regulation. Our understanding at present is that 1) TLI brings about a new balance between immune phenomena that interact to regulate the immune response; 2) in autoimmune disease the phenomena are out of balance, so to speak; and 3) TLI, perhaps in large part by favoring suppressor cells, swings the balance back in the direction of tolerance of self. This admittedly somewhat vague explanation of what takes place is more appropriate than simpler descriptions of tolerization or suppression of antibody production, because regulation of the immune response is clearly a complicated process of which only the rudiments are understood. TLI causes multiple changes, and more than one of these may be involved in any net result we observe.

Another likely example of rebalancing of the immune system is provided by the model of MRL/l mice, which was studied in my laboratory by Kotzin in collaboration with A. Theofilopoulos and F. Dixon at the Research Institute of Scripps Clinic. In addition to glomerulonephritis, these mice spontaneously develop massive lymphoid proliferation and usually die with extreme splenomegaly and lymph nodes enlarged on the order of tenfold to a hundredfold. TLI given at the time of disease onset prevents glomerulonephritis from developing in most of the mice and prolongs their lives so that 100% are still alive at an age when 92% of the nonirradiated controls are dead.

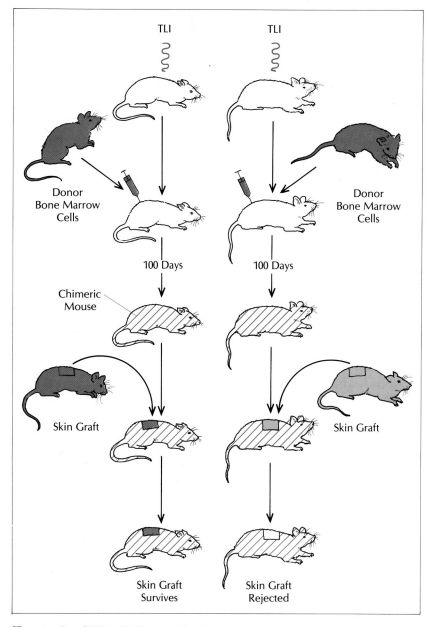

The capacity of TLI to facilitate stable chimerism was shown by Slavin. Irradiated host mice, transfused with bone marrow cells from donor mice of another strain, accepted skin grafts from the donor strain but rapidly rejected grafts from a third strain.

(Interestingly, whole-body irradiation has similar but less pronounced effects.) The most striking difference between the treated and untreated animals is that the typical pathologic lymphoproliferation is virtually eliminated in the irradiated group. It appears that the irradiated animals have suppressor T-cell function approximately equal to that of controls but helper T-cell function that is far less vigorous. Again, there has been some sort of regulatory dysfunction leading to a signal for lymphoproliferation, and radiotherapy somehow turns that signal off.

Our animal model of an inflammatory arthritis, adjuvant arthritis in rats, is an immunologic disease induced by giving the rats subcutaneous injections of *Mycobacterium butyricum* in oil. Within two weeks, the animals' joints are swollen and red, and they begin to have difficulty getting around their cages. The inflammation lasts about 60 to 100 days, by which time there is considerable ankylosis of the joints. In collaboration with David Schurman in our Division of Orthopedic Surgery, we compared TLI, local joint irradiation, the combination of the two, and untreated controls. There was a dramatic reduction in symptoms in the TLI group while the treatment went on, but arthritis scores in these rats rose to pretreatment levels shortly after TLI was completed. (This still represented considerable improvement relative to controls, which deteriorated progressively.) Local irradiation alone produced a somewhat smaller degree of improvement at first, with similar late results. Combination therapy was far and away the most successful, reducing the amount of inflammation and minimizing the ultimate joint damage as evaluated roentgenographically. The important contribution of local irradiation in this disease is probably related to the numbers and kinds of lymphocytes in the paws, which are not exposed to TLI.

With these animal studies in hand, we began to test TLI in humans with refractory rheumatoid arthritis. When the disease resists treatment by conventional agents, including nonsteroidal anti-inflammatories, penicillamine, and gold salts, the patients become candidates for treatment with cytotoxic drugs, such as azathioprine and cyclophosphamide. Since the morbidity of these drugs exceeds that expected of TLI, we began therapeutic pilot studies, first with lymphoid irradiation restricted to the subdiaphragmatic tissues and then, when that approach had apparently beneficial effects and little morbidity, with complete TLI to a dose of 2000 rad. Eleven patients have now completed TLI with follow-up sufficient for preliminary evaluation of results. Nine of them have had a marked clinical improvement in terms of joint tenderness, swelling, function, and morning stiffness. In follow-up to 20 months, there has been no obvious tendency to relapse. It must be emphasized that this is a pilot study and does not establish that TLI is effective therapy for intractable rheumatoid arthritis. To achieve that goal, we must follow this with a randomized, controlled, double-blind prospective study and obtain data for a longer follow-up period.

To summarize the status of TLI: It is a method whose use was limited for many years to the treatment of malignant disease but which is now in the process of being introduced for the management

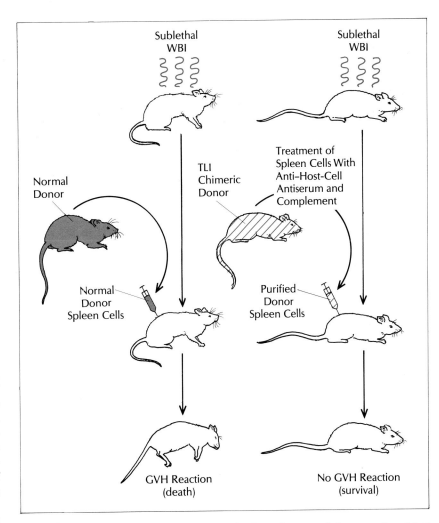

Irradiation-facilitated chimerism results in lasting tolerance of donor and recipient cells to each other. Thus, Gottlieb showed that an irradiated mouse, given spleen cells from a normal donor, dies of a graft-versus-host reaction, but if donor cells are from a TLI chimera, then purified donor cells do not produce the reaction.

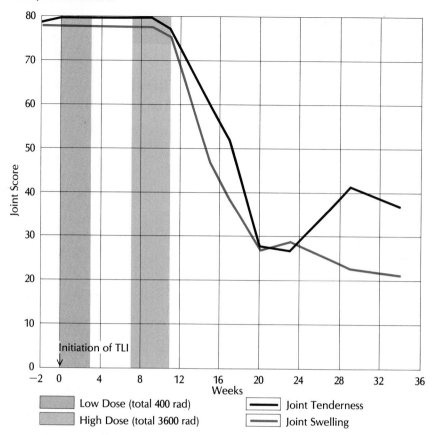

Subdiaphragmatic lymphoid irradiation has been used in treatment of refractory rheumatoid arthritis. Effects in one patient are graphed. Substantial benefit has been achieved in nine of 11 patients given TLI with a total dose of 2000 rad. (Adapted from Strober et al, Int J Radiat Oncol Biol Phys)

of unwanted immune reactions in the areas of both transplant tolerance and autoimmune disease. It induces both transient and permanent changes in the immune system and seems to favor suppressor functions at the expense of effector ones. In the case of transplant tolerance, we have a theoretical model that accounts nicely for the phenomena observed in mice, although we cannot yet satisfactorily explain everything that happens when we apply it to larger animals. In autoimmune disease, it may work by causing specific tolerance or nonspecific immunosuppression, or by a combination of these effects. Studies are under way to elucidate a better understanding of what TLI does, to use it to dissect and study the immune system, and to apply it in the management of clinical problems in organ transplantation, rheumatoid arthritis, and lupus nephritis.

Selected Readings
Index
Illustration and Data Source Credits

Selected Readings

CHAPTER 1

Taub R et al: Translocation of the c-myc gene into the immunoglobulin heavy chain locus in human Burkitt's lymphoma and murine plasmacytoma cells. Proc Natl Acad Sci USA 79:7837, 1982

Leder P: The genetics of antibody diversity. Sci Am 246:102, May 1982

Kirsch IR et al: Human immunoglobulin in heavy chain genes map to a region of translocations in malignant B lymphocytes. Science 216:301, 1982

Hieter PA et al: Evolution of human immunoglobulin κ J region genes. J Biol Chem 257:1516, 1982

Korsmeyer SJ et al: Developmental hierarchy of immunoglobulin gene rearrangements in human leukemic pre-B cells. Proc Natl Acad Sci USA 78:7096, 1981

Kirsch IR et al: Multiple immunoglobulin switch region homologies outside the heavy chain constant region locus. Nature 293:585, 1981

Leder P et al: Recombination events that activate, diversify, and delete immunoglobulin genes. Cold Spring Harbor Symp Quant Biol XLV:859, 1981

Yaoita Y, Honjo T: Detection of immunoglobulin heavy chain genes from expressed allelic chromosomes. Nature 286:850, 1980

Rogers J et al: Two mRNAs with different 3' ends encode membrane-bound and secreted form of immunoglobulin μ chain. Cell 20:303, 1980

Hozumi N, Tonegawa S: Evidence for somatic rearrangement of immunoglobulin genes coding for variable and constant regions. Proc Natl Acad Sci USA 73:3628, 1976

CHAPTER 2

Ishizaka T, Ishizaka K: Biology of immunoglobulin E: Molecular basis of reaginic hypersensitivity. Prog Allergy 19:60, 1975

Spiegelberg HL: Biological activities of immunoglobulins of different classes and subclasses. Adv Immunol 19:259, 1974

Capra JD, Kehoe JM: Hypervariable regions, idiotype and the antibody combining site. Adv Immunol 20:1, 1975

Cohn S, Porter RR: Structure and biological activity of immunoglobulins. Adv Immunol 4:287, 1964

CHAPTER 3

Benacerraf B, Katz DH: The nature and function of histocompatibility-linked immune response genes. In Immunogenetics and Immunodeficiency, Benacerraf B (Ed). Medical and Technical Publishing Co, Ltd, London, 1975

Katz DH, Benacerraf B: The function and interrelationships of T-cell receptors, Ir genes and other histocompatibility gene products. Transplant Rev 22:175, 1975

McDevitt HO et al: Ir genes and antigen recognition. In The Immune System: Genes, Receptors, Signals, Sercarz EE, Williamson A, Fox CF (Eds). Academic Press, New York, 1974

Katz DH, Benacerraf B: The regulatory influence of activated T cells on B cell responses to antigen. Adv Immunol 15:2, 1972

Katz DH: Adaptive differentiation of lymphocytes: Theoretical implications for mechanisms of cell-cell recognition and regulation of immune responses. Adv Immunol 29:137, 1980

CHAPTER 4

Möller G (Ed): Immunology and differentiation. Immunol Rev, vol 33, 1977

Evans RL et al: Detection, isolation, and functional characterization of two human T-cell subclasses bearing unique differentiation antigens. J Exp Med 145:221, 1977

Gershon RK: T-cell suppression. Contemp Top Immunobiol 3:1, 1974

CHAPTER 5

Germain RN, Benacerraf B: Helper and suppressor T cell factors. Springer Semin Immunopathol 3:93, 1980

Germain RN, Benacerraf B: A single major pathway of T-lymphocyte interactions in antigen-specific immune suppression. Scand J Immunol 13:1, 1981

Gershon KK: T cell control of antibody production. In Contemporary Topics in Immunobiology Series, vol 3, Cooper M, Warner N (Eds). Plenum Press, New York, 1974, p 1

Möller G (Ed): Suppressor T lymphocytes. Transplant Rev, vol 26, 1975

Benacerraf B, Germain RN: The immune response genes of the major histocompatibility complex. Immunol Rev 28:70, 1978

Pierce CW, Kapp JA: Suppressor T cells. In Contemporary Topics in Immunobiology Series, vol 5, Weigle WO (Ed). Plenum Press, New York, 1976, p 91

Benacerraf B et al: The I region genes in genetic regulation. ICN-UCLA Symposia on Molecular and Cellular Biology, vol 6, 1977, p 363

Murphy DB: The I-J subregion of the murine H-2 gene complex. Seminars in Immunopathology, vol 1, 1978

CHAPTER 6

Perlmann P, Cerottini J-C: Cytotoxic lymphocytes. In The Antigens, vol 5, Sela M (Ed). Academic Press, New York, 1979

Berke G: Interaction of cytotoxic T lymphocytes and target cells. Prog Allergy, vol 27, 1980

Cerottini J-C, Brunner KT; Cell-mediated cytotoxicity, allograft rejection, and tumor immunity. *In* Advances in Immunology Series, vol 18, Dixon FJ, Kunkel HG (Eds). Academic Press, New York, 1974

Engers HD, MacDonald HR: Generation of cytolytic T lymphocytes in vitro. *In* Contemporary Topics in Immunobiology Series, vol 5, Weigle WO (Ed). Plenum Press, New York, 1976

CHAPTER 7

Herberman RB, Ortaldo JR: Natural killer cells: Their role in defenses against disease. Science 214:24, 1981

Herberman RB (Ed): Natural Cell-Mediated Immunity Against Tumors. Academic Press, New York, 1980

Möller G (Ed): Natural killer cells. Immunol Rev, vol 44, 1979

Kiessling R, Haller O: Natural killer cells in the mouse: An alternative immune surveillance mechanism? Contemp Top Immunobiol 8:171, 1978

CHAPTER 8

Rosenthal AS, Shevach EM: The function of macrophages in antigen recognition by guinea pig T lymphocytes. J Exp Med 138:1194, 1973

Unanue ER: Secretory function of mononuclear phagocytes. Am J Pathol 83:395, 1976

Unanue ER: The regulation of lymphocyte functions by the macrophage. Immunol Rev 40:227, 1978

Karnovsky ML, Lazdins JK: Biochemical criteria for activated macrophages. J Immunol 121:809, 1978

Mackaness GB: The influence of immunologically committed lymphoid cells on macrophage activity in vivo. J Exp Med 129:973, 1969

Polverini PJ, Cotran RS, Gimbrone MA Jr, Unanue ER: Activated macrophages induce vascular proliferation. Nature 269:804, 1977

CHAPTER 9

Möller G (Ed): The immune response to infectious disease. Transplant Rev, vol 19, 1974

Möller G (Ed): Specificity of effector T-lymphocytes. Transplant Rev, vol 29, 1976

Dausset J, Svejgaard A (Eds): HLA and Disease. Williams & Wilkins Co, Baltimore, 1977

Notkins AL (Ed): Viral Immunology and Immunopathology. Academic Press, New York, 1975

Stutman O (Ed): T Cells. *In* Contemporary Topics in Immunobiology Series, vol 7. Plenum Press, New York, 1977

Zinkernagel RM, Doherty PC: MHC–restricted cytotoxic T cells: Studies on the biological role of polymorphic major transplantation antigens determining T-cell restriction specificity, function and responsiveness. Adv Immunol 27:51, 1979

CHAPTER 10

Louis JA, Weigle WO: A model of immunologic unresponsiveness and its relevance to autoimmunity. *In* Pathobiology Annual, Ioachim HL (Ed). Appleton-Century-Crofts, New York, 1976

Pierce CW, Kapp JA: Regulation of immune responses by suppressor T cells. *In* Contemporary Topics in Immunobiology, vol 5, Weigle WO (Ed). Plenum Press, New York, 1976

Weigle WO: Immunological unresponsiveness. *In* Advances in Immunology Series, vol 16, Dixon FJ, Kunkel HG (Eds). Academic Press, New York, 1973

Coutinho A, Möller G: Thymus-independent B-cell induction and paralysis. *In* Advances in Immunology Series, vol 21, Dixon FJ, Kunkel HG (Eds). Academic Press, New York, 1975

Howard JG, Mitchison NA: Immunological tolerance. Prog Allergy, vol 18, 1975

Ortiz-Ortiz L, Weigle WO: Cellular events in the induction of allergic encephalomyelitis in rats. J Exp Med 144:604, 1976

Weigle WO: Analysis of autoimmunity through experimental models of thyroiditis and allergic encephalomyelitis. *In* Advances in Immunology Series, vol 30, Dixon FJ, Kunkel HG (Eds). Academic Press, New York, 1980

CHAPTER 11

de Sousa M: Lymphocyte Circulation: Experimental and Clinical Aspects. John Wiley & Sons Inc, Chichester, England, 1981

de Sousa M: Ecotaxis, ecotaxopathy, and lymphoid malignancy: Terms, facts and predictions. *In* The Immunopathology of Lymphoreticular Neoplasms, Twomey JJ, Good RA (Eds). Plenum Publishing Corp, New York, 1978, chap 11

de Sousa M et al: Ecotaxis: The principle and its application to the study of Hodgkin's disease. Clin Exp Immunol 27:143, 1977

de Sousa M et al: Suggested models of ecotaxopathy in lymphoreticular malignancy. Am J Pathol 90:497, February 1978

de Sousa M: Cell traffic. *In* Receptors and Recognition, vol 2, Cuatrecasas P, Greaves MF (Eds). Chapman and Hall, London, 1976

de Sousa M: Lymphoid cell positioning: A new proposal for the mechanism of control of lymphoid cell migration. *In* Cell-Cell Recognition, Curtis ASG (Ed). Cambridge University Press, Cambridge, 1978

de Sousa M, Good RA: T- and B-cell populations in gut and gut-associated lymphoid organs: Arrangement, migration, and function. *In* Gastrointestinal Tract Cancer, Lipkin M, Good RA (Eds). Plenum Publishing Corp, New York, 1978

Blake DR et al: The importance of iron in rheumatoid arthritis. Lancet II:1142, 1981

de Sousa M et al: Migratory patterns of the Ly subsets of T lymphocytes in the mouse. *In* Function and Structure of the Immune System, Müller-Ruchholtz W, Müller-Hermelink HK (Eds). Plenum Publishing Corp, New York, 1979

de Sousa M et al: Immunologic parameters in childhood Hodgkin's disease: II. T and B lymphocytes in the peripheral blood of normal children and in the spleen and peripheral blood of children with Hodgkin's disease. Pediatr Res 12:143, 1978

CHAPTER 12

Osler AG: Complement: Mechanisms and Functions. Foundations of Immunology Series, Prentice-Hall, Inc, Englewood Cliffs, NJ, 1976

Müller-Eberhard HJ: Complement. Annu Rev Biochem 44: 697, 1975

Götz O, Müller-Eberhard HJ: The alternative pathway of complement activation. Adv Immunol 24:1, 1976

Cooper NR: The complement system. *In* Basic and Clinical Immunology, Fudenberg HH et al (Eds). Lange Medical Publications, Los Altos, Calif, 1976, p 58

Cooper NR, Ziccardi RJ: The nature and reactions of complement enzymes. *In* Proteolysis and Physiological Regulations, Ribbons DW, Breed K (Eds). Miami Winter Symposia 11, Academic Press, New York, 1976, p 167

Reid KBM, Porter RR: The structure and mechanism of activation of the first component of complement. *In* Contemporary Topics in Molecular Immunology Series, vol 4, Inman FP, Mandy WJ (Eds). Plenum Press, New York, 1975, p 1

Müller-Eberhard HJ, Schreiber RD: Molecular biology and chemistry of the alternative pathway of complement. Adv Immunol 29:1, 1980

Müller-Eberhard HJ: Complement reaction pathways. *In* Immunology 80, Progress in Immunology IV, Fougereau M, Dausset J (Eds). Academic Press, London, 1981, p 1001

Pangburn MK, Müller-Eberhard HJ: Relation of a putative thioester bond in C3 to activation of the alternative pathway and the binding of C3b to biological targets of complement. J Exp Med 152:1102, 1980

Pangburn MK, Schreiber RD, Müller-Eberhard HJ: Formation of the initial C3 convertase of the alternative complement pathway: Acquisition of C3b-like activities by spontaneous hydrolysis of the putative thioester in native C3. J Exp Med 154:856, 1981

CHAPTER 13

Fahraeus R: The suspension stability of the blood. Acta Med Scand 55:1, 1921

Gewurz H, Mold C, Sieger J, Fiedel B: C-reactive protein and the acute phase response. Adv Intern Med 27:345, 1982

Kushner I: The acute phase reactants and the erythrocyte sedimentation rate. *In* Textbook of Rheumatology, Kelley WN et al (Eds). WB Saunders Co, Philadelphia, 1981, p 669

Kushner I, Volanakis J, Gewurz H (Eds): C-Reactive Protein and the Plasma Protein Response to Tissue Injury: A Symposium, vol 389. New York Academy of Sciences, New York, 1982

Pepys MB: C-reactive protein fifty years on. Lancet I:653, 1981

Kaplan MH, Volanakis JE: Interaction of C-reactive protein complexes with the complement system: I. J Immunol 112:2135, 1974

Mold C et al: C-reactive protein is protective against *Streptococcus pneumoniae* infection in mice. J Exp Med 154:1703, 1981

Oliveira EB, Gotschlich EC, Liu T-Y: Primary structure of human C-reactive protein, J Biol Chem 254:489, 1979

CHAPTER 14

Korchak HM, Weissmann G: Changes in membrane potential of human granulocytes antecede the metabolic responses to surface stimulation. Proc Natl Acad Sci 75:3818, 1978

Hoffstein S, Weissmann G: Microfilaments and microtubules in calcium ionophore-induced secretion of lysosomal enzymes from human PMNs. J Cell Biol 78:769, 1978

Zurier RB, Hoffstein S, Weissmann G: Cytochalasin B: Effect on lysosomal enzyme release from human leukocytes. Proc Natl Acad Sci 70:844, 1973

Hoffstein S, Goldstein IM, Weissmann G: Role of microtubule assembly in lysosomal enzyme secretion from polymorphonuclear leukocytes: A re-evaluation. J Cell Biol 73:242, 1977

Zurier RB, Hoffstein S, Weissmann G: Mechanisms of lysosomal enzyme release from leukocytes. I. Effects of cyclic nucleotides and colchicine. J Cell Biol 58:27, 1973

Zurier RB et al: Mechanisms of lysosomal enzyme release from human leukocytes. II. Effects of cAMP and cGMP, autonomic agonists, and agents which affect microtubule function. J Clin Invest 53:297, 1974

Goldstein I, Hoffstein S, Gallin J, Weissmann G: Mechanisms of lysosomal enzyme release from human leukocytes: Microtubule assembly and membrane fusion induced by a component of complement. Proc Natl Acad Sci 70:2916, 1973

Goldstein IM, Cerqueira M, Lind S, Kaplan HB: Evidence that the superoxide generating system of human leukocytes is associated with the cell surface. J Clin Invest 59:249, 1977

Weissmann G, Smolen JE, Korchak HM: Release of inflammatory mediators from stimulated neutrophils. N Engl J Med 303:27, 1980

CHAPTER 15

Müller-Eberhard HJ: Chemistry and function of the complement system. Hosp Pract 12(8):33, 1977

Müller-Eberhard HJ: Complement: Molecular mechanisms, regulation and biologic function. *In* Molecular Basis of Biological Degradative Processes: Proceedings of the Dedication Symposium of the University of Connecticut, May 19–20, 1977, Berlin R et al (Eds). Academic Press, New York, 1978

Müller-Eberhard HJ: Complement. Annu Rev Biochem 44: 697, 1975

Day NK, Good RA (Eds): Biological Amplifications Systems in Immunology. Comprehensive Immunology Series, vol 2. Plenum Medical Book Co, New York, 1977

Hugli TE, Müller-Eberhard HJ: Anaphylatoxins: C3a and C5a. *In* Advances in Immunology Series, vol 26, Dixon FJ, Kunkel HG (Eds). Academic Press, New York, 1978, pp 1–53

Opferkuch W, Rother K, Schultz DR (Eds): Clinical Aspects of the Complement System. G Thieme, Stuttgart, 1978

Podack ER, Tschopp J: Polymerization of the ninth component of complement (C9): Formation of poly C9 with a tubular ultrastructure resembling the membrane attack complex of complement. Proc Natl Acad Sci USA 79:574, 1982

Podack ER, Tschopp J, Müller-Eberhard HJ: Molecular organization of C9 with the membrane attack complex of complement: Induction of circular C9 polymerization by the C5b-8 assembly. J Exp Med 156:268, 1982

Tschopp J, Müller-Eberhard HJ, Podack ER: Formation of transmembrane tubules by spontaneous polymerization of the hydrophilic complement protein C9. Nature 298:534, 1982

CHAPTER 16

Bodmer WF et al (Eds): Histocompatibility Testing 1977. Ejnar Munksgaard Forlag, Copenhagen, 1978

Terasaki PI (Ed): Histocompatibility Testing 1980. UCLA Tissue Typing Laboratory, Los Angeles, 1980

Benacerraf B, Dorf ME (Eds): The Role of the Major Histocompatibility Complex in Immunobiology. Garland Press, New York, 1980

Dausset J, Svejgaard A (Eds): HLA and Disease. Williams & Wilkins Co, Baltimore, 1977

Bodmer WF, Bodmer JG: Evolution and function of the HLA system. Br Med Bull 34:390, 1978

Ryder LP, Anderson E, Svejgaard A (Eds): HLA and Disease Registry, Third Report. Ejnar Munksgaard Forlag, Copenhagen, 1979

Engleman EG et al (Eds): Genetic control of the human immune response. J Exp Med 152(part 2):August 1980

Schaller JC, Omenn GS: The histocompatibility system and human disease. J Pediatr 88:913, 1976

CHAPTER 17

Old LJ: Cancer immunology: The search for specificity (GHA Clowes Memorial Lecture). Cancer Res 41:361, 1981

Old LJ, Stockert E: Immunogenetics of cell surface antigens of mouse leukemia. Annu Rev Genet 11:127, 1977

Oettgen HF: Host defense against cancer. In Cancer: Achievements, Challenges and Prospects for the 1980s, Burchenal JH, Oettgen HF (Eds). Grune & Stratton, New York, 1981, pp 309–330

Houghton AN, Oettgen HF, Old LJ: Malignant melanoma: Current status of the search for melanoma-specific antigens. In Immunodermatology, Safai B, Good RA (Eds). Plenum Publishing Corp, New York, 1981, pp 557–576

Livingston PO, Oettgen HF, Old LJ: Specific active immunotherapy in cancer therapy. In Immunological Aspects of Cancer Therapeutics, Mihich E (Ed). John Wiley & Sons, New York, 1981

Dippold WG et al: Cell surface antigens of human malignant melanoma: Definition of six antigenic systems with mouse monoclonal antibodies. Proc Natl Acad Sci USA 77:6114, 1980

CHAPTER 18

Siegal FP, Good RA: Human lymphocyte differentiation markers and their application to immune deficiency and lymphoproliferative diseases. Clin Haematol 6:355, 1977

Siegal FP, Filippa DA, Koziner B: Surface markers in leukemias and lymphomas. Am J Pathol 90:451, 1978

Lukes RJ, Collins RD: Immunologic characterization of human malignant lymphomas. Cancer 34:1488, 1974

Aisenberg AC, Bloch KJ, Long JC: Cell-surface immunoglobulin in chronic lymphocytic leukemia and allied disorders. Am J Med 55:184, 1973

Koziner B et al: Characterization of lymphomas in a leukemic phase by multiple differentiation markers of mononuclear cells: Correlation with clinical features and conventional morphology. Am J Med 63:556, 1977

McCaffrey R, Harrison TA, Parkman R, Baltimore D: Terminal deoxynucleotidyl transferase activity in human leukemic cells and in normal human thymocytes. N Engl J Med 292:775, 1975

Sen L, Borella L: Clinical importance of lymphoblasts with T markers in childhood acute leukemia. N Engl J Med 292:828, 1975

Brouet JC et al: Membrane markers in "histiocytic" lymphomas (reticulum cell sarcomas). J Natl Cancer Inst 56:631, 1976

Nathwani BN, Kim H, Rappaport H: Malignant lymphoma, lymphoblastic. Cancer 38:964, 1976

Fu SM, Winchester RJ, Kunkel HG: The occurrence of the HL-B alloantigens on the cells of unclassified acute lymphoblastic leukemias. J Exp Med 142:1334, 1975

Broder S et al: The Sézary syndrome: A malignant proliferation of helper T cells. J Clin Invest 58:1297, 1977

Vogler LB et al: Pre-B-cell leukemia: A new phenotype of childhood lymphoblastic leukemia. N Engl J Med 298:872, 1978

National Cancer Institute Sponsored Study of Classifications of Non-Hodgkin's Lymphomas. Summary and Description of a Working Formulation for Clinical Usage. Cancer 49:2112, 1982

Knapp W (Ed): Leukemia Markers. Academic Press, New York, 1981

CHAPTER 19

Wilson CB, Dixon FJ: The renal response to immunological injury. In The Kidney, Brenner BM, Rector FC (Eds). WB Saunders, Philadelphia, 1976, pp 838–940

Glassock RJ, Bennett CM: The glomerulopathies. In The Kidney, Brenner BM, Rector FC (Eds). WB Saunders, Philadelphia, 1976, pp 941–1078

Andres GA, McCluskey RT: Tubular and interstitial renal disease due to immunologic mechanisms. Kidney Int 7:271, 1975

Lockwood CM, Pussell B, Wilson CB, Peters DK: Plasma exchange in nephritis. Adv Nephrol 8:383, 1979

Wilson CB (Ed): Immunologic Mechanisms in Renal Disease. Contemporary Issues in Nephrology Series, vol 3, Brenner BM, Stein JH (Series Eds). Churchill Livingstone, New York, 1981

CHAPTER 20

Winslow CM, Austen KF: Enzymatic regulation of mast cell activation and secretion by adenylate cyclase and cyclic AMP-dependent protein kinases. Fed Proc 41(1):22, 1982

Caulfield JP et al: Secretion in dissociated human pulmonary mast cells. J Cell Biol 85:299, 1980

Weiss JW et al: Bronchoconstrictor effects of leukotriene C in humans. Science 216:196, 1982

Lewis RA, Austen KF: Mediation of local homeostasis and inflammation by leukotrienes and other mast-cell dependent compounds. Nature 293:103, 1981

Schwartz LB, Lewis RA, Austen KF: Tryptase from human pulmonary mast cells. J Biol Chem 256:11939, 1981

Razin E et al: Generation of leukotriene C₄ from a subclass of mast cells differentiated in vitro from mouse bone marrow. Proc Natl Acad Sci USA 79:4665, 1982

CHAPTER 21

Andrews BS et al: Spontaneous murine lupus-like syndrome: Clinical and immunopathologic comparisons in several kinds of mice. J Exp Med 148:1198, 1978

Theofilopoulos AN, Dixon FJ: Etiopathogenesis of murine SLE. Immunol Rev 55:179, 1981

Steinberg AD et al: The cellular and genetic basis of murine lupus. Immunol Rev 55:121, 1981

Creighton WD, Katz DH, Dixon FJ: Antigen-specific immunocompetency, B cell function and regulatory helper and suppressor T cell activities in spontaneously autoimmune mice. J Immunol 123:2627, 1979

Izui S et al: Association of circulating retroviral gp70-anti-gp70 immune complexes with murine systemic lupus erythematosus. J Exp Med 149:1099, 1979

Accinni L, Dixon FJ: Degenerative vascular disease and myocardial infarction in mice with lupus-like syndrome. Am J Pathol 96:477, 1979

Theofilopoulos AN et al: The influence of thymic genotype on the SLE-like disease and T cell proliferation of MRL/Mp-lpr/lpr mice. J Exp Med 153:1405, 1981

Milich DR, Gershwin ME: The pathogenesis of autoimmunity in New Zealand mice. In Immunologic Defects in Laboratory Animals, vol 2, Gershwin ME, Merchant B (Eds). Plenum Press, New York, 1981, pp 77-123

CHAPTER 22

Koffler D: Immunopathogenesis of systemic lupus erythematosus. Annu Rev Med 25:149, 1974

Kunkel HG: The immunologic approach to SLE. Arthritis Rheum 20(suppl 6):S139, July-August 1977

Haakenstad AO, Mannik M: The biology of immune complexes. In Autoimmunity, Talal N (Ed). Academic Press, New York, 1977

Tan EM, Rothfield NF: Systemic lupus erythematosus. In Immunological Diseases, vol 2, Samter M (Ed). Little, Brown & Co, Boston, 1978

Gibofsky A et al: Contrasting patterns of newer histocompatibility determinants in patients with rheumatoid arthritis and systemic lupus erythematosus. Arthritis Rheum 21(suppl 5):S134, June 1978

Decker JL et al: Systemic lupus erythematosus: Evolving concepts. Ann Intern Med 91:587, 1979

Koffler D: The immunology of rheumatoid diseases. Clin Symp 31:4, 1979

CHAPTER 23

Franklin EC, Zucker-Franklin D: Current concepts of amyloid. Adv Immunol 15:249, 1972

Glenner GG: Amyloid deposits and amyloidosis. N Engl J Med 302:1283, 1980

Glenner GG, Costa P, Frietas F (Eds): Amyloid and Amyloidosis: Proceedings of Povoa de Varzim, Portugal, September 1979. International Congress Series, vol 497, Elsevier/Excerpta Medica, New York, 1980

Isobe T, Osserman EF: Patterns of amyloidosis and their association with plasma cell dyscrasias, monoclonal immunoglobulins and Bence Jones proteins. N Engl J Med 290:473, 1974

Lavie G, Zucker-Franklin D, Franklin EC: Degradation of serum amyloid A protein by surface-associated enzymes of human blood monocytes. J Exp Med 148:1020, 1978

Rosenthal CJ, Franklin EC: Amyloidosis and amyloid protein. In Recent Advances in Clinical Immunology, Thompson R (Ed). Churchill Livingstone, Edinburgh, 1977, pp 41-76

Kyle RA, Bayrd ED: Amyloidosis: A review of 236 cases. Medicine 54:211, 1975

CHAPTER 24

Day ED, Varitek VA, Fujinami RS, Paterson PY: MBP-SF, a prominent serum factor in suckling Lewis rats that additively inhibits the primary binding of myelin basic protein (MBP) to syngeneic anti-MBP antibodies. Immunochemistry 15:1, 1978

Day ED, Varitek VA, Paterson PY: Myelin basic protein serum factor (MBP-SF) in adult Lewis rats: A method for detection and evidence that MBP-SF influences the appearance of antibody to MBP in animals developing experimental allergic encephalomyelitis. Immunochemistry 15:437, 1978

Fujinami RS, Paterson PY, Day ED, Varitek VA: Myelin basic protein serum factor (MBP-SF): An endogenous neuroantigen influencing development of experimental allergic encephalomyelitis in Lewis rats. J Exp Med 148:1716, 1978

Varitek VA, Day ED: Relative affinity of antisera for myelin basic protein (MBP) and degree of affinity heterogeneity. Mol Immunol 16:163, 1979

Varitek VA, Day ED, Paterson PY: Early loss, reappearance, and extended half-life of circulating antibodies to myelin basic protein (MBP) in passively immunized Lewis rats: Further evidence for accessible endogenous MBP neuroantigens. Mol Immunol, vol 16, 1979

Paterson PY: Autoimmune neurologic disease: Experimental animal systems and implications for multiple sclerosis. In Autoimmunity: Genetic, Immunologic, Virologic and Clinical Aspects, Talal N (Ed). Academic Press, New York, 1977, pp 643-692

Hashim G, Sharpe RD, Carvalho EF: Experimental allergic encephalomyelitis: Sequestered encephalitogenic determinant in the bovine myelin basic protein. J Neurochem 32:73, 1979

Whitaker JN: Myelin encephalitogenic protein fragments in cerebrospinal fluid of persons with multiple sclerosis. Neurology 27:911, 1977

Paterson PY: Neuroimmunologic diseases of animals and man. Rev Infect Dis 1:468, 1979

Day ED, Varitek VA, Paterson PY: Endogenous myelin basic

protein-serum factors (MBP-SFs) in Lewis rats: Evidence for their heterogeneity and reactivity with anti-MBP antibodies of different affinities. J Neurol Sci 49:1, 1981

Massanari RM, Paterson PY, Lipton HL: Potentiation of experimental allergic encephalomyelitis in hamsters with persistent measles encephalitis. J Infect Dis 139:297, 1979

Paterson PY et al: Immunologic determinants of experimental neurologic autoimmune disease and approaches to the multiple sclerosis problem. Trans Am Clin Climatol Assoc 89:109, 1977

Paterson PY, Day ED, Whitacre CC: Neuroimmunologic diseases: Effector cell responses and immunoregulatory mechanisms. Immunol Rev 55:317, 1981

Paterson PY et al: Endogenous myelin basic protein-serum factors (MBP-SFs) and anti-MBP antibodies in humans: Occurrence in sera of clinically well subjects and patients with multiple sclerosis. J Neurol Sci 52:37, 1981

Whitaker JN, Bashir RM, Chow C-HJ, Kibler RF: Antigenic features of myelin basic protein-like material in cerebrospinal fluid. J Immunol 124:1148, 1980

Wisniewski HM et al: Multiple sclerosis: Immunological and experimental aspects. In Recent Advances in Clinical Neurology, vol 3, Matthews WB, Glaser GH (Eds). Churchill Livingstone, Edinburgh, 1982, pp 95–124

Lassmann H, Kitz K, Wisniewski HM: In vivo effect of sera from animals with chronic relapsing experimental allergic encephalomyelitis on central and peripheral myelin. Acta Neuropathol (Berl) 55:297, 1981

Mertin J et al: Double-blind, controlled trial of immunosuppression in treatment of multiple sclerosis. Lancet II:949, 1980

Chapter 25

Drachman DB: Myasthenia gravis. N Engl J Med 298:136, 1978

Kahn CR: Autoantibodies to the insulin receptor: Clinical and molecular aspects. Fed Proc 38:2607, 1979

Volpé R: Immunopathology of Graves' disease. Fed Proc 38:2611, 1979

Flier JS et al: Characterization of antibodies to the insulin receptor. J Clin Invest 58:1442, 1976

Jerne NK: The immune system: A web of V-domains. Harvey Lect 70:93, 1974-5

Chapter 26

Oldstone MBA et al: Virus induced alterations in homeostasis leading to disease: Alterations in differentiated but not vital functions of infected cells in vivo. Science 218:1125, 1982

Oldstone MBA, Holmstoen J, Welsh RM Jr: Alterations of acetylcholine enzymes in neuroblastoma cells persistently infected with lymphocytic choriomeningitis virus. J Cell Physiol 91:459, 1977

Welsh RM Jr, Oldstone MBA: Inhibition of immunologic injury of cultured cells infected with lymphocytic choriomeningitis virus: Role of defective interfering virus in regulating viral antigenic expression. J Exp Med 145:1449, 1977

Oldstone MBA, Fujinami RS: Virus persistence and avoidance of immune surveillance: How measles viruses can be induced to persist in cells, escape immune assault and injure tissues. In Virus Persistence Symposium 33, Mahy BWJ, Minson AC, Darby GK (Eds). Cambridge University Press, London, 1982, pp 185–202

Oldstone MBA: Immune responses, immune tolerance and viruses. In Comprehensive Virology, vol 15, Fraenkel-Conrat H, Wagner RR (Eds). Plenum Press, New York, 1979, pp 1–36

Holland JJ et al: Defective interfering RNA viruses and the host-cell response. In Comprehensive Virology, vol 16, Fraenkel-Conrat H, Wagner RR (Eds). Plenum Press, New York, 1980, pp 137–192

Oldstone MBA: Virus neutralization and virus induced immune complex disease: Virus antibody union resulting in immunoprotection or immunologic injury—two different sides of the same coin. Prog Med Virol 19:84, 1975

Younger JS, Preble OT: Viral persistence: Evolution of viral population. In Comprehensive Virology, vol 16, Fraenkel-Conrat H, Wagner RR (Eds). Plenum Press, New York, 1980, pp 73–125

Chapter 27

Jerne NK: Towards a network theory of the immune system. Ann Immunol (Paris) 125(C):373, 1974

Walford RL: The Immunologic Theory of Aging. Williams & Wilkins Co, Baltimore, 1969

Szewczuk MR et al: Ontogeny of B lymphocyte function. VIII. Failure of thymus cells from aged donors to induce the functional maturation of B lymphocytes from immature donors. Eur J Immunol 10:918, 1980

Weksler ME, Innes JB, Goldstein G: Immunological studies of aging. IV. The contribution of thymic involution to the immune deficiencies of aging mice. J Exp Med 148:996, 1978

Goidl EA, Thorbecke GJ, Weksler ME, Siskind GW: Production of auto-idiotypic antibody during the normal immune response: Changes in the auto-anti-idiotypic antibody response and the idiotype repertoire associated with aging. Proc Natl Acad Sci USA 77:6788, 1980

Makinodan T, Kay MB: Age influence on the immune system. In Advances in Immunology Series, vol 29, Kunkel HG, Dixon FJ (Eds). Academic Press, New York, 1980, p 287

Chapter 28

Theofilopoulos AN, Dixon FJ: The biology and detection of immune complexes. Adv Immunol 28:89, 1979

Theofilopoulos AN et al: The nature of immune complexes in human cancer. J Immunol 119:657, 1977

Theofilopoulos AN, Pereira AB, Eisenberg RA, Dixon FJ: Assays for detection of complement-fixing immune complexes (Raji cell, conglutinin, and anti-C3 assay). In Manual of Clinical Immunology, Rose NR, Friedman H (Eds). American Society of Microbiology, Washington, DC, 1980

Theofilopoulos AN, Eisenberg RA, Dixon FJ: Isolation of circulating immune complexes using Raji cells: Separation of antigens from immune complexes and production of antiserum. J Clin Invest 61:1570, 1978

Zubler RH, Lambert PH: Immune complexes in clinical investigation. *In* Recent Advances in Clinical Immunology, Thompson RA (Ed). Churchill Livingstone, New York, 1977, pp 125-147

WHO Scientific Group: The Role of Immune Complexes in Disease. Technical Series 606, WHO, Geneva, 1977, p 5

Hellström KE, Hellström I: Immunologic defenses against cancer. Hosp Pract 5:45, January 1970

CHAPTER 29

Tan EM: Autoantibodies to nuclear antigens: Their immunobiology and medicine. Adv Immunol 33:167, 1982

Nakamura RM, Tan EM: New developments in antinuclear autoantibodies to nuclear antigens (ANA) in human diseases. *In* Immunologic Analysis, Nakamura RM, Dito WR, Tucker ES (Eds). Masson Publishing USA, Inc, New York, 1982, pp 1-15

Tan EM: Special antibodies for the study of systemic lupus erythematosus: An analysis. Arthritis Rheum 25:753, 1982

Fritzler MJ, Ayer LM: Anticentromere antibodies: Clinical and biological significance. J Rheumatol 9:489, 1982

Tan EM: Mixed connective tissue disease—an evolving clinical syndrome. West J Med 132:350, 1980

CHAPTER 30

Köhler G, Milstein C: Continuous cultures of fused cells secreting antibody of predefined specificity. Nature 256:495, 1975

Kennett RH, McKearn TJ, Bechtol KB (Eds): Monoclonal Antibodies. Plenum Publishing Corp, New York, 1980

Kwan S-P, Yelton DE, Scharff MD: Production of monoclonal antibodies. *In* Genetic Engineering, vol 2, Setlow JK, Hollaender A (Eds). Plenum Publishing Corp, New York, 1980

Olsson L, Kaplan HS: Human–human hybridomas producing monoclonal antibodies of predefined antigenic specificity. Proc Natl Acad Sci USA 77:5429, 1980

Yelton DE, Scharff MD: Monoclonal antibodies: A powerful tool in biology and medicine. Annu Rev Biochem 50:657, 1980

Wiktor TJ, Koprowski H: Monoclonal antibodies against rabies virus produced by somatic cell hybridization: Detection of antigenic variants. Proc Natl Acad Sci USA 75:3938, 1978

Levy R, Dilley J, Fox RI, Warnke R: A human thymus–leukemia antigen defined by hybridoma monoclonal antibodies. Proc Natl Acad Sci USA 76:6552, 1979

Reinherz EL, Kung PC, Goldstein G, Schlossman SF: Separation of functional subsets of human T cells by monoclonal antibody. Proc Natl Acad Sci USA 76:4061, 1979

CHAPTER 31

Arnon R: Chemically defined antiviral vaccines. Annu Rev Microbiol 34:593, 1980

Lerner RA et al: Chemically synthesized peptides predicted from the nucleotide sequence of the hepatitis B virus genome elicit antibodies reactive with the native envelope protein of Dane particle. Proc Natl Acad Sci USA 78:3403, 1981

Lerner RA, Sutcliffe JG, Shinnick TM: Antibodies to chemically synthesized peptides predicted from DNA sequences as probes of gene expression. Cell 23:309, 1981

Pasek M et al: Hepatitis B virus genes and their expression in *E. coli.* Nature 282:575, 1979

CHAPTER 32

Louie S, Daoust PR, Schwartz RS: Immunodeficiency and the pathogenesis of non-Hodgkin's lymphoma. Semin Oncol 7:267, 1980

Miller KB, Schwartz RS: Familial abnormalities of suppressor-cell function in systemic lupus erythematosus. N Engl J Med 301:803, 1979

Anderson JL, Bieber CP, Fowles RE, Stinson EB: Idiopathic cardiomyopathy, age, and suppressor-cell dysfunction as risk determinants of lymphoma after cardiac transplantation. Lancet II:1174, 1978

Calne RY et al: Cyclosporin A initially as the only immunosuppressant in 34 recipients of cadaveric organs: 32 kidneys, 2 pancreases, and 2 livers. Lancet II:1033, 1979

Spitler LE, Sagebiel R: A randomized trial of levamisole versus placebo as adjuvant therapy in malignant melanoma. N Engl J Med 303:1143, 1980

Terry WD: Immunotherapy of malignant melanoma. N Engl J Med 303:1174, 1980

Terman DS, Yamamoto T, Mattioli M: Extensive necrosis of spontaneous mammary adenocarcinoma after extracorporeal circulation over *Staphylococcus aureus* Cowans I: Description of acute tumoricidal response; morphologic, histologic, immunohistochemical, immunologic and serological findings. J Immunol 124:795, 1980

Penn I: Risk of lymphoma after cardiac transplantation. Lancet II:1385, 1978

CHAPTER 33

Simmons RL, Folker JE, Lower RR, Najarian JS: Transplantation. *In* Principles of Surgery, 3rd ed, Schwartz SI et al (Eds). McGraw-Hill Book Co, New York, 1978, pp 383-473

Folker JE, Simmons RL, Najarian JS: Principles of immunosuppression. *In* Davis-Christopher Textbook of Surgery, Sabiston DC (Ed). WB Saunders Co, Philadelphia, 1981, pp 496-514

Gifford RRM et al: Duration of first renal allograft as indicator of second renal allograft outcome. Surgery 88:611, 1980

Ferguson RM et al: Cyclosporin A in renal transplantation: A prospective randomized trial. Surgery 92:175, 1982

Hamburger J: Renal Transplantation: Theory and Practice, 2nd ed. Williams & Wilkins Co, Baltimore, 1981

Morris PJ (Ed): Kidney Transplantation: Principles and Practice. Grune & Stratton, New York, 1979

Katz DH: Adaptive differentiation of lymphocytes: Theoretical implications for mechanisms of cell-cell recognition and regulation of immune responses. Adv Immunol 29:138, 1979

Chess L, Schlossman SF: Human lymphocyte subpopulations. Adv Immunol 25:213, 1977

Rocklin RE, Bendtzen K, Greineder D: Mediators of immunity, lymphokines and monokines. Adv Immunol 29:56, 1980

CHAPTER 34

Onoé K et al: Humoral and cell-mediated immune responses in fully allogeneic bone marrow chimera in mice. J Exp Med 151:115, 1980

Reisner Y et al: Separation of antibody helper and antibody suppressor human T cells by using soybean agglutinin. Proc Natl Acad Sci USA 77:6778, 1980

Kapoor N et al: Reconstitution of normal megakaryocytopoiesis and immunologic functions in Wiskott-Aldrich syndrome by marrow transplantation following myeloablation and immunosuppression with busulfan and cyclophosphamide. Blood 57:692, 1981

Sorell M et al: Marrow transplantation for juvenile osteopetrosis. Am J Med 70:1280, 1981

Reisner Y et al: Transplantation for acute leukaemia using HLA-A, B nonidentical parental marrow cells fractionated with soybean agglutinin and sheep red blood cells. Lancet II: 327, 1981

O'Reilly RJ et al: Transplantation of foetal liver and thymus in patients with severe combined immunodeficiencies. *In* The Immune System: Functions and Therapy of Dysfunction, Proceedings of the Serono Symposium, vol 27, Doria G, Eshkol A (Eds). Academic Press, New York, 1980, pp 241–252

Reisner Y et al: Allogeneic hemopoietic stem cell transplantation using mouse spleen cells fractionated by lectins: In vitro study of cell fractions. Proc Natl Acad Sci USA 77:1164, 1980

O'Reilly RJ et al: Reconstitution of immunologic function in a patient with severe combined immunodeficiency following transplantation of marrow from an HLA-A, B, C nonidentical but MLC-compatible paternal donor. Transplant Proc 11: 1934, 1979

CHAPTER 35

Strober S et al: Allograft tolerance after total lymphoid irradiation. Immunol Rev 46:87, 1979

Kotzin BK, Strober S: Reversal of NZB disease with total lymphoid irradiation (TLI). J Exp Med 50:371, 1979

Kaplan HS: Hodgkin's Disease. Harvard University Press, Cambridge, 1980

Strober S et al: The treatment of intractable rheumatoid arthritis with total lymphoid irradiation. Int J Radiat Oncol Biol Phys 7:1, 1981

Index

Index

Responder strains, 29-32, 33, 38-39, 50-61
Restriction endonuclease, use of, 4
Retinoic acid, 79, 83
Rheumatic diseases, 181
Rheumatic heart disease, 115
Rheumatoid arthritis, 182, 183, 184
    antinuclear antibodies profile, 321, 322, 323, 324
    associated HLAs, 254, 281
    association with Epstein-Barr virus, 324
    complement system abnormalities in, 175
    lymphocyte distribution in, 119, 122
    in MRL/1 mice, 244
    treatment with TLI, 377, 378
Rheumatoid-arthritis-associated antigen, antibodies against, 322, 323, 324
Rheumatoid factor, 250, 303, 324
Rheumatoid factor immunoassay, 314
Rhinitis, allergic, 279
Ribonucleoprotein, antibodies against, 319, 320, 321, 322, 323
RNA splicing, 7, 10
RNA tumor virus, destruction by C1, 176
RNA virus, in leukemic T cells, 204
RNP (see Ribonucleoprotein)
Rosette reaction, 80, 81, 199, 200, 201, 202, 297-298, 365, 367

S

SAA (see Serum amyloid A component)
SAP (see Serum amyloid P component)
Schistosoma mansoni, 176
Sci-70, antibodies against, 322, 323
SCID (see Severe combined immunodeficiency)
Scleroderma, antinuclear antibodies profile, 321, 322, 323
Self markers, polymorphism of, 105
Self-tolerance (see Immunologic tolerance)
Sendai virus, immune response to, 103
Serum amyloid A component, 139, 140, 141, 142, 143, 151, 152, 262, 263, 264
Serum amyloid P component, 141, 151-152
Serum lipase, 366-367, 368
Serum sickness, 210-211, 214-215, 309, 310
Severe combined immunodeficiency, 360-363, 364-365, 366
Sézary's syndrome, cell surface markers, 203-204
Signal peptide, 6
Single-point mutation in V region, 8
Single receptor model, 101, 102
Sjögren's syndrome, 182, 254, 255
    antinuclear antibody profile, 320, 321, 322, 323
SLE (see Systemic lupus erythematosus)

Slow-reacting substance of anaphylaxis, 19, 21, 226, 231-233
Sm antigen, 247, 250
    antibodies against, 320, 321, 323
Spleen, lymphocyte distribution in, 117, 121, 124
Spleen cells, immunologic activities, 64, 66
Splenectomy, 350-351, 352
Spondylarthropathies, 181
S-protein, 171
S region, 29, 33
SRS-A (see Slow-reacting substance of anaphylaxis)
SS-A, antibodies against, 320, 321, 322, 323
SS-B, antibodies against, 320, 321, 322, 323
SSPE (see Subacute sclerosing panencephalitis)
Stem cell, 88
Steroids
    mast cells and, 228
    SLE and, 256
Streptococcal antigens, IC disease and, 216
Streptococcus pneumoniae, 144, 147, 150
Structure-function relationship, 21-22
Subacute sclerosing panencephalitis, 287-288, 290, 291
Superoxide anion, 159, 160, 162
Suppressor factors, 54-58
Suppressor T cell, 26, 32, 41, 45, 49-61
    aging and, 301, 304-306
    cell surface antigens, 50
    cellular interactions, 208
    effect of immunosuppression on, 343, 344
    effector (Ts$_2$), 54-58
    four-stage system, 57
    functions, 59-60
    genetic analysis of, 32
    induction, 50-51
    initiating (Ts$_1$), 54-58
    nonspecific, 372-374, 375, 377
    role in immunologic tolerance, 107, 116
    SLE and, 122, 240, 251, 253
    subpopulations of, 49-50, 54-58
    Ts$_3$ subpopulation, 57-58
    tumor-protective effect of, 59-60
Susceptibility
    environmental agent theory, 183
    Ir genes and, 184, 367
    MHC and, 104-105
    molecular mimicry hypothesis, 184
Syngeneic interaction, 36
Systemic lupus erythematosus, human, 85, 247-256
    antilymphocytic activity, 253
    antinuclear antibody profile, 320-322, 323
    associated HLAs, 254-255
    autoantibodies present in, 247-249, 250, 320-322, 323

central nervous system involvement, 253
    circulating immune complexes, 315
    complement deficiencies and, 171, 172, 249
    etiology, 247-248
    kidney involvement, 247-253
    lymphocyte distribution in, 122
    sex hormones and, 255-256, 280
    suppressor T-cell function and, 344
    susceptibility to, 254
    treatment, 256
Systemic lupus erythematosus, murine, 235-245

T

T cell (see also Cytolytic T cell; Helper T cell; Lymphocyte; Suppressor T cell)
    antigen recognition by, 39
    deficiency (see DiGeorge syndrome)
    differentiation, 94-96, 201, 329, 362, 364
    effect: of aging on maturation of, 297-298; of thymus on, 101-102
    immunity against intracellular parasites, 99
    interaction: with B cells, 25-26, 31-36, 310, 312; with macrophages, 27, 34, 90-91, 93, 94, 95, 99, 108
    life history, 43-47, 94-95, 96
    localization in lymph node, 118, 121, 124, 199
    population changes after TLI, 370
    proliferative diseases, 203-204, 205, 206
    restricted specificity, control of, 101-102, 103
    role in EAE, 266, 267, 270-271
    secretion products, 37, 93
    subpopulations of, 41-48, 120-121
    surface antigens, 38, 42-43, 199-200, 201
Tγ cells, 120-121
Tμ cells, 120-121
T-cell-activating factor, 93, 94
T-cell growth factor, 68, 76, 77, 78, 81, 82, 83, 194, 299, 353
T-cell proliferative response, 29
T-cell-replacing factor, 300
TCGF (see T-cell growth factor)
TDF (see Thymocyte-differentiating factor)
Terminal deoxynucleotidyltransferase (TdT), 199, 200
Testosterone (see also Hormone, sex) for treatment of C1 inhibitor deficiency, 173
(T,G)-A--L, 29, 31, 38-39
Theophylline, 164
Thromboxanes, 163
Thy-1 antigen, 42-43, 50, 189
    antiserum against, 365, 366, 367
Thymic cells, immunologic activities, 64, 66

Illustration and Data Source Credits

CHAPTER 1: 5-11, Bunji Tagawa

CHAPTER 2: 14-16, Irving Geis; 17, 18, Norman Blau; 19-23, Irving Geis

CHAPTER 3: 27, 28, 30, 31, 33, 35, 36, 38, Irving Geis

CHAPTER 4: 42-48, Irving Geis

CHAPTER 5: 50, , George V. Kelvin; 51, Nancy Lou Gahan; 52-56, George V. Kelvin; 57, nancy Lou Gahan; 58 George V. Kelvin; 59, Albert Miller

CHAPTER 6: 65-69, 72, 73, George V. Kelvin

CHAPTER 7: 77-79, 82, 84, Bunji Tagawa

CHAPTER 8: 88-90, Nancy Lou Gahan; 91, Albert Miller; 92, 94, Nancy Lou Gahan; 95, Albert Miller; 96, Nancy Lou Gahan

CHAPTER 9: 98, Nancy Lou Gahan; 100-105, George V. Kelvin; 106, Albert Miller

CHAPTER 10: 108, 109, George V. Kelvin; 110, Albert Miller; 111-115, George V. Kelvin

CHAPTER 11: 119-121, Alan D. Iselin; 123, Albert Miller; 124, 125, Alan D. Iselin

CHAPTER 12: 129 top, 130-135, George V. Kelvin; 137, Albert Miller

CHAPTER 13: 141, Albert Miller; 142, Bunji Tagawa; 143 bottom, Dana Burns; 145-149, Bunji Tagawa; 150, 152, Albert Miller

CHAPTER 14: 157, Nancy Lou Gahan; 158, Albert Miller, adapted from Korchak HM, Weissmann G: *Proc Natl Acad Sci USA* 75:3818, 1978; 160-163, Nancy Lou Gahan

CHAPTER 15: 168-171, 173, 175, Alan D. Iselin

CHAPTER 16: 178-180, 183, 184, Bunji Tagawa

CHAPTER 17: 188, 189, Alan D. Iselin; 191, Albert Miller; 193, Nancy Lou Gahan

CHAPTER 18: 199, Robert Margulies; 201, 202, Nancy Lou Gahan

CHAPTER 19: 210, 212, 213, 215, Bunji Tagawa

CHAPTER 20: 224, 226, 227, 230, 232, Bunji Tagawa

CHAPTER 21: 236, 238-242, 244, Bunji Tagawa

CHAPTER 22: 251, 252, 254, 255, Nancy Lou Gahan

CHAPTER 23: 260-262, Nancy Lou Gahan

CHAPTER 24: 266, 269, Nancy Lou Gahan; 270, Albert Miller; 274, Nancy Lou Gahan

CHAPTER 25: 276, 277, Bunji Tagawa; 278, Nancy Lou Gahan; 279, Albert Miller; 281, Bunji Tagawa

CHAPTER 26: 286-289, Nancy Lou Gahan; 292, Albert Miller; 293, Nancy Lou Gahan

CHAPTER 27: 296, Nancy Lou Gahan; 297-300, Albert Miller; 302, Nancy Lou Gahan; 303, Albert Miller; 304, 305, Nancy Lou Gahan

CHAPTER 28: 310-313, 315-317, Nancy Lou Gahan; 318, Albert Miller

CHAPTER 30: 326-328, Alan D. Iselin

CHAPTER 31: 332-334, Alan D. Iselin

CHAPTER 32: 340, 341, 344, Alan D. Iselin

CHAPTER 33: 348, 349, Bunji Tagawa; 350-352 top, Jane Henriksen; 352 bottom, 353, Nancy Lou Gahan; 354, 355, Jane Henriksen

CHAPTER 34: 361 top, Bunji Tagawa; 361 bottom, Albert Miller; 362, 364, 366-368, Bunji Tagawa

CHAPTER 35: 371-373, 375-377, Nancy Lou Gahan; 378, Albert Miller